PRINCIPLES OF
CLINICAL
PHARMACOLOGY

PRINCIPLES OF CLINICAL PHARMACOLOGY

ARTHUR J. ATKINSON, JR.

CHARLES E. DANIELS

ROBERT L. DEDRICK

CHARLES V. GRUDZINSKAS

SANFORD P. MARKEY

ACADEMIC PRESS
San Diego   London   Boston   New York
Sydney   Tokyo   Toronto

Academic Press
A Harcourt Science and Technology Company
525 B Street, Suite 1900, San Diego, California 92101-4495, USA
http://www.academicpress.com

Academic Press
Harcourt Place, 32 Jamestown Road, London NW1 7BY, UK
http://www.academic press.com

Library of Congress Catalog Card Number: 2001093791

International Standard Book Number: 0-12-066060-1

PRINTED IN THE UNITED STATES OF AMERICA
01   02   03   04   05   06   07   SB   9   8   7   6   5   4   3   2   1

Contents

CHAPTER

5

Effects of Renal Disease
on Pharmacokinetics

ARTHUR J. ATKINSON, JR.

CHAPTER

6

Pharmacokinetics in Patients
Requiring Renal Replacement
Therapy

ARTHUR J. ATKINSON, JR. AND GREGORY M. SUSLA

CHAPTER

7

Effects of Liver Disease
on Pharmacokinetics

GREGORY M. SUSLA, ARTHUR J. ATKINSON, JR.

CHAPTER

8

Noncompartmental Vs. Compartmental
Approaches to Pharmacokinetic Analysis

DAVID M. FOSTER

CHAPTER

9

Distribution Models of Drug Kinetics

PAUL F. MORRISON

CHAPTER

10

Population Pharmacokinetics

RAYMOND MILLER

PART

II

DRUG METABOLISM AND TRANSPORT

CHAPTER

11

Pathways of Drug Metabolism

SANFORD P. MARKEY

CHAPTER

12

Methods of Analysis of Drugs and Drug Metabolites

SANFORD P. MARKEY

CHAPTER

13

Clinical Pharmacogenetics

DAVID A. FLOCKHART

CHAPTER

28

Drug Discovery

ROBERT R. GORMAN

CHAPTER

29

Preclinical Drug Development

CHRIS H. TAKIMOTO AND SAMIR N. KHLEIF

CHAPTER

30

Animal Scale-up

ROBERT L. DEDRICK

CHAPTER

31

Phase 1 Clinical Studies

JERRY M. COLLINS

CHAPTER

32

Pharmacokinetic and Pharmacodynamic Considerations in the Development of Biotechnology Products and Large Molecules

PAMELA D. GARZONE

CHAPTER

33

Design of Clinical Development Programs

CHARLES GRUDZINSKAS

CHAPTER

34

Role of the FDA in Guiding Drug Development

LAWRENCE J. LESKO

Preface

The rate of introduction of new pharmaceutical products has increased rapidly over the past decade, and details learned about a particular drug become obsolete as it is replaced by newer agents. For this reason, we have chosen to focus this book on the principles that underlie the clinical use and contemporary development of pharmaceuticals. It is assumed that the reader will have had an introductory course in pharmacology and also some understanding of calculus, physiology, and clinical medicine.

This book is the outgrowth of an evening course that has been taught for the past three years at the NIH Clinical Center[1]. Wherever possible, individuals who have lectured in the course have contributed chapters corresponding to their lectures. The organizers of this course are the editors of this book and we also have recruited additional experts to assist in the review of specific chapters. Their help is acknowledged in the list of reviewers. We also acknowledge the help of William A. Mapes in preparing much of the artwork. Special thanks are due Donna Shields, Coordinator for the ClinPRAT training program at NIH, whose attention to myriad details has made possible both the successful conduct of our evening course and the production of this book. Finally, we were encouraged and patiently aided in this undertaking by Robert M. Harington and Aaron Johnson at Academic Press.

---

[1] The lecture schedule and syllabus material for the current edition of the course are available on the Internet at: http://www.cc.nih.gov/ccc/principles.

Contributing Authors

Darrell R. Abernethy, M.D., Ph.D., Clinical Director and Chief, Laboratory of Clinical Investigation, National Institute on Aging, National Institutes of Health, Baltimore, MD.

Cara L. Alfaro, Pharm. D., Clinical Pharmacy Specialist, National Institute of Mental Health, National Institutes of Health, Bethesda, MD.

Arthur J. Atkinson, Jr., M.D., Senior Advisor in Clinical Pharmacology, Warren Grant Magnuson Clinical Center, National Institutes of Health, Bethesda, MD.

Frank M. Balis, M.D., Head, Pharmacology and Experimental Therapeutics Section, Pediatric Oncology Branch, National Cancer Institute, National Institutes of Health, Bethesda, MD.

Mary J. Berg, Pharm.D., Professor, Division of Clinical and Administrative Pharmacy, University of Iowa College of Pharmacy, Iowa City, IA.

Karim Anton Calis, Pharm.D., M.P.H., Clinical Specialist, Endocrinology and Women's Health, Pharmacy Department, Warren Grant Magnuson Clinical Center, National Institutes of Health, Bethesda, MD.

Jerry M. Collins, Ph.D., Director, Laboratory of Clinical Pharmacology, Center for Drug Evaluation and Research, Food and Drug Administration, Rockville, MD.

Charles E. Daniels, R.Ph., Ph.D., Chief, Pharmacy Department, Warren Grant Magnuson Clinical Center, National Institutes of Health, Bethesda, MD.

Robert L. Dedrick, Ph.D., Chief, Drug Delivery and Kinetics Resource, Division of Bioengineering and Physical Science, Office of Research Services, Office of the Director, National Institutes of Health, Bethesda, MD.

David A. Flockhart, M.D., Ph.D., Assistant Professor of Medicine and Pharmacology and Director, Pharmacogenetics Core Laboratory and Division of Clinical Pharmacology, Georgetown University Medical Center, Washington, DC.

David M. Foster, Ph.D., Research Professor Emeritus, Department of Bioengineering, University of Washington, Seattle, WA.

Elizabeth Fox, M.D., Clinical Fellow, Pediatric Oncology Branch, National Cancer Institute, National Institutes of Health, Bethesda, MD.

Marilynn C. Frederiksen, M.D., Associate Professor and Section Head, General Obstetrics and Gynecology, Department of Obstetrics and Gynecology, Northwestern University Medical School, Chicago, IL.

Pamela D. Garzone, Ph.D., Associate Director, Clinical Pharmacology and Preclinical Studies, Cell Therapeutics, Inc., Seattle, WA.

Robert R. Gorman, Ph.D., President, Saguro Consulting, Scottsdale, AZ.

Charles V. Grudzinskas, Ph.D., Drug Development Consultant, Annapolis, MD.

Nicholas H.G. Holford, M.D., Associate Professor, Department of Pharmacology and Clinical Pharmacology, The University of Auckland, Auckland, New Zealand.

Samir N. Khleif, M.D., Senior Clinical Investigator, Developmental Therapeutics Department, Medicine Branch, National Cancer Institute, National Institutes of Health, Bethesda, MD.

Lawrence J. Lesko, Ph.D., Director, Office of Clinical Pharmacology and Biopharmaceutics, Center for Drug Evaluation and Research, Food and Drug Administration, Rockville, MD

Elizabeth S. Lowe, M.D., ClinPRAT Fellow, Pharmacology and Experimental Therapeutics Section,

Pediatric Oncology Branch, National Cancer Institute, National Institutes of Health, Bethesda, MD.

Sanford P. Markey, Ph.D., Chief, Laboratory of Neurotoxicology, National Institute of Mental Health, National Institutes of Health, Bethesda, MD.

Raymond Miller, Ph.D., Pfizer Global Research and Development, Ann Arbor, MI.

Paul Morrison, Ph.D., Physical Scientist, Drug Delivery and Kinetics Resource, Office of Research Services, Office of the Director, National Institutes of Health, Bethesda, MD.

Diane R. Mould, Ph.D., Research Associate Professor, Center for Drug Development Science, Department of Pharmacology, Georgetown University Medical Center, Washington, DC.

Carl C. Peck, M.D., Professor and Medical Director, Center for Drug Development Science, Department of Pharmacology, Georgetown University Medical Center, Washington, DC.

Stephen C. Piscitelli, Pharm. D., Coordinator, Clinical Pharmacokinetics Research Laboratory, Pharmacy Department, Warren Grant Magnuson Clinical Center, National Institutes of Health, Bethesda, MD.

Peter C. Preusch, Ph.D., Program Director, Division of Pharmacology, Physiology, and Biological Chemistry, National Institute of General Medical Sciences, National Institutes of Health, Bethesda, MD.

Catherine S. Stika, M.D., Assistant Professor, Department of Obstetrics and Gynecology, Northwestern University Medical School, Chicago, IL.

Gregory M. Susla, Pharm.D., Clinical Science Specialist, Scientific Affairs Department, Bayer Corporation, North Potomac, MD.

Chris H. Takimoto, M.D., Ph.D., Associate Professor, Division of Medical Oncology, Department of Medicine, University of Texas Health Science Center, San Antonio, TX.

Linda R. Young, Pharm.D., Assistant Professor and Director, Drug Information Center, Department of Pharmacy Practice and Pharmacoeconomics, University of Tennessee, Memphis, TN.

Invited Reviewers

The editors wish to thank the following individuals who assisted with the review of some of the chapter manuscripts.

Leif N. Bertilsson, Ph.D., Professor, Department of Medical Laboratory Sciences and Technology, Division of Clinical Pharmacology at Karolinska Institutet, Huddinge University Hospital, Stockholm, Sweden.

Peter Bungay, Ph.D., Chemical Engineer, Drug Delivery and Kinetics Resource, Division of Bioengineering and Physical Science, Office of Research Services, Office of the Director, National Institutes of Health, Bethesda, MD.

J. Richard Crout, M.D., Crout Consulting, Bethesda, MD

Nicholas H. G. Holford, M.D., Associate Professor, Department of Pharmacology and Clinical Pharmacology, The University of Auckland, Auckland, New Zealand.

Lawrence J. Lesko, Ph.D., Director, Office of Clinical Pharmacology and Biopharmaceutics, Center for Drug Evaluation and Research, Food and Drug Administration, Rockville, MD

Pamela A. Marino, Ph.D., Program Director, Division of Pharmacology, Physiology, and Biological Chemistry, National Institute of General Medical Sciences, National Institutes of Health, Bethesda, MD.

Joyce Mordenti, Ph.D., Director, Preclinical Sciences, Axys Pharmaceuticals, Inc., South San Francisco, CA

Paul Morrison, Ph.D., Physical Scientist, Drug Delivery and Kinetics Resource, Office of Research Services, Office of the Director, National Institutes of Health, Bethesda, MD.

Marcus M. Reidenberg, M.D., Professor of Pharmacology and Medicine, and Head, Division of Clinical Pharmacology, Cornell University-Weill Medical College, New York, NY.

Michael E. Rogers, Ph.D., Director, Division of Pharmacology, Physiology, and Biological Chemistry, National Institute of General Medical Sciences, National Institutes of Health, Bethesda, MD.

Introduction to Clinical Pharmacology

ARTHUR J. ATKINSON, JR.

Clinical Center, National Institutes of Health, Bethesda, Maryland

Fortunately a surgeon who uses the wrong side of the scalpel cuts his own fingers and not the patient; if the same applied to drugs they would have been investigated very carefully a long time ago. (Rudolph Bucheim, Beitrage zur Arzneimittellehre, 1849)[1]

BACKGROUND

Clinical pharmacology can be defined as the study of drugs in humans. Clinical pharmacology often is contrasted with basic pharmacology. Yet *applied* is a more appropriate antonym for *basic* [2]. In fact, many basic problems in pharmacology can only be studied in humans. This text will focus on the basic principles of clinical pharmacology. Selected applications will be used to illustrate these principles, but no attempt will be made to provide an exhaustive coverage of applied therapeutics. Other useful supplementary sources of information are listed at the end of this chapter.

Clinical pharmacology has been termed a bridging discipline because it combines elements of classical pharmacology with clinical medicine. The special competencies of individuals trained in clinical pharmacology have equipped them for productive careers in academia, the pharmaceutical industry, and governmental agencies, such as the NIH and the FDA. Reidenberg [3] has pointed out that clinical pharmacologists are concerned with both the optimal use of existing medications and the scientific study of drugs in humans. The latter area includes both evaluation of the safety and efficacy of currently available drugs and development of new and improved pharmacotherapy.

Optimizing Use of Existing Medicines

As the opening quote indicates, the concern of pharmacologists for the safe and effective use of medicine can be traced back at least to Rudolph Bucheim (1820–1879), who has been credited with establishing pharmacology as a laboratory-based discipline [1]. In the United States, Harry Gold and Walter Modell began in the 1930s to provide the foundation for the modern discipline of clinical pharmacology [4]. Their accomplishments include the invention of the double-blind design for clinical trials [5], the use of effect kinetics to measure the absolute bioavailability of digoxin and characterize the time course of its chronotropic effects [6], and the founding of *Clinical Pharmacology and Therapeutics*.

Few drugs have focused as much public attention on the problem of adverse drug reactions as thalidomide, which was first linked in 1961 to catastrophic outbreaks of phocomelia by Lenz in Germany and McBride in Australia [7]. Although thalidomide had not been approved at that time for use in the United States, this tragedy prompted passage in 1962 of the Harris–Kefauver Amendments to the Food, Drug, and Cosmetic Act. This act greatly expanded the scope of the FDA's mandate to protect the public health. The thalidomide tragedy also provided the major impetus for developing a number of NIH-funded academic centers of excellence that have shaped contemporary clinical pharmacology in this country. These U.S. centers were founded by a generation of vigorous leaders, including Ken Melmon, Jan Koch-Weser, Lou Lasagna, John Oates, Leon Goldberg, Dan Azarnoff, Tom Gaffney, and Leigh Thompson. Collin Dollery and Folke Sjöqvist established similar programs in Europe. In response to the public mandate generated by the thalidomide catastrophe, these leaders quickly reached consensus on a number of theoretically preventable causes that contribute to the high incidence of adverse drug reactions (4). These include:

1. Inappropriate polypharmacy
2. Failure of prescribing physicians to establish and adhere to clear therapeutic goals
3. Failure of medical personnel to attribute new symptoms or changes in laboratory test results to drug therapy
4. Lack of priority given to the scientific study of adverse drug reaction mechanisms
5. General ignorance of basic and applied pharmacology and therapeutic principles

The important observations also were made that, unlike the teratogenic reactions caused by thalidomide, most adverse reactions encountered in clinical practice occurred with commonly used, rather than newly introduced, drugs, and were dose related, rather than idiosyncratic (8,9).

Recognition of the considerable variation in response of patients treated with standard drug doses provided the impetus for the development of laboratory methods to measure drug concentrations in patient blood samples (9). The availability of these measurements also made it possible to apply pharmacokinetic principles to routine patient care. Despite these advances, *serious adverse drug reactions* (defined as those adverse drug reactions that require or prolong hospitalization, are permanently disabling, or result in death) recently have been estimated to occur in 6.7% of hospitalized patients (10). Although this figure has been disputed, the incidence of adverse drug reactions probably is still higher than is generally recognized (11). In addition, the majority of these adverse reactions continue to be caused by drugs that have been in clinical use for a substantial period of time (4).

The fact that most adverse drug reactions occur with commonly used drugs focuses attention on the last of the preventable causes of these reactions: the training that prescribing physicians receive in pharmacology and therapeutics. Bucheim's comparison of surgery and medicine is particularly apt in this regard (4). Most U.S. medical schools provide their students with only a single course in pharmacology that tradi-

tionally is part of the second-year curriculum, when students lack the clinical background that is needed to support detailed instruction in therapeutics. In addition, Sjöqvist (12) has observed that most academic pharmacology departments have lost contact with drug development and pharmacotherapy. As a result, students and residents acquire most of their information about drug therapy in a haphazard manner from colleagues, supervisory house staff and attending physicians, pharmaceutical sales representatives, and whatever independent reading they happen to do on the subject. This unstructured process of learning pharmacotherapeutic technique stands in marked contrast to the rigorously supervised training that is an accepted part of surgical training, in which instantaneous feedback is provided whenever a retractor, let alone a scalpel, is held improperly.

Evaluation and Development of Medicines

Leake (13) has pointed out that pharmacology is a subject of ancient interest, but a relatively new science. Reidenberg (3) recently restated Leake's listing of the fundamental problems with which the science of pharmacology is concerned:

1. The relationship between dose and biological effect
2. The localization of the site of action of a drug
3. The mechanism(s) of action of a drug
4. The absorption, distribution, metabolism, and excretion of a drug
5. The relationship between chemical structure and biological activity

These authors agree that pharmacology could not evolve as a scientific discipline until modern chemistry provided the chemically pure pharmaceutical products that are needed to establish a quantitative relationship between drug dosage and biological effect.

The modern evaluation of existing medicines and development of new drugs rests on the demonstration of therapeutic efficacy and safety through carefully controlled clinical trials that also could not be conducted in the absence of a reproducibly quantitative relationship between drug dosage and biological effect. In 1932, Paul Martini published a monograph entitled *Methodology of Therapeutic Investigation* that summarized his experience in scientific drug evaluation and probably entitles him to be considered the "first clinical pharmacologist" (14). Martini described the use of placebos, control groups, stratification, rating scales, and the "n of 1" trial design, and emphasized the need to estimate the adequacy of sample size and establish baseline conditions before beginning a trial. He also introduced the term "clinical pharmacology." Gold (5) and other academic clinical pharmacologists also have made important contributions to the design of clinical trials. Nonetheless, Sheiner (15) points out that continued improvements are needed in our approach to drug evaluation, and asserts that clinicians must regain control over clinical trials to ensure that the important questions are being addressed.

Although the expertise and resources needed to develop new drugs are primarily concentrated in the pharmaceutical industry, clinical investigators based in academia have played an important catalytic role in championing the development of a number of drugs (16). For example, dopamine was first synthesized in 1910, but the therapeutic potential of this compound was not recognized until 1963 when Leon Goldberg and his colleagues provided convincing evidence that dopamine mediated vasodilation by binding to a previously undescribed receptor (17). These investigators subsequently demonstrated the clinical utility of intravenous dopamine infusions in treating patients with hypotension or shock unresponsive to plasma volume expansion. This provided the basis for a small pharmaceutical firm to bring dopamine to market in the early 1970s.

Academically based clinical pharmacologists have a long tradition of interest in drug metabolism. Drug metabolism generally constitutes an important mechanism by which drugs are converted to inactive compounds that usually are more rapidly excreted than the parent drug. However, some drug metabolites have important pharmacologic activity. This was first demonstrated in 1935 when the antibacterial activity of prontosil was found to reside solely in its metabolite, sulfanilamide (18). Advances in analytical chemistry over the last 30 years have made it possible to measure on a routine basis plasma concentrations of drug metabolites as well as parent drugs. Further study of these metabolites has demonstrated that several of them have important pharmacologic activity that must be considered for proper clinical interpretation of plasma concentration measurements (19). In some cases, clinical pharmacologists have demonstrated that drug metabolites have pharmacologic properties that make them preferable to marketed drugs.

For example, when terfenadine (Seldane), the prototype of nonsedating antihistamine drugs, was reported to cause *torsades de pointes* and fatality in patients with no previous history of cardiac arrhythmia, Woosley and his colleagues (20) proceeded to investigate the electrophysiologic effects of both terfenadine and its carboxylate metabolite (Figure 1.1). These investigators found that terfenadine, like quinidine, an antiarrhythmic drug with known propensity to cause *torsades de pointes* in

TERFENADINE

TERFENADINE CARBOXYLATE

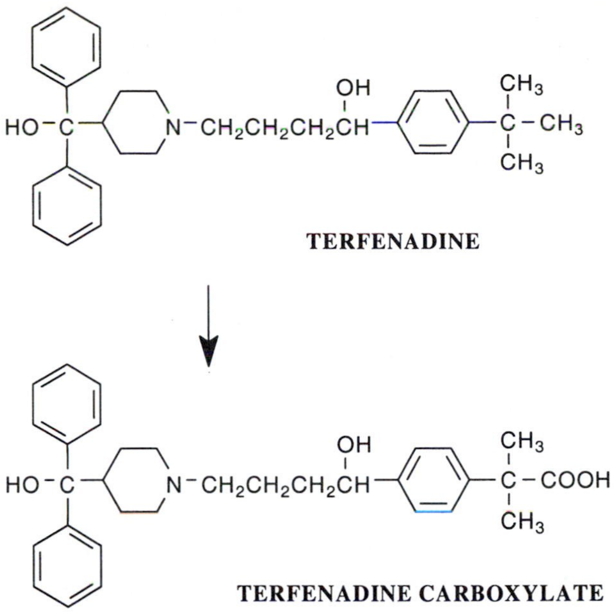

FIGURE 1.1 Chemical structures of terfenidine and its carboxylate metabolite. The acid metabolite is formed by oxidation of the *t*-butyl side chain of the parent drug.

susceptible individuals, blocked the delayed rectifier potassium current. However, terfenadine carboxylate, which actually accounts for most of the observed antihistaminic effects when patients take terfenadine, was found to be devoid of this proarrhythmic property. These findings provided the impetus for commercial development of the carboxylate metabolite as a safer alternative to terfenadine. This metabolite is now marketed as fexofenadine (Allegra).

PHARMACOKINETICS

Pharmacokinetics is defined as the quantitative analysis of the processes of drug absorption, distribution, and elimination that determine the time course of drug action. *Pharmacodynamics* deals with the mechanism of drug action. Hence, pharmacokinetics and pharmacodynamics constitute two major subdivisions of pharmacology.

Since as many as 70 to 80% of adverse drug reactions are dose related (8), our success in preventing these reactions is contingent on our grasp of the principles of pharmacokinetics that provide the scientific basis for dose selection. This becomes critically important when we prescribe drugs that have a narrow therapeutic index. Pharmacokinetics is inescapably mathematical. Although 95% of pharmacokinetic calculations required for clinical application are simple algebra, some understanding of calculus is required to fully grasp the principles of pharmacokinetics.

The Concept of Clearance

Because pharmacokinetics comprises the first few chapters of this book and figures prominently in subsequent chapters, we will pause here to introduce the clinically most important concept in pharmacokinetics: the concept of *clearance*. In 1929, Möller et al. (21) observed that, above a urine flow rate of 2 mL/min, the rate of urea excretion by the kidneys is proportional to the amount of urea in a constant volume of blood. They introduced the term clearance to describe this constant and defined urea clearance as the volume of blood that one minute's excretion serves to clear of urea. Since then, creatinine clearance has become the routine clinical measure of renal functional status and the following equation is used to calculate creatinine clearance (CL_{CR}):

$$CL_{CR} = UV/P$$

where U is the concentration of creatinine excreted over a certain period of time in a measured volume of urine (V) and P is the serum concentration of creatinine. This is really a first-order differential equation since UV is simply the rate at which creatinine is being excreted in urine (dE/dt). Hence,

$$dE/dt = CL_{CR} \cdot P$$

If instead of looking at the rate of creatinine excretion in urine, we consider the rate of change of creatinine in the body (dX/dt), we can write the following equation:

$$dX/dt = I - CL_{CR} \cdot P$$

Here I is the rate of *synthesis* of creatinine in the body and $CL_{CR} \cdot P$ is the rate of creatinine *elimination*. At steady state, these rates are equal and there is no change in the total body content of creatinine $(dX/dt = 0)$, so:

$$P = I/CL_{CR} \qquad (1.1)$$

This equation explains why it is hazardous to estimate the status of renal function solely from serum creatinine results in patients who have a reduced muscle mass and a decline in creatinine synthesis rate. For example, creatinine synthesis rate may be substantially reduced in elderly patients, so it is not unusual for serum creatinine concentrations to remain within normal limits, even though renal function is markedly impaired.

Clinical Assessment of Renal Function

In routine clinical practice, it is not practical to collect the urine samples that are needed to measure creatinine clearance directly. However, creatinine clearance in adult patients can be estimated either from a standard nomogram or from the equation of Cockcroft and Gault (22). For men, creatinine clearance can be estimated from this equation as follows:

$$CL_{CR}\,(\mathrm{mL/min}) = \frac{(140 - \mathrm{age})(\mathrm{weight\ in\ kg})}{72\,(\mathrm{serum\ creatinine\ in\ mg/dL})}$$

For women, this estimate should be reduced by 15%. This equation will overestimate glomerular filtration rate in patients with low creatinine production due to cirrhosis or cachexia and may be misleading in patients with anasarca or rapidly changing renal function. In these situations, accurate estimates of creatinine clearance can only be obtained by actually measuring urine creatinine excretion rate in a carefully timed urine specimen. By comparing Equation 1.1 with the Cockcroft and Gault equation, we see that the terms (140-age)(weight in kg)/72 simply provide an estimate of the creatinine formation rate in an individual patient.

The Cockcroft and Gault equation cannot be used to estimate creatinine clearance in pediatric patients because muscle mass has not reached the adult proportion of body weight. Therefore, Schwartz and colleagues (23,24) developed the following equation to predict creatinine clearance in these patients:

$$CL_{CR}\,(\mathrm{mL/min/1.73m^2}) = \frac{k \cdot L(\mathrm{in\ cm})}{\mathrm{plasma\ creatinine\ in\ mg/dL}}$$

where L is body length and k varies by age and sex as follows:

neonates to children 1 year of age: $k = 0.45$
children 1–13 years of age: $k = 0.55$
females 13–20 years of age: $k = 0.57$
males 13–20 years of age: $k = 0.70$

From the standpoint of clinical pharmacology, the utility of using the Cockcroft and Gault equation or other methods to estimate creatinine clearance stems from the fact that these estimates can alert healthcare workers to the presence of impaired renal function in patients whose creatinine formation rate is reduced. As discussed in Chapter 5, creatinine clearance estimates also can be used to guide dose adjustment in these patients.

Dose-related Toxicity Often Occurs When Impaired Renal Function Is Unrecognized

Failure to appreciate that a patient has impaired renal function is a frequent cause of dose-related adverse drug reactions with digoxin and other drugs that normally rely primarily on the kidneys for elimination. As shown in Table 1.1, an audit of patients with high plasma con-

TABLE 1.1 Status of Renal Function in 44 patients with Digoxin Toxicity[a]

Serum creatinine (mg/dL)	CL_{CR} (mL/min)		Percent
	≥ 50	< 50	
≤ 1.7	4	19	52
> 1.7	0	21	48

[a] Data from Piergies AA, Worwag EM, Atkinson AJ, Jr. Clin Pharmacol Ther 1994;55:353–8.

centrations of digoxin (≥ 3.0 ng/mL) demonstrated that 19 of 44, or 43% of 44 patients with digoxin toxicity had serum creatinine concentrations within the range of normal values, yet had estimated creatinine clearances less than 50 mL/min (25). Hence, assessment of renal function is essential if digoxin and many other drugs are to be used safely and effectively, and is an important prerequisite for the application of clinical pharmacologic principles to patient care. Decreases in renal function are particularly likely to be unrecognized in older patients whose creatinine clearance declines as a consequence of aging rather than overt kidney disease. It is for this reason that the Joint Commission on Accreditation of Healthcare Organizations has placed the estimation or measurement of creatinine clearance in patients of 65 years of age or older at the top of its list of indicators for monitoring the quality of medication use (26). Experience unfortunately shows that healthcare workers are only sporadic in their use of standard equations to estimate creatinine clearance. So routine provision of these estimates is probably best performed by a computerized laboratory reporting system.

References

1. Holmstedt B, Liljestrand G. Readings in pharmacology. Oxford: Pergamon; 1963.
2. Reidenberg MM. Attitudes about clinical research. Lancet 1996;347:1188.
3. Reidenberg MM. Clinical pharmacology: The scientific basis of therapeutics. Clin Pharmacol Ther 1999;66:2–8.
4. Atkinson AJ Jr., Nordstrom K. The challenge of in-hospital medication use: An opportunity for clinical pharmacology. Clin Pharmacol Ther 1996;60:363–7.
5. Gold H, Kwit NT, Otto H. The xanthines (theobromine and aminophylline) in the treatment of cardiac pain. JAMA 1937;108:2173–9.
6. Gold H, Catell McK, Greiner T, Hanlon LW, Kwit NT, Modell W, Cotlove E, Benton J, Otto HL. Clinical pharmacology of digoxin. J Pharmacol Exp Ther 1953;109:45–57.
7. Taussig HB. A study of the German outbreak of phocomelia: The thalidomide syndrome. JAMA 1962;180:1106–14.
8. Melmon KL. Preventable drug reactions—Causes and cures. N Engl J Med 1971;284:1361–8.
9. Koch-Weser J. Serum drug concentrations as therapeutic guides. N Engl J Med 1972;287:227–31.
10. Lazarou J, Pomeranz BH, Corey PN. Incidence of adverse drug reactions in hospitalized patients: A meta-analysis of prospective studies. JAMA 1998;279:1200–5.
11. Bates DW. Drugs and adverse drug reactions. How worried should we be? JAMA 1998;279:1216–7.
12. Sjöqvist F. The past, present and future of clinical pharmacology. Eur J Clin Pharmacol 1999;55:553–7.
13. Leake CD. The scientific status of pharmacology. Science 1961;134:2069–79.
14. Shelley JH, Baur MP. Paul Martini: The first clinical pharmacologist? Lancet 1999;353:1870–73.
15. Sheiner LB. The intellectual health of clinical drug evaluation. Clin Pharmacol Ther 1991;50:4–9.
16. Flowers CR, Melmon KL. Clinical investigators as critical determinants in pharmaceutical innovation. Nature Med 1997;3:136–43.
17. Goldberg LI. Cardiovascular and renal actions of dopamine: Potential clinical applications. Pharmacol Rev 1972;24:1–29.
18. Tréfouël J, Tréfouël Mme J, Nitti F, Bouvet D. Activité du p-aminophénylsulfamide sur les infections streptococciques expérimentales de la souris et du lapin. Compt Rend Soc Biol (Paris) 1935;120:756–8.
19. Atkinson AJ Jr, Strong JM. Effect of active drug metabolites on plasma level-response correlations. J Pharmacokinet Biopharm 1977;5:95–109.
20. Woosley RL, Chen Y, Freiman JP, Gillis RA. Mechanism of the cardiotoxic actions of terfenadine. JAMA 1993;269:1532–6.
21. Möller E, McIntosh JF, Van Slyke DD. Studies of urea excretion. II. Relationship between urine volume and the rate of urea excretion in normal adults. J Clin Invest 1929;6:427–65.
22. Cockroft DW, Gault MH. Prediction of creatinine clearance from serum creatinine. Nephron 1976;16:31–41.
23. Schwartz GJ, Feld LG, Langford DJ. A simple estimate of glomerular filtration rate in full-term infants during the first year of life. J Pediatr 1984;104:849–54.
24. Schwartz GJ, Gauthier B. A simple estimate of glomerular filtration rate in adolescent boys. J Pediatr 1985;106:522–6.
25. Piergies AA, Worwag EM, Atkinson AJ Jr. A concurrent audit of high digoxin plasma levels. Clin Pharmacol Ther 1994;55:353–8.
26. Nadzam DM. A systems approach to medication use. In: Cousins DM, editor. Medication use: A systems approach to reducing errors. Oakbrook Terrace (IL): Joint Commission on Accreditation of Healthcare Organizations; 1998. p. 5–17.

Additional Sources of Information

General

Hardman JG, Gilman AG, Limbird LE, editors. Goodman & Gilman's The Pharmacological basis of therapeutics. 9th ed. New York: McGraw-Hill; 1995.

This is the standard reference textbook of pharmacology. It contains good introductory presentations of the general principles of pharmacokinetics, pharmacodynamics, and therapeutics. Appendix II contains a useful tabulation of the pharmacokinetic properties of many commonly used drugs.

Carruthers SG, Hoffman BB, Melmon KL, Nierenberg, editors. Melmon and Morrelli's Clinical pharmacology. 4th ed. New York: McGraw-Hill; 2000.

This is the classic textbook of clinical pharmacology with introductory chapters devoted to general principles and subsequent chapters covering different therapeutic areas. A final section is devoted to core topics in clinical pharmacology.

Pharmacokinetics

Gibaldi M, Perrier D. Pharmacokinetics. 2nd ed. New York: Marcel Dekker; 1982.

This is a standard reference in pharmacokinetics and is the one most often cited in the "methods section" of papers that are published in journals covering this area.

Rowland M, Tozer TN. Clinical pharmacokinetics concepts and applications. 3rd ed. Baltimore: Williams & Wilkins; 1995.

This is a well-written book that is very popular as an introductory text.

Drug Metabolism

Pratt WB, Taylor P, editors. Principles of drug action: The Basis of pharmacology. 3rd ed. New York: Churchill Livingstone; 1990.

This book is devoted to basic principles of pharmacology and has good chapters on drug metabolism and pharmacogenetics.

Drug Therapy in Special Populations

Evans WE, Schentag JJ, Jusko WJ, editors. Applied pharmacokinetics: Principles of therapeutic drug monitoring. 3rd ed. Vancouver (WA): Applied Therapeutics; 1992.

This book contains detailed information that is useful for individualizing dose regimens of a number of commonly used drugs.

Drug Development

Spilker B. Guide to clinical trials. Philadelphia: Lippincott-Raven; 1996.

This book contains detailed discussions of many practical topics that are relevant to the process of drug development.

Yacobi A, Skelly JP, Shah VP, Benet LZ, editors. Integration of pharmacokinetics, pharmacodynamics, and toxicokinetics in rational drug development. New York: Plenum; 1993.

This book describes how the basic principles of clinical pharmacology currently are being applied in the process of drug development.

Journals

Clinical Pharmacology and Therapeutics
British Journal of Clinical Pharmacology
Journal of Pharmaceutical Sciences
Journal of Pharmacokinetics and Biopharmaceutics

Websites

American Society for Clinical Pharmacology and Therapeutics (ASCPT): http://www.ascpt.org/

The American Board of Clinical Pharmacology (ABCP): http://www.abcp.net/

PHARMACOKINETICS

2

Clinical Pharmacokinetics

ARTHUR J. ATKINSON, JR.

Clinical Center, National Institutes of Health, Bethesda, Maryland

Pharmacokinetics is an important tool that is used in the conduct of both basic and applied research, and is an essential component of the drug development process. In addition, pharmacokinetics is a valuable adjunct for prescribing and evaluating drug therapy. For most clinical applications, pharmacokinetic analyses can be simplified by representing drug distribution within the body by a *single compartment* in which drug concentrations are uniform (1). Clinical application of pharmacokinetics usually entails relatively simple calculations, carried out in the context of what has been termed *the target concentration strategy*. We shall begin by discussing this strategy.

THE TARGET CONCENTRATION STRATEGY

The rationale for measuring concentrations of drugs in plasma, serum, or blood is that *concentration-response* relationships are often less variable than *dose-response* relationships (2). This is true because individual variation in the processes of drug absorption, distribution, and elimination affects dose-response relationships, but not the relationship between free (nonprotein-bound) drug concentration in plasma water and intensity of effect (Figure 2.1).

Because most adverse drug reactions are dose related, therapeutic drug monitoring has been advocated as a means of improving therapeutic efficacy and reducing drug toxicity (3). Drug level monitoring is most useful when combined with pharmacokinetic-based dose selection in an integrated management plan as outlined in Figure 2.2.

This approach to drug dosing has been termed the *target concentration strategy*.

The rationale of therapeutic drug monitoring was first elucidated over 70 years ago when Otto Wuth recommended monitoring bromide levels in patients treated with this drug (4). More widespread clinical application of the target concentration strategy has been possible only because major advances have been made over the past 30 years in developing analytical methods capable of routinely measuring drug concentrations in patient serum, plasma, or blood samples, and because of increased understanding of basic pharmacokinetic principles (5). However, given the advanced state of modern chemical and immunochemical analytical methods, the greatest current challenge is the establishment of the range of drug concentrations in blood, plasma, or serum that correlate reliably with therapeutic efficacy or toxicity. This challenge is exemplified by the results shown in Figure 2.3 that are taken from the attempt by Smith and Haber (6) to correlate serum digoxin levels with clinical manifestations of toxicity. It can be seen that no patient with digoxin levels below 1.6 ng/mL was toxic and that all patients with digoxin levels above 3.0 ng/mL had evidence of digoxin intoxication. However, there is a large intermediate range between 1.6 and 3.0 ng/mL in which patients could be either nontoxic or toxic. Additional clinical information is often necessary to interpret drug concentration measurements that are otherwise equivocal. In this study, it was found that all toxic patients with serum digoxin levels less than 2.0 ng/mL had coexisting coronary heart disease, a condition known to predispose the myocardium to the toxic effects of this drug. Con-

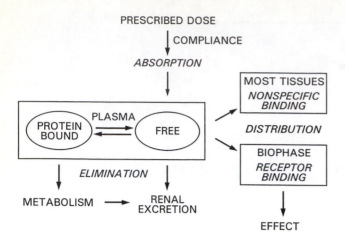

FIGURE 2.1 Diagram of factors that account for variability in observed effects when standard drug doses are prescribed. Some of this variability can be compensated for by using plasma concentration measurements to guide dose adjustments.

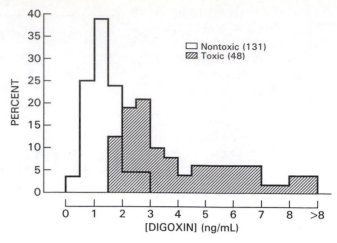

FIGURE 2.3 Superimposed frequency histograms in which serum digoxin concentrations are shown for 131 patients without digoxin toxicity and 48 patients with electrocardiographic evidence of digoxin toxicity. (Reproduced with permission from Smith TW, Haber E. J Clin Invest 1970;49:2377–86.)

versely, 4 of the 10 nontoxic patients with levels above 2.0 ng/mL were being treated with antiarrhythmic drugs that might have suppressed electrocardiographic evidence of digoxin toxicity.

In the final analysis, the digoxin level that is therapeutic for a given patient depends on the extent to which ventricular rate needs to be slowed in patients with atrial fibrillation or on the amount of additional

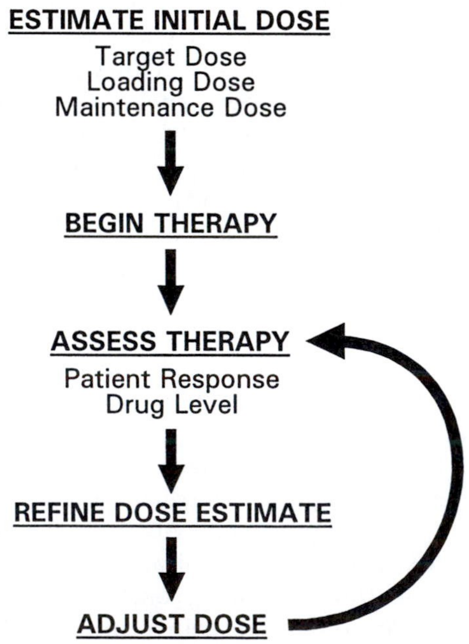

ESTIMATE INITIAL DOSE
Target Dose
Loading Dose
Maintenance Dose

↓

BEGIN THERAPY

↓

ASSESS THERAPY
Patient Response
Drug Level

↓

REFINE DOSE ESTIMATE

↓

ADJUST DOSE

FIGURE 2.2 Target concentration strategy in which pharmacokinetics and drug level measurements are integral parts of a therapeutic plan that extends from initial drug dose estimation to subsequent patient monitoring and dose adjustment.

inotropy that is needed to compensate for congestive heart failure. Since an initial maintenance dose of 0.25 mg/day is usually prescribed for patients with apparently normal renal function, this corresponds to a target level of 1.4 ng/mL. Accordingly, laboratory reports of digoxin concentration measurements are commonly accompanied by guidelines such as the following:

Usual therapeutic range	0.8–1.6 ng/mL
Possibly toxic levels	1.6–3.0 ng/mL
Probably toxic levels	> 3.0 ng/mL

However, Lee and Smith (7) have reviewed clinical conditions that may affect patient response to a given digoxin level and emphasize quite properly that digoxin concentration measurements should not be the sole criterion that is used in clinical decision making.

Despite the ambiguity in interpreting digoxin level results, it was demonstrated in a controlled study that routine availability of digoxin concentration measurements markedly reduced the incidence of toxic reactions to this drug (8). Unfortunately, controlled studies documenting the clinical benefit of plasma level monitoring are limited. In addition, one could not justify monitoring plasma levels of all prescribed drugs even if this technical challenge could be met. Thus, plasma level monitoring is most helpful for drugs that have a low therapeutic index and that have no clinically observable effects that can be easily monitored to guide dose adjustment. Generally accepted indications for measuring plasma concentrations of these drugs are:

1. To evaluate concentration-related toxicity
   - Unexpectedly slow drug elimination
   - Accidental or purposeful overdose
   - Surreptitious drug taking
   - Dispensing errors
2. To evaluate lack of therapeutic efficacy
   - Patient noncompliance with prescribed therapy
   - Poor drug absorption
   - Unexpectedly rapid drug elimination
3. To ensure that the dose regimen is likely to provide effective prophylaxis
4. To use pharmacokinetic principles to guide dose adjustment

Despite these technical advances, adverse reactions still occur frequently with digoxin, phenytoin, and many other drugs for which plasma level measurements are routinely available. The persistence in contemporary practice of dose-related toxicity with these drugs most likely reflects inadequate understanding of basic pharmacokinetic principles. This is illustrated by the following case history (5):

> In October 1981, a 39-year-old man with mitral stenosis was hospitalized for mitral valve replacement. He had a history of chronic renal failure resulting from interstitial nephritis and was maintained on hemodialysis. His mitral valve was replaced with a prosthesis and digoxin therapy was initiated postoperatively in a dose of 0.25 mg/day. Two weeks later, he was noted to be unusually restless in the evening. The following day, he died shortly after he received his morning digoxin dose. Blood was obtained during an unsuccessful resuscitation attempt, and the measured plasma digoxin concentration was 6.9 ng/mL.

CONCEPTS UNDERLYING CLINICAL PHARMACOKINETICS

Pharmacokinetics provides the scientific basis of dose selection, and the process of dose regimen design can be used to illustrate with a single-compartment model the basic concepts of *apparent distribution volume* (V_d), elimination half-life ($t_{1/2}$), and *elimination clearance* (CL_E). A schematic diagram of this model is shown in Figure 2.4 along with the two primary pharmacokinetic parameters of distribution volume and elimination clearance that characterize it.

Initiation of Drug Therapy (Concept of Apparent Distribution Volume)

Sometimes drug treatment is begun with a loading dose to produce a rapid therapeutic response. Thus, a patient with atrial fibrillation might be given a 0.75-mg intravenous loading dose of digoxin as initial

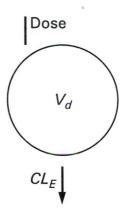

FIGURE 2.4 Diagram of a single compartment model in which the primary kinetic parameters are the apparent distribution volume of the compartment (V_d) and the elimination clearance (CL_E).

therapy to control ventricular rate. The expected plasma concentrations of digoxin are shown in Figure 2.5. Inspection of this figure indicates that the log plasma-concentration-vs.-time curve eventually becomes a straight line. This part of the curve is termed the *elimination phase*. By extrapolating this elimination-phase line back to time zero, we can estimate the plasma concentration (C_0) that would have occurred if the loading dose were instantaneously distributed throughout the body. Measured plasma digoxin concentrations lie above the back extrapolated line for several hours because distribution equilibrium actually is reached only slowly after a digoxin dose is administered. This part of the plasma level-vs.-time curve is termed the *distribution phase*. This phase reflects the underlying *multicompartmental* nature of digoxin distribution from the intravascular space to peripheral tissues.

As shown in Figure 2.5, the back-extrapolated estimate of C_0 can be used to calculate the apparent volume ($V_{d\ (extrap)}$) of a hypothetical single compartment into which digoxin distribution occurs:

$$V_{d\ (extrap)} = \text{Loading Dose}/C_0 \qquad (2.1)$$

In this case, the apparent distribution volume of 536 L is much larger than anatomically possible. This apparent anomaly occurs because digoxin has a much higher binding affinity for tissues than for plasma, and the apparent distribution volume is the volume of *plasma* that would be required to provide the observed dilution of the loading dose. Despite this apparent anomaly, the concept of distribution volume is clinically useful because it defines the relationship between plasma concentration and the total amount of drug in the body. Further complexity arises from the fact that $V_{d\ (extrap)}$ is only one of three different distribution volume estimates that we will encounter. Because

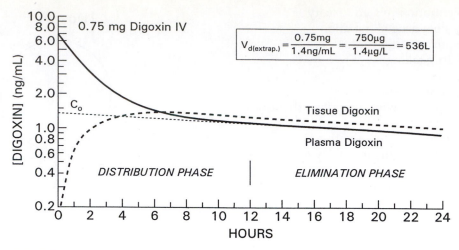

FIGURE 2.5 Simulation of plasma *(solid line)* and tissue *(broken line)* digoxin concentrations after intravenous administration of a 0.75 mg loading dose to a 70 Kg patient with normal renal function. C_0 is estimated by back extrapolation *(dotted line)* of elimination-phase plasma concentrations. V_d is calculated by dividing the administered drug dose by this estimate of C_0, as shown. Tissue concentrations are referenced to the apparent distribution volume of a peripheral compartment that represents tissue distribution. (Reproduced with permission from Atkinson AJ Jr, Kushner W. Annu Rev Pharmacol Toxicol 1979;19:105–27.)

the distribution process is neglected in calculating this volume, it represents an overestimate of the sum of the volumes of the individual compartments involved in drug distribution.

The time course of the myocardial effects of digoxin parallels its concentration profile in peripheral tissues (Figure 2.5), so there is a delay between the attainment of peak plasma digoxin concentrations and the observation of maximum inotropic and chronotropic effects. The range of therapeutic and toxic digoxin concentrations has been derived from observations made during the elimination phase, so blood should not be sampled for digoxin assay until distribution equilibrium is nearly complete. In clinical practice, this means waiting for at least 6 hours after a digoxin dose has been administered. In a recent audit of patients with measured digoxin levels of 3.0 ng/mL or more, it was found that nearly one-third of these levels were not associated with toxicity, but reflected procedural error in that blood was sampled less than 6 hours after digoxin administration (9).

For other drugs, such as thiopental (10) or lidocaine (11), the locus of pharmacologic action (termed the *biophase* in classical pharmacology) is in rapid kinetic equilibrium with the intravascular space. The distribution phase of these drugs represents their somewhat slower distribution from intravascular space to pharmacologically inert tissues, such as skeletal muscle, and serves to shorten the duration of their pharmacologic effects when single doses are administered. Plasma levels of these drugs reflect therapeutic and

toxic effects throughout the dosing interval and blood can be obtained for drug assay without waiting for the elimination phase to be reached.

Continuation of Drug Therapy (Concepts of Elimination Half-Life and Clearance)

After starting therapy with a loading dose, maintenance of a sustained therapeutic effect often necessitates administering additional drug doses to replace the amount of drug that has been excreted or metabolized. Fortunately, the elimination of most drugs is a *first-order* process in that the rate of drug elimination is directly proportional to the drug concentration in plasma.

Elimination Half-Life

It is convenient to characterize the elimination of drugs with first-order elimination rates by their *elimination half-life*, the time required for half an administered drug dose to be eliminated. If drug elimination half-life can be estimated for a patient, it is often practical to continue therapy by administering half the loading dose at an interval of one elimination half-life. In this way, drug elimination can be balanced by drug administration and a steady state maintained from the onset of therapy. Because digoxin has an elimination half-life of 1.6 days in patients with normal renal function, it is inconvenient to administer digoxin at this interval. When renal function is normal, it is customary to initiate maintenance therapy by administering

```
.25 x 2/3 = .17                                                    Dose #1
       +.25                                                        Dose #2
       .42 x 2/3 = .28
              +.25                                                 Dose #3
              .53 x 2/3 = .36
                     +.25                                          Dose #4
                     .61 x 2/3 = .41
                            +.25                                   Dose #5
                            .66 x 2/3 = .44
                                   +.25                            Dose #6
                                   .69 x 2/3 = .46
                                          +.25                     Dose #7
                                          .71
```

SCHEME 2.1

daily digoxin doses equal to one-third of the required loading dose.

Another consequence of first-order elimination kinetics is that a constant fraction of total body drug stores will be eliminated in a given time interval. Thus, if there is no urgency in establishing a therapeutic effect, the loading dose of digoxin can be omitted and 90% of the eventual steady-state drug concentration will be reached after a period of time equal to 3.3 elimination half-lives. This is referred to as the *Plateau Principle*. The classical derivation of this principle is provided later in this chapter, but for now brute force will suffice to illustrate this important concept. Suppose that we elect to omit the 0.75-mg digoxin loading dose shown in Figure 2.5 and simply begin therapy with a 0.25-mg/day maintenance dose. If the patient has normal renal function, we can anticipate that one-third of the total amount of digoxin present in the body will be eliminated each day and that two-thirds will remain when the next daily dose is administered. As shown in Scheme 2.1 (above), the patient will have digoxin body stores of 0.66 mg just after the fifth daily dose (3.3×1.6 day half-life = 5.3 days) and this is 88% of the total body stores that would have been provided by a 0.75 mg loading dose.

The solid line in Figure (2.6 shows ideal matching of digoxin loading and maintenance doses. When the digoxin loading dose (called *digitalizing dose* in clinical practice) is omitted, or when the loading dose and maintenance dose are not matched appropriately, steady-state levels are reached only asymptotically. However, the most important concept that this figure demonstrates is that *the eventual steady-state level is determined only by the maintenance dose*, regardless of the size of the loading dose. Selection of an inappropriately high digitalizing dose only subjects patients to an interval of added risk without achieving a permanent increase in the extent of digitalization. Conversely, when a high digitalizing dose is required to control ventricular rate in patients with atrial fibrillation or

flutter, a higher than usual maintenance dose also will be required.

Elimination Clearance

Just as creatinine clearance is used to quantitate the renal excretion of creatinine, the removal of drugs eliminated by first-order kinetics can be defined by an *elimination clearance* (CL_E). In fact, elimination clearance is the primary pharmacokinetic parameter that characterizes the removal of drugs that are eliminated by first-order kinetics. When drug administration is by intravenous infusion, the eventual steady-state concentration of drug in the body (C_{ss}) can be calculated from the following equation, where the drug infusion rate is given by I:

$$C_{ss} = I/CL_E \qquad (2.2)$$

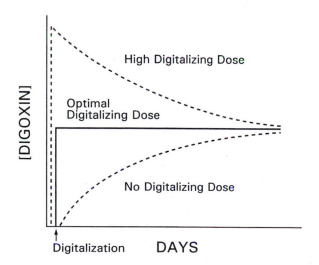

FIGURE 2.6 Expected digoxin plasma concentrations after administering perfectly matched loading and maintenance doses *(solid line)*, no initial loading dose *(bottom broken line)*, or a loading dose that is large in relation to the subsequent maintenance dose *(upper broken line)*.

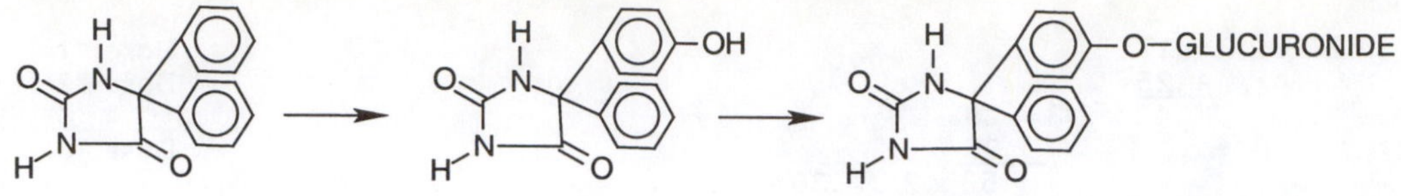

FIGURE 2.7 Metabolism of phenytoin to form *p*-HPPH and *p*-HPPH glucuronide. The first step in this enzymatic reaction sequence is rate limiting and follows Michaelis–Menten kinetics, showing progressive saturation as plasma concentrations rise within the range that is required for anticonvulsant therapy to be effective.

When intermittent oral or parenteral doses are administered at a dosing interval, τ, the corresponding equation is:

$$\bar{C}_{ss} = \frac{\text{Dose}/\tau}{CL_E} \qquad (2.3)$$

where $\bar{C}_{ss}$ is the mean concentration during the dosing interval. Under conditions of intermittent administration, there is a continuing periodicity in maximum ("peak") and minimum ('trough") drug levels so that only a quasi steady state is reached. However, unless particular attention is directed to these peak and trough levels, no distinction generally is made in clinical pharmacokinetics between the true steady state that is reached when an intravenous infusion is administered continuously and the quasi steady state that results from intermittent administration.

Since there is a directly proportionate relationship between administered drug dose and steady-state plasma level, Equations 2.2 and 2.3 provide a straightforward guide to dose adjustment for drugs that are eliminated by first-order kinetics. Thus, to double the plasma level, the dose simply should be doubled. Conversely, to halve the plasma level, the dose should be halved. It is for this reason that Equations 2.2 and 2.3 are the most clinically important pharmacokinetic equations. Note that, as is apparent from Figure 2.6, these equations also stipulate that the steady-state level is determined only by the maintenance dose and elimination clearance. The loading dose does not appear in the equations and does not influence the eventual steady-state level.

In contrast to elimination clearance, elimination half-life ($t_{1/2}$) is not a primary pharmacokinetic parameter because it is determined by distribution volume as well as by elimination clearance.

$$t_{1/2} = \frac{0.693 V_{d(area)}}{CL_E} \qquad (2.4)$$

The value of V_d in this equation is not $V_{d(extrap.)}$, but represents a second estimate of distribution volume, referred to as $V_{d(area)}$ or $V_{d(\beta)}$, that generally is estimated from measured elimination half-life and clearance. The similarity of these two estimates of distribution volume reflects the extent to which drug distribution is accurately described by a single compartment model, and obviously varies from drug to drug (12).

Drugs Not Eliminated by First-Order Kinetics

Unfortunately, the elimination of some drugs does not follow first-order kinetics. For example, the primary pathway of phenytoin elimination entails initial metabolism to form 5-(parahydroxyphenyl)-5-phenylhydantoin (*p*-HPPH), followed by glucuronide conjugation (Figure 2.7). The metabolism of this drug is not first order, but follows Michaelis–Menten kinetics because the microsomal enzyme system that forms *p*-HPPH is partially saturated at phenytoin concentrations of 10–20 µg/mL that are therapeutically effective. The result is that phenytoin plasma concentrations rise hyperbolically as dosage is increased (Figure 2.8).

For drugs eliminated by first-order kinetics, the relationship between dosing rate and steady-state plasma concentration is given by rearranging Equation 2.3 as follows:

$$\text{Dose}/\tau = CL_E \cdot \bar{C}_{ss} \qquad (2.5)$$

The corresponding equation for phenytoin is:

$$\text{Dose}/\tau = \frac{V_{max}}{K_m + \bar{C}_{ss}} \cdot \bar{C}_{ss} \qquad (2.6)$$

where V_{max} is the maximum rate of drug metabolism and K_m is the apparent Michaelis–Menten constant for the enzymatic metabolism of phenytoin.

Although phenytoin plasma concentrations show substantial interindividual variation when standard doses are administered, they average 10 µg/mL when

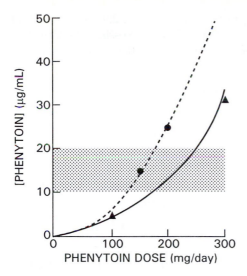

FIGURE 2.8 The lines show the relationship between dose and steady-state plasma phenytoin concentrations predicted for two patients who became toxic after initial treatment with 300 mg/day. Measured steady-state plasma concentrations are shown by the solid circles and triangles. The shaded area shows the usual range of therapeutically effective phenytoin plasma concentrations. (Reproduced with permission from Atkinson AJ Jr. Med Clin North Am 1974;58:1037–49.)

adults are treated with a 300-mg total daily dose, but rise to an average of 20 μg/mL when the dose is increased to 400 mg (13). This nonproportional relationship between phenytoin dose and plasma concentration complicates patient management and undoubtedly contributes to the many adverse reactions that are seen in patients treated with this drug. Although several pharmacokinetic approaches have been developed for estimating dose adjustments, it is safest to change phenytoin doses in small increments and to rely on careful monitoring of clinical response and phenytoin plasma levels. The pharmacokinetics of phenytoin were studied in both patients shown in Figure 2.8 after they became toxic when treated with the 300-mg/day dose that is routinely prescribed as initial therapy for adults (13). The figure demonstrates that the entire therapeutic range is traversed in these patients by a dose increment of less than 100 mg/day.

Even though many drugs in common clinical use are eliminated by drug metabolizing enzymes, relatively few of them have Michaelis–Menten elimination kinetics (e.g., aspirin and ethyl alcohol). The reason for this is that K_m for most drugs is much greater than $\bar{C}_{ss}$. Hence for most drugs, $\bar{C}_{ss}$ can be ignored in the denominator of Equation 2.6 and this equation reduces to:

$$\text{Dose}/\tau = \frac{V_{max}}{K_m} \cdot \bar{C}_{ss}$$

where the ratio V_{max}/K_m is equivalent to CL_E in Equation 2.5. Thus, for most drugs, a change in dose will change steady state plasma concentrations proportionately, a property that is termed *dose proportionality*.

Mathematical Basis of Clinical Pharmacokinetics

In the following sections we will review the mathematical basis of some of the important relationships that are used when pharmacokinetic principles are applied to the care of patients. The reader also is referred to other literature sources that may be helpful (1, 12, 14).

First-Order Elimination Kinetics

For most drugs, the amount of drug eliminated from the body during any time interval is proportional to the total amount of drug present in the body. In pharmacokinetic terms, this is called *first-order* elimination and is described by the equation:

$$dX/dt = -k\,X \tag{2.7}$$

where X is the total amount of drug present in the body at any time (t) and k is the elimination rate constant for the drug. This equation can be solved by separating variables and direct integration to calculate the amount of drug remaining in the body at any time after an initial dose:

Separating variables: $dX/X = -k\,dt$

Integrating from
zero time to time $= t$: $\int_{X_0}^{X} dX/X = -k \int_0^t dt$

$$\ln X \Big|_{X_0}^{X} = -kt \Big|_0^t$$

$$\ln \frac{X}{X_0} = -kt \tag{2.8}$$

$$X = X_0\, e^{-kt} \tag{2.9}$$

Although these equations deal with total amounts of drug in the body, the equation $C = X/V_d$ provides a general relationship between X and drug concentration (C) at any time after the drug dose is administered. Therefore, C can be substituted for X in Equations 2.7 and 2.8 as follows:

$$\ln \frac{C}{C_0} = -kt \tag{2.10}$$

$$C = C_0\, e^{-kt} \tag{2.11}$$

Equation 2.10 is particularly useful since it can be rearranged in the form of the equation for a straight line ($y = mx + b$) to give:

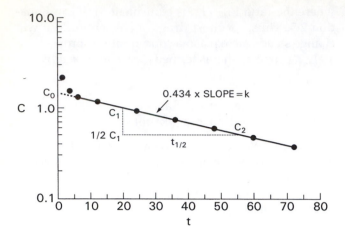

FIGURE 2.9 Plot of drug concentrations vs. time on semilogarithmic coordinates. Back extrapolation *(broken line)* of the elimination phase slope *(solid line)* provides an estimate of C_0. The elimination half-life ($t_{1/2}$) can be estimated from the time required for concentrations to fall from some point on the elimination-phase line (C_1) to $C_2 = 1/2\ C_1$, as shown by the dotted lines. In the case of digoxin, C would be in units of ng/mL and t in hours.

$$\ln C = -kt + \ln C_0 \qquad (2.12)$$

Now when data are obtained after administration of a single drug dose and C is plotted on base 10 semilogarithmic graph paper, a straight line is obtained with 0.434 times the slope equal to k ($\log x / \ln x = 0.434$) and an intercept on the ordinate of C_0. In practice, C_0 is never measured directly because some time is needed for the injected drug to distribute throughout body fluids. However, C_0 can be estimated by back-extrapolating the straight line given by Equation 2.12 (Figure 2.5).

Concept of Elimination Half-Life

If the rate of drug distribution is rapid compared with rate of drug elimination, the terminal exponential phase of a semilogarithmic plot of drug concentrations vs. time can be used to estimate the elimination half-life of a drug as, shown in Figure 2.9. Because Equation 2.10 can be used to estimate k from any two concentrations that are separated by an interval t, it can be seen from this equation that when $C_2 = 1/2\ C_1$:

$$\ln 1/2 = -kt_{1/2}$$
$$\ln 2 = kt_{1/2}$$

So:

$$t_{1/2} = \frac{0.693}{k} \quad \text{and} \quad k = \frac{0.693}{t_{1/2}} \qquad (2.13)$$

For digoxin, $t_{1/2}$ is usually 1.6 days for patients with normal renal function and $k = 0.43$ day^{-1} ($0.693/1.6 = 0.43$). As a practical point, it is easier to estimate $t_{1/2}$

from a graph such as Figure 2.9 and to then calculate k from Equation 2.13, than to estimate k directly from the slope of the elimination-phase line.

The Relationship of k to Elimination Clearance

In our introductory chapter, we pointed out that the creatinine clearance equation:

$$CL_{CR} = \frac{UV}{P}$$

could be rewritten in the form of the following first-order differential equation:

$$dX/dt = -CL_{CR} \cdot P$$

If this equation is generalized by substituting CL_E for CL_{CR}, it can be seen from Equation 2.7 that, since $P = X/V_d$:

$$k = \frac{CL_E}{V_d} \qquad (2.14)$$

Equation 2.4 is derived by substituting of CL_E/V_d for k in Equation 2.13. Although V_d and CL_E are the two primary parameters of the single compartment model, confusion arises because k is initially calculated from experimental data. However, k is influenced by changes in distribution volume as well as clearance and does not reflect just changes in drug elimination.

The Cumulation Factor

In the steady state condition, the rate of drug administration is exactly balanced by the rate of drug elimination. Gaddum (15) first demonstrated that the maximum and minimum drug levels that are expected at steady state (quasi steady state) can be calculated for drugs that are eliminated by first-order kinetics. Assume that just maintenance doses of a drug are administered without a loading dose (Figure 2.6, lowest curve). Starting with Equation 2.9:

$$X = X_0\, e^{-k\tau}$$

where X_0 is the maintenance dose and X is the amount of drug remaining in the body at time t. If τ is the dosing interval, let:

$$p = e^{-k\tau}$$

Therefore, just before the second dose:

$$X_{1(min)} = X_0\, p$$

Just after the second dose:

$$X_{2(max)} = X_0 + X_0\, p = X_0(1 + p)$$

Similarly, after the third dose

$$X_{3(max)} = X_0 + X_0\, p + X_0\, p^2 = X_0\, (1 + p + p^2)$$

and after the nth dose:

$$X_{n(max)} = X_0(1 + p + \ldots + p^{n-1})$$

or

$$X_{n(max)} = X_0 \frac{(1-p^n)}{(1-p)}$$

Since $p < 1$, as $n \to \infty$, $p^n \to 0$. Therefore,

$$X_{\infty(max)} = X_0/(1-p)$$

or, substituting for p,

$$X_{\infty(max)} = \frac{X_0}{(1-e^{-k\tau})}$$

The value of X_∞ is the maximum *total body content* of the drug that is reached during a dosing interval at steady state. The maximum *concentration* is determined by dividing this value by V_d. The *minimum* value is given by multiplying either of these maximum values by $e^{-k\tau}$.

Note that the respective maximum and minimum drug concentrations after the first dose are:

Maximum: C_0
Minimum: $C_0 e^{-k\tau}$

The expected steady-state counterparts of these initial concentration values can be estimated by multiplying them by the *cumulation factor (CF)*:

$$CF = \frac{1}{1-e^{-k\tau}} \tag{2.15}$$

The Plateau Principle

Although the time required to reach steady state cannot be calculated explicitly, the time required to reach *any specified fraction of the eventual steady state* can be estimated. For dosing regimens in which drugs are administered at a constant interval, Gaddum (15) showed that the number of drug doses *(n)* required to reach a fraction *(f)* of the eventual steady-state amount of drug in the body can be calculated as follows:

$$f = \frac{X_n}{X_\infty} = \frac{X_0\left(1-p^n\right)}{(1-p)} \cdot \frac{(1-p)}{X_0} = 1 - p^n \tag{2.16}$$

In clinical practice, $f = 0.90$ is usually a reasonable approximation of eventual steady state. Substituting this value into Equation 2.16 and solving for n:

$$0.90 = 1 - e^{-nk\tau}$$

$$e^{-nk\tau} = 0.1$$

$$n = -\frac{\ln 0.1}{k\tau}$$

$$n = \frac{2.3}{k\tau}$$

From Equation 2.13:

$$k = 0.693/t_{1/2}$$

Therefore, the time needed to reach 90% of steady state is:

$$n\tau = 3.3t_{1/2}$$

and the corresponding number of doses is:

$$n = 3.3t_{1/2} \tag{2.17}$$

Not only are drug accumulation greater and steady-state drug levels higher in patients with a prolonged elimination half-life but an important consequence of Equation 2.17 is that it takes these patients longer to reach steady state. For example, the elimination half-life of digoxin in patients with normal renal function is 1.6 days, so that 90% of the expected steady state is reached in 5 days when daily doses of this drug are administered. However, the elimination half-life of digoxin is approximately 4.3 days in functionally anephric patients, such as the one described in the case history, and 14 days would be required to reach 90% of the expected steady state. This explains why this patient's adverse reaction occurred two weeks after starting digoxin therapy.

Application of Laplace Transforms to Pharmacokinetics

The Laplace transformation method of solving differential equations falls into the area of *operational calculus* that is finding increasing utility in pharmacokinetics. Operational calculus was invented by an English engineer, Sir Oliver Heaviside (1850–1925), who had an intuitive grasp of mathematics (16). Although Laplace provided the theoretical basis for the method, some of Sir Oliver's intuitive contributions remain (e.g., the Heaviside Expansion Theorem). The idea of operational mathematics and Laplace transforms perhaps is best understood by comparison with the use of logarithms to perform arithmetic operations. This comparison is diagrammed in the flowcharts shown in the scheme on page 18.

Just as there are tables of logarithms, there are tables to aid the mathematical process of obtaining Laplace transforms ($\mathscr{L}$) and inverse Laplace transforms ($\mathscr{L}^{-1}$). Laplace transforms can also be calculated directly from the integral:

$$\mathscr{L}[F(t)] = f(s) = \int_0^\infty F(t)e^{-st}dt$$

We can illustrate the application of Laplace transforms by using them to solve the simple differential

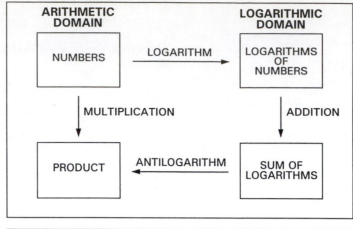

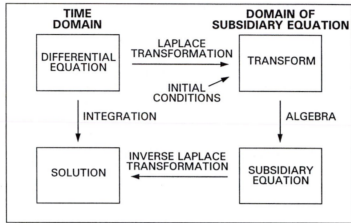

SCHEME 2.2

equation that we have used to describe the single compartment model (Equation 2.7). Starting with this equation:

$$dX/dt = -kX$$

we can use a table of Laplace transform operations
(Appendix I) to take Laplace transforms of each side of
this equation to create the *subsidiary equation:*

For X on the right side of the equation:

$$\pounds\, F(t) = f(s)$$

For *dX/dt* on the left side of the equation:

$$\pounds\, F'(t) = s\, f(s) - F(0)$$

Since $F(0)$ represents the *initial condition*, in this case
the amount of drug in the model compartment at time
zero, X_0, the subsidiary equation can be written:

$$s\, f(s) - X_0 = -k\, f(s)$$

This can be rearranged to give:

$$(s + k)\, f(s) = X_0$$

Or,

$$f(s) = \frac{X_0}{s + k}$$

A table of *inverse Laplace transforms* (Appendix I)
indicates:

$$\mathcal{L}^{-1}\, \frac{1}{s - a} = e^{at}$$

Therefore, the solution to the differential equation is:

$$X = X_0\, e^{-kt}$$

and this is the same result that we obtained as Equation 2.9.

In other words, the Laplace operation transforms the
differential equation from the time domain to another
functional domain represented by the subsidiary equation. After algebraic simplification of this subsidiary
equation, the inverse transformation is used to return

the solved equation to the time domain. We have selected a simple example to illustrate the use of Laplace transform methods. A more advanced application is given in the next chapter in which equations are derived for a two-compartment model. It will be shown subsequently that Laplace transform methods also are helpful in pharmacokinetics when convolution/deconvolution methods are used to characterize drug absorption processes.

References

1. Atkinson AJ Jr, Kushner W. Clinical pharmacokinetics. Annu Rev Pharmacol Toxicol 1979;19:105–27.
2. Atkinson AJ Jr, Reidenberg MM, Thompson WL. Clinical pharmacology. In: Greenberger N, editor. MKSAP VI Syllabus. Philadelphia, Am Col Phys; 1982. p. 85–96.
3. Koch-Weser J. Serum drug concentrations as therapeutic guides. N Engl J Med 1972;287:227–31.
4. Wuth O. Rational bromide treatment: New methods for its control. JAMA 1927;88:2013–17.
5. Atkinson AJ Jr, Ambre JJ. Kalman and Clark's Drug assay: The strategy of therapeutic drug monitoring. 2nd ed. New York: Masson; 1984.
6. Smith TW, Haber E. Digoxin intoxication: the relationship of clinical presentation to serum digoxin concentration. J Clin Invest 1970;49:2377–86.
7. Lee TH, Smith TW. Serum concentration and diagnosis of digitalis toxicity current concepts. Clin Pharmacokinet 1983;8:279–85.
8. Duhme DW, Greenblatt DJ, Koch-Weser J. Reduction of digoxin toxicity associated with measurement of serum levels. Ann Intern Med 1974;80:516–9.
9. Piergies AA, Worwag EW, Atkinson AJ Jr. A concurrent audit of high digoxin plasma levels. Clin Pharmacol Ther 1994;55:353–8.
10. Goldstein A, Aronow L. The durations of action of thiopental and pentobarbital. J Pharmacol Exp Ther 1960;128:1–6.
11. Benowitz N, Forsyth RP, Melmon KL, Rowland M. Lidocaine disposition kinetics in monkey and man. I. Prediction by a perfusion model. Clin Pharmacol Ther 1974;16:87–98.
12. Gibaldi M, Perrier D. Pharmacokinetics. 2nd ed. New York: Marcel Dekker; 1982. p. 199–219.
13. Atkinson AJ Jr. Individualization of anticonvulsant therapy. Med Clin North Am 1974;58:1037–49.
14. Rowland M, Tozer TN. Clinical pharmacokinetics: Concepts and applications. 3rd ed. Baltimore: Lea & Febiger, 1994.
15. Gaddum JH. Repeated doses of drugs. Nature 1944;153:494.
16. Van Valkenberg ME. The Laplace transformation. In: Network analysis. Englewood Cliffs, NJ: Prentice-Hall;1964. p. 159–81.

STUDY PROBLEMS

Select the *one* lettered answer or statement completion that is BEST. It may be helpful to carry out dimensional analysis by including units in your calculations. Answers are provided in Appendix II.

1. A 35-year-old woman is being treated with gentamicin for a urinary tract infection. The gentamicin plasma level is 4 µg/mL shortly after initial intravenous administration of an 80 mg dose of this drug. The distribution volume of gentamicin is:
   A. 5 L
   B. 8 L
   C. 10 L
   D. 16 L
   E. 20 L

2. A 58-year-old man is hospitalized in a cardiac intensive care following an acute myocardial infarction. He has had recurrent episodes of ventricular tachycardia that have not responded to lidocaine and an intravenous infusion of procainamide will now be administered. The patient weighs 80 kg and expected values for his procainamide distribution volume and elimination half-life are 2.0 L/kg and 3 hours, respectively.

   What infusion rate will provide a steady state plasma procainamide level of 4.0 µg/mL?
   A. 2.5 mg/min
   B. 5.0 mg/min
   C. 7.5 mg/min
   D. 10.0 mg/min
   E. 12.5 mg/min

3. A patient with peritonitis is treated with gentamicin 80 mg every 8 hours. Plasma gentamicin levels are measured during the first dosing interval. The gentamicin plasma level is 10 µg/mL at its peak after initial intravenous administration of this drug, and is 5 µg/mL when measured 5 hours later.

   The cumulation factor can be used to predict an expected steady state peak level of:
   A. 10 µg/mL
   B. 12 µg/mL
   C. 15 µg/mL
   D. 18 µg/mL
   E. 20 µg/mL

4. A 20-year-old man is hospitalized after an asthmatic attack precipitated by an upper respiratory infection fails to respond in the emergency room to two doses of subcutaneous injection of epinephrine. The patient has not been taking theophylline-containing medications for the past 6 weeks. He weighs 60 kg and you estimate that his apparent volume of theophylline distribution is 0.45 L/kg. Bronchodilator therapy includes a 5.6-mg/kg loading dose of aminophylline, infused intravenously over 20 min, followed by a maintenance infusion of 0.63 mg/kg per hour (0.50 mg/kg per hour of theophylline). Forty-eight hours later, the patient's respiratory status has improved. However, he has nausea and tachycardia, and his plasma theophylline level is 24 µg/mL.

   For how long do you expect to suspend theophylline administration in order to reach a level of

12 µg/mL before restarting the aminophylline infusion at a rate of 0.31 mg/kg per hour?

A. 5 hours
B. 10 hours
C. 15 hours
D. 20 hours
E. 25 hours

5. Digitoxin has an elimination half-life of approximately 7 days and its elimination is relatively unaffected by decreased renal function. For this latter reason, the decision is made to use this drug to control ventricular rate in a 60-year-old man with atrial fibrillation and a creatinine clearance of 25 mL/min.

   If no loading dose is administered and a maintenance dose of 0.1 mg/day is prescribed, how many days would be required for digitoxin levels to reach 90% of their expected steady state value?

A. 17 days
B. 19 days
C. 21 days
D. 23 days
E. 24 days

6. A 75-year-old man comes to your office with anorexia and nausea. Five years ago he was found to have congestive heart failure that responded to treatment with a thiazide diruetic and an angiotensin converting enzyme inhibitor. Three years ago digoxin was added to the regimen in a dose of 0.25 mg/day. This morning he omitted his digoxin dose. On hospital admission, electrocardiographic monitoring shows frequent bigeminal extrasystoles and the patient's plasma digoxin level is 3.2 ng/mL. Twenty-four hours later the digoxin level is 2.7 ng/mL. At that time you decide that it would be appropriate to let the digoxin level fall to 1.6 ng/mL before restarting a daily digoxin dose of 0.125 mg.

   For how many *more* days do you anticipate having to withhold digoxin before your target level of 1.6 ng/mL is reached?

A. 2 days
B. 3 days
C. 4 days
D. 5 days
E. 6 days

7. A 50-year-old man is being treated empirically with gentamicin and a cephalosporin for pneumonia. The therapeutic goal is to provide a maximum gentamicin level of *more than* 8 µg/mL one hour after intravenous infusion and a minimum concentration, just before dose administration, of *less than* 1 µg/mL. His estimated plasma gentamicin clearance and elimination half-life are 100 mL/min and 2 hours, respectively. Which of the following dosing regimens is appropriate?

A.   35 mg every 2 hours
B.   70 mg every 4 hours
C.   90 mg every 5 hours
D. 110 mg every 6 hours
E. 140 mg every 8 hours

8. You start a 19-year-old man on phenytoin in a dose of 300 mg/day to control generalized (grand mal) seizures. Ten days later, he is brought to an emergency room following a seizure. His phenytoin level is found to be 5 µg/mL and the phenytoin dose is increased to 600 mg/day. Two weeks later, he returns to your office complaining of drowsiness and ataxia. At that time his phenytoin level is 30 µg/mL.

   Assuming patient compliance with previous therapy, which of the following dose regimens should provide a phenytoin plasma level of 15 µg/mL (therapeutic range: 10–20 µg/mL)?

A. 350 mg/day
B. 400 mg/day
C. 450 mg/day
D. 500 mg/day
E. 550 mg/day

3

Compartmental Analysis of Drug Distribution

ARTHUR J. ATKINSON, JR.

Clinical Center, National Institutes of Health, Bethesda, Maryland

Drug distribution can be defined as the post-absorptive transfer of drug from one location in the body to another. Absorption after various routes of drug administration is not considered part of the distribution process and is dealt with separately. In most cases, the process of drug distribution is symmetrically reversible and requires no input of energy. However, there is increasing awareness that receptor-mediated endocytosis and carrier-mediated active transport also play important roles in either increasing or limiting the extent of drug distribution. The role of these processes in drug distribution will be considered in Chapter 16.

PHYSIOLOGICAL SIGNIFICANCE OF DRUG DISTRIBUTION VOLUMES

Digoxin is typical of most drugs in that its distribution volume, averaging 536 L in 70-kg subjects with normal renal function, is not readily interpreted by reference to physiologically defined fluid spaces. However, some drugs and other compounds appear to have distribution volumes that are physiologically identifiable. Thus, the distribution volumes of inulin, quaternary neuromuscular blocking drugs, and, initially, aminoglycoside antibiotics approximate expected values for extracellular fluid space (ECF). The distribution volumes of urea, antipyrine, ethyl alcohol, and caffeine also can be used to estimate total body water (TBW) (1).

Binding to plasma proteins affects drug distribution volume estimates. Initial attempts to explain the effects of protein binding on drug distribution were based on the assumption that the distribution of these proteins was confined to the intravascular space. However, "plasma" proteins distribute throughout ECF, so the distribution volume of even highly protein bound drugs exceeds plasma volume and approximates ECF in many cases (1). For example, thyroxine is 99.97% protein bound and its distribution volume of 0.15 L/kg (2) approximates recent ECF estimates of 0.16 ± 0.01 L/kg made with inulin (3). Distribution volumes are usually larger than ECF for uncharged drugs that are less tightly protein bound to plasma proteins. Theophylline is a methylxanthine, similar to caffeine, and its nonprotein-bound or free fraction distributes in TBW. The fact that theophylline is normally 40% bound to plasma proteins accounts for the fact that its 0.5-L/kg apparent volume of distribution is intermediate between expected values for ECF and TBW (Figure 3.1). The relationship between extent of plasma protein binding and theophylline V_d is given by the following equation:

$$V_d = \text{ECF} + f_u (\text{TBW} - \text{ECF}) \qquad (3.1)$$

where f_u is the fraction of unbound theophylline that can measured in plasma samples (4). An additional correction has been proposed to account for the fact interstitial fluid protein concentrations are less than those in plasma (5). However, this correction does not account for the heterogeneous nature of interstitial

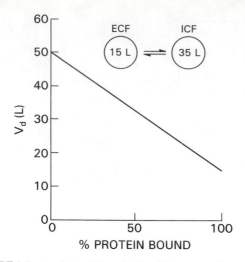

FIGURE 3.1 Analysis of theophylline V_d in terms of protein binding, ECF, and intracellular fluid (ICF) components of TBW in a hypothetical 70-kg subject. Theophylline is normally 40% bound, so its V_d approximates 35 L or 0.5 L/kg. (Reproduced with permission from Atkinson AJ Jr, Ruo TI, Frederiksen MC. Trends Pharmacol Sci 1991;12:96–101.)

TABLE 3.1   Factors Affecting Distribution of Several Lipid-Soluble Drugs

	V_d (L/kg)	f_u	Φ
Octanol/Water Partition Coefficient = 10 – 100[a]			
Phenytoin	0.64	0.08	12
Diazepam	1.10	0.013	185
Octanol/Water Partition Coefficient = 100 – >1000[a]			
Propranolol	4.30	0.13	82
Nortriptyline	18.0	0.08	572

[a] Measured at pH 7 (6).

fluid composition and entails additional complexity that may not be warranted (1).

Many lipid soluble drugs have distribution volumes that exceed expected values for TBW, or are considerably larger than ECF despite extensive binding to plasma proteins. The extensive tissue binding of these drugs increases the apparent distribution volume that is calculated by reference to drug concentrations measured in plasma water. Kurz and Fichtl (6) have found a reasonable correlation between tissue binding and the octanol/water partition coefficient of drugs and have proposed that drugs be categorized by the relative affinity of their binding to plasma proteins and to tissues. By modifying Equation 3.1 as follows:

$$V_d = \text{ECF} + \Phi f_u (\text{TBW} - \text{ECF}) \qquad (3.2)$$

standard kinetic data can be used to estimate the tissue-binding affinity (Φ) of lipid-soluble drugs. Estimates of V_d, ECF (0.16 L/kg), and TBW (0.65 L/kg) were used to calculate the tissue-binding affinities of four commonly used drugs that are compared with their octanol/water partition coefficients in Table 3.1.

Digoxin incorporates a steroid molecule (aglycone) but is relatively polar because three glycoside (sugar) groups are attached to it. It has an octanol/water partition coefficient of 18 but also binds very tightly to the enzyme Na/K-ATPase that is present in most body tissues. Since digoxin is only 25% bound to plasma proteins ($f_u = 0.75$), Equation 3.2 can be used to estimate that a 536 L distribution volume of this drug corresponds to a Φ value of 20.4.

Digoxin can be displaced from its Na/K-ATPase binding sites by concurrent administration of quinidine, causing a decrease in digoxin distribution volume (7). Sheiner et al. (8) also have shown that impairment in renal function is associated with a decrease in digoxin distribution volume (V_d) as described by the following relationship (9):

$$V_d \text{ (in L)} = 3.84 \times \text{weight (in kg)} + 3.12 \times CL_{CR} \text{ (in mL/min)}$$

This presumably reflects the same impairment in Na/K-ATPase activity that makes these patients more susceptible to toxicity when digoxin levels are ≥ 3.0 ng/mL (10).

PHYSIOLOGICAL BASIS OF MULTICOMPARTMENTAL MODELS OF DRUG DISTRIBUTION

Basis of Multicompartmental Structure

In 1937, Teorell (11) first used a multicompartmental system to model the kinetics of drug distribution. The two body distribution compartments of his model consisted of a central compartment corresponding to intravascular space and a peripheral compartment representing nonmetabolizing body tissues. Drug elimination was modeled as proceeding from the central compartment. Drug transfer between compartments is mediated by *intercompartmental clearance*, a term coined by Sapirstein et al. (12) to describe the volume-independent parameter that characterizes the rate of analyte transfer between the compartments of a kinetic model. Thus, elimination clearance and intercompartmental clearance share the property of volume independence in that they are not affected by changes in compartment volume.

Although more can be learned about the process of drug distribution when the physiological identity of the model compartments can be established, most models used in pharmacokinetics are simply mathematical constructs that are developed without regard to underlying physiology (13). The number of model compartments is defined by analysis of experimental data and corresponds to the number of exponential phases present in the plot of plasma levels vs. time. In contrast to Teorell's model, the central compartment of most two-compartment models often exceeds expected values for intravascular space, and three-compartment models are required to model the kinetics of many other drugs. The situation has been further complicated by the fact that some drugs have been analyzed with two-compartment models on some occasions and with three-compartment models on others. To some extent, these discrepancies reflect differences in experimental design. Particularly for rapidly distributing drugs, a tri-exponential plasma-level-vs.-time curve is likely to be observed only when the drug is administered by rapid intravenous injection and blood samples are obtained frequently in the immediate post-injection period.

The central compartment of a pharmacokinetic model usually is the only one that is directly accessible to sampling. When attempting to identify this compartment as intravascular space, the erythrocyte/plasma partition ratio must be incorporated in comparisons of central compartment volume with expected blood volume if plasma levels, rather than whole blood levels, are used for pharmacokinetic analysis. Models in which the central compartment corresponds to intravascular space are of particular interest because the process of distribution from the central compartment then can be identified as transcapillary exchange (Figure 3.2). In three-compartment models of this type, it might be tempting to conclude that the two peripheral compartments were connected in series (*catenary* model) and represented interstitial fluid space and intracellular water. Urea is a marker of TBW and the kinetics of its distribution can be analyzed with a three-compartment catenary model of this type. On the other hand, a three-compartment model is also required to model distribution of inulin from a central compartment that corresponds to plasma volume. This implies that interstitial fluid is kinetically heterogeneous and suggests that the *mammillary* system shown in Figure 3.2 represents the proper configuration (1,3).

The proposed physiological basis for this model is that transfer of relatively small polar compounds, like urea and inulin, occurs rapidly across fenestrated and discontinuous capillaries that are located primarily in the splanchnic vascular bed, but proceeds more slowly across less porous capillaries that have a continuous

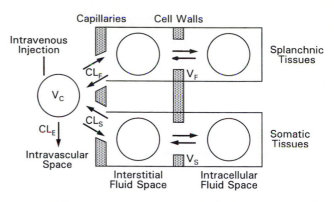

FIGURE 3.2 Multicompartmental model of the kinetics of inulin and urea distribution and elimination. After injection into a central compartment corresponding to intravascular space (V_C) both compounds distribute to rapidly (V_F) and slowly (V_S) equilibrating peripheral compartments (*rectangles*), at rates of transcapillary exchange that are characterized by intercompartmental clearances CL_F and CL_S. These peripheral compartments contain both interstitial and intracellular fluid components but transfer of urea between them is too rapid to be distinguished kinetically. Inulin is limited in its distribution to the interstitial fluid components of the peripheral compartments. (Reproduced with permission from Odeh YK, Wang Z, Ruo TI, Wang T, Frederiksen MC, Pospisil PA, Atkinson AJ Jr. Clin Pharmacol Ther 1993;53:419–25.)

basement membrane and are located primarily in skeletal muscle and other somatic tissues. Direct evidence to support this proposal has been provided by kinetic studies in which the volume of the rapidly equilibrating compartment was found to be reduced in animals whose spleen and lower intestine had been removed (14). Indirect evidence also has been provided by a study of the distribution and pharmacologic effects of *insulin,* a compound with molecular weight and extracellular distribution characteristics similar to *inulin.* Insulin distribution kinetics were analyzed together with the rate of glucose utilization needed to stabilize plasma glucose concentrations (glucose clamp) (15). Since changes in the rate of glucose infusion paralleled the rise and fall of insulin concentrations in the slowly equilibrating peripheral compartment (Figure 3.3), it was inferred that this compartment is largely composed of skeletal muscle. This *pharmacokinetic–pharmacodynamic* (PK–PD) study is also of interest because it illustrates one of the few examples in which a distribution compartment can be plausibly identified as the site of drug action or *biophase.*

Mechanisms of Transcapillary Exchange

At this time, the physiological basis for the transfer of drugs and other compounds between compartments can only be inferred for mammillary systems in which the central compartment represents intravascular space

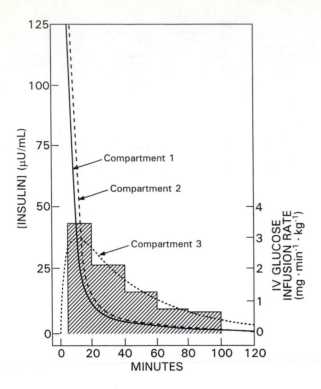

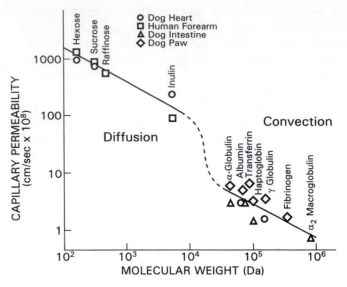

FIGURE 3.4 Plot of capillary permeability vs. molecular weight. (Reproduced with permission from Dedrick RL, Flessner MF. Prog Clin Biol Res 1989;288:429–38.)

FIGURE 3.3 Measured plasma concentrations of insulin in compartment 1 (intravascular space) after intravenous injection of a 25-mU/kg dose, and computer-derived estimates of insulin concentration in presumed splanchnic (compartment 2) and somatic (compartment 3) components of interstitial fluid space. The bar graph indicates the glucose infusion rate needed to maintain blood glucose concentrations at the basal level. (Reproduced with permission from Sherwin RS, Kramer KJ, Tobin JD, Insel PA, Liljenquist JE, Berman M, Andres R. J Clin Invest 1974;53:1481–92.)

and intercompartmental clearance can be equated with transcapillary exchange. In the case of inulin and urea, intercompartmental clearance (CL_I) can be analyzed in terms of the rate of blood flow (Q) through exchanging capillary beds and the permeability coefficient-surface area product $(P \cdot S)$ characterizing diffusion through capillary fenestrae (primarily in splanchnic capillary beds) or small pores (primarily in somatic capillary beds). The following permeability-flow equation,[1] used by Renkin (16) for analyzing transcapillary exchange across an isolated perfused hind limb preparation,

$$CL_I = Q\,(1 - e^{-P \cdot S/Q}) \qquad (3.3)$$

subsequently was adapted to multicompartmental pharmacokinetic models (17). Because CL_I is replaced by two terms, Q and $P \cdot S$, it is necessary to study both inulin and urea distribution kinetics simultaneously. In order to estimate all the parameters characterizing the transcapillary exchange of these compounds, it is also necessary to assume that the ratio of their $P \cdot S$ values is the same as the ratio of their free water diffusion coefficients. However, when this is done, there is good agreement between the sum of blood flows to the peripheral compartments and independent measures of cardiac output (1,3).

Although this approach seems valid for small, uncharged molecules, molecular charge appears to slow transcapillary exchange. Large molecular size also retards transcapillary exchange (18). Molecules considerably larger than inulin are probably transported through small-pore capillaries by convection rather than diffusion (Figure 3.4). Conversely, very lipid soluble compounds appear to pass directly though capillary walls at rates limited only by blood flow $(P \cdot S \gg Q)$. Even though theophylline is a relatively polar compound, its transcapillary exchange is also blood-flow limited and presumably occurs by car-

---

[1] There is a long history behind attempts to analyze transcapillary exchange in terms of its blood flow and diffusional permeability components. Eugene Renkin appears to be the first to have applied this equation to the transcapillary exchange of non-gaseous solutes. He was guided in this effort by Christian Bohr's derivation of the equation in the context of pulmonary gas exchange (Skand Arch Physiol 1909;22:221–80). Seymour Kety based his derivation of the equation on Bohr's prior work and also applied it to pulmonary gas exchange (Pharmacol Rev 1951;3:1–41). Renkin's derivation was not published along with his original paper (16) but was archived by the American Documentation Institute (document 4648) and serves as the basis for the derivation published in reference 17. A final independent derivation was published by Christian Crone (Acta Physiol Scand 1963;54:292–305). Renkin concludes that the equation could be eponymously termed the *Bohr/Kety/Renkin/Crone/Equation* but prefers to simply refer to it as the *flow-diffusion equation* (Renkin EM. Personal Communication. December 10, 1999).

TABLE 3.2   Classification of Transcapillary Exchange Mechanisms

1. Diffusive transfer of small molecules (< 6000 Daltons)
   * Transferred at rates proportional to their free water diffusion coefficients
       Polar, uncharged compounds (e.g., urea, inulin)
   * Transferred more slowly than predicted from free-water diffusion coefficients
       Highly charged compounds (e.g., quaternary skeletal muscle relaxants)
       Compounds with intermediate polarity that interact with capillary walls (e.g., procainamide)
   * Transferred more rapidly than predicted from free-water diffusion coefficients
       Highly lipid soluble compounds that freely penetrate endothelial cells (e.g., anesthetic gases)
       Compounds transferred by carrier-mediated facilitated diffusion (e.g., theophylline)
2. Convective transfer of large molecules (> 50,000 Daltons)

rier-mediated facilitated diffusion (19). This leads to the classification shown in Table 3.2.

Although there have been few studies designed to interpret actual drug distribution results in physiological terms, a possible approach is to administer the drug under investigation along with reference compounds such as inulin and urea. This experimental design was used to show that theophylline distributed from intravascular space to two peripheral compartments that had intercompartmental clearances corresponding to the blood flow components of urea and inulin transcapillary exchange (19). It also should be emphasized that conventional kinetic studies do not have the resolving power to identify distribution to smaller but pharmacologically important regions such as the brain in which transcapillary exchange is limited by tight-junctions or by carrier mediated active transport (e.g., P-glycoprotein).

CLINICAL CONSEQUENCES OF DIFFERENT DRUG DISTRIBUTION PATTERNS

As pointed out in Chapter 2, the process of drug distribution can account for both the slow onset of pharmacologic effect of some drugs (e.g., digoxin) and the termination of pharmacologic effect after bolus intravenous injection of others (e.g., lidocaine and thiopental). When theophylline was introduced in the 1930s, it was often administered by rapid intravenous injection to asthmatic patients. It was only after several fatalities were reported that the current practice was adopted of initiating therapy with a slow intravenous infusion, yet excessively rapid intravenous administration of theo-

phylline still contributes to the frequency of serious adverse reactions to this drug (20). The rapidity of carrier-mediated theophylline distribution to the brain and heart probably contributes to the infusion-rate dependency of these serious adverse reactions.

The impact of physiological changes on drug distribution kinetics has not been studied extensively. For example, it is known that pregnancy alters the elimination kinetics of many drugs. But physiological changes in body fluid compartment volumes and protein binding also affect drug distribution in pregnant subjects. As discussed in Chapter 22, Equation 3.1 has been used to correlate pregnancy-associated changes in theophylline distribution with this altered physiology (4). As described in Chapter 6, changes in intercompartmental clearance occur during hemodialysis and have important effects on the extent of drug removal during this procedure.

For most drugs whose plasma-level-vs-time curve demonstrates more than one exponential phase, the terminal phase primarily, but not entirely, reflects the process of drug elimination, and the initial phase or phases primarily reflect the process of drug distribution. However, the sequence of *distribution* and *elimination phases* is reversed for some drugs, and these drugs are said to exhibit *"flip-flop" kinetics*. For example, Schentag and colleagues (21) have shown that the elimination phase precedes the distribution phase of gentamicin, an aminoglycoside antibiotic, and accounts for the long terminal half-life that is seen after a course of therapy (Figure 3.5). In this case, the central compartment of drug distribution probably corresponds to ECF and the peripheral compartment primarily reflects gentamicin distribution to the kidneys. Colburn et al. (22) showed that the extent of tissue distribution is much greater in patients who have nephrotoxic reactions to gentamicin than in those whose renal function remains intact (Figure 3.6).

In technical terms, we can say that the approximation of a single-compartment model represents *misspecification* of what is really a two-compartment system for gentamicin. However, the distribution phase for this drug is not even apparent until therapy is stopped. Nonetheless, the extent to which peak and/or trough levels rise during repetitive dosing can be used to provide an important clue to extensive gentamicin accumulation in the "tissue" compartment. Most clinical pharmacokinetic calculations are made with the initial assumption that gentamicin distributes in a single compartment that roughly corresponds to ECF. If the dose and dose interval are kept constant, steady-state peak and trough levels can be predicted simply by multiplying initial peak and trough levels by the *cumulation factor (CF)*. As derived in Chapter 2,

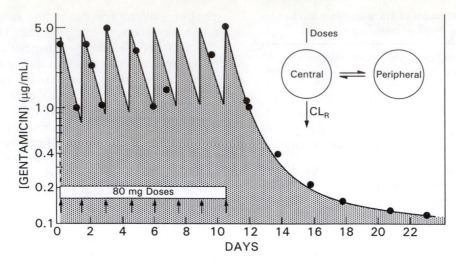

FIGURE 3.5 Serum gentamicin concentrations measured in a patient during and after a 10.5-day course of therapy (80 mg every 36 hr). Data were analyzed with the two-compartment model shown in the insert. The half-life of serum levels during therapy is primarily reflective of renal elimination. The terminal half-life seen after therapy was stopped is the actual distribution phase. (Reproduced with permission from Schentag JJ, Jusko WJ, Plaut ME, Cumbo TJ, Vance JW, Abrutyn E, JAMA 1977;238:327–9.)

$$CF = 1/(1 - e^{-k\tau}) \qquad (3.4)$$

where k is $\ln 2/t_{1/2}$ and τ is the dosing interval. If peak and trough levels initially rise more rapidly than predicted from Equation 3.4, this reflects that fact that substantial drug is accumulating in the "tissue" compartment. Of course, deterioration in renal function can also cause gentamicin peak and trough levels to increase, but usually this occurs after five or more days of therapy.

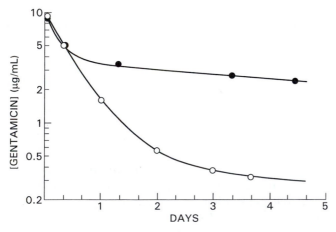

FIGURE 3.6 Decline in serum gentamicin concentrations after therapy was stopped in a patient with nephrotoxicity (●) and a patient who did not have this adverse reaction (○). Both patients had been treated with gentamicin at an 8-hour dosing interval and had nearly identical elimination-phase half-lives and peak and trough levels. (Reproduced with permission from Colburn WA, Schentag JJ, Jusko WJ, Gibalbi M. J Pharmacokinet Biopharm 1978;6:179–86.)

An important point about drugs that exhibit flip-flop kinetics is that the terminal exponential phase usually is reached only when plasma drug levels are subtherapeutic. For this reason, the half-life corresponding to this terminal exponential phase (greater than 4 days in the example shown in Figure 3.6) cannot be used in selecting an appropriate dosing interval. If the actual extent of drug accumulation is known from the ratio of steady-state/initial plasma levels, the observed cumulation factor (CF_{obs}) during repetitive dosing can be used to estimate an effective elimination rate constant (k_{eff}) by rearranging Equation 3.4 to the form:

$$k_{eff} = \frac{1}{\tau} \ln\left(\frac{CF_{obs}}{CF_{obs} - 1}\right)$$

and the effective half-life ($t_{1/2\ eff}$) can be calculated as:

$$t_{1/2eff} = \ln 2/k_{eff}$$

The effective half-life can then be used to design dose regimens for drugs that have a terminal exponential phase representing the disposition of only a small fraction of the total drug dose (23).

ANALYSIS OF EXPERIMENTAL DATA

Derivation of Equations for a Two-Compartment Model

After rapid intravenous injection, sequentially measured plasma levels may follow a pattern similar

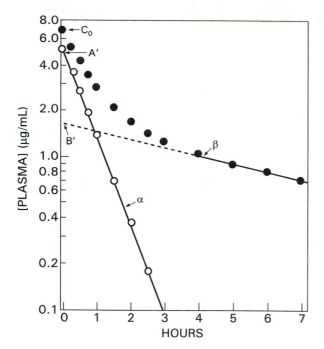

FIGURE 3.7 "Curve-peeling" technique used to estimate the coefficients and exponents of a data equation. Data points (●) are plotted on semilogarithmic coordinates and the points for the α-curve (○) are obtained by subtracting back-extrapolated β-curve values from the experimental data.

to that shown by the solid circles in Figure 3.7. For most drugs, the elimination phase is reached when the data points fall on the line marked "β." The distribution phase occurs prior to that time. In this case, the curve contains two exponential phases and can be described by the following sum of exponentials *data equation*:

$$C = A' e^{-\alpha t} + B' e^{-\beta t}$$

where A', B', α, and β are the back-extrapolated intercepts and slopes shown in the figure. The drug concentration in the central compartment at time zero (C_0) equals the sum of $A' + B'$. For convenience in the derivation that follows, we normalize the values of these intercepts:

$$A = A' V_1 / C_0 V_1 = A'/C_0$$
$$B = B' V_1 / C_0 V_1 = B'/C_0$$

Since $A + B = 1$, the administered dose also has a normalized value of 1.

Because there are two exponential terms in the data equation, the data are consistent with a two-compartment model. The assumption usually is made that both intravenous administration and subsequent drug elimination proceed via the central compartment. Accordingly, the model is drawn as shown in Figure 3.8. We are interested in obtaining values for the parameters of this model in terms of the parameters of

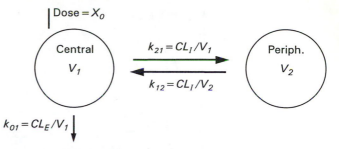

FIGURE 3.8 Schematic drawing of a two-compartment model with central and peripheral (Periph.) compartments. The number of primary model parameters (V_1, V_2, CL_E, and CL_I) that can be identified from the data cannot exceed the total number of coefficients and exponents in the data equation.

the data equation that we have defined previously. Whereas the data equation is written in the concentration units of the data, the equations for the model shown in Figure 3.8 usually are developed in terms of the amounts of drug in each compartment (X_1 and X_2), the micro-rate constants describing drug transfer between or out of compartments (k's), and a single drug dose (X_0). The model itself can be described in terms of two first-order linear differential equations (*model equations*):

$$dX_1/dt = -k_{01} X_1 - k_{21} X_1 + k_{12} X_2$$
$$dX_2/dt = k_{21} X_1 - k_{12} X_2$$

Combining terms:

$$dX_1/dt = -(k_{01} + k_{21}) X_1 + k_{12} X_2$$
$$dX_2/dt = k_{21} X_1 - k_{12} X_2$$

Laplace transforms can be used to transform this system of linear differential equations in the time domain into a system of linear equations in the Laplace domain. From the table of Laplace operations (Appendix I) we obtain:

$$s X_1 - X_1(0) = -(k_{01} + k_{21})X_1 + k_{12} X_2$$
$$s X_2 - X_2(0) = k_{21} X_1 - k_{12} X_2$$

If a single drug dose is injected intravenously, the entire administered dose is initially in compartment 1 and, because of normalization, $X_1(0)$ equals 1. The amount of drug in compartment 2 at zero time [$X_2(0)$] is 0. We can now write the following nonhomogenous linear equations:

$$(s + k_{01} + k_{21}) X_1 - k_{12} X_2 = 1$$
$$-k_{21} X_1 + (s + k_{12}) X_2 = 0$$

The method of determinants (Cramer's Rule) can be used to solve the equations for each model compartment. However, we will focus only on the solution for the central compartment, which is the one usually sampled for concentration measurements.

$$X_1 = \frac{\begin{vmatrix} 1 & -k_{12} \\ 0 & s + k_{12} \end{vmatrix}}{\begin{vmatrix} s + k_{01} + k_{21} & -k_{12} \\ -k_{21} & s + k_{12} \end{vmatrix}}$$

(3.5)

$$X_1 = \frac{s + k_{12}}{s^2 + (k_{01} + k_{21} + k_{12}) s + k_{01} k_{12}}$$

This solution is in the form of a quotient of two polynomials, $P(s)/Q(s)$. $Q(s)$ can be expressed in terms of its factors as follows:

$$X_1 = \frac{s + k_{12}}{(s + \alpha)(s + \beta)}$$

Where the roots of the polynomial $Q(s)$ are $R_1 = -\alpha$ and $R_2 = -\beta$. The Heaviside Expansion Theorem states:

$$X_i = \sum_{i=1}^{n} \frac{P(R_i)}{Q'(R_i)} e^{R_i t}$$

Since:

$$Q(s) = s^2 + (\alpha + \beta) s + \alpha\beta \qquad (3.6)$$
$$Q'(s) = 2s + \alpha + \beta$$

Therefore,

$$X_1 = \frac{k_{12} - \alpha}{-2\alpha + \alpha + \beta} e^{-\alpha t} + \frac{k_{12} - \beta}{-2\beta + \alpha + \beta} e^{-\beta t}$$

$$X_1 = \frac{k_{12} - \alpha}{\beta - \alpha} e^{-\alpha t} + \frac{k_{12} - \beta}{\alpha - \beta} e^{-\beta t}$$

(3.7)

To estimate the model parameters from the data equation, we also need to specify the rate of drug elimination from the central compartment (V_1). The rate of elimination from this compartment, dE/dt is given by the equation:

$$dE/dt = k_{01} X_1$$

So total elimination is:

$$E = k_{01} \int_0^{\infty} X_1 dt$$

Since E equals the administered dose, which has been normalized to 1,

$$k_{01} = \frac{1}{\int_0^{\infty} X_1 dt}$$

(3.8)

If X_1 is written in the form of the data equation:

$$X_1 = A e^{-\alpha t} + B e^{-\beta t} \qquad (3.9)$$

we obtain,

$$\int_0^{\infty} X_1 dt = -(A/\alpha) e^{-\alpha t} - (B/\beta) e^{-\beta t} \Big|_0^{\infty}$$

$$= A/\alpha + B/\beta$$

Substituting this result into Equation 3.5:

$$\boxed{k_{01} = \frac{1}{A/\alpha + B/\beta}}$$

(3.10)

By comparing Equations 3.5 and 3.6, it is apparent that:

$$Q(s) = s^2 + (k_{01} + k_{21} + k_{12}) s + k_{01} k_{12}$$

So from Equation 3.6:

$$\alpha + \beta = k_{01} + k_{21} + k_{12} \qquad (3.11)$$
$$\alpha\beta = k_{01} k_{12} \qquad (3.12)$$

Rearranging Equation 3.12:

$$k_{12} = \frac{\alpha\beta}{k_{01}}$$

Substituting for k_{01} (Equation 3.10):

$$\boxed{k_{12} = \beta A + \alpha B}$$

(3.13)

Equation 3.11 can be rearranged to give:

$$k_{21} = \alpha + \beta - k_{01} - k_{12}$$

$$= \alpha + \beta - \frac{\alpha\beta}{k_{12}} - k_{12}$$

$$= -\frac{k_{12}^2 - (\alpha + \beta) k_{12} + \alpha\beta}{k_{12}}$$

$$= -\frac{(k_{12} - \alpha)(k_{12} - \beta)}{k_{12}}$$

by comparing Equations 3.7 and 3.9:

$$A = \frac{k_{12} - \alpha}{\beta - \alpha}$$

so,

$$k_{12} - \alpha = -A(\alpha - \beta)$$

and:

$$B = \frac{k_{12} - \beta}{\alpha - \beta}$$

so,

$$k_{12} - \beta = -B(\alpha - \beta)$$

Therefore:

$$\boxed{k_{21} = \frac{A B (\alpha - \beta)^2}{k_{12}}}$$

(3.14)

These techniques also can be applied to develop equations for three-compartment and other commonly used pharmacokinetic models.

Calculation of Rate Constants and Compartment Volumes from Data

Values for the data equation parameters can be obtained by the technique of "curve peeling" that is illustrated in Figure 3.7. After plotting the data, the first step is to identify the terminal exponential phase of the curve, in this case termed the β-phase, and then back-extrapolate this line to obtain the ordinate intercept (B'). It is easiest to calculate the value of β by first calculating the half-life of this phase. The value for β then can be estimated from the relationship: $\beta = \ln 2/t_{1/2\beta}$. The next step is to subtract the corresponding value on the back-extrapolated β-phase line from each of the data point values obtained during the previous exponential phase. This generates the α-line from which the α-slope and A' intercept can be estimated.

After calculating the normalized intercept values A and B, the rate constants for the model can be obtained from Equations 3.10, 3.13, and 3.14. The volume of the central compartment is calculated from the ratio of the administered dose to the back-extrapolated value for C_0 (which equals $A' + B'$) as follows:

$$V_1 = \frac{\text{Dose}}{C_0}$$

Since $k_{21} = CL_I/V_1$, and $k_{12} = CL_I/V_2$,

$$k_{21} V_1 = k_{12} V_2$$

and

$$V_2 = V_1(k_{21}/k_{12})$$

The sum of V_1 and V_2 is termed the apparent volume of distribution at steady state ($V_{d\,(ss)}$) and is the third distribution volume that we have described. Note also that $CL_I = k_{21}V_1 = k_{12}V_2$.

Even though computer programs now are used routinely for pharmacokinetic analysis, most require initial estimates of the model parameters. As a result of the least-squares fitting procedures employed, these computer programs generally yield the most satisfactory results when the technique of curve peeling is used to make reasonably accurate initial estimates of parameter values.

Different Estimates of Apparent Volume of Distribution

The three estimates of distribution volume that we have encountered have slightly different properties (24). Of the three, $V_{d\,(ss)}$ has the strongest physiologic rationale for multicompartment systems of drug distribution. It is independent of the rate of both drug distribution and elimination and is the volume that is referred to in Equations 3.1 and 3.2. On the other hand, estimates of $V_{d\,(area)}$ are most useful in clinical pharmacokinetics, since it is this volume that links elimination clearance to elimination half-life in the equation:

$$t_{1/2} = \frac{0.693\,V_{d(area)}}{CL_E}$$

Because the single compartment model implied by this equation makes no provision for the contribution of intercompartmental clearance to elimination half-life, estimates of $V_{d\,(area)}$ are larger than $V_{d\,(ss)}$.

Estimates of $V_{d\,(extrap)}$ are also based on a single-compartment model in which drug distribution is assumed to be infinitely fast. However, slowing of intercompartmental clearance reduces estimates of B', the back-extrapolated β-curve intercept in Figure 3.7, to a greater extent than it prolongs elimination half-life. As a result, $V_{d\,(extrap)}$ calculated from the equation:

$$V_{d\,(extrap)} = \text{Initial Dose}/B'$$

is even larger than $V_{d\,(area)}$. Thus, when the plasma-level-vs.-time curve includes more than a single exponential component, the relationship of the three distribution volume estimates to each other is:

$$V_{d\,(extrap)} > V_{d\,(area)} > V_{d\,(ss)}$$

References

1. Atkinson, AJ Jr, Ruo TI, Frederiksen MC. Physiological basis of multicompartmental models of drug distribution. Trends Pharmacol Sci 1991;12:96–101.
2. Larsen PR, Atkinson AJ Jr, Wellman HN, Goldsmith RE. The effect of diphenylhydantoin on thyroxine metabolism in man. J Clin Invest 1970;49:1266–79.
3. Odeh YK, Wang Z, Ruo TI, Wang T, Frederiksen MC, Pospsil PA, Atkinson AJ Jr. Simultaneous analysis of inulin and $^{15}N_2$-urea kinetics in humans. Clin Pharmacol Ther 1993;53:419–25.
4. Frederiksen MC, Ruo TI, Chow MJ, Atkinson AJ Jr. Theophylline pharmacokinetics in pregnancy. Clin Pharmacol Ther 1986;40:321–8.
5. Øie S, Tozer TN. Effect of altered plasma protein binding on apparent volume of distribution. J Pharm Sci 1979;68:1203–5.
6. Kurz H, Fichtl B. Binding of drugs to tissues. Drug Metab Rev 1983;14:467–510.
7. Hager WD, Fenster P, Mayersohn M, Perrier D, Graves P, Marcus FI, Goldman S. Digoxin-quinidine interaction: Pharmacokinetic evaluation. N Engl J Med 1979;300:1238–41.
8. Sheiner LB, Rosenberg B, Marathe VV. Estimation of population characteristics of pharmacokinetic parameters from routine clinical data. J Pharmacokinet Biopharm 1977;5:445–79.
9. Benet LZ, Øie S, Schwartz JB. Appendix II. Design and optimization of dose regimens: Pharmacokinetic data. In: Hardman JG, Gilman AG, Limbird LE, editors. Goodman & Gilman's The pharmacological basis of therapeutics. 9th ed. New York: McGraw-Hill; 1995. p. 1707–92.

10. Piergies AA, Worwag EW, Atkinson AJ Jr. A concurrent audit of high digoxin plasma levels. Clin Pharmacol Ther 1994;55:353–8.

11. Teorell T. Kinetics of distribution of substances administered to the body: I. The extravascular modes of administration. Arch Intern Pharmacodyn 1937;57:205–25.

12. Sapirstein LA, Vidt DG, Mandel MJ, Hanusek G. Volumes of distribution and clearances of intravenously injected creatinine in the dog. Am J Physiol 1955;181:330–6.

13. Berman M. The formulation and testing of models. Ann NY Acad Sci 1963;108:192–4.

14. Sedek GS, Ruo TI, Frederiksen MC, Frederiksen JW, Shih S-R, Atkinson AJ Jr. Splanchnic tissues are a major part of the rapid distribution spaces of inulin, urea and theophylline. J Pharmacol Exp Ther 1989;251:963–9.

15. Sherwin RS Kramer KJ, Tobin JD, Insel PA, Liljenquist JE, Berman M, Andres R. A model of the kinetics of insulin in man. J Clin Invest 1974;53:1481–92.

16. Renkin EM. Effects of blood flow on diffusion kinetics in isolated perfused hindlegs of cats: A double circulation hypothesis. Am J Physiol 1953;183:125–36.

17. Stec GP, Atkinson AJ Jr. Analysis of the contributions of permeability and flow to intercompartmental clearance. J Pharmacokinet Biopharm 1981;9:167–80.

18. Dedrick RL, Flessner MF. Pharmacokinetic considerations on monoclonal antibodies. Prog Clin Biol Res 1989;288:429–38.

19. Belknap SM, Nelson JE, Ruo TI, Frederiksen MC, Worwag EM, Shin S-G, Atkinson AJ Jr. Theophylline distribution kinetics analyzed by reference to simultaneously injected urea and inulin. J Pharmacol Exp Ther 1987;243:963–9.

20. Camarta SJ, Weil MH, Hanashiro PK, Shubin H. Cardiac arrest in the critically ill. I. A study of predisposing causes in 132 patients. Circulation 1971;44:688–95.

21. Schentag JJ, Jusko WJ, Plaut ME, Cumbo TJ, Vance JW, Abrutyn E. Tissue persistence of gentamicin in man. JAMA 1977;238:327–9.

22. Colburn WA, Schentag JJ, Jusko WJ, Gibaldi M. A model for the prospective identification of the prenephrotoxic state during gentamicin therapy. J Pharmacokinet Biopharm 1978;6:179–86.

23. Boxenbaum H, Battle M. Effective half-life in clinical pharmacology. J Clin Pharmacol 1995;35:763–6.

24. Gibaldi M, Perrier D. Pharmacokinetics. 2nd ed. New York: Marcel Dekker;1982. p. 199–219.

STUDY PROBLEMS

1. Single dose and steady-state multiple dose plasma level-time profiles of tolrestat, an aldose reductase inhibitor, were compared. The terminal exponential phase half-life was 31.6 hours at the conclusion of multiple dose therapy administered at a 12-hour dosing interval. However, there was little apparent increase in plasma concentrations with repetitive dosing and *CF*, based on *AUC* measurements, was only 1.29. Calculate the effective half-life for this drug. (*Reference:* Boxenbaum H, Battle M. Effective half-life in clinical pharmacology. J Clin Pharmacol 1995;35:763–6.)

2. The following data were obtained in a Phase I dose-escalation tolerance study after administering a 100-mg bolus of a new drug to a normal volunteer:

Plasma Concentration Data

Time (hr)	[Plasma] (μg/mL)
0.10	6.3
0.25	5.4
0.50	4.3
0.75	3.5
1.0	2.9
1.5	2.1
2.0	1.7
2.5	1.4
3.0	1.3
4.0	1.1
5.0	0.9
6.0	0.8
7.0	0.7

a. Use two-cycle, semilogarithmic graph paper to estimate α, β, A, and B by the technique of curve peeling.

b. Draw a two-compartment model with elimination proceeding from the central compartment (V_1). Use Equations 3.10, 3.13, and 3.14 to calculate the rate constants for this model.

c. Calculate the central compartment volume and the elimination and intercompartmental clearances for this model.

d. Calculate the volume for the peripheral compartment for the model. Sum the central and peripheral compartment volumes to obtain $V_{d(ss)}$ and compare your result with the volume estimates, $V_{d(extrap)}$ and $V_{d(area)}$, that are based on the assumption that the β-slope represents elimination from a one-compartment model. Comment on your comparison.

4

Drug Absorption and Bioavailability

ARTHUR J. ATKINSON, JR.

Clinical Center, National Institutes of Health, Bethesda, Maryland

DRUG ABSORPTION

The study of drug absorption is of critical importance in developing new drugs and establishing the therapeutic equivalence of new formulations or generic versions of existing drugs. A large number of factors can affect the rate and extent of absorption of an oral drug dose. These are summarized in Figure 4.1.

Biopharmaceutic factors include drug solubility and formulation characteristics that impact the rate of drug disintegration and dissolution. From the physiologic standpoint, passive non-ionic diffusion is the mechanism by which most drugs are absorbed from solution. However, attention has been focused recently on the role that specialized small intestine transport systems play in the absorption of some drugs (1). Thus, levodopa, α-methyldopa, and baclofen are amino acid analogs that are absorbed from the small intestine by the large neutral amino acid (LNAA) transporter. Similarly, some amino-β-lactam antibiotics, captopril, and other angiotensin converting enzyme inhibitors are absorbed via an oligopeptide transporter (PEPT-1), and salicylic acid and pravastatin by a monocarboxylic acid transporter.

Absorption by passive diffusion is largely governed by the molecular size and shape, degree of ionization, and lipid solubility of a drug. Classical explanations of the rate and extent of drug absorption have been based on the pH-partition hypothesis. According to this hypothesis, weakly acidic drugs are largely unionized and lipid soluble in acid medium, and hence should be absorbed best by the stomach. Conversely, weakly basic drugs should be absorbed primarily from the more alkaline contents of the small intestine. Absorption would not be predicted for drugs that are permanently ionized, such as quaternary ammonium compounds. In reality, the stomach does not appear to be a major site for the absorption of even acidic drugs. The surface area of the intestinal mucosa is so much greater than that of the stomach that this more than compensates for the decreased absorption rate per unit area. Table 4.1 shows results that were obtained when the stomach and small bowel of rats were perfused with solutions of aspirin at two different pH values (2). Even at a pH of 3.5, gastric absorption of aspirin makes only a small contribution to the observed serum level, and the rate of gastric absorption of aspirin is less than the rate of intestinal absorption even when normalized to organ protein content. Furthermore, it is a common misconception that the pH of resting gastric contents is always 1 to 2 (3). Values exceeding pH 7 may occur after meals, and achlorhydria is common in the elderly.

Since absorption from the stomach is poor, the rate of gastric emptying becomes a prime determinant of the rate of drug absorption. Two patterns of gastric motor activity have been identified that reflect whether the subject is fed or fasting (4, 5). Fasting motor activity has a cyclical pattern. Each cycle lasts 90 to 120 minutes and consists of the following four phases:

Phase 1: A period of quiescence lasting approximately 60 minutes

Phase 2: A 40-minute period of persistent but irregular contractions that increase in intensity as the phase progresses

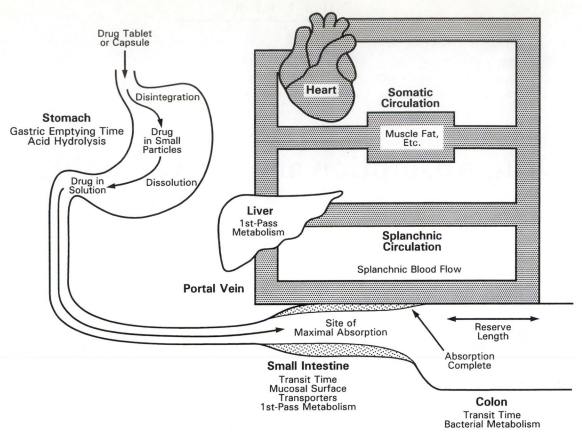

FIGURE 4.1 Summary of biopharmaceutic and physiologic processes that affect the rate and extent of absorption of an orally administered drug dose. Further explanation is provided in the text.

Phase 3: A short burst of intense contractions that are propagated distally from the stomach to the terminal ileum. These have been termed migrating motor complexes (MMC) or "housekeeper waves"

Phase 4: A short period of transition with diminished contractile activity

After feeding, the MMC are inhibited and there is uncoupling of proximal and distal gastric motility such that the resting tone of the antrum is decreased.

TABLE 4.1   Aspirin (ASA) Absorption from Simultaneously Perfused Stomach and Small Intestine[a]

pH	ASA absorption (μmol/100 mg protein/hr)		ASA serum level (mg/100 mL)
	Stomach	Small bowel	
3.5	346	469	20.6
6.5	0	424	19.7

[a] Data from Hollander D, Dadugalza VD, Fairchild PA. J Lab Clin Med 1981;98:591–8 (2).

However, solid food stimulates intense and sustained antral contractions that reduce the particle size of gastric contents. The pylorus is partially constricted and, although liquids and particles less than 1 mm in diameter can pass through to the small bowel, larger particles are retained in the stomach. Studies employing γ-scintigraphy have confirmed that, as a result of these patterns of motor activity, a tablet taken in the fasting state will generally leave the stomach in less than 2 hours but may be retained in the stomach for more than 10 hours if taken following a heavy meal (6).

Slow gastric emptying may not only retard drug absorption but, in some cases, may lead to less complete drug absorption as well. Thus, penicillin is degraded under acid conditions and levodopa is decarboxylated by enzymes in the gastric mucosa. Accordingly, patients should be advised to take these medications before meals. On the other hand, the prolonged gastric residence time that follows feeding may be needed to optimize the bioavailability of saquinavir and other drugs that are either poorly soluble or are prepared in formulations that have a slow rate of disintegration (7). Concurrent administration of drugs that modify gastric motility may also affect drug absorption. Hence, metoclopramide stimulates gastric emptying and has been shown to increase the rate of acetaminophen absorption, whereas propantheline delays gastric emptying and retards acetaminophen absorption (8).

Transit through the small intestine is more rapid than generally has been appreciated. Small intestinal transit time averages 3 ± 1 hours ($\pm$ SE), is similar for large and small particles, and is not appreciably affected by fasting or fed state (6). Rapid transit through the small intestine may reduce the bioavailability of compounds that either are relatively insoluble or are administered as sustained release formulations that have an absorption window with little reserve length. *Reserve length* is defined as the anatomical length over which absorption of a particular drug can occur, less the length at which absorption is complete (Figure 4.1) (9). Digoxin is an important example of a compound that has marginal reserve length. Consequently, the extent of absorption of one formulation of this drug is influenced by small bowel motility, being decreased when co-administered with metoclopramide and increased when an atropinic was given shortly before the digoxin dose (10).

Mucosal integrity of the small intestine also may affect the bioavailability of drugs that have little reserve length. Thus, the extent of digoxin absorption was found to be less than one-third of normal in patients with *D*-xylose malabsorption due to sprue, surgical resection of the small intestine, or intestinal hypermotility (11). Splanchnic blood flow is another factor that can affect the rate and extent of drug absorption (12), but only a few clinical studies have been designed to demonstrate its significance (13). Administered drug also may be lost in transit from the intestine to the systemic circulation. Thus, digoxin is metabolized to inactive dihydro compounds by *Eubacterium lentum,* a constituent of normal bacterial flora in some individuals (14). In addition to their effects on gastrointestinal motility, drug–drug and food–drug interactions can have a direct effect on drug absorption (15).

Once absorbed, drugs can be metabolized before reaching the systemic circulation, either in their first pass through the intestinal mucosa or after delivery by the portal circulation to the liver. Hepatic first-pass metabolism of a number of drugs has been well studied and in many cases reflects the activity of cytochrome P450 enzymes (16). These enzymes are also located at the apex of mature enterocytes, and studies in anhepatic patients have demonstrated that intestinal CYP3A4 may account for as much as half of the first-pass metabolism of cyclosporine that normally is observed (17). P-Glyco-

TABLE 4.2   Drugs with Extensive First-Pass Metabolism or Intestinal P-Glycoprotein Transport

Aldosterone	Morphine
Cyclosporine	Nortriptyline
Isoproterenol	Organic nitrates
Lidocaine	Propranolol

protein, which shares considerable substrate specificity with CYP3A4, is also localized on the luminal membrane of intestinal epithelial cells, and may act in concert with intestinal CYP3A4 to reduce the net absorption of a variety of lipophilic drugs (18). Listed in Table 4.2 are some commonly used drugs that have extensive first-pass metabolism or intestinal P-glycoprotein transport. As a result of these processes, effective oral doses of these drugs are substantially higher than intravenously administered doses.

BIOAVAILABILITY

Bioavailability is the term most often used to characterize drug absorption. This term has been defined as the relative amount of a drug administered in a pharmaceutical product that enters the systemic circulation in an unchanged form, and the rate at which this occurs (19). Implicit in this definition is the concept that a comparison is being made. If the comparison is made between an oral and an intravenous formulation of a drug, which by definition has 100% bioavailability, the *absolute bioavailability* of the drug is measured. If the comparison is made between two different oral formulations, then the *relative bioavailability* of these formulations is determined. As shown in Figure 4.2, three indices of drug bioavailability usually are estimated: the maximum drug concentration in plasma (C_{max}), the time needed to reach this maximum (t_{max}), and the area under the plasma or serum-concentration-vs.-time curve (*AUC*). Generally there is also an initial lag period (t_{lag}) that occurs before drug concentrations are measurable in plasma.

The *AUC* measured after administration of a drug dose is related to the extent of drug absorption in the following way. Generalizing from the analysis of creatinine clearance that we presented in our first chapter, the first-order differential equation describing rate of drug elimination from a single-compartment model is:

$$dE/dt = CL \cdot C$$

where dE/dt is the rate of drug elimination, CL is the elimination clearance, and C is the concentration of

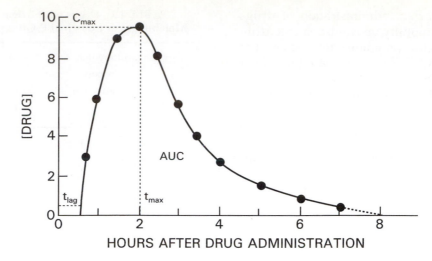

FIGURE 4.2 Hypothetical plasma concentration-vs.-time curve after a single oral drug dose. Calculation of the area under the plasma level-vs.-time curve (AUC) requires extrapolation of the elimination phase curve beyond the last measurable plasma concentration, as shown by the broken line.

drug in the compartment. Separating variables and integrating yields the result:

$$E = CL \int_0^\infty C \, dt \tag{4.1}$$

where E is the total amount of drug eliminated in infinite time. By mass balance, E must equal the amount of the drug dose that is bioavailable. The integral is simply the AUC. Thus, for an oral drug dose (D_{oral}):

$$D_{oral} \cdot F = CL \cdot AUC_{oral} \tag{4.2}$$

where F is the fraction of the dose that is absorbed and AUC_{oral} is the AUC resulting from the administered oral dose.

Absolute Bioavailability

In practice, absolute bioavailability usually is measured by sequentially administering single intravenous and oral doses (D_{IV} and D_{oral}) of a drug and comparing their respective $AUCs$. Extent of absorption of the oral dose can be calculated by modifying Equation 4.2 as follows:

$$\% \, Absorption = \frac{CL \cdot D_{IV} \cdot AUC_{oral}}{CL \cdot D_{oral} \cdot AUC_{IV}} \times 100$$

$$= \frac{D_{IV} \cdot AUC_{oral}}{D_{oral} \cdot AUC_{IV}} \times 100$$

A two-formulation, two-period, two-sequence crossover design is usually used to control for administration sequence effects. $AUCs$ frequently are estimated using the linear trapezoidal method, the log trapezoidal method, or a combination of the two (20). Alternatively,

bioavailability can be assessed by comparing the amounts of unmetabolized drug recovered in the urine after giving the drug by the intravenuous and oral routes. This follows directly from Equation 4.1, since urinary excretion accounts for a constant fraction of total drug elimination when drugs are eliminated by first-order kinetics.

In either case, the assumption usually is made that the elimination clearance of a drug remains the same in the interval between drug doses. This problem can be circumvented by administering an intravenous dose of the stable-isotope-labeled drug at the same time that the test formulation of unlabeled drug is given orally. Although the feasibility of this technique was first demonstrated in normal subjects (21), the method entails only a single study and set of blood samples and is ideally suited for the evaluation of drug absorption in patients, as shown in Figure 4.3(13).

In this case, a computer program employing a least-squares fitting algorithm was used to analyze the data in terms of the pharmacokinetic model shown in Figure 4.4. The extent of N-acetylprocainamide (NAPA) absorption was calculated from model parameters representing the absorption rate (k_a) and nonabsorptive loss (k_o) from the gastrointestinal tract, as follows:

$$\% \, Absorption = \frac{k_a}{k_a + k_o} \times 100$$

The extent of absorption also was assessed by comparing the 12-hour urine recovery of NAPA and NAPA-^{13}C. A correction was made to the NAPA recovery to compensate for the lag in NAPA absorption that was

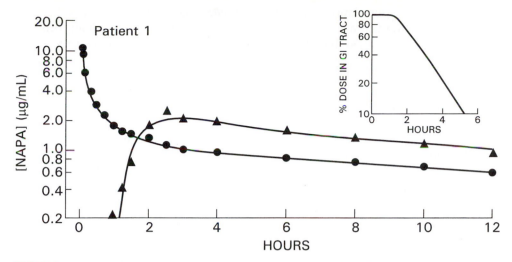

FIGURE 4.3 Kinetic analysis of plasma concentrations resulting from the intravenous injection of NAPA-^{13}C *(circles)* and the simultaneous oral administration of a NAPA tablet *(triangles)*. The solid lines are a least-squares fit of the measured concentrations shown by the data points. The calculated percentage of the oral dose remaining in the gastrointestinal (GI) tract is plotted in the insert. (Reproduced with permission from Atkinson AJ, Jr, et al. Clin Pharmacol Ther 1989;46:182–9.)

observed after the oral dose was administered. The results of these two methods of assessing extent of absorption are compared in Table 4.3. The discrepancy was less than 2% for all but one of the subjects.

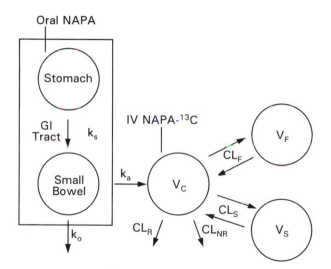

FIGURE 4.4 Multicompartment system used to model the kinetics of NAPA absorption, distribution, and elimination. NAPA labeled with ^{13}C was injected intravenously (IV) to define the kinetics of NAPA disposition. NAPA distribution from intravascular space (V_C) to fast (V_F) and slow (V_S) equilibrating peripheral compartments is characterized by the intercompartmental clearances CL_F and CL_S. NAPA is cleared from the body by both renal (CL_R) and nonrenal (CL_{NR}) mechanisms. A NAPA tablet was administered orally with the intravenous dose to analyze the kinetics of NAPA absorption from the gastrointestinal (GI) tract. After an initial delay that consisted of a time lag (not shown) and presumed delivery of NAPA to the small bowel (k_s), the rate and extent of NAPA absorption were determined by k_a and k_o, as described in the text. (Reproduced with permission from Atkinson AJ, Jr, et al. Clin Pharmacol Ther 1989;46:182–9.)

Slow and incomplete absorption of procainamide has been reported in patients with acute myocardial infarction and has been attributed to decreased splanchnic blood flow (22). Decreased splanchnic blood flow also may reduce the bioavailability of NAPA, the acetylated metabolite of procainamide. Although an explicit relationship between CL_F and k_a is not shown in Figure 4.4, splanchnic blood flow is proposed as a major determinant of CL_F, and it is noteworthy that the extent of NAPA absorption in patients was well correlated with CL_F estimates ($R = 0.89$, $P = 0.045$). This illustrates how a model-based approach can provide important insights into patient factors affecting drug absorption.

Relative Bioavailability

If the bioavailability comparison is made between two oral formulations of a drug, then their relative bioavailability is measured. Two formulations generally are regarded as being *bioequivalent* if the 90% con-

TABLE 4.3 Comparison of Bioavailability Estimates

Patient number	Kinetic analysis (%)	NAPA recovery in urine[a] (%)
1	66.1	65.9
2	92.1	92.1
3	68.1	69.9
4	88.2	73.1
5	75.7	75.6

[a] Corrected for absorption lag time.

fidence interval of the ratios of the population average estimates of *AUC* and C_{max} for the test and reference formulations lie within a preestablished bioequivalence limit, usually 80 to 125% (23). Bioequivalence studies are needed during clinical investigation of a new drug product to ensure that different clinical trial batches and formulations have similar performance characteristics. They also are required when significant manufacturing changes occur after drug approval. Following termination of marketing exclusivity, generic drugs that are introduced are expected to be bioequivalent to the innovator's product. Population average metrics of the test and reference formulations have traditionally been compared to calculate an *average bioequivalence*. However, more sophisticated statistical approaches have been advocated to compare full population distributions or estimate intraindividual differences in bioequivalence (23).

Although *therapeutic equivalence* is assured if two formulations are bioequivalent, the therapeutic equivalence of two bioinequivalent formulations can be judged only within a specific clinical context (19). Thus, if we ordinarily treat streptococcal throat infections with a 10-fold excess of penicillin, a formulation having half the bioavailability of the usual formulation would be therapeutically equivalent since it still would provide a five-fold excess of antibiotic. On the other hand, bioinequivalence of cyclosporine formulations, and of other drugs that have a narrow therapeutic index, could have serious therapeutic consequences.

In Vitro Prediction of Bioavailability

The introduction of combinatorial chemistry and high throughput biological screens has placed increasing stress on the technology that traditionally has been used to assess bioavailability. Insufficient time and resources are available to conduct formal *in vivo* kinetic studies for each candidate compound that is screened. Consequently, there is a clear need to develop *in vitro* methods that can be integrated into biological screening processes as reliable predictors of bioavailability. For reformulation of some immediate release compounds it even is possible that *in vitro* data will suffice and that the requirement for repeated *in vivo* studies can be waived (24).

An important part of this development effort has been the establishment of a theoretical basis for drug classification that focuses on three critical biopharmaceutical properties: drug solubility relative to drug dose, dissolution rate of the drug formulation, and the intestinal permeability of the drug (25). Drug solubility can be measured *in vitro* and related to the volume of fluid required to dissolve the drug dose completely.

In vitro dissolution tests have been standardized and are widely used for manufacturing quality control and in the evaluation of new formulations and generic products. However, proper selection of the apparatus and dissolution medium for these tests needs to be based on the physical chemistry of the drug and on the dosage form being evaluated (26). For immediate release products, a dissolution specification of 85% dissolved in less than 15 minutes has been proposed as sufficient to exclude decreases in bioavailability due to dissolution-rate limitations. Based on these considerations, the following biopharmaceutic drug classification has been established (25).

Class I—High Solubility–High Permeability Drugs

Drugs in this class are well absorbed, but their bioavailability may be limited either by first-pass metabolism or by P-glycoprotein-mediated efflux from the intestinal mucosa. *In vitro–in vivo* correlations of dissolution rate with the rate of drug absorption are expected if dissociation is slower than gastric emptying rate. If dissociation is sufficiently rapid, gastric emptying will limit absorption rate.

Class II—Low Solubility–High Permeability Drugs

Poor solubility may limit the extent of absorption of high drug doses. The rate of absorption is limited by dissolution rate and generally is slower than for drugs in Class I. *In vitro–in vivo* correlations are tenuous in view of the many formulation and physiological variables that can affect the dissolution profile.

Class III—High Solubility–Low Permeability Drugs

Intestinal permeability limits both the rate and extent of absorption for this class of drugs and intestinal reserve length is marginal. Bioavailability is expected to be variable but, if dissolution is 85% complete in less than 15 minutes, this variability will reflect differences in physiological variables such as intestinal permeability and intestinal transit time.

Class IV—Low Solubility–Low Permeability Drugs

Effective oral delivery of this class of drugs presents the most difficulties, and reliable *in vitro–in vivo* correlations are not expected.

The rapid evaluation of the intestinal membrane permeability of drugs represents a continuing challenge. Human intubation studies have been used to measure jejunal effective permeability of a number of drugs, and these measurements have been compared with the extent of drug absorption. It can be seen from Figure 4.5 that the expected fraction absorbed exceeds

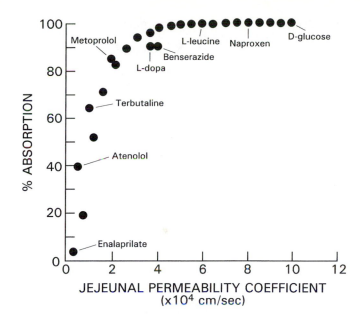

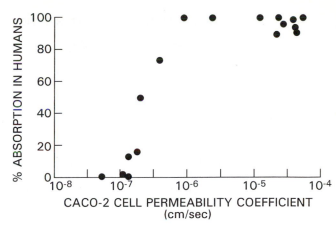

FIGURE 4.5 Relationship between jejunal permeability measured by intestinal intubation and extent of absorption of a series of compounds. (Reproduced with permission from Amidon GL, Lennerös H, Shah VP, Crison JR: Pharm Res 1995;12:413–20.)

FIGURE 4.6 Relationship for a series of 20 compounds between apparent permeability coefficients in a Caco-2 cell model and the extent of absorption after oral administration to humans. (Reproduced with permission from Artursson P, Karlsson J: Biochem Biophys Res Commun 1991;175:880–5.)

95% for drugs with a jejunal permeability of more than 2–4×10^{-4} cm/sec (25).

Although human intubation studies are even more laborious than formal assessment of absolute bioavailability, they have played an important role in validating *in vitro* methods that have been developed. The most commonly used *in vitro* method is based on measurement of drug transfer across a monolayer of cultured Caco-2 cells derived from a human colorectal carcinoma. Artursson and Karlsson (27) found that the apparent permeability of 20 drugs measured with the Caco-2 cell model was well correlated with the extent of drug absorption in human subjects, and that drugs with permeability coefficients exceeding 1×10^{-6} cm/sec were completely absorbed (Figure 4.6).

However, Caco-2 cells, being derived from colonic epithelium, have a lower paracellular permeability than jejunal mucosa, and the activity of drug metabolizing enzymes, transporters, and efflux mechanisms in these cells does not always reflect what is encountered *in vivo*. In addition, the Caco-2 cell model provides no assessment of the extent of hepatic first-pass metabolism. Despite these shortcomings, this *in vitro* model is well suited to the demands of biological screening programs and further methodological improvements can be expected (28). At some point, *in silico* methods, such as those based on the calculation of the dynamic polar surface area of candidate drug molecules, may enable predic-

tions of drug absorption to be incorporated into the initial drug design process (29).

KINETICS OF DRUG ABSORPTION AFTER ORAL ADMINISTRATION

After drug administration by the oral route, some time passes before any drug appears in the systemic circulation. This lag time (t_{lag}) reflects the time required for disintegration and dissolution of the drug product and the time for the drug to reach the absorbing surface of the small intestine. After this delay, the plasma-drug-concentration-vs.-time curve shown in Figure 4.2 reflects the combined operation of the processes of drug absorption and of drug distribution and elimination. The peak concentration, C_{max}, is reached when drug entry into the systemic circulation no longer exceeds drug removal by distribution to tissues, metabolism, and excretion. Thus, drug absorption is not completed when C_{max} is reached.

In the last two chapters we analyzed the kinetic response to a bolus injection of a drug, an input that can be represented by a single impulse. Similarly, the input resulting from administration of an oral or intramuscular drug dose, or a constant intravenous infusion, can be regarded as a series of individual impulses, $G(\theta)d\theta$, where $G(\theta)$ describes the rate of absorption over a time increment between θ and $\theta + d\theta$. If the system is linear and the parameters are time invariant (30), we can think of the plasma response $[X(t)]$ observed at time t as resulting from the sum or integral over each absorption increment occurring at prior time θ $[G(\theta)d\theta$ where $0 \leq \theta \leq t]$ reduced by the

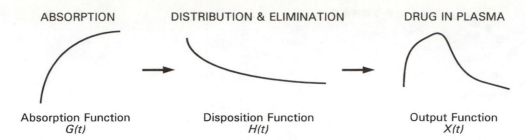

ABSORPTION   DISTRIBUTION & ELIMINATION   DRUG IN PLASMA

Absorption Function   Disposition Function   Output Function
        G(t)   H(t)   X(t)

FIGURE 4.7 The processes of drug absorption and disposition (distribution and elimination) interact to generate the observed time-course of drug in the body. Similarly, the output function can be represented as an interaction between absorption and disposition functions.

fractional drug disposition that occurs between θ and t $[H(t - \theta)]$, that is:

$$X(t) = \int_0^t G(\theta) \cdot H(t - \theta)d\theta$$

The function $H(t)$ describes drug disposition after intravenous bolus administration of a unit dose at time t. The interplay of these functions and associated physiological processes is represented schematically in Figure 4.7. This expression for $X(t)$ is termed the *convolution* of $G(t)$ and $H(t)$ and can be represented as:

$$X(t) = G(t) * H(t)$$

where the operation of convolution is denoted by the symbol $*$. The operation of convolution in the time domain corresponds to multiplication in the domain of the subsidiary algebraic equation given by Laplace transformation. Thus, in Laplace transform notation:

$$x(s) = g(s) \cdot h(s)$$

In the disposition model shown in Figure 4.8, the kinetics of drug distribution and elimination are represented by a single compartment with first-order elimination as described by the equation:

$$dH/dt = -kH$$

Since:

$$\mathscr{L}F(t) = f(s)$$

and:

$$\mathscr{L}F'(t) = sf(s) - F_0$$

$$sh(s) - H_0 = -kh(s)$$

H_0 is a unit impulse function, so $h(s)$ is given by:

$$h(s) = \frac{1}{s + k} \tag{4.3}$$

Although the absorption process is quite complex, it often follows simple first-order kinetics. To obtain the appropriate absorption function, consider absorption under circumstances where there is no elimination (31). This can be diagrammed as shown in Figure 4.9. In this absorption model, drug disappearance from the gut is described by the equation:

$$\frac{dM}{dt} = -aM$$

So:

$$M = M_0 e^{-at}$$

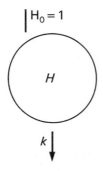

FIGURE 4.8 Disposition model representing the elimination of a unit impulse drug dose ($H_0 = 1$) from a single body compartment. Drug in this compartment (H) is removed as specified by the first-order elimination rate constant k.

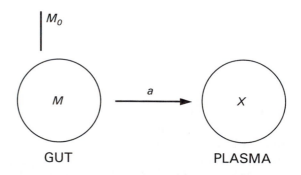

FIGURE 4.9 Model representing the absorption of a drug dose (M_0) from a gut compartment to a plasma compartment. The first-order absorption constant a determines the rate at which drug remaining in the gut (M) is transferred to plasma (X).

But the rate of drug appearance in plasma is:

$$\frac{dM}{dt} = aM$$

The absorption function is defined as this rate, so $G(t)$ is:

$$G(t) = a\,M_0\,e^{-at}$$

By definition:

$$g(s) = \int_0^\infty G(t)\,e^{-st}\,dt$$

So:

$$g(s) = a\,M_0\int_0^\infty e^{-at}\,e^{-st}\,dt$$

$$g(s) = -\frac{a\,M_0}{s+a}\,e^{-(s+a)t}\Big|_0^\infty$$

Therefore:

$$g(s) = \frac{aM_0}{s+a} \qquad (4.4)$$

Multiplication of Equations 4.3 and 4.4 gives:

$$x(s) = g(s)\cdot h(s) = \frac{a\,M_0}{s+a}\cdot\frac{1}{s+k}$$

and

$$X(t) = \mathcal{L}^{-1}\frac{aM_0}{(s+a)(s+k)}$$

The table of inverse Laplace transforms shows that there are two solutions for this equation. Usually, $a \neq k$ and:

$$X(t) = \frac{a\,M_0}{k-a}\left(e^{-at} - e^{-kt}\right) \qquad (4.5)$$

In the special case, where $a = k$:

$$X(t) = a\,M_0\,t\,e^{-kt} \qquad (4.6)$$

Time to Peak Level

The time needed to reach the peak level (t_{max}) can be determined by differentiating $X(t)$.
For $a \neq k$:

$$X'(t) = \left[\frac{a\,M_0}{k-a}\right]\left(-ae^{-at} + ke^{-kt}\right)$$

At the peak level, $X'(t) = 0$. Therefore:

$$k\,e^{-kt_{max}} = ae^{-at_{max}} \qquad (4.7)$$

$$a/k = e^{(a-k)t_{max}}$$

and

$$t_{max} = \frac{1}{a-k}\ln\,(a/k) \qquad (4.8)$$

The absorption half-life is another kinetic parameter that can be calculated as $\ln 2/a$.

Value of Peak Level

The value of the peak level (C_{max}) can be estimated by substituting the value for t_{max} back into the equation for $X(t)$. For $a \neq k$, we can use Equation 4.7 to obtain:

$$e^{-at_{max}} = \frac{k}{a}\,e^{-kt_{max}}$$

Substituting this result into Equation 4.5:

$$X_{max} = \frac{a\,M_0}{k-a}\left(\frac{k}{a}-1\right)e^{-kt_{max}}$$

Hence:

$$X_{max} = M_0\,e^{-kt_{max}}$$

But from Equation 4.8:

$$-k\,t_{max} = \frac{k}{k-a}\,\ln\left(a/k\right)$$

So:

$$e^{-kt_{max}} = (a/k)^{k/(k-a)}$$

Therefore:

$$X_{max} = M_0\,(a/k)^{k/(k-a)} \qquad (4.9)$$

The maximum plasma concentration would then be given by: $C_{max} = X_{max}/V_d$, where V_d is the distribution volume. It can be seen from Equations 4.8 and 4.9 that C_{max} and t_{max} are complex functions of both the absorption rate, a, and the elimination rate, k, of a drug.

Use of Convolution/Deconvolution to Assess *In Vitro–In Vivo* Correlations

Particularly for extended release formulations, the simple characterization of drug absorption in terms of AUC, C_{max} and t_{max} is inadequate and a more comprehensive comparison of *in vitro* test results with *in vivo* drug absorption is needed (32). Both $X(t)$, the output function after oral absorption, and $H(t)$, the disposition function, can be obtained from experimental data and the absorption function, $G(t)$ estimated by the process of *deconvolution*. This process is the inverse of convolution and, in the Laplace domain, $g(s)$ can be obtained by dividing the trans-

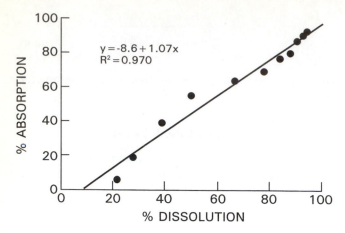

FIGURE 4.10 Linear regression comparing the extent of drug dissolution and oral absorption at common time points. (Reproduced with permission from Rackley RJ: Examples of *in vitro–in vivo* relationships with a diverse range of quality. In: Young D, Devane JG, Butler J, editors. *In vitro–in vivo* correlations. New York: Plenum Press; 1997. p. 1–15.)

form of the output function, *x(s)*, by the transform of the disposition function, *h(s)*:

$$g(s) = \frac{x(s)}{h(s)}$$

Since this approach requires that *X(t)* and *H(t)* be defined by explicit functions, deconvolution is usually performed using numerical methods (33). Alternatively, the absorption function can be obtained from a pharmacokinetic model, as shown by the insert in Figure 4.3 (13). Even when this approach is taken, numerical deconvolution methods may be helpful in developing the appropriate absorption model (21). As a second step in the analysis, linear regression commonly is used to compare the time course of drug absorption with dissolution test results at common time points, as shown in Figure 4.10 (34). The linear relationship in this figure, with a slope and a coefficient of determination (R^2) of nearly one, would be expected primarily for Class I drugs. The nonzero intercept presumably reflects the time lag in gastric emptying.

Another approach is to convolute a function representing *in vitro* dissolution with the disposition function in order to predict the plasma-level-vs.-time curve following oral drug administration. Obviously, correlations will be poor if there is substantial first-pass metabolism of the drug or if *in vivo* conditions, such as intestinal transit time, are not reflected in the dissolution test system.

References

1. Tsuji A, Tamai I. Carrier-mediated intestinal transport of drugs. Pharm Res 1996;13:963–77.
2. Hollander D, Dadugalza VD, Fairchild PA. Intestinal absorption of aspirin: Influence of pH, taurocholate, ascorbate, and ethanol. J Lab Clin Med 1981;98:591–8.
3. Meldrum SJ, Watson BW, Riddle HC, Sladen GE. pH profile of gut as measured by radiotelemetry capsule. Br Med J 1972;2:104–6.
4. Wilding IR, Coupe AJ, Davis SS. The role of γ-scintigraphy in oral drug delivery. Adv Drug Del Rev 1991;7:87–117.
5. Rees WDW, Brown CM. Physiology of the stomach and duodenum. In: Haubrich WS, Schaffner F, Berk JE, editors. Bockus gastroenterology. Philadelphia: WB Saunders; 1995. p. 582–614.
6. Davis SS, Hardy JG, Fara JW. Transit of pharmaceutical dosage forms through the small intestine. Gut 1986;27:886–92.
7. Kenyon CJ, Brown F, McClelland, Wilding IR. The use of pharmacoscintigraphy to elucidate food effects observed with a novel protease inhibitor (saquinavir). Pharm Res 1998;15:417–22.
8. Nimmo I, Heading RC, Tothill P, Prescott LF. Pharmacological modification of gastric emptying: Effects of propantheline and metoclopromide on paracetamol absorption. Br Med J 1973;1:587–9.
9. Higuchi WI, Ho NFH, Park JY, Komiya I. Rate-limiting steps in drug absorption. In: Prescott LF, Nimmo WS, editors. Drug absorption. Sydney: ADIS Press; 1981. p. 35–60.
10. Manninen V, Melin J, Apajalahti A, Karesoja M. Altered absorption of digoxin in patients given propantheline and metoclopramide. Lancet 1973;1:398–9.
11. Heizer WD, Smith TW, Goldfinger SE. Absorption of digoxin in patients with malabsorption syndromes. N Engl J Med 1971;285:257–9.
12. Winne D. Influence of blood flow on intestinal absorption of xenobiotics. Pharmacology 1980;21:1–15.
13. Atkinson AJ Jr, Ruo TI, Piergies AA, Breiter HC, Connelly TJ, Sedek GS, Juan D, Hubler GL, Hsieh A-M. Pharmacokinetics of N-acetylprocainamide in patients profiled with a stable isotope method. Clin Pharmacol Ther 1989;46:182–9.
14. Dobkin JF, Saha JR, Butler VP Jr, Neu HC, Lindenbaum J. Digoxin-inactivating bacteria: Identification in human gut flora. Science 1983;220:325–7.
15. Welling PG. Interactions affecting drug absorption. Clin Pharmacokinet 1984;9:404–34.
16. Watkins PB. Drug metabolism by cytochromes P450 in the liver and small bowel. Gastroenterol Clin N Amer 1992;21:511–26.
17. Kolars JC, Merion RM, Awni WM, Watkins PB. First-pass metabolism of cyclosporine by the gut. Lancet 1991;338:1488–90.
18. Hall SD, Thummel KE, Watkinson PB, Lown KS, Benet LZ, Paine MF, Mayo RR, Turgeon DK, Bailey DG, Fontana RJ, Wrighton SA. Molecular and physical mechanisms of first-pass extraction. Drug Metab Dispos 1999;27:161–6.
19. Koch-Weser J. Bioavailability of drugs. N Engl J Med 1974;291:233-7, 503–6.
20. Yeh KC, Kwan KC. A comparison of numerical integrating algorithms by trapezoidal, Lagrange, and spline approximation. J Pharmacokinet Biopharm 1978;6:79–98.
21. Strong JM, Dutcher JS, Lee W-K, Atkinson AJ Jr. Absolute bioavailability in man of N-acetylprocainamide determined by a novel stable isotope method. Clin Pharmacol Ther 1975;18:613–22.

22. Koch-Weser J. Pharmacokinetics of procainamide in man. Ann NY Acad Sci 1971;179:370–82.

23. Patnaik RN, Lesko LJ, Chen ML, Williams RL, the FDA Individual Bioequivalence Working Group. Individual bioequivalence: New concepts in the statistical assessment of bioequivalence metrics. Clin Pharmacokinet 1997;33:1–6.

24. Biopharmaceutic Classification Working Group, Biopharmaceutics Coordinating Committee, CDER. Waiver of in vivo bioavailability and bioequivalence studies for immediate-release solid oral dosage forms based on a biopharmaceutics classification system. Guidance for Industry, Rockville: FDA; 2000. (Internet at http://www.fda.gov/cder/guidance/index.htm.)

25. Amidon GL, Lenneräs H, Shah VP, Crison JR. A theoretical basis for a biopharmaceutic drug classification: The correlation of *in vitro* drug product dissolution and *in vivo* bioavailability. Pharm Res 1995;12:413–20.

26. Rohrs BR, Skoug JW, Halstead GW. Dissolution assay development for *in vitro–in vivo* correlations: Theory and case studies. In: Young D, Devane JG, Butler J, editors. In vitro–in vivo correlations. New York: Plenum Press; 1997. p. 17–30.

27. Artursson P, Karlsson J. Correlation between oral drug absorption in humans and apparent drug permeability coefficients in human intestinal epithelial (Caco-2) cells. Biochem Biophys Res Commun 1991;175:880–5.

28. Artursson P, Borchardt RT. Intestinal drug absorption and metabolism in cell cultures: Caco-2 and beyond. Pharm Res 1997;14:1655–8.

29. Palm K, Luthman K, Ungell A-L, Strandlund G, Artursson P. Correlation of drug absorption with molecular surface properties. J Pharm Sci 1996;85:32–9.

30. Sokolnikoff IS, Redheffer RM. Mathematics of physics and modern engineering. 2nd ed. New York: McGraw-Hill; 1966. p. 224.

31. Atkinson AJ Jr, Kushner W. Clinical pharmacokinetics. Annu Rev Pharmacol Toxicol 1979;19:105–27.

32. Langenbucher F, Mysicka J. *In vitro* and *in vivo* deconvolution assessment of drug release kinetics from oxprenolol Oros preparations. Br J Clin Pharmacol 1985;19: 151S–62S.

33. Vaughan DP, Dennis M. Mathematical basis of point-area deconvolution method for determining *in vivo* input functions. J Pharm Sci 1978;67:663–5.

34. Rackley RJ. Examples of *in vitro–in vivo* relationships with a diverse range of quality. In: Young D, Devane JG, Butler J, editors. *In vitro–in vivo* correlations. New York: Plenum Press; 1997. p. 1–15.

STUDY PROBLEMS

1. An approach that has been used during drug development to measure the absolute bioavailability of a drug is to administer an initial dose intravenously in order to estimate the area under the plasma-level-vs.-time curve from zero to infinite time *(AUC)*. Subjects then are begun on oral therapy. When steady state is reached, the *AUC* during a dosing interval $(AUC_{0 \to \tau})$ is measured. The extent of absorption of the oral formulation is calculated from the following equation:

$$\% \text{ Absorption} = \frac{D_{IV} \cdot AUC_{0 \to \tau(oral)}}{D_{oral} \cdot AUC_{IV}} \times 100$$

   This approach requires AUC to equal $AUC_{0 \to \tau}$ if the same doses are administered intravenously and orally and the extent of absorption is 100%. Derive the proof for this equality.

2. When a drug is administered by constant intravenous administration, this zero-order input can be represented by a "step function." Derive the appropriate absorption function and convolute it with the disposition function to obtain the output function. (*Clue:* Remember that the absorption function is the *rate* of drug administration.)

3. A 70-kg patient is treated with an intravenous infusion of lidocaine at a rate of 2 mg/min. Assume a single-compartment distribution volume of 1.9 L/kg and an elimination half-life of 90 minutes.

   a. Use the output function derived in Problem 2 to predict the expected steady-state plasma lidocaine concentration.

   b. Use this function to estimate the time required to reach 90% of this steady state level.

   c. Express this 90% equilibration time in terms of number of elimination half-lives.

Effects of Renal Disease
on Pharmacokinetics

ARTHUR J. ATKINSON, JR.

Clinical Center, National Institutes of Health, Bethesda, Maryland

Although drugs are developed to treat patients who have diseases, relatively little attention has been given to the fact that these diseases themselves exert important effects that affect patient response to drug therapy. In the idealized scheme of contemporary drug development shown in Figure 5.1, the pertinent information would be generated in pharmacokinetic and pharmacodynamic (PK/PD) studies in special populations that are carried out concurrently with Phase II and Phase III clinical trials (1). Additional useful information can be obtained by using population pharmacokinetic methods to analyze data obtained in the large-scale Phase III trials themselves (2). However, a review of labeling in the *Physicians' Desk Reference* indicates that there often is scant information available to guide dose selection for individual patients (3).

Illness, aging, sex, and other patient factors may have important effects on *pharmacodynamic* aspects of patient response to drugs. For example, patients with advanced pulmonary insufficiency are particularly sensitive to the respiratory depressant effects of narcotic and sedative drugs. In addition, these patient factors may affect the *pharmacokinetic* aspects of drug elimination, distribution, and absorption. Even when the necessary pharmacokinetic and pharmacodynamic information is available, appropriate dose adjustments often are not made for patients with impaired renal function because assessment of this function usually is based solely on serum creatinine measurements without concomitant estimation of creatinine clearance (4).

Because there is a large population of functionally anephric patients who are maintained in relatively stable condition by hemodialysis, a substantial number of pharmacokinetic studies have been carried out in these individuals. Patients with intermediate levels of impaired renal function have not been studied to the same extent, but studies in these patients are recommended in current FDA guidelines (5).

EFFECTS OF RENAL DISEASE
ON DRUG ELIMINATION

The effects of decreased renal function on drug elimination have been examined most extensively. This is appropriate since only elimination clearance (CL_E) and drug dose determine the steady state concentration of drug in the body (C_{ss}). This is true whether the drug is given by constant intravenous infusion (I), in which case:

$$C_{ss} = I/CL_E \qquad (5.1)$$

or by intermittent oral or parenteral doses, in which case the corresponding equation is:

$$\bar{C}_{ss} = \frac{Dose/\tau}{CL_E} \qquad (5.2)$$

where $\bar{C}_{ss}$ is the mean concentration during the dosing interval τ.

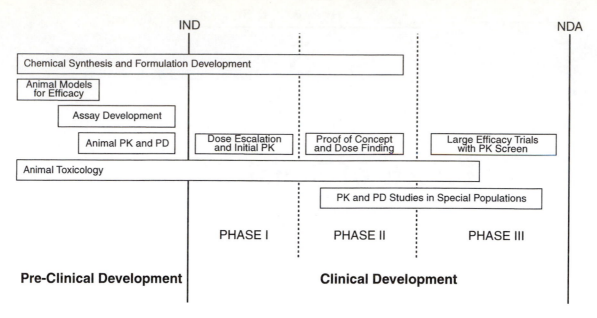

FIGURE 5.1   Timing of pharmacokinetic (PK) and pharmacodynamic (PD) studies during different phases of drug development.

For many drugs, CL_E consists of additive renal (CL_R) and nonrenal (CL_{NR}) components, as indicated by the following equation:

$$CL_E = CL_R + CL_{NR} \qquad (5.3)$$

Nonrenal clearance is usually equated with drug metabolism, but also could include hemodialysis and other methods of drug removal. In fact, even the metabolic clearance of a drug frequently consists of additive contributions from several parallel metabolic pathways. The characterization of drug metabolism by a clearance term usually is appropriate, since the metabolism of most drugs usually can be described by first-order kinetics within the range of therapeutic drug concentrations.

Dettli (6) proposed that the additive property of *elimination rate constants* representing parallel elimination pathways provides a way of either using Equation 5.3 or constructing nomograms to estimate the dose reductions that are appropriate for patients with impaired renal function. This approach also can be used to estimate *elimination clearance*, as illustrated for cimetidine in Figure 5.2. In implementing this approach, creatinine clearance (CL_{CR}) usually is estimated from the Cockcroft and Gault equation (8), although recently a more accurate prediction method has been proposed (9). Calculations or nomograms for many drugs can be made after consulting tables in Appendix II of Goodman and Gilman (10) or other reference sources to obtain values of CL_E and the fractional dose eliminated by renal excretion (% urinary excretion) in normal subjects.

Schentag et al. (11) obtained slightly lower estimates of cimetidine percentage urinary excretion in normal subjects and of CL_E in patients with duodenal ulcer and in older normal subjects than shown in Figure 5.2, which is based on reports by previous investigators who studied only young subjects (12). Nonetheless, there is apparent internal discrepancy in the labeling for cimetidine. Under "Dosage Adjustment for Patients with Impaired Renal Function," the label states that "Patients with creatinine clearance less than 30 cc/min who are being treated for prevention of upper gastrointestinal bleeding should receive half the recommended dose." However, under "Pharmacokinetics" it indicates that "following i.v. or i.m. administration, approximately 75% of the drug is recovered from the urine after 24 hours as the parent compound" (13). Since only one-fourth of the dose is eliminated by nonrenal mechanisms, it can be inferred that functionally anephric patients who receive half the usual cimetidine dose will have potentially toxic blood levels that are twice those recommended for patients with normal renal function.

When dose adjustments are needed for patients with impaired renal function, they can be made by reducing the drug dose or by lengthening the dosing interval. Either approach, or a combination of both, may be employed in practice. For example, once the expected value for CL_E has been estimated, the daily drug dose can be reduced in proportion to the quotient of the expected clearance divided by the normal clearance. This will maintain the average drug concentra-

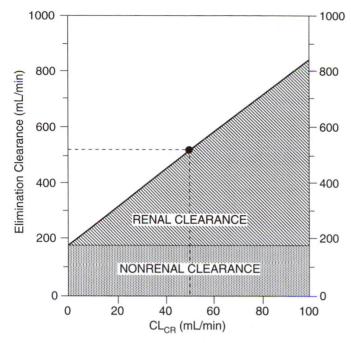

FIGURE 5.2 Nomogram for estimating cimetidine elimination clearance (CL_E) for a 70-kg patient with impaired renal function. The right-hand ordinate indicates cimetidine CL_E measured in young adults with normal renal function, and the left-hand ordinate indicates expected cimetidine CL_E in a functionally anephric patient, based on the fact that 23% of an administered dose is eliminated by nonrenal routes in normal subjects. The dotted line connecting these points can be used to estimate cimetidine CL_E from creatinine clearance (CL_{CR}). For example, a 70-kg patient with CL_{CR} of 50 mL/min (large dot) would be expected to have a cimetidine CL_E of 517 mL/min, and to respond satisfactorily to doses that are 60% of those recommended for patients with normal renal function. (Reproduced with permission from Atkinson AJ Jr, Craig RM. Therapy of peptic ulcer disease. In: Molinoff PB, editor. Peptic ulcer disease. Mechanisms and management. Rutherford, NJ: Healthpress Publishing Group, Inc.; 1990 p. 83–112.)

tion at the usual level, regardless of whether the drug is administered by intermittent doses or by continuous infusion. On the other hand, it is often convenient to administer doses of drugs that have a short elimination half-life at some multiple of their elimination half-life. The multiple that is used is determined by the therapeutic index of the drug. The expected half life can be calculated from the following equation:

$$t_{1/2} = \frac{0.693\, V_{d(area)}}{CL_E} \qquad (5.4)$$

and the usual dose can be administered at an interval equal to the same multiple of the increased half-life. Dose-interval adjustment is usually necessary when safety and efficacy concerns specify a target range for both peak and trough plasma levels or when selection of drug doses is limited.

The reliability of the Dettli method of predicting drug clearance depends on two critical assumptions:

1. The nonrenal clearance of the drug remains constant when renal function is impaired.
2. CL_E declines in a linear fashion with CL_{CR}.

There are several important exceptions to the first assumption that will be considered when we discuss the effects of impaired renal function on drug metabolism. Nonetheless, this approach is widely used for individualizing drug dosage for patients with impaired renal function. In addition, Equations 5.3 and 5.4 provide a useful tool for hypothesis generation during drug development when pharmacokinetic studies are planned for subjects with impaired renal function (Figure 5.1).

Mechanisms of Renal Excretion of Drugs

Important mechanisms involved in the renal excretion of drugs have been reviewed by Reidenberg (14) and are shown in Table 5.1. Glomerular filtration affects all drugs of small molecular size and is *restrictive* in the sense that it is limited by drug binding to plasma proteins. On the other hand, renal tubular secretion is *nonrestrictive* since both protein bound and free drug concentrations in plasma are available for elimination. In fact, the renal tubular secretion of para-aminohippurate is rapid enough that its elimination clearance is used to estimate renal blood flow. Competition by drugs for renal tubular secretion is an important cause of drug–drug interactions.

Net drug elimination also may be affected by drug reabsorption by non-ionic passive diffusion and by active transport mechanisms. These renal tubular mechanisms can be analyzed by stop-flow and other standard methods used in renal physiology, but detailed studies are seldom performed. For most drugs, all that has been done has been to correlate renal drug clearance with the reciprocal of serum creatinine or with creatinine clearance. Even though creatinine clearance primarily reflects glomerular filtration rate, it serves as a rough guide to the renal clearance of drugs that have extensive renal tubular secretion or reabsorption. This is a consequence of the glomerulo-tubular balance that is maintained in damaged nephrons by intrinsic tubule and peritubular capillary adaptations that parallel reductions in single nephron glomerular filtration rate (GFR) (15). For this reason, CL_E usually declines fairly linearly with reductions in CL_{CR}. However, some discrepancies can be expected. For example, Reidenberg et al. (16) have shown that renal secre-

TABLE 5.1   Important Mechanisms of Renal Elimination of Drugs

I. Glomerular filtration

- Affects all drugs and metabolites of appropriate molecular size
- Influenced by protein binding (f_u = free fraction)
  Drug filtration rate = GFR $\times f_u \times$ [drug]

II. Renal tubular secretion

- Not influenced by protein binding
- May be affected by competition with other drugs, etc.
  Examples:

Active drugs:	Acids—penicillin
	Bases—Procaine amide
Metabolites:	Glucuronides, hippurates, etc.

III. Reabsorption by non-ionic diffusion

- Affects weak acids and weak bases
- Only important if excretion of free drug is major elimination path
  Examples:

Weak acids:	Phenobarbital
Weak bases:	Quinidine

IV. Active reabsorption

- Affects ions, not proved for other drugs
  Examples:

Halides:	Fluoride, bromide
Alkaline metals:	Lithium

TABLE 5.2   Effect of Renal Disease on Drug Metabolism

I. Oxidations		Normal or increased
Example:	Phenytoin	
II. Reductions		Slowed
Example:	Hydrocortisone	
III. Hydrolyses		
• Plasma esterase		Slowed
Example:	Procaine	
• Plasma peptidase		Normal
Example:	Angiotensin	
• Tissue peptidase		Slowed
Example:	Insulin	
IV. Syntheses		
• Glucuronide formation		Normal
Example:	Hydrocortisone	
• Acetylation		Slowed
Example:	Procainamide	
• Glycine conjugation		Slowed
Example:	PAS[a]	
• O-Methylation		Normal
Example:	Methyldopa	
• Sulfate conjugation		Normal
Example:	Acetaminophen	

[a] Para-aminosalicylic acid

tion of some basic drugs declines with aging more rapidly than GFR. In addition, studies with *N*-1-methylnicotinamide, an endogenous marker of renal tubular secretion, have demonstrated some degree of glomerulo-tubular imbalance in patients with impaired renal function (17).

Despite the paucity of detailed studies, it is possible to draw some general mechanistic conclusions from renal clearance values:

- If renal clearance *exceeds* drug filtration rate (Table 5.1), there is net renal tubular secretion of the drug.
- If renal clearance *is less than* drug filtration rate, there is net renal tubular reabsorption of the drug.

Effects of Impaired Renal Function on Drug Metabolism

Most drugs are not excreted unchanged by the kidneys but first are biotransformed to metabolites that are then excreted. Renal failure not only may retard the excretion of these metabolites, which in some cases have important pharmacologic activity, but, in some cases, alters the metabolic clearance of drugs (14, 18). The impact of impaired renal function on drug metabolism is dependent on the metabolic pathway, as indicated in Table 5.2. In most cases, it is unclear how much impairment in renal function needs to be present before drug metabolism is affected. However, clinical experience suggests, for example, that creatinine clearance must fall below 25 mL/min before the acetylation rate of procainamide is impaired.

EFFECTS OF RENAL DISEASE ON DRUG DISTRIBUTION

Impaired renal function is associated with important changes in the binding of some drugs to *plasma proteins*. In some cases the *tissue binding* of drugs is also affected.

Plasma Protein Binding of Acidic Drugs

Reidenberg and Drayer (19) have stated that protein binding in serum from uremic patients is decreased for every acidic drug that has been studied. Most acidic drugs bind to the bilirubin binding site on albumin but there are also different binding sites that play a role.

TABLE 5.3   **Effect of Impaired Renal Function on Phenytion Kinetics**

	Normal subjects (n = 4)	Uremic patients (n = 4)
Percent unbound (f_u)	12%	26%
Distribution volume ($V_{d(area)}$)	0.64 L/kg	1.40 L/kg
Hepatic clearance (CL_H)	2.46 L/hr	7.63 L/hr
Intrinsic clearance (CL_{int})	20.3 L/hr	29.9 L/hr

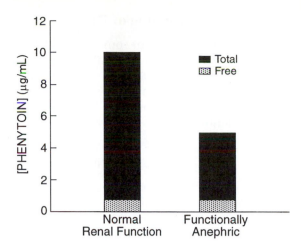

FIGURE 5.3   Comparison of free and total plasma phenytoin levels in a patient with normal renal function and a functionally anephric patient who have identical CL_{int} and are both treated with a 300-mg daily phenytoin dose. Although free phenytoin levels are 0.8 µg/mL in both patients, phenytoin is only 84% bound (16% free) in the functionally anephric patient, compared to 92% bound (8% free) in the patient with normal renal function. For that reason total phenytoin levels in the functionally anephric patient are only 5 µg/mL, whereas they are 10 µg/mL in the patient with normal renal function.

The reduced binding that occurs when renal function is impaired has been variously attributed to reductions in serum albumin concentration, structural changes in the binding sites, or displacement of drugs from albumin binding sites by organic molecules that accumulate in uremia. As described in Chapter 3, reductions in the protein binding of acidic drugs result in increases in their distribution volume. In addition, the elimination clearance of *restrictively eliminated* drugs is increased. However, protein binding changes do not affect distribution volume or clearance estimates when they are referenced to unbound drug concentrations For restrictively eliminated drugs, the term *intrinsic clearance* is used to describe the clearance that would be observed in the absence of any protein binding restrictions. As discussed in Chapter 7, the clearance of restrictively eliminated drugs, when referenced to total drug concentrations, simply equals the product of the unbound fraction of drug (f_u) and this intrinsic clearance (CL_{int}):

$$CL = f_u \cdot CL_{int} \qquad (5.5)$$

Phenytoin is an acidic, restrictively eliminated drug that can be used to illustrate some of the changes in drug distribution and elimination that occur in patients with impaired renal function. In patients with normal renal function, 92% of the phenytoin in plasma is protein bound. However, the percentage that is unbound or "free" rises from 8% in these individuals to 16%, or more, in hemodialysis-dependent patients. In a study comparing phenytoin pharmacokinetics in normal subjects and uremic patients, Odar-Cederlöf and Borgå (20) administered a single low dose of this drug so that first-order kinetics were approximated. The results shown in Table 5.3 can be inferred from their study. The uremic patients had an increase in distribution volume that was consistent with the observed decrease in phenytoin binding to plasma proteins. The three-fold increase in hepatic clearance that was observed in these patients also was primarily the result of decreased phenytoin protein binding. Although

intrinsic hepatic clearance also appeared to be increased in the uremic patients, the difference did not reach statistical significance at the $P = 0.05$ level.

A major problem arises in clinical practice when only total (protein bound + free) phenytoin concentrations are measured and used to guide therapy of patients with severely impaired renal function. The decreases in phenytoin binding that occur in these patients result in commensurate decreases in total plasma levels (Figure 5.3). Even though therapeutic and toxic pharmacologic effects are correlated with unbound rather than total phenytoin concentrations in plasma, the decrease in total concentrations can mislead physicians to increase phenytoin doses inappropriately. Fortunately, rapid ultrafiltration procedures are available that make it possible to measure free phenytoin concentrations in these patients on a routine basis.

Plasma Protein Binding of Basic and Neutral Drugs

The protein binding of basic drugs tends to be normal or only slightly reduced (19). In some cases, this may reflect the facts that these drugs bind to α_1–acid glycoprotein and that concentrations of this glycoprotein are higher in hemodialysis-dependent patients than in patients with normal renal function.

Tissue Binding of Drugs

The distribution volume of some drugs also can be altered when renal function is impaired. As described in Chapter 3, Sheiner et al. (21) have shown that impaired renal function is associated with a decrease in digoxin distribution volume that is described by the following equation:

$$V_d \text{ (in L)} = 3.84 \cdot \text{weight (in kg)} + 3.12 \, CL_{CR} \text{ (in mL/min)}$$

This presumably reflects a reduction in tissue levels of Na/K-ATPase, an enzyme that represents a major tissue-binding site for digoxin (22). In other cases in which distribution volume is decreased in patients with impaired renal function, the relationship between the degree of renal insufficiency and reduction in distribution volume has not been characterized nor have plausible mechanisms been proposed.

EFFECTS OF RENAL DISEASE ON DRUG ABSORPTION

The bioavailability of most drugs that have been studied has not been found to be altered in patients with impaired renal function. However, the absorption of *D*-xylose, a marker compound used to evaluate small intestinal absorptive function, was slowed (0.555 hr⁻¹ vs. 1.03 hr⁻¹) and less complete (48.6% vs. 69.4%) in patients with chronic renal failure than in normal subjects (23). Although these results were statistically significant, there was considerable interindividual variation in both patients and normal subjects. This primary absorptive defect may explain the fact that patients with impaired renal function have *reduced* bioavailability of furosemide (24) and pindolol (25). However, it also is possible that impaired renal function will result in *increased* bioavailability of drugs exhibiting first-pass metabolism when the function of drug metabolizing enzymes is compromised. Studies with orally administered propranolol have suggested this, but absolute bioavailability was not measured (26).

The paucity of reliable bioavailability data in patients with impaired renal function underscores the cumbersome nature of most absolute bioavailability studies in which oral and intravenous drug doses are administered on two separate occasions. The validity of these studies rests on the assumption that the kinetics of drug distribution and elimination remain unchanged in the interval between the two studies, an assumption that obviously is more tenuous for patients than for normal subjects. As discussed in Chapter 4, these shortcomings can be overcome by conducting a single study in which an intravenous formulation of the stable isotope labeled drug is administered simultaneously with the oral drug dose (27).

The simultaneous administration technique was used to study a 64-year-old man with a creatinine clearance of 79 ml/min who was started on *N*-acetylprocainamide (NAPA) therapy for ventricular arrhythmias (Figure 4.3). The oral NAPA dose was 66% absorbed in this patient, compared to 91.6% ± 9.2% when this method was used to assess NAPA absorption in normal subjects. Although this approach is ideally suited for studies of drug absorption in various patient populations, the required additional chemical synthesis of stable isotope-labeled drug and mass spectrometric analysis of patient samples have precluded its widespread adoption.

References

1. Yacobi A, Batra VK, Desjardins RE, Faulkner RD, Nicolau G, Pool WR, Shah A, Tonelli AP. Implementation of an effective pharmacokinetics research program in industry. In: Yacobi A, Skelly JP, Shah VP, Benet LZ, editors. Integration of pharmacokinetics, pharmacodynamics, and toxicokinetics in rational drug development. New York: Plenum; 1993. p. 125–35.

2. Peck CC. Rationale for the effective use of pharmacokinetics and pharmacodynamics in early drug development. In: Yacobi A, Skelly JP, Shah VP, Benet LZ, editors. Integration of pharmacokinetics, pharmacodynamics, and toxicokinetics in rational drug development. New York: Plenum; 1993. p. 1–5.

3. Spyker DA, Harvey ED, Harvey BE, Harvey AM, Rumack BH, Peck CC, Atkinson AJ Jr, Woosley RL, Abernethy DR, Cantilena LR. Assessment and reporting of clinical pharmacology information in drug labeling. Clin Pharmacol Ther 2000;67:196–200.

4. Piergies AA, Worwag EM, Atkinson AJ Jr. A concurrent audit of high digoxin plasma levels. Clin Pharmacol Ther 1994;55:353–8.

5. CDER, CBER. Pharmacokinetics in patients with impaired renal function—Study design, data analysis, and impact on dosing and labeling. Guidance for Industry, Rockville: FDA; 1998. (Internet at http://www.fda.gov/cder/guidance/index.htm.)

6. Dettli L. Individualization of drug dosage in patients with renal disease. Med Clin North Am 1974;58:977–85.

7. Atkinson AJ Jr, Craig RM. Therapy of peptic ulcer disease. In: Molinoff PB, editor. Peptic ulcer disease. Mechanisms and management. Rutherford, NJ: Healthpress Publishing Group, Inc.; 1990. p. 83–112.

8. Cockroft DW, Gault MH. Prediction of creatinine clearance from serum creatinine. Nephron 1976;16:31–41.

9. Levey AS, Bosch JP, Breyer Lewis J, Greene T, Rogers N, Roth D. A more accurate method to estimate glomerular filtration rate from serum creatinine: A new prediction equation. Ann Intern Med 1999;130:461–70.

10. Benet LZ, Øie S, Schwartz JB. Appendix II. Design and optimization of dose regimens: Pharmacokinetic data. In: Hardman JG, Gilman AG, Limbird LE, editors. Goodman & Gilman's The pharmacological basis of therapeutics. 9th ed, New York: McGraw-Hill; 1995. p. 1707–92.

11. Schentag JJ, Cerra FB, Calleri GM, Leising ME, French MA, Bernhard H. Age, disease, and cimetidine disposition in healthy subjects and chronically ill patients. Clin Pharmacol Ther 1981;29:737–43.

12. Grahnén A, von Bahr C, Lindström B, Rosén A. Bioavailability and pharmacokinetics of cimetidine. Eur J Clin Pharmacol 1979;16:335–40.

13. Physician's Desk Reference. 54th ed. Montvale, NJ: Medical Economics; 2000. p. 3043–6.

14. Reidenberg MM. Renal function and drug action. Philadelphia: WB Saunders; 1971.

15. Brenner BM. Nephron adaptation to renal injury or ablation. Am J Physiol 1985;249:F324–37.

16. Reidenberg MM, Camacho M, Kluger J, Drayer DE. Aging and renal clearance of procainamide and acetylprocainamide. Clin Pharmacol Ther 1980;28:732–5.

17. Maiza A, Waldek S, Ballardie FW, Daley-Yates PT. Estimation of renal tubular secretion in man, in health and disease, using endogenous N-1-methylnicotinamide. Nephron 1992;60:12–16.

18. Reidenberg MM. The biotransformation of drugs in renal failure. Am J Med 1977;62:482–5.

19. Reidenberg MM, Drayer DE. Alteration of drug-protein binding in renal disease. Clin Pharmacokinet 1984;9(suppl 1):18–26.

20. Odar-Cederlöf I, Borgå O. Kinetics of diphenylhydantoin in uremic patients: Consequences of decreased plasma protein binding. Eur J Clin Pharmacol 1974;7:31–7.

21. Sheiner LB, Rosenberg B, Marathe VV. Estimation of population characteristics of pharmacokinetic parameters from routine clinical data. J Pharmacokinet Biopharm 1977;5:445–79.

22. Aronson JK, Grahame-Smith DG. Altered distribution of digoxin in renal failure—A cause of digoxin toxicity? Br J Clin Pharmacol 1976;3:1045–51.

23. Craig RM, Murphy P, Gibson TP, Quintanilla A, Chao GC, Cochrane C, Patterson A, Atkinson AJ Jr. Kinetic analysis of D-xylose absorption in normal subjects and in patients with chronic renal failure. J Lab Clin Med 1983;101:496–506.

24. Huang CM, Atkinson AJ Jr, Levin M, Levin NW, Quintanilla A. Pharmacokinetics of furosemide in advanced renal failure. Clin Pharmacol Ther 1974;16:659–66.

25. Chau NP, Weiss YA, Safar ME, Lavene DE, Georges DR, Milliez P. Pindolol availability in hypertensive patients with normal and impaired renal function. Clin Pharmacol Ther 1977; 22: 505–10.

26. Bianchetti G, Graziani G, Brancaccio D, Morganti A, Leonetti G, Manfrin M, Sega R, Gomeni R, Ponticelli C, Morselli PL. Pharmacokinetics and effects of propranolol in terminal uraemic patients and in patients undergoing regular dialysis treatment. Clin Pharmacokinet 1976; 1: 373–84.

27. Atkinson AJ Jr, Ruo TI, Piergies AA, Breiter HC, Connely TJ, Sedek GS, Juan D, Hubler GL, Hsieh A-M. Pharmacokinetics of N-acetylprocainamide in patients profiled with a stable isotope method. Clin Pharmacol Ther 1989; 46: 182–9.

STUDY PROBLEM

The following pharmacokinetic data for *N*-acetylprocainamide (NAPA) were obtained in a Phase I study* in which procainamide and NAPA kinetics were compared in volunteers with normal renal function:

Elimination half-life: 6.2 hrs
Elimination clearance: 233 mL/min
% renal excretion: 85.5%

a. Use these results to predict the elimination half-life of NAPA in functionally anephric patients, assuming that nonrenal clearance is unchanged in these individuals.

b. Create a nomogram similar to that shown in Figure 5.2 to estimate the elimination clearance of NAPA that would be expected for a patient with a creatinine clearance of 50 mL/min. Assume that a creatinine clearance of 100 mL/min is the value for individuals with normal renal function.

c. If the usual starting dose of NAPA is 1 g every 8 hours in patients with normal renal function, what would be the equivalent dosing regimen for a patient with an estimated creatinine clearance of 50 mL/min if the dose is decreased but the 8-hour dosing interval is maintained?

d. If the usual starting dose of NAPA is 1 g every 8 hours in patients with normal renal function, what would be the equivalent dosing regimen for a patient with an estimated creatinine clearance of 50 mL/min if the 1-g dose is maintained but the dosing interval is increased?

* Dutcher JS, Strong JM, Lucas SV, Lee W-K, Atkinson AJ Jr. Procainamide and N-acetylprocainamide kinetics investigated simultaneously with stable isotope methodology. Clin Pharmacol Ther 1977; 22: 447–57.

6

Pharmacokinetics in Patients Requiring Renal Replacement Therapy

ARTHUR J. ATKINSON, JR. AND GREGORY M. SUSLA

Clinical Center, National Institutes of Health, Bethesda, Maryland

Although measurements of drug recovery in the urine enable reasonable characterization of the renal clearance of most drugs, analysis of drug elimination by the liver is hampered by the types of measurements that can be made in routine clinical studies. Hemodialysis and hemofiltration are considered at this point in the text because they provide an unparalleled opportunity to measure blood flow to the eliminating organ, drug concentrations in blood entering and leaving the eliminating organ, and recovery of eliminated drug in the dialysate or ultrafiltrate. The measurements that can be made in analyzing drug elimination by different routes are compared in Table 6.1.

Hemodialysis is an area of long-standing interest to pharmacologists. The pioneer American pharmacologist, John Jacob Abel, can be credited with designing the first artificial kidney (1). He conducted extensive studies in dogs to demonstrate the efficacy of hemodialysis in removing poisons and drugs. European scientists were the first to apply this technique to humans and Kolff sent a rotating-drum artificial kidney to the United States when World War II ended (2, 3). Repetitive use of hemodialysis for treating patients with chronic renal failure finally was made possible by the development of techniques for establishing long-lasting vascular access in the 1960s. By the late 1970s, continuous peritoneal dialysis had become a therapeutic alternative for these patients and offered the advantages of simpler, nonmachine-dependent home therapy and less hemodynamic stress (4). In 1977, continuous

arteriovenous hemofiltration (CAVH) was introduced as a method for removing fluid from diuretic-resistant patients, whose hemodynamic instability made them unable to tolerate conventional intermittent hemodialysis (5). Since then, this and related techniques have become the preferred treatment modality for critically ill patients with acute renal failure. Several variations of these techniques have been developed that use hemodialysis and/or hemofiltration to remove both solutes and fluid, and some of these are listed in Table 6.2 (6). All these methods can affect pharmacokinetics, but we will focus on conventional intermittent hemodialysis and selected aspects of continuous renal replacement therapy in this chapter.

KINETICS OF INTERMITTENT HEMODIALYSIS

Solute Transfer Across Dialyzing Membranes

In Abel's artificial kidney, blood flowed through a hollow cylinder of dialyzing membrane that was immersed in a bath of dialysis fluid. However, in modern hollow-fiber dialysis cartridges, there is a continuous countercurrent flow of dialysate along the outside of the dialyzing membrane that maximizes the concentration gradient between blood and dialysate. Mass transfer across the dialyzing membrane occurs by diffusion and ultrafiltration. The rate of transfer has

51

TABLE 6.1   Measurements Made in Assessing Drug Elimination by Different Routes

Measurements	Renal elimination	Hepatic elimination	Hemo-dialysis
Blood flow	$+^a$	$+^a$	+
Afferent blood concentration	+	+	+
Efferent blood concentration	0	0	+
Recovery of eliminated drug	+	0	+

^{a} Not actually measured in routine pharmacokinetic studies.

been analyzed with varying sophistication by a number of investigators (7). A simple approach is that taken by Eugene Renkin who neglected ultrafiltration and nonmembrane diffusive resistance and likened this transfer process to mass transfer across capillary walls (see Chapter 3) (8). Renkin expressed dialysis clearance (Cl_D) as:

$$Cl_D = Q(1 - e^{-P \cdot S/Q}) \qquad (6.1)$$

where Q is blood flow through the dialyzer and $P \cdot S$ is the permeability coefficient-surface area product of the dialyzing membrane, defined by Fick's First Law of Diffusion as:

$$P \cdot S = DA/\lambda$$

In this equation, A is the surface area, λ is the thickness of the dialyzing membrane, and D is the diffusivity of a given solute in the dialyzing membrane. Solute diffusivity is primarily determined by molecular weight. Nonspherical molecular shape may also affect the diffusivity of larger molecules.

Renkin used Equation 6.1 to estimate permeability coefficients for several solutes from flow and clearance measurements made on the Kolff-Brigham artificial

kidney (Figure 6.1). This theoretical analysis seems reasonably consistent with the experimental results. The broken line indicates that clearance can never exceed dialyzer blood flow, a result that is obvious from inspection of Equation 6.1 (i.e., $e^{-P \cdot S/Q}$ is never less than zero).

An analysis of relative dialysis clearance and dialyzer permeability coefficent-surface area products that was made for the closely related compounds procainamide (PA) and N-acetylprocainamide (NAPA) is summarized in Table 6.3. Dialyzer clearance measurements of PA (CL_{PA}) and NAPA (CL_{NAPA}) made by Gibson et al. (9) were used together with Equation 6.1 to calculate $P \cdot S$ values for PA $(P \cdot S_{PA})$ and NAPA $(P \cdot S_{NAPA})$. The ratio of these $P \cdot S$ values is also shown since this ratio indicates the relative diffusivity of PA and NAPA. The utility of Renkin's approach is confirmed by the fact that the mean $P \cdot S$ ratio of 1.28 ± 0.23 ($\pm$ SD) is in close agreement with the diffusion coefficient ratio of 1.23 that was obtained for PA and NAPA by the porous plate method of McBain and Liu (10).

Calculation of Dialysis Clearance

Currently, the efficiency of hemodialysis is expressed in terms of *dialysis clearance*. Dialysis clearance (Cl_D) is usually estimated from the Fick equation as follows:

$$Cl_D = Q\left[\frac{A - V}{A}\right] \qquad (6.2)$$

where A is the solute concentration entering (arterial) and V the solute concentration leaving (venous) the dialyzer. The terms in brackets collectively describe

TABLE 6.2   Summary of Selected Renal Replacement Therapies

Procedure	Abbreviation	Diffusion	Convection	Vascular access	Replacement fluid
Intermittent hemodialysis	HD	++++	+	Fistula or vein–vein	No
Intermittent high-flux dialysis	HFD	+++	++	Fistula or vein–vein	No
Continuous ambulatory peritoneal dialysis	CAPD	++++	+	None	No
Continuous arteriovenous hemofiltration	CAVH	0	++++	Artery–vein	Yes
Continuous venovenous hemofiltration	CVVH	0	++++	Vein–vein	Yes
Continuous arteriovenous hemodialysis	CAVHD	++++	+	Artery–vein	Yes
Continuous venovenous hemodialysis	CVVHD	++++	+	Vein–vein	Yes
Continuous arteriovenous hemodiafiltration	CAVHDF	+++	+++	Artery–vein	Yes
Continuous venovenous hemodiafiltration	CVVHDF	+++	+++	Vein–vein	Yes

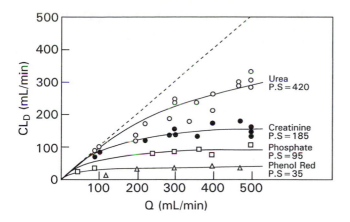

FIGURE 6.1 Plot of dialysis clearance (CL_D) vs. dialyzer blood flow (Q). The theoretical curves were fit to experimental data points to obtain estimates of the permeability coefficient-surface area product ($P \cdot S$) for each solute. Flow-limited clearance is indicated by the broken line. The data were generated with a Kolff-Brigham type hemodialysis apparatus. (Reproduced with permission from Renkin EM: Tr Am Soc Artific Organs 1956;2:102–5.)

what is termed the *extraction ratio* (E). As a general principle, clearance from an eliminating organ can be thought of as the product of organ blood flow and extraction ratio.

Single pass dialyzers are now standard for patient care and clearance calculations suffice for characterizing their performance. However, recirculating dialyzers were used in the early days of hemodialysis. Dialysis bath solute concentration (Bath) had to be

TABLE 6.3   Dialyzer Permeability Coefficient-Surface Area Products for PA and NAPA

Column	CL_{PA} (mL/min)	CL_{NAPA} (mL/min)	$P \cdot S_{PA}$ (mL/min)	$P \cdot S_{NAPA}$ (mL/min)	RATIO $P \cdot S_{PA}/P \cdot S_{NAPA}$
Dow 4	79.9	55.3	102.0	64.7	1.58
Dow 5	114.6	89.9	170.2	119.4	1.43
Gambro 17	50.8	33.3	58.6	36.4	1.61
Ultra-flow II	78.5	63.8	99.7	76.8	1.30
Ultra-flow 145	63.4	50.4	76.3	58.1	1.31
Vivacell	37.1	27.8	41.0	29.9	1.37
Ex 23	50.4	50.4	58.1	58.1	1.00
Ex 25	71.6	62.6	88.6	75.1	1.18
Ex 29	81.4	78.0	104.5	98.9	1.06
Ex 55	51.8	53.9	60.0	62.8	0.93
				Mean ± SD	1.28 ± 0.23

[a] Clearance data obtained by Gibson TP, et al. (9) with dialyzer blood flow set at 200 mL/min and single pass dialysate flow at 400 mL/min.

considered in describing the performance of recirculating dialyzers and was included in the equation for calculating *dialysance* (D), as shown in the following equation (7):

$$D = Q \left[\frac{A - V}{A - \text{Bath}} \right]$$

Considerable confusion surrounds the proper use of Equation 6.2 to calculate dialysis clearance. There is general agreement that *blood clearance* is calculated when Q is set equal to blood flow and A and V are expressed as blood concentrations. In conventional practice, *plasma clearance* is obtained by setting Q equal to plasma flow and expressing A and V as plasma concentrations. In fact, this estimate of plasma clearance is only the same as plasma clearance calculated by standard pharmacokinetic techniques when the solute is totally excluded from red blood cells.

This dilemma is best avoided by calculating dialysis clearance from the same equation that is used to determine renal clearance: $CL = UV/P$. If the product UV equals the amount of solute recovered in the dialysis bath per unit time and if P is the concentration of drug in plasma delivered to the dialyzer, an estimate of plasma clearance (CL_P) is obtained that is *pharmacokinetically consistent* with other plasma clearance estimates. If the blood concentration (B) is substituted for P, a valid estimate of blood clearance (CL_B) is obtained. The term *recovery clearance* has been coined for these clearance estimates, and they are regarded as the "gold standard" of dialysis clearance estimates (11). We can use these recovery clearances to examine the *effective* flow of plasma (Q_{EFF}) that is needed if Equation 6.2 is to yield an estimate of dialysis clearance that is consistent with the corresponding recovery clearance value.

Since $CL_B = Q_B E$ and $CL_B = UV/B$, it follows that:

$$UV/E = Q_B \cdot B$$

But $CL_P = UV/P$. Therefore,

$$CL_P/E = Q_B \cdot B/P$$

However, $CL_P = Q_{EFF} \cdot E$. Therefore,

$$Q_{EFF} = Q_B \cdot B/P$$

For drugs like NAPA that partition preferentially into red blood cells and are fully accessible to the dialyzer from both plasma and erythrocytes, the effective plasma flow will not be less than but will *exceed* measured blood flow (12).

Some authorities argue that it is improper to combine organ *blood* flow and *plasma* concentrations in

Equation 6.2 (7, 11). However, in many cases the ratio of red cell/plasma drug concentrations remains constant over a wide concentration range so the same estimate of extraction ratio is obtained regardless of whether plasma concentrations or blood concentrations are measured.

As shown in Figure 6.2, pharmacokinetic models can be constructed that incorporate all the measurements made during hemodialysis (12). For this purpose it is convenient to rearrange Equation 6.2 to the form:

$$V = [(Q_{PK} - CL_D)/Q_{PK}] \cdot A \qquad (6.3)$$

where Q_{PK} is the pharmacokinetically calculated flow of blood or plasma through the dialysis machine. Since CL_D is calculated from the recovery of drug in dialysis bath fluid, an estimate of Q_{PK} can be obtained from the observed ratio of V/A (Equation 6.3 and Figure 6.2).

In a study of NAPA hemodialysis kinetics, blood flow measured through the dialyzer averaged 195 mL/min (12). When evaluated by paired t test this was significantly less than Q_{PK}, which averaged 223 mL/min. However, Q_{PK} was similar to estimates of Q_{EFF} that averaged 217 mL/min. In this case, NAPA concentrations in erythrocytes were 1.5 times as high as in plasma, and this preferential distribution of drug into red blood cells enhanced drug removal by hemodialysis. Unfortunately, most studies of pharmacokinetics during hemodialysis have not incorporated the full range of readily available measurements.

Hemodynamic Changes During Dialysis

Few studies of pharmacokinetics during hemodialysis have considered the impact of hemodynamic changes that may affect the efficiency of this procedure. The fall in both A and V drug concentrations that occurs during hemodialysis is generally followed by a post-dialysis rebound, as shown for NAPA in Figure 6.3. However, if no change in drug distribution is assumed, two discrepancies are likely to be found when hemodialysis kinetics are modeled rigorously:

1. The total amount of drug recovered from the dialysis fluid is less than would be expected from the drop in plasma concentrations during hemodialysis.
2. The extent of the rebound in plasma levels is less than would be anticipated.

The only single parameter change that can resolve these discrepancies is a reduction in the intercompartmental clearance for the slowly equilibrating compartment (CL_S). This is illustrated in the bottom panel of Figure 6.3, and in this study the extent of reduction in CL_S was found to average 77% during hemodialysis (12). This figure also shows that a reduction in CL_S persisted for some time after hemodialysis was completed

The hemodynamic basis for these changes in CL_S was investigated subsequently in a dog model (13). Urea and inulin were used as probes and were injected simultaneously two hours before dialysis. The pharmacokinetic model shown in Figure 6.2 was used for data analysis and representative results are shown in Figure 6.4. During hemodialysis, CL_S for urea and inulin fell on average to 19% and 63% of their respective pre-dialysis values and it was estimated that the efficiency of urea removal was reduced by 10%. In the 2 hours after dialysis, urea CL_S averaged only 37% of pre-dialysis values but returned to its pre-dialysis level for inulin. Compartmental blood flow and permeability coefficient-surface area products of the calculated intercompartmental clearances were calculated as described in Chapter 3 from the permeability-flow equation derived by Renkin (14). During and after dialysis, blood flow to the slow equilibrating compartment (Q_S) on average was reduced to 10% and 20%, respectively, of pre-dialysis values. The permeability coefficient-surface area product did not change significantly. There were no changes in either fast compartment blood flow or permeability coefficient-surface area product. Measurements of plasma renin activity in these dogs with intact kidneys (lower panel of Figure 6.4) suggest that these hemodynamic changes, both during and after

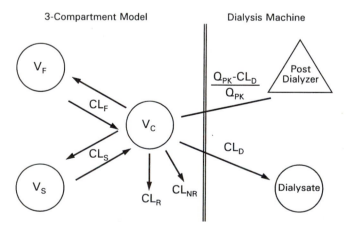

FIGURE 6.2 Multicompartmental system for modeling pharmacokinetics during hemodialysis. Drug is delivered to the dialysis machine from the central compartment (V_C) and represents A in the Fick equation. The dialysis machine is modeled by a compartment representing drug recovery in dialysis bath fluid and a proportionality *(triangle)* representing the drug concentration in blood returning to the patient.

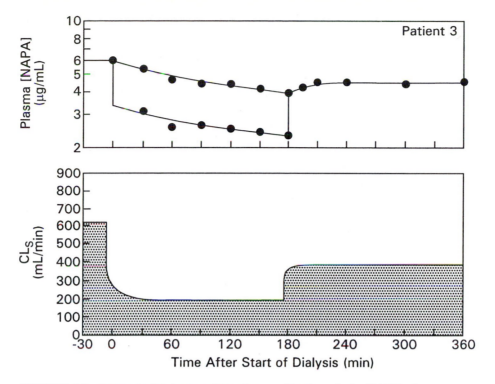

FIGURE 6.3 Computer-fitted curves from pharmacokinetic analysis of NAPA plasma concentrations (•) measured before, during and after hemodialysis. NAPA plasma concentrations entering *(A)* and leaving *(V)* the artificial kidney are shown during dialysis. The bottom panel shows changes occurring in slow compartment intercompartmental clearance *(CL$_S$)* during and after dialysis. (Reproduced with permission from Stec GP, Atkinson AJ Jr, Nevin MJ, Thenot J-P, Gibson TP, Ivanovich P, del Greco F. Clin Pharmacol Ther 1979;26:618–28.)

hemodialysis, were mediated at least in part by the renin–angiotensin system.

Since the slow equilibrating compartment is largely composed of skeletal muscle, it is not surprising that the hemodynamic changes associated with hemodialysis result in the skeletal muscle cramps that have been estimated to complicate more than 20% of hemodialysis sessions. Plasma volume contraction appears to be the initiating event that triggers blood pressure homeostatic responses. Those patients who are particularly prone to cramps appear to have a sympathetic nervous system response to this volume stress that is not modulated by activation of a normal renin angiotensin system (15).

KINETICS OF CONTINUOUS RENAL REPLACEMENT THERAPY

Hemofiltration is a prominent feature of many continuous renal replacement therapies (Table 6.2). However, continuous hemodialysis can also be employed to accelerate solute removal (16). The contribution of both processes to extracorporeal drug clearance will be considered separately in the context of continuous renal replacement therapy.

Clearance by Continuous Hemofiltration

Hemofiltration removes solutes by convective mass transfer down a hydrostatic pressure gradient (17, 18). As plasma water passes through the hemofilter membrane, solute is carried along by solvent drag. Convective mass transfer thus mimics the process of glomerular filtration. The pores of hemofilter membranes are larger than those of dialysis membranes and permit passage of solutes having a molecular weight of up to 50 kDa. Accordingly, a wider range of compounds will be removed by hemofiltration than by hemodialysis. Since large volumes of fluid are removed, fluid replacement solutions need to be administered at rates exceeding 10 L/day (19). This fluid can be administered either before (predilution mode) or after (postdilution mode) the hemofilter. In contemporary practice, roller pumps are used to generate the hydrostatic driving force for ultrafiltration, and the need for arterial catheterization has been obvi-

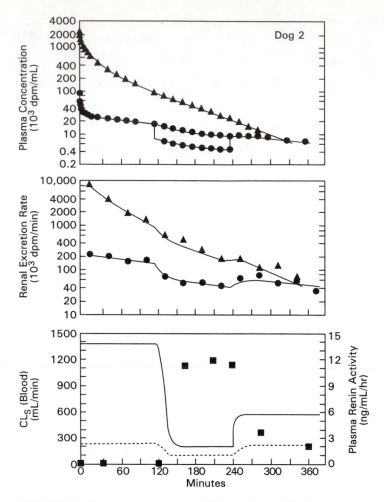

FIGURE 6.4   Kinetic analysis of urea ^{14}C (●) and inulin ^{3}H (▲) plasma concentrations *(upper panel)* and renal excretion rates *(middle panel)* before, during, and after dialysis of a dog with intact kidneys. Inulin was not dialyzable but urea concentrations entering and leaving the dialyzer are both shown. The lower panel shows CL_S estimates for urea (—) and inulin (---), and measured plasma renin activity (■). (Reproduced with permission from Bowsher DJ, Krejcie TC, Avram MJ, Chow MJ del Greco F, Atkinson AJ Jr. J Lab Clin Med 1985;105:489–97.)

ated by the placement of double-lumen catheters into a large vein (18).

Albumin and other drug-binding proteins do not pass through the filtration membrane, so only unbound drug in plasma water is removed by ultra-filtration. In addition, albumin and other negatively charged plasma proteins exert a Gibbs-Donnan effect that retards the transmembrane convection of some polycationic drugs such as gentamicin (20, 21). The situation with regard to erythrocyte drug binding is less clear. However, urea removal is enhanced when replacement fluid is administered in the predilution mode because it can diffuse down its concentration gradient from red blood cells into the diluted plasma water before reaching the hemofilter (19). The extent

to which a solute is carried in the ultrafiltrate across a membrane is characterized by its *sieving coefficient*. An approximate equation for calculating sieving coefficients *(SC)* is:

$$SC = \frac{UF}{A} \qquad (6.4)$$

where *UF* is the solute concentration in the ultrafiltrate and *A* is the solute concentration in plasma water entering the hemofilter (22).

The convective clearance of solute across an ultrafilter *(CL$_{UF}$)* is given by the product of *SC* and the rate at which fluid crosses the ultrafilter *(UFR)*:

$$CL_{UF} = SC \cdot UFR \qquad (6.5)$$

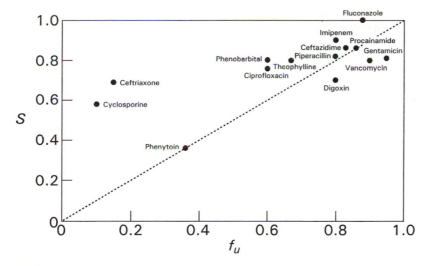

FIGURE 6.5 Relationship between free fraction (f_u) and hemofiltration sieving coefficient *(SC)* for selected drugs. The line of identity *(broken line)* indicates what would be expected if *SC* were equal to f_u. (See text for further details.)

Since *UFR* can not exceed blood flow through the hemofilter, that establishes the theoretical upper limit for CL_{UF}. The major determinants of *SC* are molecular size and the unbound fraction of a compound in plasma water. Values of *SC* may range from 0 for macromolecules that do not pass through the pores of the hemofilter membrane to 1 for small molecule drugs that are not protein bound. Although less information has been accumulated about the ultrafiltration clearance of drugs than about their dialysis clearance, in many cases the unbound fraction of drug in plasma water can be used to approximate *SC*.

Measured values of *SC* and fraction of unbound drug in plasma (f_u) are compared for several drugs in Figure 6.5. Values of f_u and *SC* were taken from data published by Golper and Marx (21) with the following exceptions. For both theophylline (23) and phenytoin (24), measurements of f_u are much higher in serum from uremic patients than in serum from normal subjects and agree more closely with experimental values of *SC*. Accordingly, uremic patient f_u values for theophylline (23) and phenytoin (24) were chosen for the figure, as well as values of *SC* that were obtained in clinical studies of ceftazidime (25), ceftriaxone (26), ciprofloxacin (27), cyclosporine (28) and phenytoin (24). The fact that *SC* values for gentamicin and vancomycin are less than expected on the basis of their protein binding reflects the retarding Gibbs–Donnan effect referred to previously (20, 21). On the other hand, *SC* values for cyclosporine and ceftazidime are considerably greater than expected from f_u measurements. Hence, factors other than plasma protein binding may affect the sieving of some drugs during hemofiltration (29).

Clearance by Continuous Hemodialysis

Some of the renal replacement therapies listed in Table 6.2 incorporate continuous hemodialysis, or a combination of continuous hemofiltration and hemodialysis. Continuous hemodialysis differs importantly from conventional intermittent hemodialysis in that the flow rate of dialysate is much lower than countercurrent blood flow through the dialyzer. As a result, concentrations of many solutes in dialysate leaving the dialyzer (C_d) will have nearly equilibrated with their plasma concentrations in blood entering the dialyzer (C_p) (16, 30). The extent to which this equilibration is complete is referred to as the dialysate saturation (S_d) and is calculated as the following ratio:

$$S_d = \frac{C_d}{C_p}$$

In contrast with intermittent hemodialysis in which dialyzer blood flow is rate limiting, diffusive drug clearance during continuous renal replacement therapy is limited by dialysate flow (Q_d), which typically is only 25 mL/min. Accordingly, diffusive drug clearance (CL_D) is calculated from the equation:

$$CL_D = Q_d \cdot S_d \qquad (6.6)$$

Equation 6.6 is a nonmechanistic description of clearance that does not incorporate the factors of molecular size or protein binding that account for incomplete equilibration of plasma and dialysate solute concentrations. Dialysate saturation also becomes progressively less complete as dialysate flow approaches blood flow (16).

Extracorporeal Clearance During Continuous Renal Replacement Therapy

Extracorporeal clearance during continuous renal replacement therapy (CL_{EC}) can be regarded as the sum of convective and hemodialytic clearance (16, 30):

$$CL_{EC} = SC \cdot UFR + Q_d \cdot S_d \qquad (6.7)$$

Unfortunately, ultrafiltration rate (UFR) tends to decrease with time, falling rather rapidly during the first 6 hours of therapy and reaching about half of its original value in approximately 20 hours (16). Conversely, drug adsorption to the dialyzer membrane may decrease during therapy, resulting in an increase in the sieving coefficient (SC) (31). For these reasons, estimates of extracorporeal drug clearance during continuous renal replacement therapy are most reliable when made from measurements of drug recovery in dialysate, as discussed for conventional hemodialysis. Where the total volume of dialysate recovered during treatment time t_d is V_{UF}, extracorporeal clearance of drug from plasma can be calculated as follows:

$$CL_{EC} = (C_d \cdot V_{UF})/(C_p \cdot t_d) \qquad (6.8)$$

CLINICAL CONSIDERATIONS

From the clinical standpoint, the two main pharmacokinetic considerations regarding renal replacement therapy deal with the use of these therapeutic modalities to treat drug toxicity and, more frequently, the need to administer supplemental drug doses to patients whose impaired renal function necessitates intervention. Because elimination clearances are additive, total solute clearance during renal replacement therapy (CL_T), can be expressed as the sum of extracorporeal clearance (CL_{EC}), and the patient's renal clearance (CL_R) and nonrenal clearance (CL_{NR}):

$$CL_T = CL_{EC} + CL_R + CL_{NR} \qquad (6.9)$$

Other factors besides extracorporeal clearance determine the extent of drug removal by renal replacement therapy. These are summarized in Table 6.4. As yet, there has been no attempt to analyze the interaction of all these factors with sufficient rigor to provide precise guidelines for clinical practice. However, extensive protein binding and large distribution volume are the most important factors limiting the extent to which most drugs are removed by hemodialysis or hemofiltration. The interaction between distribution volume and total clearance will impact elimination half-life as follows:

TABLE 6.4   Factors Affecting the Extent of Drug Removal by Renal Replacement Therapy

Characteristics of hemodialysis or hemofiltration

Extracorporeal clearance ($CL_{EC} = CL_D + CL_{UF}$)

Duration of hemodialysis or hemofiltration

Patient characteristics

Distribution volume of drug

Drug binding to plasma proteins

Drug partitioning into erythrocytes

Reduction in intercompartmental clearance

$$t_{1/2} = \frac{0.693 V_d}{CL_T}$$

For this reason, neither conventional intermittent hemodialysis nor continuous renal replacement therapy will significantly enhance the removal of drugs such as digoxin that have large distribution volumes.

Reduction in intercompartmental clearance during hemodialysis may result in a greater than expected fall in drug concentrations in plasma and rapidly equilibrating tissues, since hemodynamic changes during hemodialysis may effectively sequester a substantial amount of drug in skeletal muscle. This tourniquet-like effect, and its persistence in the postdialysis period, may be useful in treating patients with central nervous system or cardiovascular toxic reactions to drugs (32). Although intercompartmental clearance has not been studied during continuous renal replacement therapy, these modalities produce less hemodynamic instability and would be expected to provoke a smaller cardiovascular homeostatic response.

Drug Dosing Guidelines for Patients Requiring Renal Replacement Therapy

Drug doses need to be increased or supplemented for patients requiring renal replacement therapy only if CL_{EC} is substantial when compared to $CL_R + CL_{NR}$ (Equation 6.9). Levy (33) has proposed that supplementation is needed only when CL_{EC} is greater than 30% of $CL_R + CL_{NR}$. Several approaches will be considered that can be used to make appropriate drug dose adjustments for patients requiring renal replacement therapy.

Perhaps the simplest approach is to guide dosage using standard reference tables, such as those published by Aronoff and colleagues (34). These tables are based on published literature and suggest drug dose reductions for patients with various levels of renal impairment, as well as for patients requiring conventional hemodialysis, chronic ambulatory peritoneal dialysis, and continuous renal replacement therapy. Although less data is available for patients treated with continuous renal replacement therapy than with conventional intermittent hemodialysis, *UFR* generally ranges from 10 to 16 mL/min during hemofiltration without extracorporeal blood pumping, and from 20 to 30 mL/min when blood pumps are used (21). Accordingly, for many drugs, the dose recommendation for patients treated with continuous renal replacement therapy is considered simply to be that which is appropriate for patients with a glomerular filtration rate of 10 to 50 mL/min.

A second approach is to calculate supplemental doses to replace drug lost during hemodialysis or continuous renal replacement therapy by directly measuring drug loss by extracorporeal removal or by estimating this loss from drug levels measured in plasma (21, 22). In the latter case, the supplemental dose (D_{sup}) can be estimated from a plasma level measured at the conclusion of dialysis or at a convenient interval during continuous renal replacement therapy ($C_{measured}$):

$$D_{sup} = (C_{target} - C_{measured})\, V_d$$

When used in the setting of conventional hemodialysis, this method is likely to overestimate the supplemental dose that is needed because the hemodynamic changes that occur during hemodialysis persist for some time after hemodialysis (12). On the other hand, it is relatively easy to make repeated plasma level measurements of some drugs, and to use these to

refine supplemental dose estimates (21). Theoretically, the most reliable estimate of extracorporeal drug loss is based on actual measurement of the drug that is removed in dialysate. Unfortunately, it is often inconvenient to measure large volumes of dialysate, and many routine drug assay laboratories are not prepared to assay drug concentrations in this fluid.

A third approach is to use the principles previously discussed to calculate a maintenance dose multiplication factor (*MDMF*) that can be used to augment the dose that would be appropriate in the absence of renal replacement therapy (31). For continuous renal replacement therapy, *MDMF* is given simply by the following ratio of clearances:

$$MDMF = \frac{CL_{EC} + CL_R + CL_{NR}}{CL_R + CL_{NR}} \qquad (6.10)$$

The relative time on (t_{ON}) and off (t_{OFF}) extracorporeal therapy during a dosing interval also must be taken into account for conventional hemodialysis and other intermittent interventions. In this situation:

$$MDMF = \frac{(CL_{EC} + CL_R + CL_{NR})t_{ON}}{(CL_R + CL_{NR})(t_{ON} + t_{OFF})}$$
$$+ \frac{(CL_R + CL_{NR})t_{OFF}}{(CL_R + CL_{NR})(t_{ON} + t_{OFF})}$$

$$MDMF = \left(\frac{CL_{EC}}{CL_R + CL_{NR}}\right)\left(\frac{t_{ON}}{t_{ON} + t_{OFF}}\right) + 1 \qquad (6.11)$$

Estimates of *MDMF* for several drugs are listed in Table 6.5. With the exception of vancomycin, baseline

TABLE 6.5   Estimated Drug Dosing Requirements for Patients Needing Renal Replacement Therapy

Drug	$CL_{(aneph.)}$ (mL/min)	Intermittent hemodialysis				Continuous renal replacement therapy							
		Mode	CL_D (mL/min)	*MDMF*	Ref.	MODE	SC	UFR (mL/min)	CL_{UF} (mL/min)	CL_{HD} (mL/min)	CL_{EC} (mL/min)	*MDMF*	Ref.
Ceftazidime	11.2	HD	43.6	1.6	36	CAVHD	0.86	7.5	6.5	6.6	13.1	2.2	25
Ceftriazone	7.0	HD	11.8	1.0	37	CVVH	0.69	24.1	16.6		16.6	3.4	26
Ciprofloxacin	188[a]	HD	40.0	1.0	38	CAVHD/ CVVHD	0.76	7.2	4.8	7.3	12.1	2.4	27
Cyclosporine	463	HD	0.31	1.0	39	CAVH	0.58	4.4	2.6		2.6	1.0	28
Gentamicin	15.3	HFD	116	2.0	40	CAVHD				5.2	1.3	45
Phenytoin	83[b]	HD	12.0	1.0	41	CAVH	0.36	2.8	1.0		1.0	1.0	24
Theophylline	57.4	HD	77.9	1.1	42	CAVHD			23.3		23.3	1.4	44
Vancomycin	6	HFD	106	3.9	43	CVVH	0.89	26.2	23.3		23.3	4.9	46

[a] Calculated from CL/F with F assumed to be 60% as in normals.

[b] Elimination of this drug follows Michaelis–Menten kinetics. Apparent clearance will be lower when plasma levels are higher than those obtained in this study.

drug clearance values for functionally anephric patients (CL_{aneph}) are taken from either the intermittent hemodialysis or the continuous renal replacement references that are cited. In the first two weeks after the onset of acute renal failure, vancomycin CL_{aneph} falls from approximately 40 mL/min to the value of 6.0 mL/min that is found in patients with chronic renal failure (35). This latter value is included in Table 6.5. The abbreviations used for treatment modality are defined in Table 6.2. In the studies of intermittent hemodialysis, CL_{EC} was calculated by the recovery method except for the studies of ceftazidime (36), ceftriaxone (37), and ciprofloxacin (38) in which this clearance was estimated from the reduction in elimination half-life during dialysis. Equation 6.11 was used to estimate $MDMF$ for a dialysis time of 4 hours during a single 24-hour period. In the studies of continuous renal replacement therapy, CL_{EC} was calculated from drug recovery in ultrafiltrate/dialysate in all but the case report of theophylline removal by CAVHD (44). In this study, CL_{EC} was estimated from the change in theophylline clearance before and during extracorporeal therapy. Dialysate flow also was not specified in this report. However, the CL_{EC} values for ceftazidime (25), ciprofloxacin (27), and gentamicin (45) all were obtained with a dialysate flow rate of 1 L/hr. Estimates of $MDMF$ were made from Equation 6.10.

It is apparent from Table 6.5 that drug dose adjustments generally are required more frequently for patients receiving continuous renal replacement therapy than for those requiring intermittent hemodialysis. In addition, it is evident that drug dosing need not be altered with any modality for phenytoin, cyclosporine, and other drugs that are extensively bound to plasma proteins. As in treating other patients with impaired renal function, maintenance drug doses for patients receiving renal replacement therapy can be adjusted by increasing the dosing interval as well as by reducing the drug dose. An estimate of the increased dosing interval (τ') can be made by dividing the usual maintenance dosing interval (τ) by $MDMF$ (31). Finally, it should be noted that plasma level measurements of gentamicin, theophylline, and vancomycin are routinely available and can be used to provide a more accurate assessment of dosing requirements when these drugs are used to treat patients requiring renal replacement therapy.

Extracorporeal Therapy of Patients with Drug Toxicity

Intensive supportive therapy is all that is required for the majority of patients suffering from dose-related drug toxicity, and drug removal by extracorporeal methods generally is indicated only for those patients whose condition deteriorates despite institu-

tion of these more conservative measures (47). However, a decision to intervene with extracorporeal therapy may be prompted by other clinical and pharmacologic considerations that are listed in Table 6.6. For example, most intoxications with phenobarbital can be managed by a combination of supportive care and minimization of renal tubular reabsorption of this drug by forced diuresis and urine alkalinization. However, extracorporeal therapy is indicated if the serum phenobarbital level exceeds 100 µg/mL (47). A number of low molecular weight alcohols are converted to toxic metabolites. For example, methanol is converted to formate, which causes metabolic acidosis and retinal injury (48). Clinical evidence of this toxicity is delayed for 12 to 18 hours. During this time conversion of methanol to formate can be inhibited by administering ethyl alcohol. However, hemodialysis effectively removes both methanol and formate and is indicated when plasma or serum methanol levels exceed 50 mg/dL (47). Since clinical risk is more specifically related to the presence of serum formate levels in excess of 20 mg/dL, these may provide an even better indicator of the need to institute hemodialysis (49).

Although hemodialysis is effective in removing phenobarbital, methanol, and other low molecular weight compounds that have a relatively small distribution volume and are not extensively protein bound, the technique of hemoperfusion has greater efficiency in treating patients with a wide range of intoxications (47, 48). Hemoperfusion entails passage of blood in an extracorporeal circuit through a sorbent column of activated charcoal or resin. Because hemoperfusion relies on the physical process of adsorption and the blood comes in direct contact with sorbent particles, it is not limited in its efficiency by protein binding and compounds with molecular weights as high as 40 kDa can be adsorbed. Several

TABLE 6.6 Considerations for Extracorporeal Treatment of Drug Intoxications

General clinical considerations

Clinical deterioration despite intensive supportive therapy

Severe intoxication indicated by depression of midbrain function or measured plasma or serum level

Condition complicated by pneumonia, sepsis, or other coexisting illness

Pharmacologic considerations

Extracorporeal intervention can increase drug elimination significantly

Drug clearance is slow due to pharmacologic properties of intoxicant or patient's impaired renal or hepatic function

Intoxicant has a toxic metabolite or has toxic effects that are delayed

TABLE 6.7 Comparison of Hemodialysis and Hemoperfusion Efficiency[a]

Intoxicant	Hemo-dialysis	Charcoal hemoper-fusion	Resin hemoper-fusion
Acetaminophen	++[b]	++	+++
Acetylsalicylic Acid	++	++	
Amobarbital	++	++	+++
Phenobarbital	++	++	+++
Theophylline	++	+++	+++
Tricyclic Antidepressants	++	++	+++

[a] Calculated for blood flow of 200 mL/min (based on data from Winchester JF (48)).

[b] ++ = extraction ratio 0.2 – 0.5, +++ = extraction ratio > 0.5.

common intoxicants are listed in Table 6.7 along with the relative efficiency with which they can be removed by hemodialysis and hemoperfusion. Additional practical considerations are that only hemodialysis may be available in certain clinical settings and that hemodialysis also provides an opportunity to correct acidosis and electrolyte imbalances that may occur in conjunction with some intoxications.

Complications of hemoperfusion include platelet and leukocyte depletion, hypocalcemia, and a mild reduction in body temperature (48). In many cases, these complications are outweighed by the fact that intoxicants are removed more rapidly by hemoperfusion than by hemodialysis. However, an additional consideration is that hemoperfusion clearance tends to decline during therapy as column efficiency declines, presumably reflecting saturation of adsorbent sites (50). In addition, intercompartmental clearance from skeletal muscle and other slowly equilibrating tissues can limit the extent of drug removal by hemoperfusion and result in a rebound of blood levels and possible toxicity at the conclusion of this procedure (51). In some instances, alternative therapies have been developed that are even more efficient than hemoperfusion. For example, digoxin-specific antibody fragments (Fab) now are available for treating severe intoxication with either digoxin or digitoxin (52). In most patients, initial improvement is observed within 1 hour of Fab administration and toxicity is resolved completely within 4 hours.

References

1. Abel JJ, Rowntree LG, Turner BB. On the removal of diffusible substances from the circulating blood of living animals by dialysis. J Pharmacol Exp Ther 1914;5:275–317.
2. Kolff WJ. First clinical experience with the artificial kidney. Ann Intern Med 1965;62:608–19.
3. Uribarri J. Past, present and future of end-stage renal disease therapy in the United States. Mt Sinai J Med 1999;66:14–9.
4. Baillie GR, Eisele G. Continuous ambulatory peritoneal dialysis: A review of its mechanics, advantages, complications, and areas of controversy. Ann Pharmacother 1992;26:1409–20.
5. Kramer P, Wigger W, Rieger J, Matthaei D, Scheler F. Arteriovenous haemofiltration: A new and simple method for the treatment of overhydrated patients resistant to diuretics. Klin Wochenschr 1977;55:1121–2.
6. Ronco C, Bellomo R. Continuous renal replacement therapies: The need for a standard nomenclature. Contrib Nephrol 1995;116:28–33.
7. Henderson LW. Hemodialysis: Rationale and physical principles. In: Brenner BM, Rector FC Jr, editors. The kidney. Philadelphia: WB Saunders; 1976. p. 1643–71.
8. Renkin EM. The relation between dialysance, membrane area, permeability and blood flow in the artificial kidney. Tr Am Soc Artific Organs 1956;2:102–5.
9. Gibson TP, Matusik E, Nelson LD, Briggs WA. Artificial kidneys and clearance calculations. Clin Pharmacol Ther 1976;20:720–6.
10. McBain JW, Liu TH. Diffusion of electrolytes, non-electrolytes and colloidal electrolytes. J Am Chem Soc 1931;53:59–74.
11. Gibson TP. Problems in designing hemodialysis drug studies. Pharmacotherapy 1985;5:23–9.
12. Stec GP, Atkinson AJ Jr, Nevin MJ, Thenot J-P, Ruo TI, Gibson TP, Ivanovich P, del Greco F. N-Acetylprocainamide pharmacokinetics in functionally anephric patients before and after perturbation by hemodialysis. Clin Pharmacol Ther 1979;26:618–28.
13. Browsher DJ, Krejcie TC, Avram MJ, Chow MJ, del Greco F, Atkinson AJ Jr. Reduction in slow intercompartmental clearance of urea during dialysis. J Lab Clin Med 1985;105:489–97.
14. Renkin EM. Effects of blood flow on diffusion kinetics in isolated perfused hindlegs of cats: A double circulation hypothesis. Am J Physiol 1953;183:125–36.
15. Sidhom OA, Odeh YK, Krumlovsky FA, Budris WA, Wang Z, Pospisil PA, Atkinson AJ Jr. Low dose prazosin in patients with muscle cramps during hemodialysis. Clin Pharmacol Ther 1994;56:445–51.
16. Sigler MH, Teehan BP. Solute transport in continuous hemodialysis: A new treatment for acute renal failure. Kidney Int 1987;32:562–71.
17. Bressolle F, Kinowski J-M, de la Coussaye JE, Wynn N, Eledjam J-J, Galtier M. Clinical pharmacokinetics during continuous haemofiltration. Clin Pharmacokinet 1994;26:457–71.
18. Meyer MM. Renal replacement therapies Critical Care Clin 2000;16:29–58.
19. Golper TA. Continuous arteriovenous hemofiltration in acute renal failure. Am J Kidney Dis 1985;6:373–86.
20. Golper TA, Saad A-M A. Gentamicin and phenytoin in vitro sieving characteristics through polysulfone hemofilters: Effect of flow rate, drug concentration and solvent systems. Kidney Int 1986;30:937–43.
21. Golper TA, Marx MA. Drug dosing adjustments during continuous renal replacement therapies. Kidney Int 1998;53(suppl 66):165–8.
22. Golper TA, Wedel SK, Kaplan AA, Saad A-M, Donta ST, Paganini EP. Drug removal during continuous arteriovenous hemofiltration: theory and clinical observations. Intern J Artif Organs 1985;8:307–12.
23. Vanholder R, Van Landschoot N, De Smet R, Schoots A, Ringoir S. Drug protein binding in chronic renal failure: Evaluation of nine drugs. Kidney Int 1988;33:996–1004.
24. Lau AH, Kronfol NO. Effect of continuous hemofiltration on phenytoin elimination. Ther Drug Monitor 1994;16:53–7.

25. Davies SP, Lacey LF, Kox WJ, Brown EA. Pharmacokinetics of cefuroxime and ceftazidime in patients with acute renal failure treated by continuous arteriovenous haemodialysis. Nephrol Dial Transplant 1991;6:971–6.

26. Kroh UF, Lennartz H, Edwards DJ, Stoeckel K. Pharmacokinetics of ceftriaxone in patients undergoing continuous venovenous hemofiltration. J Clin Pharmacol 1996;36:1114–9.

27. Davies SP, Azadian BS, Kox WJ, Brown EA. Pharmacokinetics of ciprofloxacin and vancomycin in patients with acute renal failure treated by continuous haemodialysis. Nephrol Dial Transplant 1992;7:848–54.

28. Cleary JD, Davis G, Raju S. Cyclosporine pharmacokinetics in a lung transplant patient undergoing hemofiltration. Transplantation 1989;48:710–12.

29. Lau AH, Pyle K, Kronfol NO, Libertin CR. Removal of cephalosporins by continuous arteriovenous ultrafiltration (CAVU) and hemofiltration (CAVH). Int J Artif Organs 1989;12:379–83.

30. Schetz M, Ferdinande P, Van den Berghe G, Verwaest C, Lauwers P. Pharmacokinetics of continuous renal replacement therapy. Intensive Care Med 1995;21:612–20.

31. Reetze-Bonorden P, Böhler J, Keller E. Drug dosage in patients during continuous renal replacement therapy: Pharmacokinetic and therapeutic considerations. Clin Pharmacokinet 1993;24:362–79.

32. Atkinson AJ Jr, Krumlovsky FA, Huang CM, del Greco F. Hemodialysis for severe procainamide toxicity. Clinical and pharmacokinetic observations. Clin Pharmacol Ther 1976;20:585–92.

33. Levy G. Pharmacokinetics in renal disease. Am J Med 1977;62:461–5.

34. Aronoff GR, Berns JS, Brier ME, Golper TA, Morrison G, Singer I, Swan SK, Bennett WM. Drug prescribing in renal failure: Dosing guidelines for adults. 4th ed. Philadelphia: American College of Physicians;1999.

35. Macias WL, Mueller BA, Scarim KS. Vancomycin pharmacokinetics in acute renal failure: Preservation of nonrenal clearance. Clin Pharmacol Ther 1991;50:688–94.

36. Ohkawa M, Nakashima T, Shoda R, Ikeda A, Orito M, Sawaki M, Sugata T, Shimamura M, Hirano S, Okumura K. Pharmacokinetics of ceftazidime in patients with renal insufficiency and in those undergoing hemodialysis. Chemotherapy 1985;31:410–16.

37. Ti T-Y, Fortin L, Kreeft JH, East DS, Ogilvie RI, Somerville PJ. Kinetic disposition of intravenous ceftriaxone in normal subjects and patients with renal failure on hemodialysis or peritoneal dialysis. Antimicrob Agents Chemother 1984;25:83–7.

38. Singlas E, Taburet AM, Landru I, Albin H, Ryckelinck JP. Pharmacokinetics of ciprofloxacin tablets in renal failure; influence of haemodialysis. Eur J Clin Pharmacol 1987;31:589–93.

39. Venkataramanan R, Ptachcinski RJ, Burckart GJ, Yang SL, Starzl TE, van Theil DH. The clearance of cyclosporine by hemodialysis. J Clin Pharmacol 1984;24:528–31.

40. Amin NB, Padhi ID, Touchette MA, Patel RV, Dunfee TP, Anandan JV. Characterization of gentamicin pharmacokinetics in patients hemodialyzed with high-flux polysulfone membranes. Am J Kidney Dis 1999;34:222–7.

41. Martin E, Gambertoglio JG, Adler DS, Tozer TN, Roman LA, Grausz H. Removal of phenytoin by hemodialysis in uremic patients. JAMA 1977;238:1750–3.

42. Kradjan WA, Martin TR, Delaney CJ, Blair AD, Cutler RE. Effect of hemodialysis on the pharmacokinetics of theophylline in chronic renal failure. Nephron 1982;32:40–4.

43. Touchette MA, Patel RV, Anandan JV, Dumler F, Zarowitz BJ. Vancomycin removal by high-flux polysulfone hemodialysis membranes in critically ill patients with end-stage renal disease. Am J Kidney Dis 1995;26:469–74.

44. Urquhart R, Edwards C. Increased theophylline clearance during hemofiltration. Ann Pharmacother 1995;29:787–8.

45. Ernest D, Cutler DJ. Gentamicin clearance during continuous arteriovenous hemodiafiltration. Crit Care Med 1992;20:586–9.

46. Boereboom FTJ, Ververs FFT, Blankestijn PJ, Savelkoul THE, van Dijk A. Vancomycin clearance during continuous venovenous haemofiltration in critically ill patients. Intensive Care Med 1999;25:1100–4.

47. Blye E, Lorch J, Cortell S. Extracorporeal therapy in the treatment of intoxication. Am J Kidney Dis 1984;3:321–38.

48. Winchester JF. Active methods for detoxification. In: Haddad LM, Shannon MW, Winchester JF, editors. Clinical management of poisoning and drug overdose. 3rd ed. Philadelphia: WB Saunders; 1998. p. 175–88.

49. Osterloh JD, Pond SM, Grady S, Becker CE. Serum formate concentrations in methanol intoxication as a criterion for hemodialysis. Ann Intern Med 1986;104:200–3.

50. Shah G, Nelson HA, Atkinson AJ Jr, Okita GT, Ivanovich P, Gibson TP. Effect of hemoperfusion on the pharmacokinetics of digitoxin in dogs. J Lab Clin Med 1979;93:370–80.

51. Gibson TP, Atkinson AJ Jr. Effect of changes in intercompartment rate constants on drug removal during hemoperfusion. J Pharm Sci 1978;67:1178–9.

52. Antman E, Wenger TL, Butler VP Jr, Haber E, Smith TW. Treatment of 150 cases of life-threatening digitalis intoxication with digoxin-specific Fab antibody fragments: Final report of a multicenter study. Circulation 1990;81:1744–52.

7

Effect of Liver Disease on Pharmacokinetics

GREGORY M. SUSLA AND ARTHUR J. ATKINSON, JR.

Clinical Center, National Institutes of Health, Bethesda, Maryland

HEPATIC ELIMINATION OF DRUGS

Hepatic clearance (CL_H) may be defined as the volume of blood perfusing the liver that is cleared of drug per unit time. Usually, hepatic clearance is equated with nonrenal clearance and is calculated as total body clearance (CL_E) minus renal clearance (CL_R).

$$CL_H = CL_E - CL_R \qquad (7.1)$$

Accordingly, these estimates may include a component of extrahepatic nonrenal clearance.

The factors that affect hepatic clearance include blood flow to the liver (Q), the fraction of drug not bound to plasma proteins (f_u), and intrinsic clearance (CL_{int}) (1, 2). Intrinsic clearance is simply the clearance that would be observed in the absence of blood flow and protein binding restrictions. As discussed in Chapter 2, hepatic clearance usually can be considered to be a first-order process. In those cases, intrinsic clearance represents the ratio of V_{max}/K_m, and this relationship has been used as the basis for correlating *in vitro* studies of drug metabolism with *in vivo* results (3). However, for phenytoin and several other drugs the Michaelis–Menten equation is needed to characterize intrinsic clearance.

The well-stirred model, shown in Figure 7.1, is the model of hepatic clearance that is used most commonly in pharmacokinetics. If we apply the Fick equation (see Chapter 6) to this model, hepatic clearance can be defined as follows (2):

$$CL_H = Q \left[\frac{C_a - C_v}{C_a} \right] \qquad (7.2)$$

The ratio of concentrations defined by the terms within the brackets is termed the extraction ratio *(ER)*. An expression for the extraction ratio also can be obtained by applying the following mass balance equation to the model shown in Figure 7.1:

$$V \frac{dCa}{dt} = QC_a - QC_v - f_u \, CL_{int} \, C_v$$

At steady state:

$$Q \, (C_a - C_v) = f_u \, CL_{int} \, C_v \qquad (7.3)$$

Also:

$$QC_a = (Q + f_u \, CL_{int}) \, C_v \qquad (7.4)$$

Since:

$$ER = \frac{C_a - C_v}{C_a}$$

Equation 7.3 can be divided by Equation 7.4 to define extraction ratio in terms of Q, f_u, and CL_{int}.

$$ER = \frac{f_u \, CL_{int}}{Q + f_u \, CL_{int}} \qquad (7.5)$$

By substituting this expression for extraction ratio into Equation 7.2, hepatic clearance can be expressed as:

$$CL_H = Q \left[\frac{f_u \, CL_{int}}{Q + f_u \, CL_{int}} \right] \qquad (7.6)$$

63

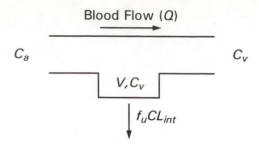

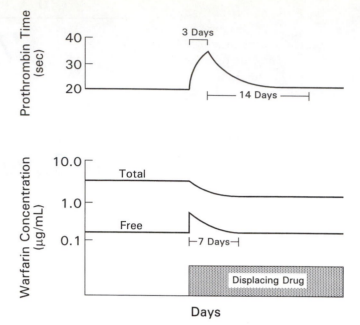

FIGURE 7.1 The well-stirred model of hepatic clearance in which the liver is viewed as a single compartment having a volume (V) and blood flow (Q). Drug concentrations reaching the liver via the hepatic artery and portal vein are designated by C_a, and those in emergent hepatic venous blood by C_v. Drug concentrations within the liver are considered to be in equilibrium with those in emergent venous blood. Intrinsic clearance (CL_{int}) acts to eliminate the fraction of drug not bound to plasma proteins (f_u).

FIGURE 7.2 Time course of an interaction in which warfarin, a restrictively metabolized drug, is displaced from its plasma protein binding sites. Although free warfarin concentrations rise initially as a result of the interaction, they subsequently return to pre-interaction levels. As a result, the increase in prothrombin time is only transient. Because f_u is increased, total (bound plus free) warfarin levels remain depressed as long as treatment with the displacing drug is continued. (Reproduced with permission from Atkinson AJ Jr, Reidenberg MM, Thompson WL. Clinical pharmacology. In: Greenberger N, editor. MKSAP VI Syllabus. Philadelphia: Am Col Phys; 1982. p. 85–96.)

Two limiting cases arise when $f_u\,CL_{int} \ll Q$ and when $f_u\,CL_{int} \gg Q$ (2). In the former instance Equation 7.5 can be simplified to

$$CL_H = f_u\,CL_{int} \tag{7.7}$$

Hepatic clearance is termed *restrictive* in this case, since it is limited by protein binding. This situation is analogous to the elimination of drugs by glomerular filtration. Drugs that are restrictively eliminated have extraction ratios < 0.3.

When $f_u\,CL_{int} \gg Q$, Equation 7.5 can be reduced to:

$$CL_H = Q \tag{7.8}$$

In this case, hepatic clearance is *flow limited*, similar to the renal tubular excretion of para-aminohippurate. Because protein binding does not affect their clearance, drugs whose hepatic clearance is flow limited are said to be *nonrestrictively* eliminated and have extraction ratios > 0.7.

In addition to the well-stirred model that is the basis for Equation 7.6, several other kinetic models of hepatic clearance have been developed (4). However, the following discussion will be based on the relationships defined by Equation 7.6, and the limiting cases represented by Equations 7.7 and 7.8.

Restrictively Metabolized Drugs (ER < 0.3)

The product of f_u and CL_{int} is small relative to liver blood flow (usually about 1500 mL/min) for drugs that are restrictively metabolized. Although the extraction ratio of these drugs is less than 0.3, hepatic metabolism often constitutes their principle pathway of elimination and they frequently have long elimina-

tion-phase half-lives (e.g., diazepam: $t_{1/2} = 43$ hr). The hepatic clearance of these drugs is affected by changes in their binding to plasma proteins, by induction or inhibition of hepatic drug metabolizing enzymes, and by age, nutrition, and pathological factors. However, as indicated by Equation 7.7, their hepatic clearance is not affected significantly by changes in hepatic blood flow.

Effect of Changes in Protein Binding on Hepatic Clearance

It usually is assumed that the free drug concentration in blood is equal to the drug concentration to which hepatic drug metabolizing enzymes are exposed. Although protein binding would not be anticipated to change hepatic clearance significantly for restrictively metabolized drugs that have $f_u > 80\%$, displacement of highly bound ($f_u < 20\%$) drugs from their plasma protein binding sites will result in a significant increase in their hepatic clearance. However, steady state concentrations of unbound drug will be unchanged as long as there is no change in CL_{int}. This occurs in some drug interactions, as diagrammed in Figure 7.2. This situation is also encountered in pathological conditions in which plasma proteins or plasma protein binding are decreased, as described in Chapter 5 for phenytoin kinetics in patients with impaired renal function. Since pharmacological effects are related to concentrations of unbound drug, pure displacement-type drug interactions put patients at risk for only a brief period of time. Similarly, dose adjustments are not needed for patients whose protein binding is impaired. In fact, as pointed out in Chapter 5, measurement of total rather than unbound drug levels in these patients actually may lead to inappropriate dose increases.

Effect of Changes in Intrinsic Clearance on Hepatic Drug Clearance

Both hepatic disease and drug interactions can alter the intrinsic clearance of restrictively eliminated drugs. Drug interactions will be considered in more detail in Chapter 14. The effects of liver disease on drug elimination will be discussed later in this chapter. Although a number of probe drugs have been used to characterize hepatic clearance, analysis of the factors influencing the intrinsic clearance of drugs is hampered by the fact that, in contrast to the use of creatinine clearance to assess renal function, there are no simple measures that can be applied on a routine clinical basis to assess hepatic clearance.

Drugs with an Intermediate Extraction Ratio ($0.3 < ER < 0.7$)

Few drugs exhibit an intermediate extraction ratio. Evaluation of the hepatic clearance of these drugs requires consideration of all of the parameters included in Equation 7.6. Disease-associated or drug-induced alterations in protein binding, hepatic blood flow, or intrinsic clearance may alter hepatic clearance significantly.

Nonrestrictively Metabolized Drugs ($ER > 0.70$)

The product of f_u and CL_{int} is large relative to liver blood flow for drugs that are nonrestrictively metabolized. These drugs characteristically have short elimination-phase half-lives (e.g., propranolol: $t_{1/2} = 3.9$ hr), and changes in hepatic blood flow have a major effect on their hepatic clearance (Equation 7.8). Accordingly, hemodynamic changes, such as congestive heart failure, that reduce liver blood flow will reduce the hepatic clearance of these drugs and may necessitate

appropriate adjustments in intravenous dosage. Changes in hepatic blood flow will also affect the first-pass metabolism of oral doses of nonrestrictively metabolized drugs, but the effects of this on patient exposure are not intuitively obvious.

First-Pass Metabolism

Because nonrestrictively metabolized drugs have an extraction ratio that exceeds 0.7, they undergo extensive first-pass metabolism, which reduces their bioavailability after oral administration (Chapter 4). If there is no loss of drug due to degradation or metabolism within the gastrointestinal tract or to incomplete absorption, the relationship between bioavailability (F) and extraction ratio is given by the following equation:

$$F = 1 - ER \qquad (7.9)$$

Because Equation 7.8 implies that $ER = 1$ for nonrestrictively metabolized drugs, yet the oral route of administration can be used for many drugs in this category (e.g., $F > 0$ for morphine and propranolol), it is apparent that Equation 7.9 represents only a rough approximation. By using Equation 7.5 to substitute for ER in Equation 7.9, we obtain a more precise estimate of the impact of first pass metabolism on bioavailability:

$$F = \frac{Q}{Q + f_u CL_{int}} \qquad (7.10)$$

Considering the case in which a drug is eliminated only by hepatic metabolism, Equation 4.2 from Chapter 4 can be rewritten as follows:

$$D_{oral} \cdot F = CL_H \cdot AUC_{oral}$$

Using Equations 7.6 and 7.10 to substitute respectively for CL_H and F, yields the result that:

$$D_{oral} = f_u CL_{int} \cdot AUC_{oral} \qquad (7.11)$$

It can be seen from Equation 7.11 that oral doses of nonrestrictively metabolized drugs should not need to be adjusted in response to changes in hepatic blood flow. Equation 7.11 also forms the basis for using AUC_{oral} measurements to calculate so-called "oral clearance" as an estimate of $f_u CL_{int}$. However, if renal excretion contributes to drug elimination, it will reduce AUC_{oral} and lead to overestimation of $f_u CL_{int}$ unless the contribution of renal clearance is accounted for (2).

Biliary Excretion of Drugs

Very few drugs are taken up by the liver and without further metabolism excreted into bile. On the other hand, many polar drug metabolites, such as glucuronide conjugates, are eliminated by biliary excretion. In order for compounds to be excreted in bile they must first pass the fenestrated endothelium that lines the hepatic sinusoids, then cross both the luminal and canalicular membrane surfaces of hepatocytes. Passage across these two hepatocyte membrane surfaces is often facilitated by active transport systems that will be discussed in Chapter 16. Consequently, chemical structure, polarity, and molecular weight are important determinants of the extent to which compounds are excreted in bile (5). In general, polar compounds with a molecular weight greater than 400 Da are excreted in bile, whereas those with a lower molecular weight tend to be eliminated preferentially by renal excretion. However, 5-fluorouracil has a molecular weight of only 130 Da, yet is excreted in bile with a bile/plasma concentration ratio of 2.0 (5). Nonetheless, biliary excretion of parent drug and metabolites accounts for only 2 to 3% of the elimination of an administered 5-fluorouracil dose in patients with normal renal function (6).

Compounds that enhance bile production stimulate biliary excretion of drugs normally eliminated by this route, whereas biliary excretion of these drugs will be decreased by compounds that decrease bile flow or pathophysiologic conditions that cause cholestasis (7). Route of administration may also influence the extent of drug excretion into bile. Oral administration may cause a drug to be extracted by the liver and excreted into bile to a greater degree than if the intravenous route were used.

Enterohepatic Circulation

Drugs excreted into bile traverse the biliary tract to reach the small intestine where they may be reabsorbed. Drug metabolites that reach the intestine also may be converted back to the parent drug and be reabsorbed. This is particularly true for some glucuronide conjugates that are hydrolyzed by β-glucuronidase present in intestinal bacteria. The term *enterohepatic circulation* refers to this cycle in which a drug or metabolite is excreted in bile and then reabsorbed from the intestine as the parent drug.

Studies in animals have demonstrated that biliary clearance actually may exceed plasma clearance for some drugs and species with extensive enterohepatic circulation (8). Interruption of enterohepatic circulation reduces both the area under the plasma level-vs.-time curve and the elimination-phase half-life. Enterohepatic circulation also increases the total exposure of the intestinal mucosa to potentially toxic drugs. Thus, the intestinal toxicity of indomethacin is most marked in those species that have a high ratio of biliary to renal drug excretion (8).

Enterohepatic circulation may result in a second peak in the plasma level-vs.-time curve. In one study of cyclosporine pharmacokinetics, patients exhibited an initial peak in this curve 3.1 ± 2.0 hours after an oral dose was administered (9). In addition, a second peak was observed in 36% of the patients 5.6 ± 1.8 hours after the dose. In one patient with an ileostomy, it was shown that there was a peak in indomethacin concentrations in ileostomy drainage that occurred shortly before the second peak. The occurrence of this large peak of drug concentrations in intestinal fluid appears to reflect intermittent gallbladder contraction and pulsatile delivery of bile to the intestine since this double peak phenomenon is not encountered in species that lack a gallbladder (8).

EFFECTS OF LIVER DISEASE ON PHARMACOKINETICS

Liver disease in humans encompasses a wide range of pathological disturbances that can lead to a reduction in liver blood flow, extrahepatic or intrahepatic shunting of blood, hepatocyte dysfunction, quantitative and qualitative changes in serum proteins, and changes in bile flow. Different forms of hepatic disease may produce different alterations in drug absorption, disposition, and pharmacologic effect. The pharmacokinetic or pharmacodynamic consequences of a specific hepatic disease may differ between individuals or even within a single individual over time. Each of the major determinants of hepatic clearance, CL_{int}, f_u, Q, and vascular architecture may be independently altered.

Although there are numerous causes of hepatic injury, it appears that the hepatic response to injury is a limited one and that the functional consequences are determined more by the extent of the injury than by the cause. At this time there is no generally available test that can be used to correlate changes in drug absorption and disposition with the degree of hepatic impairment.

Acute Hepatitis

Acute hepatitis is an inflammatory condition of the liver that is caused by viruses or hepatotoxins. In acute viral hepatitis, inflammatory changes in the hepatocyte are generally mild and transient, although they can be chronic (chronic active hepatitis) and severe, resulting in cirrhosis or death. Blaschke and Williams and their colleagues (10–13) have conducted informative studies of the effects of acute viral hepatitis on drug disposition. These investigators used a longitudinal study design in which each of a small number of

TABLE 7.1 Pharmacokinetics of Some Drugs During and After Acute Viral Hepatitis

| | f_u | | V_d | | CL_H | | CL_{int} | | |
	During	After	During (L/kg)	After (L/kg)	During (mL/hr/kg)	After (mL/hr/kg)	During (mL/hr/kg)	After (mL/hr/kg)	Ref.
Phenytoin[a]	0.126[b]	0.099	0.68[b]	0.63	0.0430	0.0373	0.352	0.385	10
Tolbutamide	0.087[b]	0.068	0.15	0.15	26[b]	18	300	260	11
Warfarin	0.012	0.012	0.09	0.21	6.1	6.1	519	514	12
Lidocaine	0.56	0.49	3.1	2.0	13.0	20.0	23.2[c]	40.8[c]	13

[a] A low dose of phenytoin was administered so that first-order kinetics would be approximated.
[b] Difference in studies during and after recovery from acute viral hepatitis was significant at $P < 0.05$ by paired t-test.
[c] Protein binding results for individual patients were not given so CL_{int} was estimated from average values.

patients was studied initially during the time that they had acute viral hepatitis and subsequently after recovery (Table 7.1). The drugs that were administered included phenytoin (10), tolbutamide (11), warfarin (12) and lidocaine (13). The most consistent significant finding was that the plasma protein binding of both phenytoin and tolbutamide was reduced during acute hepatitis. For both drugs, this was partly attributed to drug displacement from protein binding sites by elevated bilirubin levels. As a result of these changes, the distribution volume of phenytoin increased slightly during hepatitis (see Chapter 3). Although no significant change was noted in the average values of either phenytoin CL_H or CL_{int}, CL_{int} was reduced by approximately 50% in the two patients with the greatest evidence of hepatocellular damage. On the other hand, the reduction in tolbutamide binding to plasma proteins had no observable effect on distribution volume or CL_{int} but did result in an increase in CL_H. No consistent changes were observed in warfarin kinetics during acute viral hepatitis. However, prothrombin time was prolonged to a greater extent than expected in two of the five patients, reflecting impaired synthesis of Factor VII. Lidocaine kinetics also were not altered consistently during acute viral hepatitis, although clearance decreased in four of the six patients who were studied.

In general, drug elimination during acute viral hepatitis is either normal or only moderately impaired. Observed changes tend to be variable and related to the extent of hepatocellular damage incurred. If the acute hepatitis resolves, drug disposition returns to normal. Drug elimination is likely to be impaired most significantly in patients who develop chronic hepatitis B virus-related liver disease, but even then only late in the evolution of this disease (14). This stands in marked contrast to the severity of acute hepatitis that can be caused by hepatotoxins. For example, Prescott and Wright (15) found that liver damage can occur

within 2 to 3 hours after ingestion of an acetaminophen overdose. The elimination-phase half-life of acetaminophen averaged only 2.7 hours in patients without liver damage, but ranged from 4.3 to 7.7 hours (mean = 5.8 hr) in four patients with liver damage and from 4.3 to 13.9 hours (mean = 7.7 hr) in three patients with both liver and kidney damage resulting from acetaminophen toxicity. These authors observed that a fatal outcome was likely in patients whose acetaminophen elimination half-life exceeded 10 to 12 hours.

Chronic Liver Disease and Cirrhosis

Chronic liver disease is usually secondary to chronic alcohol abuse or chronic viral hepatitis. Alcoholic liver disease is most common and begins with the accumulation of fat vacuoles within hepatocytes and hepatic enlargement. There is a decrease in cytochrome P450 content per weight of tissue, but this is compensated for by the increase in liver size so that drug metabolism is not impaired (16). Alcoholic fatty liver may be accompanied or followed by alcoholic hepatitis, in which hepatocyte degeneration and necrosis become evident. In neither of these conditions is there significant diversion of blood flow past functioning hepatocytes by functional or anatomic shunts.

Cirrhosis occurs most frequently in the setting of alcoholic liver disease and represents the final common pathway of a number of chronic liver diseases. The development of cirrhosis is characterized by the appearance of fibroblasts and collagen deposition. This is accompanied by a reduction in liver size and the formation of nodules of regenerated hepatocytes. As a result, total liver content of cytochrome P450 is reduced in these patients. Initially, fibroblasts deposit collagen fibrils in the sinusoidal space, including the space of Disse (16). Collagen deposition not only produces characteristic bands of connective scar tissue but forms a basement membrane devoid of microvilli along the sinusoidal surface of the hepatocyte. The collagen barrier between the hepatocyte and sinusoid, in conjunction with alterations in the sinusoidal membrane of the hepatocyte, results in functional shunting of blood past the remaining hepatocyte mass. This can interfere significantly with the hepatic uptake of oxygen, nutrients, and plasma constituents, including drugs and metabolites.

The deposition of fibrous bands also disrupts the normal hepatic vascular architecture and increases vascular resistance and portal venous pressure This reduces portal venous flow that normally accounts for 70% of total liver blood flow (17). However, the decrease in portal venous flow is compensated for by an increase in hepatic artery flow so that total blood flow reaching the liver is maintained at the normal value of 18 mL/min·kg in patients with either chronic viral hepatitis or cirrhosis (18). The increase in portal venous pressure also leads to the formation of extrahepatic and intrahepatic shunts. Extrahepatic shunting occurs through the extensive collateral network that connects the portal and systemic circulations (17). Important examples include collaterals at the gastroesophageal junction, which can dilate to form varices, and the umbilical vein. In a study of cirrhotic patients with bleeding esophageal varices, an average of 70% of mesenteric and 95% of splenic blood flow was found to be diverted through extrahepatic shunts (19). Intrahepatic shunting results both from intrahepatic vascular anastamoses that bypass hepatic sinusoids and from the functional sinusoidal barrier caused by collagen deposition. In one study, the combination of anatomic and functional intrahepatic shunting averaged 25% of total liver blood flow in normal subjects, but was increased to 33% in patients with chronic viral hepatitis and to 52% in cirrhotic patients (18).

Pharmacokinetic Consequences of Liver Cirrhosis

The net result of chronic hepatic disease that leads to cirrhosis is that pathophysiologic alterations may result in both decreased hepatocyte function, with as much as a 50% decrease in cytochrome P450 content, and/or shunting of blood away from optimally functioning hepatocytes. Accordingly, cirrhosis affects drug elimination and the absorption of nonrestrictively eliminated drugs more than any other form of liver disease. An important consequence of these changes is that the clearance of drugs that are nonrestrictively eliminated in subjects with normal liver function no longer approximates hepatic blood flow but is influenced to a greater extent by hepatic intrinsic clearance (20).

Influence of Portosystemic Shunting

When portosystemic shunting is present, total hepatic blood flow (Q) equals the sum of perfusion flow (Q_p) and shunt flow (Q_s). Portocaval shunting will impair the efficiency of hepatic extraction and reduce the extraction ratio, as indicated by the following modification of Equation 7.5 (21).

$$ER = \frac{f_u\,CL_{int}}{Q + f_u\,CL_{int}} \cdot \frac{Q_p}{Q} \qquad (7.12)$$

The corresponding impact on hepatic clearance is given by the following equation:

$$CL_H = Q_p\left[\frac{f_u\,CL_{int}}{Q + f_u\,CL_{int}}\right] \qquad (7.13)$$

As a result, portocaval shunting will reduce hepatic clearance of nonrestrictively metabolized drugs, but will have little impact on the clearance of restrictively eliminated drugs.

Similarly, restrictively metabolized drugs exhibit little first-pass metabolism even in subjects with normal liver function, and portocaval shunting will have little impact on their bioavailability. On the other hand, portocaval shunting will decrease the extraction ratio and increase the bioavailability of nonrestrictively metabolized drugs as follows:

$$F = 1 - \frac{f_u\,CL_{int}}{Q + f_u\,CL_{int}} \cdot \frac{Q_p}{Q} \qquad (7.14)$$

For example, if the extraction ratio of a completely absorbed but nonrestrictively metabolized drug falls from 0.95 to 0.90, the bioavailability will double from 0.05 to 0.10. Because this increase in absorption is accompanied by a decrease in elimination clearance, total exposure following oral administration of nonrestrictively eliminated drugs will increase to an even greater extent than the increase in bioavailability, as shown in Table 7.2 for meperidine (22), pentazocine (22), and propranolol (23). Cirrhosis is also associated with a reduction in propranolol binding to plasma proteins, so this also contributes to the increased exposure following either intravenous or oral doses of this drug (see the following section). Accordingly, the relative exposure estimates for propranolol in Table 7.2 are based on comparisons of area under the plasma-level-vs.-time curve of nonprotein-bound plasma concentrations. The increase in drug exposure resulting from these changes may result in unexpected increases in intensity of pharmacologic response or in toxicity

TABLE 7.2   Impact of Cirrhosis on Bioavailability and Relative Exposure to Doses of Nonrestrictively Eliminated Drugs

	Absolute bioavailability		Relative exposure cirrhotics/control		
	Controls (%)	Cirrhotics (%)	IV	Oral	Ref.
Meperidine	48	87	1.6	3.1	22
Pentazocine	18	68	2.0	8.3	22
Propranolol	38	54	1.5[a]	2.0[a]	23

[a] These estimates also incorporate the 55% increase in propranolol free fraction that was observed in cirrhotic patients.

Consequences of Decreased Protein Binding

Hypoalbuminemia frequently accompanies chronic liver disease and may reduce drug binding to plasma proteins (24). In addition, endogenous substances such as bilirubin and bile acids accumulate and may displace drugs from protein binding sites. Reductions in protein binding will tend to increase the hepatic clearance of restrictively metabolized drugs. For drugs that have low intrinsic clearance and tight binding to plasma proteins it is possible that liver disease results in a decrease in CL_{int} but also an increase in f_u. The resultant change in hepatic clearance will depend on changes in both these parameters. Thus, hepatic disease generally produces no change in warfarin clearance, a decrease in diazepam clearance, and an increase in tolbutamide clearance. However, as discussed in Chapter 5, unbound drug concentrations will not be affected by decreases in the protein binding of restrictively metabolized drugs. Therefore, no dosage alterations are required for these drugs when protein binding is the only parameter that is changed.

Although reduced protein binding will not affect the clearance or total (bound plus free) plasma concentration of nonrestrictively eliminated drugs, it will increase the plasma concentration of free drug. This may increase the intensity of pharmacological effect that is observed at a given total drug concentration (24). Therefore, even in the absence of changes in other pharmacokinetic parameters, a reduction in the plasma protein binding of nonrestrictively eliminated drugs will necessitate a corresponding reduction in drug dosage.

As previously discussed in the context of renal disease (Chapter 5), reduced protein binding will increase the distribution volume referenced to total drug concentrations and this will tend to increase elimination-phase half-life (24).

TABLE 7.3   Differential Alterations of Cytochrome P-450 Enzyme Content in Cirrhosis

		Percent change in cirrhosis	
Enzyme	Representative substrate	Guengerich and Turvy (25)	George et al. (26)
CYP 1A2	Theophylline	↓53%[a]	↓71%[b]
CYP 2C19	Omeprazole	↑95%	↓43%
CYP 2E1	Acetaminophen	↓59%[a]	↓19%
CYP 3A	Midazolam	↓47%	↓75%[c]

[a] $P < .05$.
[b] $P < .005$.
[c] $P < .0005$.

Consequences of Hepatocellular Changes

The liver content of cytochrome P450 enzymes is decreased in patients with cirrhosis. In these patients, intrinsic clearance is the main determinant of the systemic clearance of lidocaine and indocyanine green, two drugs that have nonrestrictive metabolism in subjects with normal liver function. However, cirrhosis does not reduce the function of different drug metabolizing enzymes uniformly. As can be seen from the results of the two *in vitro* studies summarized in Table 7.3, CYP1A2 content is consistently reduced in cirrhosis (25,26). Significant reductions in CYP2E1 and CYP3A also have been found by some investigators. Although CYP2C19 appears to be somewhat more resilient in these *in vitro* studies, content of this enzyme was markedly reduced in patients with cholestatic types of cirrhosis (26). More recent studies in patients with liver disease, in whom the presence or absence of cholestasis was not noted, have indicated that clearance of S-mephenytoin, a CYP2C19 probe, was decreased by 63% in patients with mild cirrhosis and by 96% in patients with moderate cirrhosis (27). On the other hand, administration of debrisoquine to these patients indicated normal function of CYP2D6. Glucuronide conjugation of morphine, and presumably of other drugs, is relatively well preserved in patients with mild and moderate cirrhosis, but morphine clearance was 59% reduced in patients whose cirrhosis was severe enough to have caused previous hepatic encephalopathy (28).

USE OF THERAPEUTIC DRUGS IN PATIENTS WITH LIVER DISEASE

A number of clinical classification schemes and laboratory measures have been proposed as a means of guiding dose adjustments in patients with liver disease, much as creatinine clearance has been used to guide dose adjustments in patients with impaired

TABLE 7.4 Pugh Modification of Child's Classification of Liver Disease Severity[a]

Assessment parameters	Assigned score		
	1 point	2 points	3 points
Encephalopathy grade	0	1 or 2	3 or 4
Ascites	Absent	Slight	Moderate
Bilirubin (mg/dL)	1–2	2–3	> 3
Albumin (gm/dL)	> 3.5	2.8–3.5	< 2.8
Prothrombin time (seconds > control)	1–4	4–10	> 10

Classification of clinical severity

Clinical severity	Mild	Moderate	Severe
Total points	5–6	7–9	> 9

Encephalopathy grade

Grade 0 Normal consciousness, personality, neurological examination, EEG

Grade 1 Restless, sleep disturbed, irritable/agitated, tremor, impaired hand writing, 5 cps waves on EEG

Grade 2 Lethargic, time-disoriented, inappropriate, asterixis, ataxia, slow triphasic waves on EEG

Grade 3 Somnolent, stuporous, place-disoriented, hyperactive reflexes, rigidity, slower waves on EEG

Grade 4 Unrousable coma, no personality/behavior, decerebrate, slow 2–3 cps delta waves on EEG

[a] Adapted from Pugh et al. Br J Surg 1973;60:646–9 (29), and CDER, CBER. Draft Guidance for Industry, Rockville, FDA, 1999. (Internet at http://www.fda.gov/cder/guidance/index.htm.)

renal function. The Pugh modification of Child's classification of liver disease severity (Table 7.4) is the classification scheme that is used most commonly in studies designed to formulate drug dosing recommendations for patients with liver disease (29,30). Because patients with only mild or moderately severe liver disease usually are enrolled in these studies, there is relatively little data from patients with severe liver disease, in whom both pharmacokinetic changes and altered pharmacologic response are expected to be most pronounced. The administration of narcotic, sedative, and psychoactive drugs to patients with severe liver disease is particularly hazardous because these drugs have the potential to precipitate life-threatening hepatic encephalopathy.

Effects of Liver Disease on the Hepatic Elimination of Drugs

A number of probe drugs have been administered to normal subjects and to patients to evaluate hepatic clear-

ance. In one such test, a 1-mg/kg dose of lidocaine is administered intravenously and plasma concentrations of its *N*-dealkylated metabolite, monoethyl-glycinexylidide (MEGX), are measured either 15 or 30 minutes later. Testa et al. (31) found that a 30-minute post-dose MEGX concentration of 50 ng/ml provided the best discrimination between chronic hepatitis and cirrhosis (sensitivity: 93.5%, specificity: 76.9%). These authors concluded that both hepatic blood flow and the CYP3A4 pathway responsible for metabolizing lidocaine to MEGX were well preserved in patients with mild and moderate chronic hepatitis. However, MEGX levels fell significantly in patients with cirrhosis and were well correlated with the clinical stage of cirrhosis. Because no single probe drug estimates the activity of all drug-metabolizing enzymes, the strategy has been developed of simultaneously administering a combination of probes (32). As many as five probe drugs have been administered in this fashion to provide a profile of CYP1A2, CYP2E1, CYP3A, CYP2D6, CYP2C19, and *N*-acetytransferase activity (33). The method was evaluated to exclude the possibility of a significant metabolic interaction between the individual probes. Unfortunately, tests with probe drugs are too cumbersome for routine clinical use. Nevertheless, clinical studies in which the clearance of probe drugs has been examined in patients with different gradations of liver disease suggest the approximate relationships that are shown in Figure 7.3. However, even when the metabolic pathway for a given drug is known, prediction of hepatic drug clearance in individual patients is complicated further by the effects of pharmacogenetic variation and drug interactions

Bergquist et al. (34) have presented examples in which several laboratory tests that are commonly used to assess liver function provide a more reliable indication of impaired drug metabolic clearance than this clinical classification scheme (Table 7.5). Serum albumin concentrations were of greatest predictive value for two of the drugs shown in the table. However, this marker was not correlated with the hepatic clearance of lansoprazole, and a combination of all three laboratory tests was better correlated with hepatic clearance of atorvastatin than serum albumin alone. Serum concentrations of AST or ALT were not correlated with hepatic drug clearance, as might be expected from the fact that these enzymes reflect hepatocellular damage rather than hepatocellular function.

Equation 7.13 emphasizes the central point that changes in perfusion and protein binding, as well as intrinsic clearance, will affect the hepatic clearance of a number of drugs. The intact hepatocyte theory has been proposed as a means of simplifying this complexity (35). This theory is analogous to the intact nephron

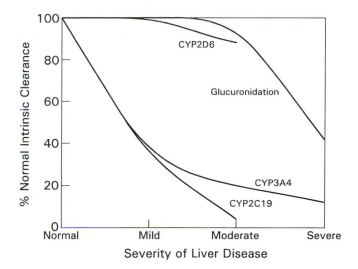

FIGURE 7.3 Schematic diagram showing the effects of various stages of liver disease severity on the intrinsic clearance of drugs mediated by representative metabolic pathways. Estimates for glucuronidation (28), CYP2D6 (27), CYP3A4 (31) and CYP2C19 (27) pathways are based on the literature sources indicated in parentheses.

theory (see Chapter 5) in that it assumes that the increase in portocaval shunting parallels the loss of functional cell mass, and that the reduced mass of normally functioning liver cells is perfused normally. Other theories have been proposed to account for the effects of chronic liver disease on hepatic drug clearance and it currently is not clear which, if any, of these theories is most appropriate (36). However, what is apparent from studies in patients with significantly impaired liver function is that the intrinsic clearance of some drugs that normally are nonrestrictively metabolized is reduced to the extent that $f_u CL_{int}$ now becomes rate limiting and clearance is no longer approximated by hepatic perfusion rate (20). It also is apparent from Equation 7.14 that the presence of portosystemic shunting and hepatocellular damage will significantly

TABLE 7.5   Correlation of Laboratory Test Results with Impaired Hepatic Clearance[a]

Drug	Enzyme(s)	Laboratory test		
		Albumin	PT[b]	Bilirubin
"A"	CYP2C9	X		
"B"	Not given	X		
Atorvastatin	CYP3A4	X	X	X
Lansoprazole	CYP3A4 + CYP 2C19		X	

[a] Data from Bergquist et al. Clin Pharmacol Ther 1999;62:365–76.
[b] Prothrombin time.

increase the bioavailability of drugs that normally have extensive first pass hepatic metabolism.

Effects of Liver Disease on the Renal Elimination of Drugs

Drug therapy in patients with advanced cirrhosis is further complicated by the fact that renal blood flow and glomerular filtration rate are frequently depressed in these patients in the absence of other known causes of renal failure. This condition, termed the *hepatorenal syndrome,* occurs in a setting of marked hemodynamic change and is a functional abnormality that reverses following successful liver transplantation. Ginès et al. (37) monitored 234 patients with cirrhosis, ascites, and a glomerular filtration rate (GFR) of more than 50 mL/min. These authors found that this syndrome developed within 1 year in 18%, and within 5 years in 39%, of these patients. Although Pugh score was of no predictive value, high plasma renin activity, low serum sodium concentrations, and small liver size were independent predictors of the onset of the hepatorenal syndrome. Baseline GFR also was of predictive value, but serum creatinine and creatinine clearance, either measured or calculated from the Cockcroft and Gault equation (Chapter 5), overestimated renal function in this group of patients (38). This overestimation reflects the fact that the rate of creatinine synthesis is depressed in these patients, so serum creatinine concentrations may remain within the normal range even when inulin clearance falls as low as 10 mL/min. As a result, many patients with cirrhosis and ascites have a normal serum creatinine concentration but a GFR of less than 60 mL/min.

The need for caution in estimating drug dosage for patients with the hepatorenal syndrome is exemplified by carbenicillin, an antipseudomonal, semisynthetic penicillin that is excreted primarily by the kidneys with biliary excretion normally accounting for less than 20% of total elimination. The decline in renal function that is associated with severe liver disease prolongs the elimination half-life of this drug from 1 hour in subjects with normal renal and liver function to approximately 24 hours (39). Although studies in patients with hepatorenal syndrome were not reported, similar half-life prolongations have been described in patients with combined renal and hepatic functional impairment who were treated with the newer but pharmacokinetically similar antipseudomnal penicillins piperacillin (40) and mezlocillin (41). Consequently, it is advisable to consider reducing doses even for drugs that are eliminated to a significant extent by renal excretion when treating patients with cirrhosis that is severe enough to be accompanied by ascites.

Effects of Liver Disease on Patient Response

The relationship between drug concentration and response can also be altered in patients with advanced liver disease. Of greatest concern is the fact that customary doses of sedatives may precipitate the disorientation and coma that are characteristic of portal-systemic or hepatic encephalopathy. Experimental hepatic encephalopathy is associated with increased γ-aminobutyric acid-mediated inhibitory neurotransmission, and there has been some success in using the benzodiazepine antagonist flumazenil to reverse this syndrome (42). This provides a theoretical basis for the finding that brain hypersensitivity, as well as impaired drug elimination, is responsible for the exaggerated sedative response to diazepam that is exhibited by some patients with chronic liver disease (43). Bakti et al. (44) conducted a particularly well-controlled demonstration of benzodiazepine hypersensitivity by showing that CNS performance in cirrhotic patients was impaired when compared to subjects with normal liver function at a time when plasma concentrations of unbound triazolam were the same in both groups. Changes in the CSF/serum concentration ratio of cimetidine have been reported in patients with liver disease, suggesting an increase in blood–brain barrier permeability that also could make these patients more sensitive to the adverse CNS effects of a number of other drugs (45).

Although cirrhotic patients frequently are treated with diuretic drugs to reduce ascites, they exhibit a reduced responsiveness to loop diuretics that cannot be overcome by administerinig larger doses and is presumably related to the pathophysiology of increased sodium retention that contributed to the development of ascites (46). In addition, decreases in renal function, which are often unrecognized in these patients (38), may lead to decreased delivery of loop diuretics to their renal tubular site of action. Because hyperaldosteronism is prevalent in these patients and spironolactone is not dependent on glomerular filtration for efficacy, it should be the mainstay of diuretic therapy in this clinical setting (47).

When diuretic therapy does result in effective fluid removal in cirrhotic patients, it is associated with a very high incidence of adverse reactions. In one study of diuretic therapy in cirrhosis, furosemide therapy precipitated the hepatorenal syndrome in 12.8% and hepatic coma in 11.6% of the patients (48). Although daily doses of this drug did not differ, patients who had adverse drug reactions received total furosemide doses that averaged 1384 mg, whereas patients without adverse reactions received lower total doses that averaged 743 mg. Accordingly, when spironolactone therapy does not provide an adequate diuresis, only small frequent doses of loop diuretics should be added to the spironolactone regimen (47). Cirrhotic patients also appear to be at an increased risk of developing acute renal failure after being treated with angiotensin converting enzyme inhibitors and nonsteroidal anti-inflammatory drugs (49).

Modification of Drug Therapy in Patients with Liver Disease

It is advisable to avoid using certain drugs in patients with advanced liver disease. For example, angiotensin-converting enzyme inhibitors and nonsteroidal anti-inflammatory drugs should be avoided because of their potential to cause acute renal failure. Paradoxically, administration of captopril to cirrhotic patients with ascites actually impairs rather than promotes sodium excretion (50). Since coagulation disorders are common in patients with advanced cirrhosis, alternatives should be sought for therapy with β-lactam antibiotics that contain the N-methylthiotetrazole side chain (e.g., cefotetan) that inhibits γ-carboxylation of vitamin K-dependent clotting factors (49).

It also is prudent to reduce the dosage of a number of other drugs that frequently are used to treat patients with liver disease (51). Particular attention has been focused on drugs whose clearance is significantly impaired in patients with moderate hepatic impairment, as assessed in Table 7.5 (30). Even greater caution should be exercised in using these drugs to treat patients with severely impaired liver function. Table 7.6 lists several drugs whose dose should be reduced by 50% in treating patients with moderate hepatic impairment. Most of the drugs in this table have first-pass metabolism that is greater than 50% in normal subjects but is substantially reduced when liver function is impaired. Drug exposure to standard doses is further increased by what is generally a substantial decrease in elimination clearance. Although not routinely evaluated in most studies of patients with liver disease, drug binding to plasma proteins also may be reduced in these patients and may contribute to exaggerated responses. Formation of pharmacologically active metabolites is another complicating factor that deserves consideration. For example, losartan has an active metabolite, EXP3174, that is primarily responsible for the extent and duration of pharmacological effect in patients treated with this drug (57). Although standard doses produce plasma concentrations of losartan that are four to five times higher in patients with cirrhosis than those observed in normal subjects, plasma levels of EXP3174 are only increased by a fac-

TABLE 7.6 Some Drugs Requiring at Least a 50% Dose Reduction in Patients with Moderate Cirrhosis

	Normal	Parameter Values or Changes in Cirrhosis			
	F (%)	F (%)	Clearance	f_u	Ref.
Analgesic Drugs					
Morphine	47	100	↓59%		28
Meperidine	47	91	↓46%		22
Pentazocine	17	71	↓50%		22
Cardiovascular drugs					
Propafenone	21	75	↓24%	↑213%	52
Verapamil	22	52	↓51%	No change	53
Nifedipine	51	91	↓60%	↑93%	54
Nitrendipine	40	54	↓34%	↑43%	55
Nisoldipine	4	15	↓42%		56
Losartan	33	66	↓50%		57–59
Other					
Omeprazole	56	98	↓89%		60
Tacrolimus	27	36	↓72%		61, 62

tor of 1.5 to 2.0 (59). This provided the rationale for reducing the usual losartan dose by only half in a trial in which this drug was used to reduce portal pressure in patients with cirrhosis and esophageal varices (63).

References

1. Rowland M, Benet LZ, Graham GG. Clearance concepts in pharmacokinetics. J Pharmacokinet Biopharm 1973;1:123–36.
2. Wilkinson GR, Shand DG. A physiological approach to hepatic drug clearance. Clin Pharmacol Ther 1975;18:377–90.
3. Rane A, Wilkinson GR, Shand DG. Prediction of hepatic extraction ratio from *in vitro* measurement of intrinsic clearance. J Pharmacol Exp Ther 1977;200:420–4.
4. Roberts MS, Donaldson JD, Rowland M. Models of hepatic elimination: Comparison of stochastic models to describe residence time distributions and to predict the influence of drug distribution, enzyme heterogeneity, and systemic recycling on hepatic elimination. J Pharmacokinet Biopharm 1988;16:41–83.
5. Rollins DE, Klaassen CD. Biliary excretion of drugs in man. Clin Pharmacokinet 1979;4:368–79.
6. Heggie GD, Sommadossi J-P, Cross DS, Huster WJ, Diasio RB. Clinical pharmacokinetics of 5-fluorouracil and its metabolites in plasma, urine, and bile. Cancer Res 1987;47:2203–6.
7. Siegers C-P, Bumann D. Clinical significance of the biliary excretion of drugs. Prog Pharmacol Clin Pharmacol 1991;8:537–49.
8. Duggan DE, Hooke KF, Noll RM, Kwan KC. Enterohepatic circulation of indomethacin and its role in intestinal irritation. Biochem Pharmacol 1975;24:1749–54.
9. Kahan BD, Ried M, Newburger J. Pharmacokinetics of cyclosporine in human renal transplantation. Transplant Proc 1983;15:446–53.
10. Blaschke TF, Meffin PJ, Melmon KL, Rowland M. Influence of acute viral hepatitis on phenytoin kinetics and protein binding. Clin Pharmacol Ther 1975;17:685–91.
11. Williams RL, Blaschke TF, Meffin PJ, Melmon KL, Rowland M. Influence of acute viral hepatitis on disposition and plasma binding of tolbutamide. Clin Pharmacol Ther 1977;21:301–9.
12. Williams RL, Schary WL, Blaschke TF, Meffin PJ, Melmon KL, Rowland M. Influence of acute viral hepatitis on disposition and pharmacologic effect of warfarin. Clin Pharmacol Ther 1976;20:90–7.
13. Williams RL, Blaschke TF, Meffin PJ, Melmon KL, Rowland M. Influence of viral hepatitis on the disposition of two compounds with high hepatic clearance: Lidocaine and indocyanine green. Clin Pharmacol Ther 1976;20:290–9.
14. Villeneuve JP, Thibeault MJ, Ampelas M, Fortunet-Fouin H, LaMarre L, Côté J, Pomier-Layrargues G, Huet P-M. Drug disposition in patients with HB$_s$Ag-positive chronic liver disease. Dig Dis Sci 1987;32:710–4.
15. Prescott LF, Wright N. The effects of hepatic and renal damage on paracetamol metabolism and excretion following overdosage. A pharmacokinetic study. Br J Pharmacol 1973;49:602–13.
16. Sotaniemi EA, Niemelä O, Risteli L, Stenbäck F, Pelkonen RO, Lahtela JT, Risteli J. Fibrotic process and drug metabolism in alcoholic liver disease. Clin Pharmacol Ther 1986;40:46–55.
17. Boyer TD, Henderson JM. Portal hypertension and bleeding esophageal varices. In: Zakim D, Boyer TD, editors. Hepatology: A textbook of liver disease. Philadelphia: WB Saunders; 1996.p.720–63.
18. Iwasa M, Nakamura K, Nakagawa T, Watanabe S, Katoh H, Kinosada Y, Maeda H, Habara J, Suzuki S. Single photon emission computed tomography to determine effective hepatic blood flow and intrahepatic shunting. Hepatology 1995;21:359–65.
19. Lebrec D, Kotelanski B, Cohn JN. Splanchnic hemodynamics in cirrhotic patients with esophageal varices and gastrointestinal bleeding. Gastroenterology 1976;70:1108–11.
20. Huet P-M, Villeneuve J-P. Determinants of drug disposition in patients with cirrhosis. Hepatology 1983;3:913–18.
21. McLean A, du Souich P, Gibaldi M. Noninvasive kinetic approach to the estimation of total hepatic blood flow and shunting in chronic liver disease—A hypothesis. Clin Pharmacol Ther 1979;25:161–6.
22. Neal EA, Meffin PJ, Gregory PB, Blaschke TF. Enhanced bioavailability and decreased clearance of analgesics in patients with cirrhosis. Gastroenterology 1979;77:96–102.
23. Wood AJJ, Kornhauser DM, Wilkinson GR, Shand DG, Branch RA. The influence of cirrhosis on steady-state blood concentrations of unbound propranolol after oral administration. Clin Pharmacokinet 1978;3:478–87.
24. Blaschke TF. Protein binding and kinetics of drugs in liver diseases. Clin Pharmacokinet 1977;2:32–44.
25. Guengerich FP, Turvy CG. Comparison of levels of several human microsomal cytochrome P-450 enzymes and epoxide hydrolase in normal and disease states using immunochemical analysis of surgical liver samples. J Pharmacol Exp Ther 1991;256:1189–94.
26. George J, Murray M, Byth K, Farrell GC. Differential alterations of cytochrome P450 proteins in livers from patients with severe chronic liver disease. Hepatology 1995;21:120–8.
27. Adedoyin A, Arns PA, Richards WO, Wilkinson GR, Branch RA. Selective effect of liver disease on the activities of specific metabolizing enzymes: Investigation of cytochromes P450 2C19 and 2D6. Clin Pharmacol Ther 1998;64:8–17.
28. Hasselström J, Eriksson S, Persson A, Rane A, Svensson O, Säwe J. The metabolism and bioavailability of morphine in patients with severe liver cirrhosis. Br J Clin Pharmacol 1990;29:289–97.

29. Pugh RNH, Murray-Lyon IM, Dawson JL, Pietroni MC, Williams R.. Transection of the oesophagus for bleeding oesophageal varices. Br J Surg 1973;60:646–9.

30. CDER, CBER. Pharmacokinetics in patients with impaired hepatic function: Study design, data analysis, and impact on dosing and labeling. Draft Guidance for Industry, Rockville, FDA, 1999. (Internet at http://www.fda.gov/cder/guidance/index.htm.)

31. Testa R, Caglieris S, Risso D, Arzani L, Campo N, Alvarez S, Giannini E, Lantieri PB, Celle G. Monoethylglycinexylidide formation measurement as a hepatic function test to assess severity of chronic liver disease. Am J Gastroenterol 1997;92:2268–73.

32. Breimer DD, Schellens JHM. A 'cocktail' strategy to assess *in vivo* oxidative drug metabolism in humans. Trends Pharmacol Sci 1990;11:223–5.

33. Frye RF, Matzke GR, Adedoyin A, Porter JA, Branch RA. Validation of the five-drug "Pittsburgh cocktail" approach for assessment of selective regulation of drug-metabolizing enzymes. Clin Pharmacol Ther 1997;62:365–76.

34. Bergquist C, Lindergård J, Salmonson T. Dosing recommendations in liver disease. Clin Pharmacol Ther 1999;66:201–4.

35. Wood AJJ, Villeneuve JP, Branch RA, Rogers LW, Shand DG. Intact hepatocyte theory of impaired drug metabolism in experimental cirrhosis in the rat. Gastroenterology 1979;76:1358–62.

36. Tucker GT. Alteration of drug disposition in liver impairment. Br J Clin Pharmacol 1998;46:355.

37. Ginès A, Escorsell A, Ginès P, Saló J, Jiménez W, Inglada L, Navasa M, Clària J, Mimola A, Arroyo V, Rodés J. Incidence, predictive factors, and prognosis of the hepatorenal syndrome in cirrhosis with ascites. Gastroenterology 1993;105:229–36.

38. Papadakis MA, Arieff AI. Unpredictability of clinical evaluation of renal function in cirrhosis: prospective study. Am J Med 1987;82:945–52.

39. Hoffman TA, Cestero R, Bullock WE. Pharmacodynamics of carbenicillin in hepatic and renal failure. Ann Intern Med 1970;73:173–8.

40. Green L, Dick JD, Goldberger SP, Anelopulos CM. Prolonged elimination of piperacillin in a patient with renal and liver failure. Drug Intell Clin Pharm 1985;19:427–9.

41. Cooper BE, Nester TJ, Armstrong DK, Dasta JF. High serum concentrations of mezlocillin in a critically ill patient with renal and hepatic dysfunction. Clin Pharm 1986;5:764–6.

42. Ferenci P, Grimm G, Meryn S, Gangl A. Successful long-term treatment of portal-systemic encephalopathy by the benzodiazepine antagonist flumazenil. Gastroenterology 1989;96:240–3.

43. Branch RA, Morgan MH, James J, Read AE. Intravenous administration of diazepam in patients with chronic liver disease. Gut 1976;17:975–83.

44. Bakti G, Fisch HU, Karlaganis G, Minder C, Bircher J. Mechanism of the excessive sedative response of cirrhotics to benzodiazepines: model experiments with triazolam. Hepatology 1987;7:629–38.

45. Schentag JJ, Cerra FB, Calleri GM, Leising ME, French MA, Bernhard H. Age, disease, and cimetidine disposition in healthy subjects and chronically ill patients. Clin Pharmacol Ther 1981;29:737–43.

46. Brater DC. Resistance to loop diuretics: why it happens and what to do about it. Drugs 1985;30:427–43.

47. Brater DC. Use of diuretics in cirrhosis and nephrotic syndrome. Semin Nephrol 1999;19:575–80.

48. Naranjo CA, Pontigo E, Valdenegro C, González G, Ruiz I, Busto U. Furosemide-induced adverse reactions in cirrhosis of the liver. Clin Pharmacol Ther 1979;25:154–60.

49. Westphal J-F, Brogard J-M. Drug administration in chronic liver disease. Drug Safety 1997;17:47–73.

50. Daskalopoulos G, Pinzani M, Murray N, Hirschberg R, Zipser RD. Effects of captopril on renal function in patients with cirrhosis and ascites. J Hepatol 1987;4:330–6.

51. Rodighiero V. Effects of liver disease on pharmacokinetics: An update. Clin Pharmacokinet 1999;37:399–431.

52. Lee JT, Yee Y-G, Dorian P, Kates RE. Influence of hepatic dysfunction on the pharmacokinetics of propafenone. J Clin Pharmacol 1987;27:384–9.

53. Somogyi A, Albrecht M, Kliems G, Schäfer K, Eichelbaum M. Pharmacokinetics, bioavailability and ECG response of verapamil in patients with liver cirrhosis. Br J Clin Pharmacol 1981;12:51–60.

54. Kleinbloesem CH, van Harten J, Wilson JPH, Danhof M, van Brummelen P, Breimer DD. Nifedipine: Kinetics and hemodynamic effects in patients with liver cirrhosis after intravenous and oral administration. Clin Pharmacol Ther 1986;40:21–8.

55. Dylewicz P, Kirch W, Santos SR, Hutt HJ, Mönig H, Ohnhaus EE. Bioavailability and elimination of nitrendipine in liver disease. Eur J Clin Pharmacol 1987;32:563–8.

56. van Harten J, van Brummelen P, Wilson JHP, Lodewijks MTM, Breimer DD. Nisoldipine: kinetics and effects on blood pressure in patients with liver cirrhosis after intravenous and oral administration. Eur J Clin Pharmacol 1988;34:387–94.

57. Lo M-W, Goldberg MR, McCrea JB, Lu H, Furtek CI, Bjornsson TD. Pharmacokinetics of losartan, an angiotensin II receptor antagonist, and its active metabolite EXP3174 in humans. Clin Pharmacol Ther 1995;58:641–9.

58. Goa KL, Wagstaff AJ. Losartan potassium. A review of its pharmacology, clinical efficacy and tolerability in the management of hypertension. Drugs 1996;51:820–45.

59. McIntyre M, Caffe SE, Michalak RA, Reid JL. Losartan, an orally active angiotensin (AT$_1$) receptor antagonist: A review of its efficacy and safety in essential hypertension. Pharmacol Ther 1997;74:181–94.

60. Andersson T, Olsson R, Regårdh C-G, Skänberg I. Pharmacokinetics of [^{14}C]omeprazole in patients with liver cirrhosis. Clin Pharmacokinet 1993;24:71–8.

61. Venkataramanan R, Jain A, Cadoff E, Warty V, Iwasaki K, Nagase K, Drajack A, Imventarza O, Todo S, Fung JJ, Starzl TE. Pharmacokinetics of FK 506: Preclinical and clinical studies. Transplant Proc 1990;22(suppl 1):52–6.

62. Jain AB, Venkataramanan R, Cadoff E, Fung JJ, Todo S, Krajack A, Starzl TE. Effect of hepatic dysfunction and T tube clamping on FK 506 pharmacokinetics and trough concentrations. Transplant Proc 1990;22(suppl 1):57–9.

63. Schneider AW, Kalk JF, Klein CP. Effect of losartan, an angiotensin II receptor antagonist, on portal pressure in cirrhosis. Hepatology 1999;29:334–9.

Noncompartmental vs. Compartmental Approaches to Pharmacokinetic Analysis

DAVID M. FOSTER

Department of Bioengineering, University of Washington, Seattle, Washington

INTRODUCTION

From previous chapters, it is clear that the evaluation of pharmacokinetic parameters is an essential part of understanding how drugs function in the body. To estimate these parameters, studies are undertaken in which transient data are collected. These studies can be conducted in animals at the pre-clinical level, through all stages of clinical trials, and can be data rich or sparse. No matter what the situation, there must be some common means by which to communicate the results of the experiments. Pharmacokinetic parameters serve this purpose. Thus, in the field of pharmacokinetics, the definitions and formulas for the parameters must be agreed upon, and the methods used to calculate them understood. This understanding includes assumptions and domains of validity, for the utility of the parameter values depends on them. This chapter will focus on the assumptions and domains of validity for the two commonly used methods—noncompartmental and compartmental analysis. Compartmental models have been presented in earlier chapters. This chapter will expand on this, and compare the two methods.

Pharmacokinetic parameters fall basically into two categories. One category is qualitative or descriptive—that is, observational parameters requiring no formula for calculation. Examples would include the maximal observed concentration of a drug or the amount of drug excreted in the urine during a given time period.

The other category is quantitative—parameters that require a mathematical formalism for calculation. Examples here would include mean residence times, clearance rates, and volumes of distribution. Estimation of terminal slopes would also fall into this category. This chapter will be concerned only with parameters requiring a mathematical formalism.

The quantitative parameters require not only a mathematical formalism but data from which to estimate them. As noted, the two most common methods used for pharmacokinetic estimation are noncompartmental and compartmental analysis. A recent comparison of the two methods has been given by Gillespie (1). Comparisons regarding the two methodologies as applied to metabolic studies have been provided by DiStefano III (2) and Cobelli and Toffolo (3). Covell et al. (4) have given an extensive theoretical comparison of the two methods.

Under what circumstances can the two methods be used to estimate the pharmacokinetic parameters of interest? The answer to this question is the subject of this chapter. To begin, one must start with a definition of kinetics since it is through this definition that one can introduce mathematical and statistical analyses to study the dynamic characteristics of a system. This can be used to define specific parameters of interest that can be estimated from data. From the definition of kinetics, the types of equations that can be used to provide a mathematical description of the system can be

75

given. The assumptions underlying noncompartmental analysis and estimation techniques for the different parameters for different experimental input-output configurations can then be discussed. One can then move to compartmental analysis and understand that the models set in full generality are very difficult to solve. With appropriate assumptions that are commonly made in pharmacokinetic studies, a simpler set of compartmental models will evolve. These models are easy to solve, and it will be seen that all parameters estimated using noncompartmental analysis can be recovered from these compartmental models. Under conditions when the two methods should, in theory, yield the same estimates, differences can be attributed to the numerical techniques used (e.g., sums of exponentials vs. trapezoidal integration). With this knowledge, the circumstances under which the two methods will provide the same or different estimates of the pharmacokinetic parameters can be discussed. Thus, it is not the point of this chapter to favor one method over another; it is the intent to describe the assumptions and consequences of using either method.

Most of the theoretical details of the material covered in this chapter can be found in Covell et al. (4), Jacquez and Simon (5), and Jacquez (6). Of particular importance to this chapter is the material covered in Covell et al. (4) in which the relationship between the calculation of kinetic parameters from statistical moments and the same parameters calculated from the rate constants of a linear, constant coefficient compartmental model are derived. Jacquez and Simon (5) discuss in detail the mathematical properties of systems that depend on local mass balance; this forms the basis for understanding compartmental models and the simplifications that result from certain assumptions about a system under study. Berman (7) gives examples using metabolic turnover data while the examples provided in Gibaldi and Perrier (8) and Rowland and Tozer (9) are more familiar to clinical pharmacologists.

KINETICS, PHARMACOKINETICS, AND PHARMACOKINETIC PARAMETERS

Kinetics and the Link to Mathematics

Substances in a biological system are constantly undergoing change. These changes can include transport (e.g., transport via the circulation or transport into or out from a cell) or transformation (e.g., biochemically changing from one substance to another). These changes and the concomitant outcomes form the basis for the system in which the substance interacts. How can one formalize these changes, and once formalized,

how can one describe their quantitative nature? Dealing with these questions involves an understanding and utilization of concepts related to kinetics.

The *kinetics* of a substance in a biological system are its spatial and temporal distribution in that system. The kinetics are the result of several complex events including entry into the system, and subsequent distribution, which may entail circulatory dynamics, transport into and from cells, and elimination, which usually requires biochemical transformations. Together these events characterize the substance and the system in which it resides.

While the substance can be an element such as calcium or zinc, or a compound such as amino acids, proteins, or sugars that exist normally in the body, in this chapter, it will be assumed to be a drug that is not normally present in the system. Thus, in this chapter, the *pharmacokinetics* of a drug are defined as its spatial and temporal distribution in a system. Unlike substances normally present, input into the system (i.e., the drug) will be from exogenous sources only. In addition, unless otherwise noted, the system will be the whole body. It should be noted that this definition of pharmacokinetics differs somewhat from the more conventional definition given in Chapter 1. The reason for this is seen in the following section.

From the spatial component of the definition, location in the system is important. From the temporal component of the definition is the fact that the amount of substance at a specific location is changing with time. The combination of temporal and spatial components leads to partial derivatives:

$$\frac{\partial}{\partial t}, \frac{\partial}{\partial x}, \frac{\partial}{\partial y}, \frac{\partial}{\partial z} \qquad (8.1)$$

which, mathematically, reflect change in time and space. Here t is time, and a location in the system in three dimensions is represented by the coordinates (x, y, z).

If one chooses to use partial derivatives to provide a description of the kinetics of a drug in the body, then expressions for each of $\frac{\partial}{\partial t}, \frac{\partial}{\partial x}, \frac{\partial}{\partial y}$ and $\frac{\partial}{\partial z}$ must be written. That is, a system of partial differential equations must be specified. Writing these equations involves a knowledge of physical chemistry, irreversible thermodynamics, and circulatory dynamics. Such equations will require parameters that can be either deterministic (known) or stochastic (contain statistical uncertainties). Although such equations can be written for specific systems, defining and then estimating the unknown parameters is in most cases impossible because of the difficulty in obtaining data to resolve the spatial components of the system. In pharmacokinetic applications, partial differential equations are used to describe distributed systems models. Such models are discussed in Chapter 9.

How does one resolve the difficulty associated with partial differential equations? The most common way is to reduce the system into a finite number of components. This can be accomplished by lumping together processes based on time, location, or a combination of the two. One thus moves from partial derivatives to ordinary derivatives where space is not taken directly into account. Reducing the system results in the compartmental models discussed later in this chapter. The lumping also forms the basis for the noncompartmental models discussed in the next section, although the reduction is much simpler than for compartmental models.

One can now recognize why conventional definitions of pharmacokinetics are a little different from the definition given in this chapter. The conventional definitions make references to events other than temporal and spatial distribution. These events are, in fact, consequences of a drug's kinetics, and thus the two should be separated. The processes of drug absorption, distribution, metabolism, and elimination relate to parameters that can only be estimated from a mathematical model describing the kinetics of the drug. The point is that to understand the mathematical basis of pharmacokinetic parameter estimation, the separation between kinetics per se and using kinetic data to estimate the parameters needs to be kept in mind.

Using the definition of pharmacokinetics given in terms of spatial and temporal distributions, one can easily progress to a description of the underlying assumptions and mathematics of noncompartmental and compartmental analysis and, from there, proceed to the processes involved in estimating the pharmacokinetic parameters. This will permit a better understanding of the domain of validity of noncompartmental vs. compartmental parameter estimation.

The Pharmacokinetic Parmaters

What is desired from the pharmacokinetic parameters is a quantitative measure of how a drug behaves in the system. To estimate these parmaeters, one must design an experiment to collect transient data that can then be used to estimate the parmeters of interest.

To design such an experiment, the system must contain at least one *accessible pool,* that is, the system must contain a "pool" that is available for drug input and data collection. As we will seen, this pool must have certain properties. If the system contains an accessible pool, this implies that parts of the system are not accessible for test input and/or data collection. This

divides the system into accessible and nonaccessible pools. A drug (or drug metabolite) in this pool interacts with other components of the system. The difference between noncompartmental and compartmental models is the way in which the nonaccessible portion of the system is described.

The pharmacokinetic parameters defined in the following section characterize both the accessible pool and the system parameters—that is, parameters that characterize the accessible and nonaccessible pools together. This situation is illustrated by the two models shown in Figure 8.1. Panel A normally accommodates the situation in which the accessible pool is plasma, and input and sampling occur in this pool. Panel B accommodates extravascular input (e.g., oral or subcutaneous injection), but it can also accommodate the situation in which the input is intravascular and only urine data are collected. Thus, the schematic in Figure 8.1 describes the experimental situation for most pharmacokinetic studies.

Accessible Pool Parameters

The pharmacokinetic parameters descriptive of the accessible pool are as follows. These definitions apply both to noncompartmental and compartmental models. How they relate to the situation where there are two accessible pools will be discussed for the individual cases.

Volume of distribution: V_a (units: volume). The volume of the accessible pool is a volume in which the drug upon introduction into the system intermixes uniformly (kinetically homogeneous) and instantaneously.

Clearance rate: CL_a (units: volume/time). This is the rate at which the accessible pool is irreversibly cleared of drug per unit time.

Elimination rate constant: k_e (units: 1/time). This is the fraction of drug that is irreversibly cleared from the accessible pool per unit time. (In some literature, this is referred to as the fractional clearance or fractional catabolic rate.)

Mean residence time: MRT_a (units: time). This is the average time a drug spends in the accessible pool during all passages through the system before being irreversibly cleared.

System Parameters

The pharmacokinetic parameters descriptive of the system are defined in this section. Although these definitions apply both to the noncompartmental and compartmental models, some modification will be needed for two accessible pool models as well as compartmental models.

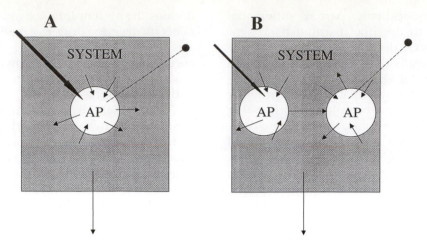

FIGURE 8.1   Panel A: A system in which an accessible pool (AP) is available for test input *(bold arrow)* and sampling *(dashed line with bullet)*. Loss of material from the system is indicated by the arrow leaving the system box. Material exchanging between the accessible pool and the rest of the system is indicated by the small arrows leaving and entering the accessible pool. The pharmacokinetic parameters estimated from kinetic data characterize the accessible pool and the system in which the accessible pool is embedded. Panel B: A system in which there are two accessible pools one of which is available for test input *(bold arrow)* and a second that is available for sampling *(dashed line with bullet)*; the test input is transported to the second accessible pool as indicated by the transfer arrow. Other transfer arrows are as explained in Panel A.

Total equivalent volume of distribution: V_{tot} (units: volume). This is the total volume of the system seen from the accessible pool; it is the volume in which the total amount of drug would be distributed assuming the concentration of material throughout the system is uniform and equal to the concentration in the accessible pool.

System mean residence time: MRT_s (units: time). This is the average time the drug spends in the system before leaving the system for the last time.

Mean residence time outside the accessible pool: MRT_o (units: time). This is the average time the drug spends outside the accessible pool before leaving the system for the last time.

Bioavailability: F (units: dimensionless). This is the fraction of drug that appears in a second accessible pool following administration in a first accessible pool.

Absorption rate constant: k_a (units: 1/time). This is the fraction of drug that appears per unit time in a second accessible pool following administration in a first accessible pool.

Moments

Moments of a function will play an essential role in estimating specific pharmacokinetic parameters. The modern use of moments in the analysis of pharmacokinetic data and the notions of noncompartmental or integral equation analysis can be traced to Yamaoka et al. (10), although these authors correctly

point out that the formulas were known since the late 1930s.

The moments of a function are defined as follows; how they are used will be described later. Suppose $C(t)$ is a real-valued function defined on the interval $(0, \infty)$; in this chapter, $C(t)$ will be used to denote a functional description of a set of pharmacokinetic data. The zeroth, first, and second moments of $C(t)$, denoted S_0, S_1 and S_2, are defined:

$$S_0 = \int_0^\infty C(t)dt = AUC \qquad (8.2)$$

$$S_1 = \int_0^\infty t \cdot C(t)dt = AUMC \qquad (8.3)$$

$$S_2 = \int_0^\infty t^2 \cdot C(t)dt \qquad (8.4)$$

In these equations, the first and second moments, S_0 and S_1, are also defined as *AUC*, "area under the curve," and *AUMC*, "area under the first moment curve." *AUC* and *AUMC* are the more common expressions in pharmacokinetics and will be used in the following. The second moment, S_2, is rarely used and will not be discussed in this chapter.

The following discussion will describe how *AUC* and *AUMC* are estimated, how they are used to estimate specific pharmacokinetic parameters (including the assumptions), and what their relationship is to specific pharmacokinetic parameters estimated from compartmental models. Both moments, however, are used for other purposes. For example, *AUC* acts as a surrogate for exposure, and values of *AUC* for different dos-

A   B

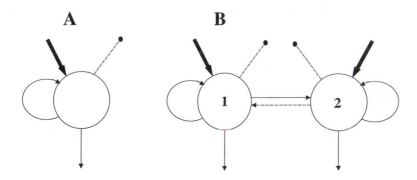

FIGURE 8.2 The single *(Panel A)* and two *(Panel B)* accessible pool models. See text for explanation.

ing schemes have been used to justify assumptions of linearity of the system in which a drug distributes. These uses will not be reviewed.

NONCOMPARTMENTAL ANALYSIS

The Noncompartmental Model

The noncompartmental model provides a framework to introduce and use statistical moment analysis to estimate pharmacokinetic parameters. There are basically two forms of the noncompartmental model: the single accessible pool model and the two accessible pool model. These are schematized in Figure 8.2.

What is the relationship between the situation described in Figure 8.1 and the two models shown in Figure 8.2? Consider first the single accessible pool model shown in Figure 8.2, Panel A. The accessible pool here, denoted by the circle into which drug is input (*bold arrow*) and from which samples are taken (*dotted line with bullet*) is the same as that shown in the corresponding panel of Figure 8.1. The entire interaction of the accessible pool with the rest of the system is indicated by the arrow leaving and returning to the accessible pool. This is called the *recirculation-exchange* arrow, and encompasses all interactions the drug has in the system outside of the accessible pool. Notice that a drug introduced into this pool has two routes by which it can leave the accessible pool. One is via recirculation-exchange, and the other is via irreversible loss, denoted by the arrow leaving the accessible pool. As indicated in Figure 8.2, Panel A, drug can only enter and leave the accessible pool. Drug can neither enter nor leave the system along the recirculation-exchange arrow. This is called the equivalent sink and source constraint, and is fundamental in understanding the domain of validity of the pharmacokinetic parameters estimated from this model (2). The single accessible pool model is used primarily

when the accessible pool is plasma, and the drug is administered directly into plasma.

The situation depicted in Figure 8.2, Panel B, the two accessible pool model, derives in a similar fashion from the model shown in Panel B in Figure 8.1. The difference between the single and two accessible pool models is the following. While both pools have recirculation-exchange arrows, material can flow from pool 1 to pool 2. This model is used to describe extravascular drug input or a situation in which both plasma and urine data are collected.

Note that there is a dotted arrow from pool 2 to pool 1 in Figure 8.2, Panel B. This indicates that exchange can occur in this direction also. Although analysis of this exchange is frequently incorporated in metabolic kinetic studies, there are relatively few examples in pharmacokinetics where this has been studied. It is essential to note that this arrow is not equivalent to an arrow in a multicompartmental model! This arrow represents transfer of material from pool 1 to pool 2 by whatever routes exist; it can be a composite of many activities, including delays.

The two accessible pool model accommodates a more complex experimental format than the single pool model. For example, one could have inputs into both pools and samples from both as well. However, in most pharmacokinetic studies with the two accessible pool model, pool 2 is plasma and input is only into pool 1. In this situation, the pharmacokinetic parameters depend on bioavailability and can only be estimated up to a proportionality constant.

Kinetic Parameters of the Noncompartmental Model

The kinetic parameters of the noncompartmental model are those defined previously for the accessible pool and system. However, the formulas depend on the experimental protocol, especially on the route by which the drug is administered. In this chapter, only the canonical inputs will be considered—that is, the bolus (or multiple boluses) or constant infusion (or multiple constant infusions). References will be given for those interested in more complex protocols.

The relationships among the accessible pool parameters in the noncompartmental model are are given in the following equations.

$$k_e = \frac{CL_a}{V_a} \tag{8.5}$$

$$MRT_a = \frac{1}{k_e} \tag{8.6}$$

Equation 8.5 can be rearranged to yield

$$k_e \cdot V_a = CL_a \tag{8.5'}$$

In addition, Equations 8.5 and 8.6 can be combined to yield the more familiar

$$V_a = MRT_a \cdot CL_a \tag{8.7}$$

The relationships among the system parameters for the noncompartmental model are:

$$V_{tot} = MRT_s \cdot CL_a \tag{8.8}$$

$$MRT_o = MRT_s - MRT_a \tag{8.9}$$

The Single Accessible Pool Model

Assume a single bolus injection of drug whose amount is denoted by d or a constant infusion of drug whose infusion rate is u over the time domain [0, t]. Then:

Bolus	Infusion	
$V_a = \dfrac{d}{C(0)}$	$V_a = \dfrac{u}{\dot{C}(0)}$	(8.10)
$CL_a = \dfrac{d}{AUC}$	$CL_a = \dfrac{u}{\bar{C}}$	(8.11)
$MRT_a = \dfrac{AUMC}{AUC}$	$MRT_s = \dfrac{\int_0^\infty [\bar{C} - C(t)]dt}{\bar{C}}$	(8.12)

In these formulas, $C(0)$ is the concentration of drug in the system at time zero, $\dot{C}(0)$ is the first derivative of $C(t)$ evaluated at time zero, and $\bar{C}$ is the steady-state value for the concentration of drug in the accessible pool following a constant infusion into that pool.

The remaining single accessible pool parameters, k_e, V_{tot}, and MRT_o can be calculated for either method of input using Equations 8.5, 8.6, and 8.9.

Although these formulas are for the single input format, formulas also exist for generic inputs including multiple boluses or infusions. If $u(t)$ is a generic input function, the formulas for V_a, CL_a, and MRT are:

$$V_a = \frac{u(0)}{\dot{C}(0)} \tag{8.13}$$

$$CL_a = \frac{\int_0^\infty u(t)dt}{AUC} \tag{8.14}$$

$$MRT_s = \frac{\int_0^\infty t \cdot C(t)dt}{AUC} - \frac{\int_0^\infty t \cdot u(t)dt}{\int_0^\infty u(t)dt} \tag{8.15}$$

What is the origin of these formulas? That is, how are Equations 8.10–8.12, and 8.13–8.15 obtained? The answer is not obvious. Weiss (11) presents an excellent description of mean residence times and points out that, besides an accessible pool that must be available for test input and measurement, the system must be linear and time-invariant for the equations to be valid. The notions of linearity and time-invariance will be discussed in more detail below. For a formal derivation of these equations, the reader is referred to Weiss (11), Covell et al. (4), or Cobelli et al. (12). An understanding of the derivations is absolutely essential to understanding the domain of validity of the pharmacokinetic parameters obtained by noncompartmental methods no matter what method of evaluating the integrals or extrapolations is employed.

The Two Accessible Pool Model

The two accessible pool model presents problems in estimating the pharmacokinetic parameters characterizing this situation. This is largely because the desired parameters such as clearance, volumes, and residence times cannot be estimated from a single input (into the first pool)–single output (samples from the second pool) experiment. To deal with this situation, recall first the notion of absolute bioavailability originally discussed in Chapter 4. Let D_{oral} be the total dose of drug input into the first accessible pool, and let D_{iv} be the dose into the second accessible pool, assumed to be plasma. Let $AUC\{2\}$ be the area under the concentration-time curve in the second accessible pool following the dose D_{oral} (this is AUC_{oral} in the notation of Chapter 4), and let AUC_{iv} be the area under the concentration-time curve in the second accessible pool following the bolus dose D_{iv} (in a separate experiment). The absolute bioavailability is defined:

$$F = \frac{AUC\{2\}}{AUC_{iv}} \cdot \frac{D_{iv}}{D_{oral}} \tag{8.16}$$

The following parameters can be calculated from data following a bolus injection into the first accessible pool. Let $CL\{2\}$ and $V\{2\}$ respectively be the clearance from and volume of the second accessible pool, and let $CL\{2,rel\}$ and $V\{2,rel\}$ be the "relative" clearance from and volume of the second accessible pool. Then

$$MRT\{2,1\} = \frac{\int_0^\infty tC\{2\}(t)dt}{\int_0^\infty C\{2\}(t)dt} \qquad (8.17)$$

$$CL\{2,rel\} = \frac{CL\{2\}}{F} = \frac{D_{oral}}{AUC\{2\}} \qquad (8.18)$$

$$V\{2,rel\} = \frac{V\{2\}}{F} = CL\{2,rel\} \cdot MRT\{2,1\} \qquad (8.19)$$

$MRT\{2,1\}$ is the mean residence time of drug in the second accessible pool following introduction of drug into the first accessible pool.

Clearly this situation is not as rich in information as the single accessible pool situation. Of course the parameters $CL\{2\}$ and $V\{2\}$ can be calculated in the event that F is known or when a separate intravenous dose is administered. Information on other input formats or the situation when there is a two input-four output experiment can be found in Cobelli et al. (12).

Estimating the Kinetic Parameters of the Noncompartmental Model

For the canonical input of drug, what information is needed? For the bolus input, an estimate of the drug concentration at time zero, $C(0)$, is needed in order to estimate V_a. For a constant infusion of drug, an estimate of $\dot{C}(0)$ is needed to estimate V_a, and an estimate of the plateau value $\bar{C}$ is needed to estimate clearance and the system mean residence time.

The most important estimates, however, involve AUC and $AUMC$. These integrals are from time zero to time infinity while an experiment is over a finite time domain $[0, t_n]$ where t_n is the time of the last measurable datum. In addition, it is rarely the case that the first datum is obtained at time zero. Hence, assuming that the time of the first measurable datum is t_1, one must divide the integral as follows to estimate AUC and $AUMC$:

$$AUC = \int_0^\infty C(t)dt = \int_0^{t_1} C(t)dt + \int_{t_1}^{t_n} C(t)dt + \int_{t_n}^\infty C(t)dt \qquad (8.20)$$

$$AUMC = \int_0^\infty t \cdot C(t)dt = \int_0^{t_1} t \cdot C(t)dt +$$
$$\int_{t_1}^{t_n} t \cdot C(t)dt + \int_{t_n}^\infty t \cdot C(t)dt \qquad (8.21)$$

Estimating AUC and AUMC Using Sums of Exponentials

For the single accessible pool model, following a bolus injection of amount D into the pool, the pharmacokinetic data can be described by a sum of exponentials equation of the general form shown in Equation (8.22).

$$C(t) = A_1 e^{-\lambda_1 t} + \dots + A_n e^{-\lambda_n t} \qquad (8.22)$$

In this and subsequent equations, the A_i are called *coefficients* and the λ_i are *exponentials* (in mathematical parlance, they are called *eigenvalues*). Following a constant infusion into the accessible pool, Equation 8.22 changes to Equation 8.23 with the restriction that the sum of the coefficients equals zero reflecting the fact that no drug is present in the system at time zero.

$$C(t) = A_0 + A_1 e^{-\lambda_1 t} + \dots + A_n e^{-\lambda_n t} \qquad (8.23)$$
$$A_0 + A_1 + \dots + A_n = 0$$

What is the advantage of using sums of exponentials to describe pharmacokinetic data in the situation of the single accessible pool model following a bolus or constant infusion? The reason is that the integrals required to estimate the pharmacokinetic parameters are very easy to calculate!

For the bolus injection, from Equation 8.22,

$$AUC = \int_0^\infty C(t)dt = \frac{A_1}{\lambda_1} + \dots + \frac{A_n}{\lambda_n} \qquad (8.24)$$

$$AUMC = \int_0^\infty t \cdot C(t)dt = \frac{A_1}{\lambda_1^2} + \dots + \frac{A_n}{\lambda_n^2} \qquad (8.25)$$

In addition, for the bolus injection,

$$C(0) = A_1 + \dots + A_n \qquad (8.26)$$

provides an estimates for $C(0)$. Thus, with a knowledge of the amount in the bolus, D, all pharmacokinetic parameters can be estimated.

For the constant infusion, the steady state concentration, $\bar{C}$ can be seen from Equation 8.23 to equal A_0. An estimate for $\dot{C}(0)$ can be obtained

$$\dot{C}(0) = -A_1\lambda_1 - \dots - A_n\lambda_n \qquad (8.27)$$

and since the estimate for $\bar{C}$ is A_0,

$$\int_0^\infty [\bar{C} - C(t)]dt = \frac{A_1}{\lambda_1} + \dots + \frac{A_n}{\lambda_n} \qquad (8.28)$$

Thus, all the pharmacokinetic parameters for the constant infusion can easily be estimated.

An advantage of using sums of exponentials is that error estimates for all the pharmacokinetic parameters can also be obtained as part of the fitting process; this is not the case for most of the so-called numerical techniques (see the following section). In addition, for multiple inputs (i.e., multiple boluses or infusions) sums of exponentials can be used over each experimental time period for a specific bolus or infusion recognizing that the exponentials, the λ_i, remain the same. The reason is that the exponentials are system parameters and do not depend on a particular mode of introducing drug into the system (13).

Estimating AUC and AUMC Using Other Functions

Although sums of exponentials may seem the logical function to use to describe $C(t)$ and hence estimate AUC

and *AUMC*, the literature is full of other recommendations for estimating *AUC* and *AUMC* [see, for example, Yeh and Kwan (14) or Purves (15)]. These include the trapezoidal rule, the log-trapezoidal rule, a combination of the two, splines, and Lagrangians, among others. All result in formulas for calculations over the time domain of the data, and are left with the problem of estimating the integrals $\int_{t_n}^{\infty} C(t)dt$ and $\int_{t_n}^{\infty} t \cdot C(t)dt$. The difficulty of estimating $\int_{0}^{t_1} C(t)dt$ and $\int_{0}^{t_1} t \cdot C(t)dt$ and estimating a value for $C(0), \dot{C}(0)$, or $\bar{C}$ is rarely discussed.

There are two problems with this approach. First, estimating *AUMC* is very difficult. Although one hopes that the experiment has been designed so that $\int_{t_n}^{\infty} C(t)dt$ contributes 5% or less to *AUC*, $\int_{t_n}^{\infty} C(t)dt$ can contribute as much as 50% or more to *AUMC* and hence estimates of *AUMC* are subject to large errors. The second problem is that it is extremely difficult to obtain error estimates for *AUC* and *AUMC* that will translate into error estimates for the pharmacokinetic parameters derived from them. As a result, it is normal practice in individual studies to ignore error estimates for these parameters and hence the pharmacokinetic parameters that rely on them. One tries to circumvent the statistical nature of the problem by conducting repeated studies and basing the statistics on averages and standard errors of the mean.

Estimating $\int_{t_1}^{t_n} C(t)dt$ and $\int_{t_1}^{t_n} t \cdot C(t)dt$

In what follows, some comments will be made on the commonly used functional approaches to estimating $\int_{t_1}^{t_n} C(t)dt$ and $\int_{t_1}^{\infty} t \cdot C(t)dt$ (i.e., the trapezoidal rule, or a combination of the trapezoidal and log-trapezoidal rule) (15, 16). Other methods such as splines and Lagrangians will not be discussed. The interested reader is referred to Yeh and Kwan (14) and Purves (15).

Suppose $[(y_{obs}(t_i),t_i)]_{i=1}^{n}$ is a set of pharmacokinetic data. For example, this can be n plasma samples starting with the first measurable sample being at time t_1 and the last measurable sample at time t_n. If $[t_{i-1}, t_i]$ is the ith interval, then the *AUC* and *AUMC* for this interval calculated using the trapezoidal rule are:

$$AUC_{i-1}^{i} = \frac{1}{2}[y_{obs}(t_i) + y_{obs}(t_{i-1})](t_i - t_{i-1}) \qquad (8.29)$$

$$AUMC_{i-1}^{i} = \frac{1}{2}[t_i \cdot y_{obs}(t_i) + t_{i-1} \cdot y_{obs}(t_{i-1})](t_i - t_{i-1}) \qquad (8.30)$$

For the log-trapezoidal rule, the formulas are:

$$AUC_{i-1}^{i} = \frac{1}{\ln\left(\dfrac{y_{obs}(t_i)}{y_{obs}(t_{i-1})}\right)}[y_{obs}(t_i) + y_{obs}(t_{i-1})](t_i - t_{i-1}) \qquad (8.31)$$

$$AUMC_{i-1}^{i} = \frac{1}{\ln\left(\dfrac{y_{obs}(t_i)}{y_{obs}(t_{i-1})}\right)} [t_i \cdot y_{obs}(t_i) + t_{i-1} \cdot y_{obs}(t_{i-1})](t_i - t_{i-1}) \qquad (8.31)$$

One method by which *AUC* and *AUMC* can be estimated from t_1 to t_n is to use the trapezoidal rule and add up the individual terms AUC_{i-1}^{i} and $AUMC_{i-1}^{i}$. If one chooses this approach, then it is possible to obtain an error estimate for *AUC* and *AUMC* using the method proposed by Katz and D'Argenio (17). Other approaches use a combination of the trapezoidal and log-trapezoidal formulas. The idea here is that the trapezoidal approximation is a good approximation when $y_{obs}(t_i) \geq Y_{obs}(t_{i-1})$ (i.e., when the data are rising), and the log-trapezoidal rule is a better approximation when $Y_{obs}(t_i) < Y_{obs}(t_{i-1})$ (i.e., the data are falling). The rationale is that the log-trapezoidal formula takes into account some of the curvature in the falling portion of the curve. If a combination of the two formulas is used, it is not possible to obtain an error estimate for *AUC* and *AUMC* from t_1 to t_n using the quadrature method of Katz and D'Argenio.

The software system WinNonlin (18) uses a combination of the trapezoidal and log-trapezoidal formulas to estimate *AUC* and *AUMC* and the formulas resulting from them. As a result, no statistical information is available.

Extrapolating from t_n to Infinity

One now has to deal with estimating $\int_{t_n}^{\infty} C(t)dt$ and $\int_{t_n}^{\infty} t \cdot C(t)dt$. The most common way to estimate these integrals is to assume that the data decay monoexponentially beyond the last measurement at time t_n. Such a function can be written:

$$y(t) = A_z e^{-\lambda_z t} \qquad (8.33)$$

Here the exponent λ_z characterizes the terminal decay and is used to calculate the half-life of the terminal decay

$$t_{z,1/2} = \frac{\ln(2)}{\lambda_z} \qquad (8.34)$$

Estimates for the integrals can be based on the last datum [i.e., assuming the monoexponential decay is from the last datum $y_{obs}(t_n)$]:

$$AUC_{extrap-dat} = \int_{t_n}^{\infty} C(t)dt = \frac{y_{obs}(t_n)}{\lambda_z} \qquad (8.35)$$

$$AUMC_{extrap-dat} = \int_{t_n}^{\infty} t \cdot C(t)dt = \frac{t_n \cdot y_{obs}(t_n)}{\lambda_z} + \frac{y_{obs}(t_n)}{\lambda_z^2} \qquad (8.36)$$

or from the model calculated "last datum":

$$AUC_{extrap-calc} = \int_{t_n}^{\infty} C(t)dt = \frac{A_z e^{-\lambda_z t_n}}{\lambda_z} \qquad (8.37)$$

$$AUMC_{extrap-calc} = \int_{t_n}^{\infty} t \cdot C(t)dt = \frac{t_n \cdot A_z e^{-\lambda_z t_n}}{\lambda_z} + \frac{A_z e^{-\lambda_z t_n}}{\lambda_z^2} \qquad (8.38)$$

There are a variety of ways that one can estimate λ_z. Most rely on the fact that the last two or three data decay exponentially, and thus Equation 8.33 can be fitted to these data. Various options for including or excluding other data have been proposed [e.g., Gabrielsson and Weiner (16), Marino et al. (19)]. These will not be discussed here. What is certain is that all parameters and area estimates will have statistical information since they are obtained by fitting Equation 8.33 to the data.

It is of interest to note that an estimate for λ_z could differ from λ_n, the terminal slope of a multiexponential function describing the pharmacokinetic data. The reason is that all data are considered in estimating λ_n as opposed to a finite (terminal) subset used to estimate λ_z. Thus, a researcher checking both methods should not be surprised if there are slight differences.

Estimating AUC and AUMC from Zero to Infinity

Estimating AUC and $AUMC$ from zero to infinity is now simply a matter of adding the two components (i.e., the AUC and $AUMC$) over the time domain of the data and the extrapolation from the last datum to infinity. The zero time value is handled in a number of ways. For the bolus injection, it can be estimated using a modification of the methodology used to estimate λ_z. In this way, statistical information on $C(0)$ would be available. Otherwise, if an arbitrary value is assigned, no such information is available.

Error estimates for the pharmacokinetic parameters will be available only if error estimates for AUC and $AUMC$ are calculated. In general, this will not be the case when numerical formulas are used over the time domain of the data. Performing studies on several individuals and obtaining averages and standard errors of the mean on these individuals essentially begs the question. With all the limitations, it is somewhat surprising that sums of exponentials are not used as the function of choice, especially since the canonical inputs, boluses and infusions, are the most common ways to introduce a drug into the system.

COMPARTMENTAL ANALYSIS

Definitions and Assumptions

As noted in the introduction, it is very difficult to use partial differential equations to describe the kinetics of a

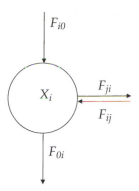

FIGURE 8.3 The ith compartment of an n-compartment model. See text for explanation.

drug. A convenient way to deal with this situation is to lump portions of the system into discrete entities and then discuss movement of material among these entities. These lumped portions of the system essentially contain the same material whose kinetics share a similar time frame. Thus, the lumping is a combination of known physiology and biochemistry on the one hand, and the time frame of a particular experiment on the other.

Compartmental models are the mathematical result of such lumping. A *compartment* is an amount of material that is kinetically homogeneous. *Kinetic homogeneity* means that material introduced into a compartment mixes instantaneously, and that each particle in the compartment has the same probability as all other particles in the compartment of leaving the compartment along the various exit pathways from the compartment. A *compartmental model* consists of a finite number of compartments with specified interconnections, inputs, and losses.

Let $X_i(t)$ be the mass of a drug in the ith compartment. The notation for input, loss, and transfers is summarized in Figure 8.3. Because this notation describes the compartment in full generality it is a little different from that used in earlier chapters. This difference is necessary to understand how one passes to the linear compartmental model. In Figure 8.3, the F_{pq} describe mathematically the mass transfer of material among compartments interacting with the ith compartment (F_{ji} is transfer of material from compartment i to compartment j, F_{ij} is the transfer of material from compartment j to compartment i), the new input F_{i0} (this corresponds to X_0 in Chapter 4) and loss to the environment F_{i0} from compartment i. The mathematical expression describing the rate of change for $X_i(t)$ is derived from the mass balance equation:

$$\frac{dX_i(t)}{dt} = \frac{dX_i}{dt} = \sum_{\substack{j=0 \\ j \neq i}}^{n} F_{ij} - \sum_{\substack{j=0 \\ j \neq i}}^{n} F_{ji} \qquad (8.39)$$

There are several important features to understand about the F_{ij} that derive from the fact the compartmental model is being used to describe a biological system and hence conservation of mass must be obeyed. First, the F_{ij} must be nonnegative for all times t (assumed to be between time zero and infinity). In fact, the F_{ij} can be either stochastic (have uncertainty associated with them) or deterministic (the form known exactly). In this chapter, the F_{ij} will be assumed to be deterministic, but can be functions of the X_i and/or time t. [Readers interested in stochastic compartmental models can find references to numerous articles in Covell et al. (4)]. Second, as pointed out by Jacquez and Simon (5), if $X_i = 0$ then $F_{ji} = 0$ for all $j \neq i$ and hence $dX_i/dt \geq 0$. An important consequence of this, as shown by these authors, is that the F_{ji}, with the exception of F_{i0} which remains unchanged, can be written:

$$F_{ji}(\vec{X}, \vec{p}, t) = k_{ji}(\vec{X}, \vec{p}, t) \cdot X_i(t) \qquad (8.40)$$

The function F_{i0} is either a constant or a function of t alone. The k_{ji} written in this format are called the *fractional transfer functions*. Equation 8.40 is a subtle but important step in moving from the general compartment model to the linear, constant coefficient model because it shows explicitly that the fractional transfers can be functions and not necessarily constants, and that, as functions, the mass terms can be split out from the fractional transfer term. In Equation 8.40, $\vec{X} = (X_1, ..., X_n)$ is a notation for compartmental masses (mathematically it is called a vector), $\vec{p}$ is a descriptor of other elements such as pH and temperature that control the system, and t is time. Written in this format, Equation 8.39 becomes

$$\frac{dX_i}{dt} = -\left(\sum_{\substack{j=0 \\ j \neq i}}^{n} k_{ji}(\vec{X}, \vec{p}, t) \right) X_i(t) \qquad (8.41)$$

$$+ \sum_{\substack{j=1 \\ j \neq i}}^{n} k_{ij}(\vec{X}, \vec{p}, t) X_j(t) + F_{i0}$$

Define

$$k_{ii}(\vec{X}, \vec{p}, t) = -\left(\sum_{\substack{j=0 \\ j \neq i}}^{n} k_{ji}(\vec{X}, \vec{p}, t) \right) \qquad (8.42)$$

and write

$$K(\vec{X}, \vec{p}, t) = \begin{bmatrix} k_{11} & k_{12} & \cdots & k_{1n} \\ k_{21} & k_{22} & \cdots & k_{2n} \\ \vdots & \vdots & \ddots & \vdots \\ k_{n1} & k_{n2} & \cdots & k_{nn} \end{bmatrix} \qquad (8.43)$$

where in the previous definition the individual terms of the matrix, for convenience, do not contain the $(\vec{X},$ $\vec{p}, t)$. The matrix $K(\vec{X}, \vec{p}, t)$ is called the *compartmental matrix*. This matrix is key to deriving many kinetic parameters and in making the link between compartmental and noncompartmental analysis.

There are several reasons for going first to this level of generality for the n-compartment model. First, it points out clearly that the theories of noncompartmental and compartmental models are very different. Although the theory underlying noncompartmental models relies more on statistical theory, especially in developing residence time concepts [see, e.g., Weiss (11)], the theory underlying compartmental models is really the theory of ordinary, first-order differential equations in which, because of the nature of the compartmental model applied to biological applications, there are special features in the theory. These are reviewed in detail in Jacquez and Simon (5), who also refer to the many texts and research articles on the subject.

Second, this gets at the complexity involved in postulating the structure of a compartmental model to describe the kinetics of a particular drug. As illustrated by the presentation in Chapter 3, it is very difficult to postulate a model structure in which the model compartments have physiological relevance as opposed simply to representing the mathematical construct X_i, especially when one is dealing with the single input–single output experiment. This will be discussed in more detail. However, while the most general compartmental model must be appreciated in its application in interpreting kinetic data, the fact is that such models are not often used. The most common models are the linear, constant coefficient compartmental models described in the next section. In this discussion, it will be assumed that all systems are open (i.e., drug introduced into the system will eventually leave the system). This means that some special situations discussed by Jacquez and Simon (5) do not have to be considered (i.e., compartmental models with submodels from which material cannot escape).

Linear, Constant Coefficient Compartmental Models

Suppose the compartmental matrix is a constant matrix—that is, all k_{ij} are constants. In this situation, one can write K instead of $K(\vec{X}, \vec{p}, t)$ to indicate that the elements of the matrix no longer depend on $(\vec{X}, \vec{p}, t)$. As will be seen, there are several important features of the K matrix that will be used in recovering pharmacokinetic parameters of interest. In addition, as described in Jacquez and Simon (5) and Covell et al. (4), the solution to the compartmental equations (a system of linear, constant coefficient equations) involves sums of exponentials.

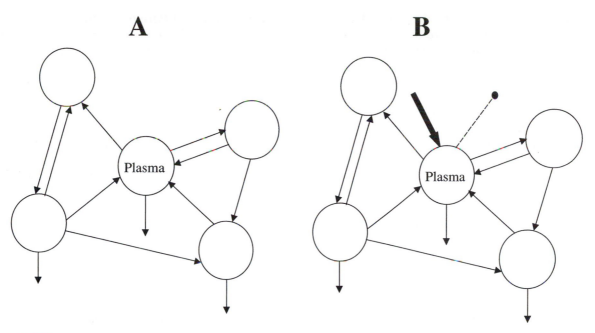

A

B

FIGURE 8.4   *Panel A:* A compartmental model of drug behavior in the body. *Panel B:* An experimental protocol on the model in Panel A showing drug administration *(bold arrow)* and plasma sampling *(dashed line with bullet).*

What is needed for the compartmental matrix to be constant? Recall that the individual elements of the matrix k_{ij} ($\vec{X}$, $\vec{p}$, t) are functions of several variables. For the k_{ij} ($\vec{X}$, $\vec{p}$, t) to be constant, $\vec{X}$ and $\vec{p}$ must be constant (actually, this assumption can be relaxed, but, for the purposes of this chapter, constancy will be assumed) and the k_{ij} ($\vec{X}$, $\vec{p}$, t) cannot depend explicitly on time—that is, the k_{ij} ($\vec{X}$, $\vec{p}$, t) are time invariant. Notice with this concept that the time-invariant k_{ij} ($\vec{X}$, $\vec{p}$, t) can assume different values depending on the constant values for $\vec{X}$ and $\vec{p}$. This leads naturally to the concept of the steady state.

Under what circumstances are compartmental models linear, constant coefficient? This normally depends on a particular experimental design. The reason is that most biological systems, including those in which drugs are analyzed, are inherently nonlinear. However, the assumption of linearity holds reasonably well over the dose range studied for most drugs, and most pharmacokinetic studies have been carried out under stable conditions of minimal physiological perturbation.

Parameters Estimated from Compartmental Models

Experimenting on Compartmental Models: Input and Measurements

In postulating a compartmental model such as that shown in Figure 8.4 Panel A, one is actually making a statement concerning how the system is believed to behave. To know if a particular model structure can predict the behavior of a drug in the body, one must be able to obtain kinetic data from which the parameters characterizing the system of differential equations can be estimated; the model predictions can then be compared against the data. Experiments are designed to generate the data; the experiment must then be reproduced on the model. This is done by specifying inputs and samples, as shown in Panel B of Figure 8.4. More specifically, the input specifies the F_{i0} terms in the differential equations, and the samples provide the measurement equations that link the model's predictions, which are in units normally of drug mass, with the samples, which are usually in concentration units.

To emphasize this point, once a model structure is postulated, the compartmental matrix is known since it depends only on the transfers and losses. The input, the F_{i0}, comes from the experimental input and thus is determined by the investigator. In addition, the units of the differential equation, (i.e., the units of the X_i) are determined by the units of the input. The point is that if the parameters of the model can be estimated from the data from a particular experimental design [i.e., if the model is a priori identifiable, see Carson et al. (20), Cobelli et al. (12)], then the specific form of the input is not important. Thus, the data from a bolus or constant infusion should be equally rich from an information point of view.

The final point to make in dealing with experiments on the model relates to the measurement variable(s). The units of the X_i are determined by the experimental input vector, and are usually mass. The units of the data are normally concentration. No matter what the units of the data, there must be a measurement equation linking the X_i involved in the measurement with the data. For example, if the measurement was taken from compartment 1 and the units of the data are concentration, one would need to write the measurement equation

$$C_1(t) = \frac{X_1}{V_1} \qquad (8.44)$$

Here V_1 is the volume of compartment 1, and is a parameter to be estimated from the data.

Clearly, once a compartmental structure is postulated, there are many experimental protocols and measurement variables that can be accommodated. One just needs to be sure that the parameters characterizing the compartmental matrix, K, and the parameters characterizing the measurement variables can be estimated from the data generated by the experiment.

Nonlinearities in Compartmental Models

Some fractional transfer functions of compartmental models may actually be functions, (i.e., the model may actually be nonlinear). The most common example is when a transfer or loss is saturable. Here a Michaelis–Menten type of transfer function can be defined, as was shown in Chapter 2 for the elimination of phenytoin. In this case, loss from compartment 1 is concentration dependent and saturable, and one can write

$$CL_1 = k_{01} \cdot V_1 = \frac{V_{max}}{K_m + C_1} \qquad (8.45)$$

where V_{max} and K_m are parameters that can be estimated from the pharmacokinetic data. In the differential equation dX_1/dt, this will result in the term

$$-k_{01} \cdot X_1 = -\frac{V_{max}}{K_m + C_1} \cdot C_1 \qquad (8.45)$$

In addition, an example of a function-dependent transfer function is given in Chapter 6 in which hemodynamic changes during and after hemodialysis reduce the intercompartmental clearance of N-acetylprocainamide between the intravascular space and a peripheral compartment.

If one has pharmacokinetic data and knows that the situation calls for nonlinear kinetics, then compartmental models, no matter how difficult to postulate, are really required. Noncompartmental models cannot deal with the time-varying situation.

Calculating Model Parameters from a Compartmental Model

Realizing the full generality of the compartmental model, consider now only the limited situation of linear, constant coefficient models. What parameters can be calculated from a model? The answer to this question can be addressed in the context of Figure 8.5.

Model Parameters

Once a specific multicompartmental structure has been developed to explain the pharmacokinetics of a particular drug, the parameters characterizing this model are the components of the compartmental matrix, K, and the volume parameters associated with the individual measurements. The components of the compartmental matrix are the rate constants k_{ij}. Together, these constitute the primary *mathematical* parameters of the model. The primary *physiological* parameters of clearance and distribution volume are secondary from a mathematical standpoint. For this reason, the mathematical parameters of compartmental models need to be reparameterized in order to recover these physiological parameters (e.g., see Figure 3.8). Although this works relatively well for simple models, it becomes a very difficult exercise once one moves to more complex models.

The next question is whether the parameters characterizing a model can be estimated from a set of pharmacokinetic data. The answer to the question has two parts. The first is called *a priori identifiability*. This answers the question: given a particular model structure and experimental design, if the data are "perfect", can the model parameters be estimated? The second is *a posteriori identifiability*. This answers the question: given a particular model structure and a set of pharmacokinetic data, can the model parameters be estimated within reasonable degree of statistical precision?

A priori identifiability is a critical part of model development. Although the answer to the question for many of the simpler models used in pharmacokinetics is well known, the general answer, even for linear, constant coefficient models, is more difficult (12). Figure 8.6 illustrates the situation with some specific model structures; the interested reader is referred to Cobelli et al. (12) for precise details. The model shown in Panel A is a standard two-compartment model with input and sampling from a "plasma" compartment. There are three k_{ij} and a volume term to be estimated. This model can be shown to be a priori identifiable. The model shown in Panel B has four k_{ij} and a volume term to be estimated. These parameters cannot be estimated from a single set of pharmacokinetic data, no matter how information rich they are. In fact, there is an infinite number of values for

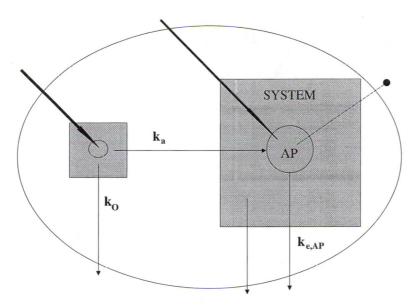

FIGURE 8.5 The system model shown on the right contains an accessible pool embedded in an arbitrary multicompartmental model indicated by the shaded box. The drug can be introduced directly into this pool as indicated by the bold arrow. The drug can also be introduced into a second compartment indicated by the circle in the small, shaded box. Drug can move from this compartment as denoted by the arrow passing through the shaded small box and large box into the accessible pool. The rate is denoted k_a. Material also can be lost from the small box; this is denoted k_o. Finally, material has two ways by which it can leave the system. One is directly from the accessible pool, $k_{e, AP}$, and the other is from nonaccessible pools denoted by the arrow leaving the large box. That both small and large boxes exist in a larger system is denoted by the ellipse surrounding the individual components of the system. See text for additional explanation.

the k_{ij} and volume term that will produce the same fit of the data. If one insists on using this model structure, then some constraint will have to be placed on the parameters, such as fixing the volume or defining a relationship among the k_{ij}. The model shown in Panel C, while a priori identifiable, will have a different compartmental matrix from the model in Panel A, and hence, as discussed previously, some of the pharmacokinetic parameters will be different between the two models.

Two commonly used three-compartment models are shown in Panels D and E. Of the two peripheral compartments, one exchanges rapidly and one slowly with the central compartment. The model shown in Panel D is a priori identifiable; the model shown in Panel E is not. The model in Panel E will have two different compartmental matrices that will produce the same fit of the data. The reason is that the loss is from a peripheral compartment.

Finally, the model shown in Panel F, a model very commonly used to describe the pharmacokinetics of drug absorption, is not a priori identifiable. Again, there are two values for the compartmental K matrix that will produce the same fit to the data.

A posteriori identifiability is linked to the theory of optimization in mathematics because one normally uses a software package that has an optimization (data fitting) capability to estimate parameter values for a multicompartmental model from a set of pharmacokinetic data. One obtains an estimate for the parameter values, an estimate for their errors, and a value for the correlation (or covariance) matrix. The details of optimization and how to deal with the output from an optimization routine are beyond the scope of this chapter, and the interested reader is referred to Cobelli et al. (12). The point to be made here is that the output from these routines is crucial in assessing the goodness-of-fit—that is, how well the model performs when compared to the data, since inferences about a drug's pharmacokinetics will be made from these parameter values.

Residence Time Calculations

The notion of residence times can be very important in assessing the pharmacokinetics of a drug. The information about residence times available from a linear, constant coefficient compartmental model is very rich, and will be reviewed in the following comments.

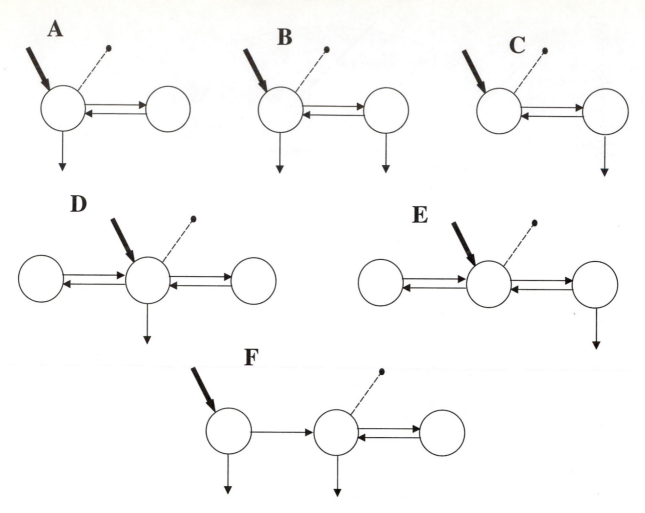

FIGURE 8.6   Examples of multicompartmental models. See text for explanation.

Residence time calculations are a direct result of manipulating the compartmental matrix K. Let $\theta = -K^{-1}$ be the negative inverse of the compartmental matrix, and let ϑ_{ij} be the ijth element of θ. The matrix θ is called the *mean residence time* matrix. The information given concerning the interpretation of this matrix comes from Covell et al. (4) and Cobelli et al. (12). Further detail is beyond the scope of this chapter and the interested reader is directed to these two references.

As explained in Covell et al. (4) and Cobelli et al. (12), the elements of the mean residence time matrix have important probabilistic interpretations. First, the generic element ϑ_{ij} represents the average time a drug particle entering the system in compartment j spends in compartment i before irreversibly leaving the system by any route. Second, the ratio $\vartheta_{ij}/\vartheta_{jj}$, $i \neq j$, equals the probability that a drug particle in compartment j will eventually reach compartment i. Finally, if a compartmental model has loss from a single compartment only, say compartment 1, then it can be shown that $k_{01} = 1/\vartheta_{11}$. Clearly, if one is analyzing pharmacokinetic data using compart-

mental models in which the K matrix is constant, this information can be critical in assessing the behavior of a particular drug.

However, more can be said about the ϑ_{ij} that is important in comparing compartmental and noncompartmental models. Suppose there is a generic input into compartment 1 only, F_{10} (remember in this situation F_{10} can be a function). Then it can be shown that the area under $X_i(t)$, the drug mass in the ith compartment, equals:

$$\int_0^\infty X_i(t)dt = \vartheta_{i1}\int_0^\infty F_{10}\,dt \qquad (8.47)$$

whence:

$$\vartheta_{i1} = \frac{\int_0^\infty X_i(t)dt}{\int_0^\infty F_{10}dt} \qquad (8.48)$$

More generally, suppose F_{j0} is an arbitrary input into compartment j, and $X_i^j(t)$ is the amount of drug in compartment i following an initial administration in compartment j. Then:

$$\vartheta_{ij} = \frac{\int_0^\infty X_i^j(t)dt}{\int_0^\infty F_{j0}dt} \qquad (8.49)$$

This equation shows that ϑ_{ij} equals the area under the model predicted drug mass curve in compartment i resulting from an input compartment j, normalized to the dose.

The use of the mean residence time matrix can be a powerful tool in pharmacokinetic analysis with a compartmental model, especially if one is dealing with a model of the system in which physiological and/or anatomical correlates are being assigned to specific compartments (2). Modeling software tools such as SAAM II (21) automatically calculate the mean residence time matrix from the compartmental matrix, making the information easily available.

NONCOMPARTMENTAL VERSUS COMPARTMENTAL MODELS

In comparing noncompartmental with compartmental models, it should now be clear that this is not a question of declaring one method better than the other. It is a question of 1) what information is desired from the data, and 2) what is the most appropriate method to obtain this information. It is hoped that the reader of this chapter will be enabled to make an informed decision on this issue.

This discussion will rely heavily on the following sources. First, the publications of DiStefano and Landaw (22, 23) deal with issues related to compartmental versus single accessible pool noncompartmental models. Second, Cobelli and Toffolo (3) discuss the two accessible pool noncompartmental model. Finally, Covell et al. (4) provide the theory to demonstrate the link between noncompartmental and compartmental models in estimating the pharmacokinetic parameters.

Models of Data vs. Models of System

Suppose one has a set of pharmacokinetic data. The question is how to obtain information related to the disposition of the drug in question from the data. DiStefano and Landaw (22) deal with this question by making the distinction between models of data and models of system. Understanding this distinction is useful in understanding the differences between compartmental and noncompartmental models.

As discussed, the noncompartmental model divides the system into two components: an accessible pool and nonaccessible pools. The kinetics of the nonaccessible pools are lumped into the recirculation-exchange arrows. From this, as has been discussed, we can esti-

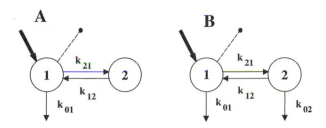

FIGURE 8.7 Two two-compartment models in which drug is administered into plasma compartment 1; samples are taken from this compartment. See text for explanation.

mate pharmacokinetic parameters describing the accessible pool and system.

What happens in the compartmental model framework? Here the most common way to deal with pharmacokinetic data is to fit them first by a sum of exponentials since, in a linear, constant coefficient system, the number of exponential phases in the plasma level-vs.-time curve equals the number of compartments in the model.

Consider the situation in which plasma data are obtained following a bolus injection of the drug. Then the data can be described by:

$$C(t) = A_1 e^{-\lambda_1 t} + A_2 e^{-\lambda_2 t} \qquad (8.50)$$

These data can be equally well fitted by the standard two-compartment model shown in Panel A in Figure 8.7. While the model in Panel A will produce an identical fit to the data as Equation 8.50, and while, as seen in the following, all pharmacokinetic parameters recovered from this model will equal those calculated using the noncompartmental formulas, the model serves only as a descriptor of the data. That is, no comment is being made about a physiological, biochemical and/or anatomical significance to the extravascular compartment 2. This is what DiStefano and Landaw would call a model of data because little to nothing is being said about the system into which the drug is administered.

Suppose, on the other hand, additional information is known about the disposition of the drug. For example, suppose it is known that a major tissue in the body is where virtually all the drug is taken up extravascularly, and that it is known from independent experiments approximately what fraction of the drug is metabolized in that compartment. Now, given that the plasma data can be fitted by a sum of two exponentials, one can start to develop a system model for the drug. In particular, one can write an equation in which the loss rate constants k_{01} and k_{02} are related through a knowledge of how much of the drug is metabolized in the tissue; compartment 2 can thus be associated with the tissue.

It is interesting how people react to such modeling techniques. First, one has used the fact that the data support a two-compartment model, and the fact that a relationship between the loss rate constants can be written based on a priori knowledge. A physiological significance can thus be associated with the compartments and the k_{ij} that goes beyond the model of data previously discussed. A criticism of such a statement is that the model does not contain all elements of the system in which the drug is known to interact. If this critique is justified, then one has to design a new experiment to uncover information on these parts of the system. One may have to change the sampling schedule to resolve more components in the data, or one may have to design a different series of input-output experiments. One even may have to conduct a study in which marker compounds for known physiological spaces are co-administered with the study drug (24).

This is not a shortcoming of the modeling approach, but illustrates how a knowledge of compartmental modeling can be a powerful tool for understanding the pharmacokinetics of a drug. Such an understanding is not available from noncompartmental models or when compartmental models are used only as models of data. Thus, predicting detailed events in nonaccessible portions of the system model is the underlying rationale for developing models of systems—remembering, of course, that such predictions are only as good as the assumptions in the model.

The Equivalent Sink and Source Constraints

When are the parameter estimates from the non-compartmental model equal to those from a linear, constant coefficient compartmental model? As DiStefano and Landaw (22) explain, they are equal when the equivalent sink and source constraints are valid. The equivalent source constraint means that all drug enters the same accessible pools; this is almost universally the case in pharmacokinetic studies. The equivalent sink constraint means that irreversible loss of drug can occur only from the accessible pools. If any irreversible loss occurs from the nonaccessible part of the system, this constraint is not valid. For the single accessible pool model, for example, the system mean residence time and the total equivalent volume of distribution will be underestimated (22).

The equivalent sink constraint is illustrated in Figure 8.8. In Panel A, the constraint holds and hence the parameters estimated either from the noncompartmental model (*left figure*) or multicompartmental model (*right figure*) will be equal. If the multicompartmental model is a model of the system, then of course the information about the drug's disposition will be much richer since many more specific parameters can be estimated to describe each compartment.

In Panel B, the constraint is not satisfied, and the noncompartmental model is not appropriate. As previously described, if used, it will underestimate certain pharmacokinetic parameters. On the other hand, the multicompartmental model shown in the right panel can account for sites of loss from nonaccessible compartments providing a richer source of information about the drug's disposition.

Recovering Pharmacokinetic Parameters from Compartmental Models

Assume a linear, constant-coefficient compartmental model in which compartment 1 is the accessible compartment into which the drug is administered and from which samples are taken. Following a bolus injection of the drug, the volume V_1 will be estimated as a parameter of the model. V_1 thus will correspond to V_a for the noncompartmental model. The clearance rate from compartment 1, CL_1, is equal to the product of V_1 and k_{01}:

$$CL_1 = V_1 \cdot k_{01} \qquad (8.51)$$

If the only loss is from compartment 1, then k_{01} equals k_e, and one has

$$CL_a = CL_1 = V_1 \cdot k_{01} = V_a \cdot k_e \qquad (8.52)$$

showing the equivalence of the two methods. From the residence time matrix,

$$\vartheta_{11} = \frac{\int_0^\infty X_1(t)dt}{Dose} = k_{01} \qquad (8.53)$$

hence, the mean residence time in compartment 1, MRT_1, equals the reciprocal of k_{01}. Again if the only loss from the system is via compartment 1, then MRT_1 equals MRT_a

Similar results hold for the constant infusion or generic input—that is, the parameters can be shown to be equal if the equivalent sink and source constraints are valid. Again, the interested reader is referred to Cobelli and Toffolo (3) or Covell et al. (4) for details and for consideration of the situation in which the equivalent source and sink constraints are not valid.

CONCLUSION

In conclusion, noncompartmental models and linear, constant coefficient models have different domains of validity. When the domains are identical, then the pharmacokinetic parameters estimated by

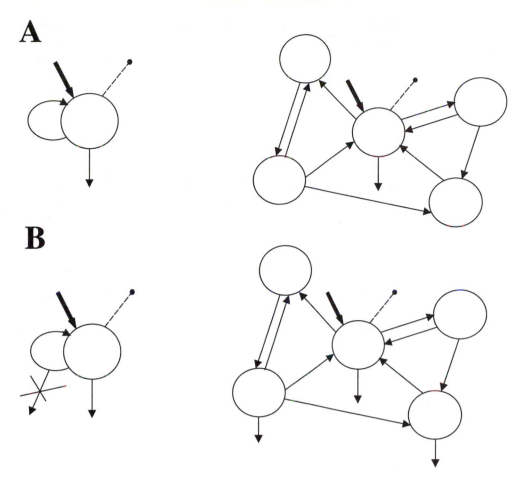

FIGURE 8.8 *Panel A:* A single accessible pool model *(left figure)* and a multicompartmental model showing a structure for the recirculation/exchange arrow *(right figure)*. *Panel B:* A single accessible pool model with an irreversible loss from the recirculation/exchange arrow *(left figure)* and a multicompartmental model showing a structure for the recirculation exchange arrow that includes loss from peripheral compartments *(right figure)*. See text for additional explanation.

either method should, in theory, be equal. If they are not, then differences are due to the methods used to estimate them.

Information provided in this chapter should make it easier for a researcher to choose a particular method and to have greater confidence in evaluating reported results of pharmacokinetic analyses.

References

1. Gillespie WR. Noncompartmental versus compartmental modeling in clinical pharmacokinetics. Clin Pharmacokinet 1991;20:253–62.
2. DiStefano JJ III. Noncompartmental versus compartmental analysis: Some bases for choice. Am J Physiol 1982;243:R1–6.
3. Cobelli C, Toffolo G. Compartmental versus noncompartmental modeling for two accessible pools. Am J Physiol 1984;247:R488–96.
4. Covell DG, Berman M, DeLisi C. Mean residence time—theoretical development, experimental determination, and practical use in tracer analysis. Math Biosci 1984;72:213–44.
5. Jacquez JA, Simon CP. Qualitative theory of compartmental systems. Journal Citation 1993;35;43–79.
6. Jacquez JA. Compartmental analysis in biology and medicine. 3rd ed. Ann Arbor: BioMedware; 1996.
7. Berman M. Kinetic analysis of turnover data. Prog Biochem Pharmacol 1979;15:67–108.
8. Gibaldi M, Perrier D. Pharmacokinetics. 2nd ed. New York: Marcel Dekker; 1982
9. Rowland M, Tozer TN. Clinical pharmacokinetics: concepts and applications. 3rd ed. Baltimore: Williams & Wilkins; 1995
10. Yamaoka K, Nakagawa T, Uno T. Statistical moments in pharmacokinetics. J Pharmacokinet Biopharm 1978;6:547–58.
11. Weiss M. The relevance of residence time theory to pharmacokinetics. Eur J Clin Pharmacol 1992;43:571–9.
12. Cobelli C, Foster DM, Toffolo G. Tracer kinetics in biomedical research. New York: Kluwer Academic/Plenum Press; 2000.
13. Berman M, Schonfeld R. Invariants in experimental data on linear kinetics and the formulation of models. J Appl Physics 1956;27:1361–70.
14. Yeh KC, Kwan KC. A comparison of numerical integration algorithms by trapezoidal, Lagrange and spline approximation. J Pharmacokinet Biopharm. 1978;6:79–98.

15. Purves RD. Optimum numerical integration methods for estimation of area-under-the-curve and area-under-the-moment-curve. J Pharmacokinet Biopharm 1992;20:211–26.

16. Gabrielsson J, Weiner D. Pharmacokinetic/pharmacodymanic data/analysis: Concepts and applications, 2nd ed. Stockholm: The Swedish Pharmaceutical Press; 1997.

17. Katz D, D'Argenio DZ. Experimental design for estimating integrals by numerical quadrature, with applications to pharmacokinetic studies. Biometrics 1983;39:621–8.

18. User's guide for version 1.5 of WinNonlin. Apex, NC: Scientific Consulting; 1997.

19. Marino AT, DiStefano JJ III, Landaw EM. DIMSUM: An expert system for multiexponential model discrimination. Am J Physiol 1992;262:E546–56.

20. Carson ER, Cobelli C, Finkelstein L. Mathematical modeling of metabolic and endocrine systems. Model formulation, identification and validation. New York: Wiley; 1983.

21. SAAM II User Guide. Seattle, WA: SAAM Institute; 1998.

22. DiStefano JJ, III, Landaw EM. Multiexponential, multicompartmental and noncompartmental modeling I: Methodological limitations and physiological interpretations. Am J Physiol 1984;246:R651–64.

23. Landaw EM, DiStefano JJ III. Multiexponential, multicompartmental and noncompartmental modeling II. Data analysis and statistical considerations. Am J Physiol 1984;246:R665–76.

24. Belknap SM, Nelson JE, Ruo TI, Frederiksen MC, Worwag EM, Shin S-G, Atkinson AJ Jr. Theophylline distribution kinetics analyzed by reference to simultaneously injected urea and inulin. J Pharmacol Exp Ther 1987; 243: 963–9.

9

Distributed Models of Drug Kinetics

PAUL F. MORRISON

Division of Bioengineering and Physical Science, Office of Research Services, National Institutes of Health, Bethesda, Maryland

INTRODUCTION

The hallmark of distributed models of drug kinetics is their ability to describe not only the time dependence of drug distribution in tissue but also its detailed spatial dependence. Previous discussion has mostly revolved around methods meant to characterize the time history of a drug in one or more spatially homogeneous compartments. In these earlier approaches, the end results of pharmacokinetic modeling were time-dependent concentrations, $C(t)$, of the drug or metabolite of interest for each body compartment containing one or more organs or tissue types. In these situations, the agent is also delivered homogeneously and reaches a target organ, either via blood capillaries whose distribution is assumed to be homogeneous throughout the organ or via infusion directly into that organ followed by instantaneous mixing with the extravascular space. In contrast, distributed pharmacokinetic models require that neither the tissue architecture nor the delivery source be uniform throughout the organ. The end results of this type of modeling are organ concentration functions (for each drug or metabolite) that depend on two independent variables, one describing spatial dependence and the other time dependence—that is, $C(\vec{r}, t)$ where $\vec{r}$ is a spatial vector to a given location in an organ. As might be expected, the pharmacokinetic analysis and equations needed to incorporate spatial dependence in this function require a more complicated formalism than used previously with compartment models.

It is the goal of this chapter to describe the general principles behind distributed models and to provide an introduction to the formalisms employed with them. Emphasis will be placed on the major physiological, metabolic, and physical factors involved. Following this, we will present several examples in which distributed kinetic models are necessary. These will include descriptions of drug delivery to the tissues forming the boundaries of the peritoneal cavity following intraperitoneal infusion, to the brain tissues comprising the ventricular walls following intraventricular infusion, and to the parenchymal tissue of the brain following direct interstitial infusion. The chapter will end by identifying still other applications in which distributed kinetic models are required.

GENERAL PRINCIPLES

The central issue with distributed models is to answer the question: What is the situation that leads to a spatially dependent distribution of drug in a tissue and how is this distribution described quantitatively?

The situation leading to spatial dependence involves the delivery of an agent to a tissue from a geometrically nonuniform source followed by movement of the agent away from the source along a path on which local clearance or binding mechanisms deplete it, thus causing its concentration to vary with location. Several modes of drug delivery lead to this situation. The most common is the delivery of an agent from a spatially restricted source to a homogeneous tissue. One such example is the slow infusion of drugs directly into the interstitial space of tissues via implanted needles or catheters. The infused drug concentration drops due to local clearances as the drug moves out radially from the catheter tip. Another example is the delivery of drugs from solutions bathing the surface of a target organ in which the drug concentration drops with increasing penetration depth and residence time in the tissue. Modes of drug delivery in which either the source or target tissue are nonuniform are also encountered. One such example is the intravenous delivery of drugs to tumor tissue. In this case, especially in larger tumors, the distribution of capillaries is often highly heterogeneous and microvasculature is completely absent in the necrotic core. Certain tumors are also characterized by cystic inclusions and channeling through the interstitial space, all of which lead to drug concentrations that are spatially dependent throughout the target tissue. Still another example is the intravenous delivery of very tight binding proteins (e.g., high-affinity antibody conjugates) to a homogeneous tissue. In this case, the concentration of protein between adjacent capillaries often exhibits a spatially dependent profile, even though the capillary bed itself is homogeneously distributed. Such profiles arise because the tight binding causes the concentration fronts, spreading out from capillaries into the space between them, to be extremely steep; if intravascular concentrations are sufficiently low relative to binding capacity, these fronts may move slowly, thus producing time-dependent spatial concentration profiles (1).

The formalisms required to describe these time and spatially dependent concentration profiles, as introduced in Chapter 8, are essentially microscopic mass balances expressed as partial differential equations. As previously noted, the ordinary differential equations used to describe well-mixed compartments are no longer sufficient since they only account for the time-dependence of concentration. To see how these equations are formulated, and to visualize the underlying physiology and metabolism, consider the specific example of drug delivery from a solution across a tissue interface (e.g., as might occur during continuous intraperitoneal infusion of an agent). Figure 9.1 A shows a typical concentration profile that might develop across an interface. The region to the left of the y-axis corresponds to the region containing the peritoneal infusate at drug concentration C_{inf}, while the region at the right corresponds to the tissue in contact with the infusate. Small circles show capillaries and they are assumed to be homogeneously distributed. In this figure, x is the distance from the fluid-tissue interface. The box is a typical differential volume element in the tissue. The transport of drug from the infusate into the tissue in this example is taken to be purely diffusional—that is, no convection (pressure driven flow) is present. The mathematical model

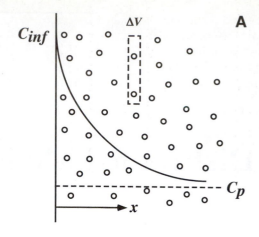

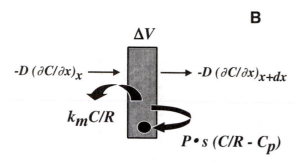

FIGURE 9.1 *Panel A:* Representative concentration profile that develops in tissue when delivering a drug across a fluid-tissue interface. Differential volume element ΔV is indicated by box and circles denote capillaries. C_{inf} is the concentration of infusate solution in contact with the tissue surface. C_p is the plasma concentration. *Panel B:* Elements contributing to the mass balance over ΔV. $-D(\partial C/\partial x)_x$ is the diffusive (Fickian) flux entering the volume element at x and $-D(\partial C/\partial x)_{x+dx}$ is the outgoing flux at $x + dx$. Other terms denote metabolic rate constant (k_m) and microvascular permeability coefficient-surface area product $(P \cdot s)$.

leading to an expression for the concentration profile is a differential mass balance over the volume element ΔV:

$$\underset{\substack{\text{rate of conc}\\\text{change in }\Delta V}}{\frac{\partial C}{\partial t}} = \underset{\substack{\text{net diffusion}\\\text{in }\Delta V}}{D\frac{\partial^2 C}{\partial x^2}} - \underset{\substack{\text{metabolism}\\\text{in }\Delta V}}{\frac{k_m}{R}C}$$

$$- \underset{\substack{\text{net transport}\\\text{across microvasculature}}}{P \cdot s\left(\frac{C}{R} - C_p\right)} \qquad (9.1)$$

This equation says that the change in total drug concentration within ΔV over a small increment of time (left-hand term; see Figure 9.1B) is equal to the sum of all the mass fluxes generating this change, namely, the net change in mass due to diffusion into and out of ΔV (first right-hand term) less mass loss due to metabolism within ΔV (second right-hand term) less net mass loss across the microvasculature within ΔV (third right-hand term). $C = C(x,t)$ in this equation is the tissue concentration of bound plus free drug, R is a constant of proportionality that relates C to the free extracellular concentration of drug C_e, that is:

$$C = RC_e \qquad (9.2)$$

k_m/R is the metabolic rate constant,[1] $P \cdot s$ is the product of permeability coefficient and surface area per volume of tissue accounting for passive movement across the microvasculature, and C_p is the free plasma concentration of drug. The parameter s is analogous to S in Chapter 3 that refers to the surface area of an entire capillary bed. D is the apparent tissue diffusion constant and is equal to $\varphi_e D_e/R$, where φ_e is the extracellular volume fraction of the tissue and D_e is the diffusion constant within just the extracellular space. For nonbinding substances distributed solely in the extracellular space of a tissue, $R = \varphi_e$ and $D = D_e$. For nonbinding substances that partition equally into the intra- and extracellular spaces, $R = 1$ and $D = \varphi_e D_e$.

Formulation of the model is completed by the specification of initial and boundary conditions. The initial condition, the state of the system just before exposing the interface to drug (the beginning of the intraperitoneal infusion in our example), is that the tissue concentration is everywhere zero—that is, $C(x, 0) = 0$. At all times at the fluid–tissue interface, the extracellular concentration equals the infusate concentration, that is:

$$C_e(0, t) = C(0, t)/R = C_{inf}$$

where C_{inf} is the constant infusate (peritoneal) concentration. Far from the interface, the concentration of drug $[C(\infty, t)]$ is determined by the tissue's transport balance with the plasma. If the plasma concentration is zero, then $C(\infty, t) = 0$.

With these initial and boundary conditions, the solution to Equation 9.1 is (3):

$$\frac{C(x,t)}{RC_{inf}} = \frac{1}{2}exp\left[-\frac{x}{\sqrt{k/D}}\right] erfc\left[\frac{x}{\sqrt{4Dt}} - \sqrt{kt}\right]$$
$$+ \frac{1}{2}exp\left[\frac{x}{\sqrt{k/D}}\right] erfc\left[\frac{x}{\sqrt{4Dt}} + \sqrt{kt}\right] \qquad (9.3)$$

where $k = (k_m + P \cdot s)/R$ and $erfc$ is the complementary error function (available in standard spreadsheet programs). If no reaction or microvascular loss is present, then this solution simplifies to:

$$\frac{C(x,t)}{RC_{inf}} = erfc\left[\frac{x}{\sqrt{4Dt}}\right] \qquad (9.4)$$

When reaction or microvascular loss is present, the steady state limit of Equation 9.3 is just

$$\frac{C(x)}{RC_{inf}} = exp\left[-x\sqrt{k/D}\right] \qquad (9.5)$$

In the special steady state case where the plasma concentration is constant *but not zero*, as may happen when a large intraperitoneal infusion delivers sufficient mass to raise the plasma concentration to a level consistent with a mass balance between intraperitoneal delivery and whole body clearance, a generalized form of Equation 9.5 applies, that is:

$$\frac{\dfrac{C(x)}{R} - \dfrac{P \cdot s}{P \cdot s + k_m}C_p}{C_{inf} - \dfrac{P \cdot s}{P \cdot s + k_m}C_p} = exp\left[-x\sqrt{k/D}\right] \qquad (9.5')$$

where C_p is now the constant plasma concentration.

Equation 9.4 provides a relationship between time and the distance at which a particular concentration is achieved. When clearance rates are small relative to diffusion rates, it states that the distance from the surface (penetration depth) at which a particular concentration C is achieved advances as the square root of time. In other words, to double the penetration of a compound, the exposure time must quadruple. Equation 9.5 states that, given sufficient time and negligible plasma concentration, most compounds will develop a semilogarithmic concentration profile whose slope is determined by the ratio of the clearance rate to the diffusion constant. This result is very useful and we will refer to it repeatedly.

One implication of these results is that drug can be delivered to a tissue layer near the exposed surface of an organ but its penetration depth depends strongly on the rate of metabolism of the agent. Another is that the delivery of non- or slowly metabolized substances across surfaces for purposes of systemic drug administration (e.g., intraperitoneal administration) is domi-

---

[1] When drug exchanges rapidly between the intracellular (ICS) and extracellular (ECS) spaces and also equilibrates rapidly between bound and free forms, it can be shown (2) that $R = \varphi_e(1 + K_e B_e) + (1 - \varphi_e)(1 + K_i B_i)K_\pi$. Here φ_e is the extracellular volume fraction, K_e and K_i are affinity constants for binding, and B_e and B_i are binding capacities in the ECS and ICS, respectively. K_π is the equilibrium ratio of the free intracellular concentration to the free extracellular concentration ($K_\pi = 0$ for substances confined solely to the ECS). Similarly, $k_m = \varphi_e k_e + (1-\varphi_e)k_i K_\pi$ where k_e and k_i are fundamental rate constants describing the rates of metabolism in the individual ECS and ICS regions.

nated by distributed microvascular uptake in the tissue layer underlying the surface. In the particular case of intraperitoneal administration, the barrier to uptake of drug into the circulation is thus the resistence to transfer across distributed capillary walls and not, as assumed in the early literature, the resistence to transfer across the thin peritoneal membrane that is relatively permeable.

Distributed pharmacokinetics is characterized not only by spatially dependent concentration profiles but also by dose-response relationships that become spatially dependent. For example, biological responses such as cell kill are often quantified as functions of area-under-the-concentration curve (AUC). In compartment models, response is frequently correlated with the area under the plasma concentration curve where:

$$AUC = \int_0^\infty C_p(t)\, dt \qquad (9.6)$$

or, alternatively, with the AUC formed by integration over the tissue concentration C(t). With distributed pharmacokinetics, however, the response within each local region of the tissue will vary according to its local exposure to drug. The appropriate correlate of response in this case is thus a spatially dependent AUC formed over the local tissue concentration, that is:

$$AUC(x) = \int_0^\infty C(x, t)\, dt \qquad (9.7)$$

The use of distributed pharmacokinetic models to estimate expected concentration profiles associated with different modes of drug delivery requires that various input parameters be available. The most commonly required parameters, as seen in Equation 9.1, are diffusion coefficients, reaction rate constants, and capillary permeabilities. As will be encountered later, hydraulic conductivities are also needed when pressure-driven rather than diffusion-driven flows are involved. Diffusion coefficients (i.e., the D_e parameter previously defined) are available by extrapolation from known values for reference substances. Diffusion constants in tissue are known to be proportional to their aqueous value, which in turn is proportional to a power of the molecular weight. Hence,

$$D_e = \lambda^2 \alpha D_{aqueous}^{37\,^\circ C} \propto \lambda^2 \alpha (MW)^{-0.6} \qquad (9.8)$$

in which λ accounts for the tortuosity of the diffusion path in tissue, α accounts for any additional diffusional drag of the interstitial matrix over that of pure water, and MW is the molecular weight of the diffusing species. The 0.6 exponent applies to most small molecular weight species. The diffusion constant for a substance of arbitrary molecular weight can be obtained from the ratio of Equation 9.8 for the desired substance to that for a reference substance—that is, from:

$$\left(\frac{D_e}{D_{e,\, ref}} \right) = \left(\frac{MW_{ref}}{MW} \right)^{0.6} \qquad (9.9)$$

Reference values are available for many substances but the one available for a wide variety of tissues is sucrose. In the macromolecular range (> 40 kDa), albumin values are available in the literature and the exponent increases from 0.6 to nearly unity.

Capillary permeability coefficient-surface area product values ($P \cdot s$) are also available from molecular weight scaling of reference values (4, 5). In the small molecular weight range shown in Figure 3.4, a relationship very similar to Equation 9.9 is valid, that is:

$$\left(\frac{P \cdot s}{P \cdot s_{ref}} \right) = \left(\frac{MW_{ref}}{MW} \right)^{0.63} \qquad (9.10)$$

The similarity of the diffusion and permeability scaling relationships leads to the prediction that, for slowly metabolized substances, the *steady state* concentration profiles that develop in a tissue following diffusion across an interface (as in Figure 9.1) are nearly independent of molecular weight. This follows from Equation 9.5 since nearly identical molecular weight scaling factors for k (proportional to $P \cdot s$ in this case) and D appear in both the numerator and denominator of the k/D argument. Hence, one would predict that the penetration depths of inulin (MW 5000 Da) and urea (MW 60 Da) would be similar within the interstitial fluid space.

Reaction rate parameters required for the distributed pharmacokinetic model generally come from independent experimental data. One source is the analysis of rates of metabolism of cells grown in culture. However, the parameters from this source are potentially subject to considerable artifact since cofactors and cellular interactions may be absent *in vitro* that are present *in vivo*. Published enzyme activities are a second source but these are even more subject to artifact. A third source is previous compartmental analysis of a tissue dosed uniformly by intravenous infusion. If a compartment in such a study can be closely identified with the organ or tissue later considered in distributed pharmacokinetic analysis, then its compartmental clearance constant can often be used to derive the required metabolic rate constant.

EXAMPLE 1: THE INTRAPERITONEAL ADMINISTRATION OF AGENTS

Some aspects of this mode of delivery have already been introduced as part of our discussion of general principles, but now the focus will narrow to two specific chemical agents and the use of one of them in the treatment of ovarian cancer.

The goal of ovarian cancer chemotherapy is to achieve sufficient penetration of the surfaces of tumor nodules to allow effective treatment. These nodules lie on the serosal surfaces of the peritoneum, are not invasive, and are not associated with high probabilities of metastasis. When the cancer is diagnosed early, or the larger nodules are removed surgically in more advanced disease, the residual nodules in 73% of the cases have maximum diameters of <5 mm (6). Collectively, these characteristics suggest that, if complete irrigation of the serosal surfaces can be achieved, ovarian tumors may be good candidates for treatment by peritoneal infusion.

The present drug of choice for this purpose is cisplatin, (cis-diamminedichloroplatinum II), or its analog carboplatin. Early compartmental models predicted a substantial pharmacokinetic advantage of intraperitoneal over intravenous delivery (7), and a later Phase III trial (6) confirmed that a comparative survival advantage could be achieved with intraperitoneal administration of cisplatin.

The effectiveness of cisplatin depends on its ability to penetrate target tissue. Therefore, we need to estimate its penetration depth from a distributed model such as that represented by Equation 9.1. However, this is difficult to do with ovarian tumor because the permeabilities and reaction rates are not available. Hence, a first estimate is made for penetration of normal peritoneal cavity tissues by EDTA, a molecule of similar molecular weight to cisplatin. The steady state concentration profiles of EDTA should resemble those of cisplatin in normal peritoneal tissues because both compounds are cleared primarily by permeation through the fenestrated capillaries in these tissues, and the small molecular weight-related differences in $P \cdot s$ and D should cancel out in Equations 9.5 and 9.5'. By first focusing on EDTA, experimental data also become available for assessing the ability of the distributed model to account for them.

EDTA concentration profiles were determined experimentally from data such as those shown in Figure 9.2 (8). In these experiments, a ^{14}C-EDTA solution was infused into the peritoneal cavity of a rat. After 1 hour of exposure (sufficient time to establish steady state profiles in the tissues), the animal was sacrificed, frozen, and sectioned for autoradiography. The upper panel of Figure 9.2 displays a transverse section across the rat in which a cross section of the large intestine is identified. This cross section is magnified in the lower panel and a grid is shown from which the concentration profile was estimated by quantitative autoradiog-

raphy. Concentration profiles for most of the peritoneal viscera were obtained in this manner, and the aggregated profiles for the stomach, small intestine, and large intestine are shown as the circles in Figure 9.3. The concentrations in this figure are all expressed relative to the infusate concentration. Because the mass of EDTA that was infused was sufficiently large to distribute throughout the entire body of the rat, the plasma concentration at the end of the experiment could not be neglected. It is shown as the single data point labeled "Plasma," and is expressed as the ratio of the actual plasma concentration to the infusate concentration. Because EDTA distributes only in the extracellular space, the deep tissue concentration only approaches the "Plasma" concentration reduced by the extracellular volume fraction φ_e.

The steady state formalism of Equation 9.5', which includes the effects of a constant plasma concentration, should describe these data. Noting from EDTA's distribution into the extracellular space that $R = \varphi_e$ and from its negligible metabolism that $P \cdot s/(P \cdot s + k_m) \rightarrow 1$, Equation 9.5' can be simplified to:

$$\frac{C(x) - \varphi_e C_p}{\varphi_e C_{inf} - \varphi_e C_p} = exp\left[-x\sqrt{k/D}\right] \quad (9.11)$$

When this equation is fit to the data of Figure 9.3 using φ_e and $\sqrt{k/D}$ as fitting parameters, the solid line results. The value of φ_e so obtained is reasonable (an extracellular volume fraction of 0.27), and the permeability derived from the $\sqrt{k/D}$ term $(= \sqrt{P \cdot s/(\varphi_e D_e)})$ agrees with that expected from molecular weight correlations. The theory largely accounts for the data, although it tends to overestimate the concentrations at the deepest penetration, perhaps because vascularity increases as one passes toward the lumenal side of the organs. However, the fit is sufficiently good to conclude that the theory has captured most of the relevant physiology and that it can be used to account for or, given availability of parameters, predict the observed results.

As a predictor of the concentration of cisplatin in normal peritoneal tissues, these data indicate a steady state penetration depth (distance to half the surface layer concentration) of about 0.1 mm (100 μ). If this distance applied to tumor tissue, penetration even to three or four times this depth would make it difficult to effectively dose tumor nodules of 1- to 2-mm diameter. Fortunately, crude data are available from proton-induced X-ray emission studies of cisplatin transport into intraperitoneal rat tumors that indicate that the penetration into tumor is deeper and in the range of 1 to 1.5 mm (9). Such distances are obtained from Equations 9.5 or 9.5' only if k is much smaller than in normal peritoneal tissues—that is, theory suggests that low

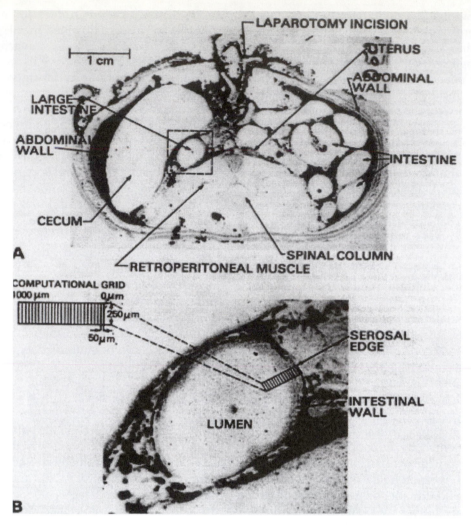

FIGURE 9.2 *Panel A:* Autoradiogram of a cross section of peritoneal cavity from a study of transport from the peritoneal cavity to plasma. *Panel B:* Close-up of dashed area in Panel A. (Reproduced from Flessner MF, et al. Am J Physiol 1985;248:F425–35.)

permeability coefficient-surface area products in tumor (e.g., due to a developing microvasculature and a lower capillary density) may be responsible for the deeper tumor penetration.

EXAMPLE 2: THE INTRAVENTRICULAR ADMINISTRATION OF AGENTS

Another example of a situation in which distributed pharmacokinetics plays an important role is in the infusion of drug solutions into the lateral ventricles or cisternal space of the brain. Drugs that have been delivered this way include chemotherapeutic agents for the treatment of tumors, antibacterial and antiviral agents for the treatment of infection, and neurotrophic factors for the treatment of neurodegenerative disease.

The principle reason for using this route of administration is to deliver drugs behind the blood-brain-barrier (BBB) by taking advantage of the fact that no equivalent barrier exists at the interface between the ventricular fluid space and the interstitial space of the brain parenchyma. That the BBB is often a major problem to be overcome is suggested by the image of Figure 9.4. This figure shows a longitudinal cross section of an autoradiogram of a rat that was sacrificed 5 minutes after an intravenous injection of ^{14}C-histamine (10). While the compound has distributed throughout most organs of the body, the brain and spinal cord remain white in this image, indicating no significant delivery of histamine to the central nervous system. With intraventricular delivery of agents, high brain interstitial fluid levels can be achieved while the BBB allows drug to be released to the plasma and systemic

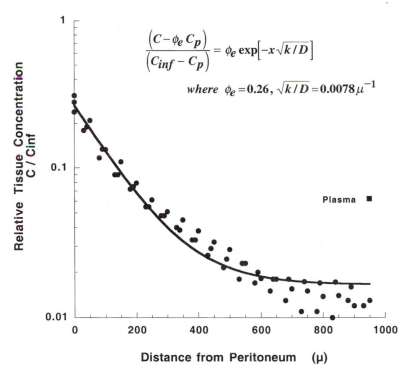

$$\frac{\left(C - \phi_e\, C_p\right)}{\left(C_{inf} - C_p\right)} = \phi_e \exp\!\left[-x\sqrt{k/D}\,\right]$$

$$\text{where}\quad \phi_e = 0.26,\ \sqrt{k/D} = 0.0078\,\mu^{-1}$$

FIGURE 9.3   Profile of ^{14}C-EDTA concentrations (expressed relative to C_{inf}) in gastrointestinal tissues following intraperitoneal infusion. Equation 9.5′ *(inset)* was used to fit the experimental tissue (●) and plasma (■) concentration data as shown by the *solid line.*

tissues only by bulk flow of cerebrospinal fluid through the arachnoid villi.

The distribution of agent into the brain parenchyma following intraventricular delivery is exemplified by the profile shown in Figure 9.5. In this case, ^{14}C-sucrose was continuously infused by an osmotic minipump into the lateral ventricle of a rat for 1 to 7 days (steady state profiles were obtained by day 1) (11). From quantitative autoradiography of coronal tissue slices, the tissue concentration was determined, expressed relative to the tissue concentration at the ventricular interface (C_0), and plotted semilogarithmically. The plasma concentration of labeled sucrose is negligible in this experiment. Analysis of the data with Equation 9.5 shows that it closely accounts for observation. First, in agreement with theory, the concentration profile exhibits strict linearity on a semilogarithmic plot. Second, the parametric fitting process results in a $\sqrt{k/D}$ estimate that, in turn, yields a brain capillary permeability value of 2×10^{-8} cm/sec that is consistent with permeability–molecular weight correlations obtained by a variety of experimental techniques (4, 12). The theoretical fit to the data

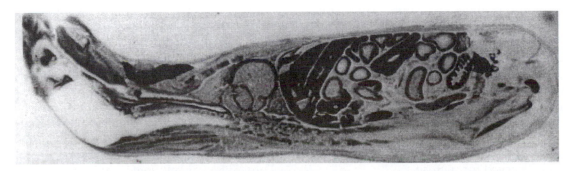

FIGURE 9.4   Autoradiogram showing a sagittal cross section of a rat 5 minutes after an intravenous injection of ^{14}C-histamine. (Reproduced with permission from Pardridge WM, et al. Ann Intern Med 1986;105:82–95.)

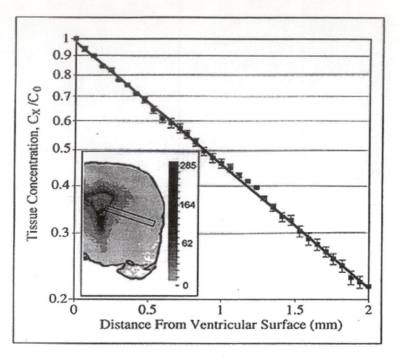

FIGURE 9.5 Concentration profile of ^{14}C-sucrose in rat caudate following intraventricular infusion to steady state (expressed relative to average tissue concentration at tissue surface C_0). Inset shows the autoradiogram of a coronal brain section and the rectangle used to generate the concentration profile. (Reproduced with permission from Groothuis DR, et al. J Neurosurg 1999;90:321–31.)

appears as the solid line in Figure 9.5, and the excellent goodness-of-fit strongly supports the simple diffusion-reaction model used to estimate penetration distances in the brain.

Of significance is that sucrose penetration of brain tissue is much deeper than EDTA penetration of normal peritoneal tissues. The penetration distance for sucrose in the brain is 1 mm versus one-tenth that distance in the organs of the peritoneal cavity. This is a reflection of the nearly 100-fold lower capillary permeability of the BBB relative to that of peritoneal organs. Other small molecules (MW < 500 Da) that undergo negligible metabolism in the brain would be subject to similarly low permeabilities and would exhibit similar penetration depths. On the other hand, many molecules are subject to metabolism and cannot penetrate into the tissue as deeply as sucrose before undergoing reaction. The exact magnitude of the penetration depth (Γ) varies with the metabolic rate constant and can be derived from Equation 9.5 as:

$$\Gamma = (\ln 2)/\sqrt{k/D} \qquad (9.12)$$

but for metabolized compounds Γ always tends to be less than that observed for sucrose.

What sort of penetration depth is expected for macromolecules? As with small molecules the depth is again determined by Equation 9.12, but some differences emerge. Were both k and D for nonmetabolized macromolecules (for which $k = P \cdot s/R$) given as mere extensions of the molecular weight functions for the smaller compounds, the penetration depth would remain independent of molecular weight. However, unmetabolized macromolecules (MW > 10 kDa) have been observed to penetrate more deeply at steady state than their nonmetabolized small molecular weight counterparts such as sucrose (on the order of two- to three-fold deeper in visceral or muscle tissues). The primary reason is that capillary $P \cdot s$ values for macromolecules are relatively smaller. $P \cdot s$ for macromolecules is related to molecular weight by a power formula of the form:

$$P \cdot s = A(MW)^{-0.6} \qquad (9.13)$$

where the exponent is similar to that for small molecules, but A is nearly 10-fold lower (5). Since the penetration depth Γ is inversely proportional to the square root of this coefficient, the depth for unmetabolized macromolecules will be about three-fold larger than for small unmetabolized compounds. As with small molecules, steady state penetration depths are on the order of a few millimeters at best.

One other important difference exists between small and macromolecular weight molecules: the time

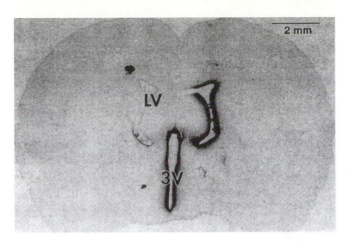

FIGURE 9.6 Autoradiogram showing the distribution of ^{125}I-BDNF in the vicinity of the intraventricular foramen in rat brain following a 20-hr intraventricular infusion. (Reproduced with permission from Yan Q, et al. Exp Neurol 1994;27:23–36.)

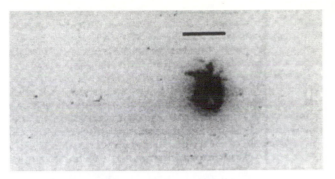

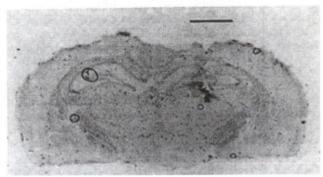

FIGURE 9.7 Autoradiogram *(top)* and unstained photograph *(bottom)* obtained from a coronal section of rat brain 48 hr after implantation of an ^{125}I-NGF-loaded polymer. Bars = 2.5 mm. (Reproduced with permission from Krewson CE, et al. Brain Res 1995;680:196–206.)

required to achieve steady state concentration profiles across an interface. Maximum penetration is obtained by unmetabolized molecules and the time to steady state is largely controlled by the rate of diffusion through the tissue. For sucrose in brain, this time is approximately 4 hours. However, for a macromolecule of 67 kDa, the diffusion constant decreases 19-fold (13, 14) leading to a corresponding 19-fold increase in the time required to achieve the steady state profile (c.f. Equation 9.4). The 4 hours required for sucrose thus increases to 3 days or more. For both small molecules and macromolecules, these times will greatly decrease as metabolism begins to play a greater role, but only at the cost of a much reduced penetration depth.

Examples of the effects of binding and rapid reaction with macromolecules are demonstrated in Figures 9.6 and 9.7. Figure 9.6 shows the distribution of brain-derived-neurotrophic-factor, ^{125}I-BDNF (MW ~ 17 kDa) following 20 hours of intraventricular infusion into the brain of a rat (15). The penetration depth is very shallow (~ 0.2 mm), far less than the few millimeter distance theoretically obtainable at steady state from an unmetabolized and unbound molecule of this size. Part of the reason for the shallow penetration is that the infusion time is, at most, a third of the time required for unmetabolized and unbound molecules to reach this theoretical distance. An even more important factor is that BDNF receptors, whose mRNA (trkB) is known from *in situ* hybridization analyses to be present on neurons and glia, bind BDNF and further retard progress to steady state (15). Figure 9.7 shows the distribution of nerve-growth-factor, ^{125}I-NGF (MW ~ 14 kDa) 48 hours after the implantation of a poly(ethylene-covinyl acetate) disk (2 mm diameter

× 0.8 mm thickness) containing this neurotrophic factor (16). The upper panel shows the location of radioactivity in a coronal brain section, including the 0.8-mm wide contribution from the disk in this view. In this image, the maximum observable extent of diffusion out from the disk is about 0.4 mm on either side of the disk, corresponding to a penetration depth of 0.25 mm (16). This is a steady-state penetration depth since the same distribution shown in Figure 9.7 is also observed after 7 days of infusion. Therefore, the shallow penetration of this protein is due neither to slow diffusion nor to the presence of NGF receptors since none are present in this region (16), but rather is attributable to degradative metabolic processes that result in an NGF half-life of approximately 30 min.

EXAMPLE 3: DIRECT INTERSTITIAL INFUSION OF AGENTS

As has been seen with the examples of intraperitoneal and intraventricular infusion, tissue penetration depths of only a few millimeters are generally achievable by diffusive transport across an interface. If the goal of therapy is to dose entire tissue masses such as glioblastomas or structures of the basal ganglia, mil-

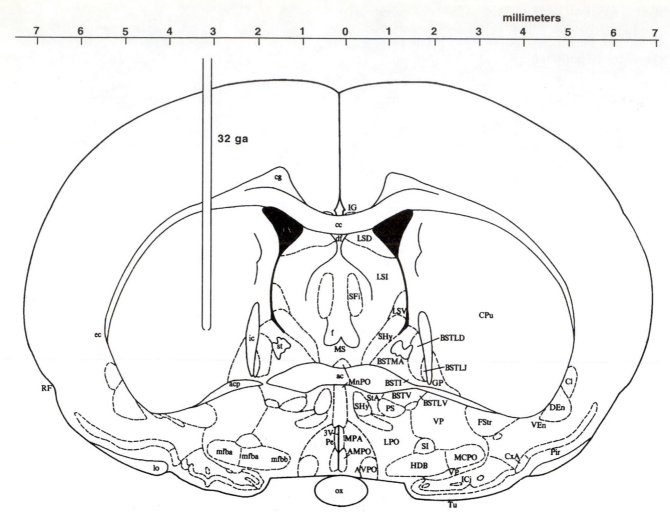

FIGURE 9.8 Schematic drawing of direct interstitial infusion showing a 32-gauge infusion cannula placed in the center of the rat caudate-putamen.

limeter penetrations are insufficient and another mode of drug delivery is required. A mode capable of achieving multicentimeter instead of multimillimeter depths is direct interstitial infusion (17, 18). It is the description of the distributed pharmacokinetics of this modality that is next examined.

In direct interstitial infusion, a narrow-gauge cannula is inserted into tissue and infusate is pumped through it directly into the interstitial space of a target tissue. Figure 9.8, for example, shows a 32-gauge cannula placed stereotactically into the center of the caudate nucleus of a rat. This type of drug delivery uses volumetric flow rates ranging from 0.01 μL/min to 4.0 μL/min. The lower end of this range corresponds to flows provided by osmotic minipumps while the upper end corresponds to flows provided by microinjection (syringe) pumps. For small molecular weight compounds, the lowest flow rates allow all transport to occur by diffusion, even near the

tip of the cannula. At higher flow rates, sufficiently high fluid velocities are generated so that pressure-driven bulk flow processes (convection) dominate most transport for both small molecules and macromolecules. Delivery of mass to a tissue thus involves the outward radial flow of infused drug solution from the cannula tip, and the concentration of drug changes along that radial path as the drug is progressively exposed to clearance processes. A distributed model is required to quantitatively describe this spatially dependent concentration profile.

Low-Flow Microinfusion Case

The simplest model describing this mode of drug delivery applies to the low volumetric flow range for small molecules—for example, cisplatin delivered at 0.9 μL/hour (19). The model is a differential mass balance for a typical shell volume surrounding the cannula tip. Deriving it in the same fashion as Equation 9.1, except taking the spherical geometry of the distribution into account, it is:

$$\frac{\partial C}{\partial t} = D\frac{1}{r^2}\frac{\partial}{\partial r}r^2\frac{\partial C}{\partial r} - \frac{k_m}{R}C -$$

rate of conc   net diffusion   metabolism
change in ΔV in ΔV in ΔV

$$P\cdot s\left(\frac{C}{R} - C_p\right) \qquad (9.14)$$

net transport
across microvasculature

All parameters have the same definitions as used previously. The initial condition is that drug concentration in the tissue is everywhere zero. The boundary conditions are, first, that the drug concentration remains zero at all times far from the cannula tip and, second, that the mass outflow from the cannula be equal to the diffusive flux through the tissue at the cannula tip—that is, that:

$$C(x,0) = 0 \quad \text{and} \quad qC_{inf} = -4\pi r_0^2 D\left.\frac{\partial C}{\partial r}\right|_{r_o} \quad (9.15)$$

where q is the volumetric flow rate, C_{inf} is the infusate concentration, and r_0 is the radius of the cannula. The steady state solution to this model is:

$$C(r) = \frac{qC_{inf}}{4\pi Dr}\exp\left(-r\sqrt{k/D}\right) \qquad (9.16)$$

where, again, $k = (k_m + P \cdot s)/R$ and $D = \varphi_e D_e/R$. For cisplatin, $R = 1$. Equation 9.16 is the radial concentration profile of drug about a cannula tip in homogeneous tissue. It is similar in form to Equation 9.5, including the same parameter dependence of the argument of the exponential, but differs by an extra r factor in the denominator that causes the concentration to drop off faster with distance. For cisplatin, the time to achieve this steady state profile 4 mm distant from the cannula tip is about 3 hours. Figure 9.9 shows the measured steady state concentration profile of cisplatin in normal rat brain achieved after 160 hours of infusion at 0.9 µL/hr. The solid line is the theoretical fit to the data showing that the r-damped exponential of Equation 9.16 accounts well for the data. The penetration depth is on the order of 0.6 mm, several fold deeper than observed with EDTA penetration across the peritoneal interface because of the much lower brain capillary permeability, but generally of the same order of magnitude.

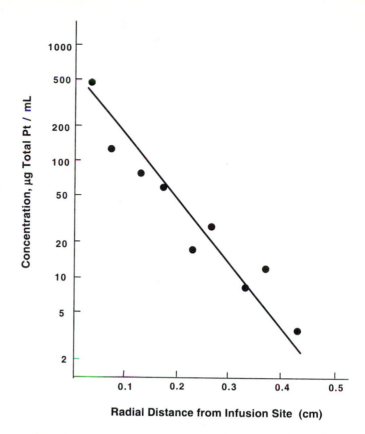

FIGURE 9.9 Concentration profile of cisplatin in rat brain following slow infusion at 0.9 µL/hr for 160 hr. *Solid line* is fit of Equation 9.16 to data (•). (Reproduced from Morrison PF, Dedrick RL. J Pharm Sci 1986;75:120–9.)

High-Flow Microinfusion Case

The submillimeter penetration distances found to hold for transport across tissue interfaces or for low-flow microinfusion are insufficiently large to provide effective dosing for many targets. For example, some brain structures such as the human putamen or cortex have centimeter-scale dimensions. Likewise, highly invasive glioblastoma multiforma tumors of the brain are characterized by protrusions of tumor that extend for centimeter distances along vascular and fiber pathways. This mismatch of low-flow microinfusion penetration distance with target dimension provides a rationale for raising the volumetric infusion rate with the intent of increasing the velocity with which materials move through the interstitium. This retards their exposure to capillary or metabolic clearance mechanisms and increases their penetration depth. In the next few paragraphs, simple estimators of the concentration profiles and distribution volumes that result from high-flow microinfusion will be developed for brain from an appropriate distributed drug model (17).

At its core, the distributed model for high-flow microinfusion is once again a differential mass balance on the drug solute in the infusate. However, because the pumps used in this method generate relatively high fluid velocities, transport of molecules through tissue is not just diffusive but also advective (i.e., pressure driven). This necessitates additional model equations so that these velocities may be computed. Once again, because of the spatial and time dependence involved, they take the form of partial differential equations. If the tissue is recognized as a porous medium, then these velocities may be computed from Darcy's Law, which states that the fluid velocity is proportional to the local pressure gradient, that is:

$$v = -\kappa \frac{\partial p}{\partial r} \tag{9.17}$$

where κ is defined as the hydraulic conductivity, v is the average fluid velocity in the tissue at position r, and p is the hydrostatic pressure. This equation can be combined with another describing the differential mass balance of water in the brain—that is, the continuity equation,

$$\frac{\partial \rho}{\partial t} = \frac{1}{r^2} \frac{\partial}{\partial r} r^2 \rho v - \Sigma$$

in which ρ is the density of water (infusate), and Σ is the sum of any source and sink terms. If the brain is considered an incompressible fluid medium and water losses across the microvascular are negligible (17), then the water density is invariant with time and Σ is negligible so that the continuity equation reduces to just:

$$0 = \frac{1}{r^2} \frac{\partial}{\partial r} r^2 v \tag{9.18}$$

Equations 9.17 and 9.18 can then be combined to generate a single differential equation in pressure; combined with the pressure boundary conditions that 1) pressure is zero at the brain boundary and that 2) the volumetric flow of infusate q equals the flow across the tissue interface at the cannula tip (i.e., $q = 4\pi r_0^2 v = -4\pi r_0^2 [\kappa(\partial p/\partial r)]$ at $r = r_0$), this pressure equation yields the simple result that:

$$v = \frac{q}{4\pi r^2} \tag{9.19}$$

The distributed model is completed by forming a differential mass balance for the drug solute in a manner completely analogous to that shown previously in deriving Equation 9.14 except for the inclusion of an additional term describing advective flow:

$$\underset{\substack{\text{rate of conc} \\ \text{change in } \Delta V}}{\frac{\partial C}{\partial t}} = \underset{\substack{\text{net diffusion} \\ \text{in } \Delta V}}{D \frac{1}{r^2} \frac{\partial}{\partial r} r^2 \frac{\partial C}{\partial r}} - \underset{\substack{\text{net convective} \\ \text{flow in } \Delta V}}{\frac{1}{Rr^2} \frac{\partial}{\partial r} r^2 v C}$$

$$- \underset{\substack{\text{metabolism} \\ \text{in } \Delta V}}{\frac{k_m}{R} C} - \underset{\substack{\text{net transport} \\ \text{across microvasculature}}}{P \cdot s \left(\frac{C}{R} - C_p \right)} \tag{9.20}$$

As with low-flow microinfusion, the initial condition is that drug concentration in the tissue is everywhere zero, and the outer boundary condition is that the drug concentration remains zero at all times far from the cannula tip. The boundary condition at the cannula tip (at r_0) differs in that the mass outflow from the cannula is equal to the advective (not diffusive) flux at the cannula tip—that is, that:

$$q\, C_{inf} = -4\pi r_0^2 \left(v\, C \right) \big|_{r=r_0} \tag{9.21}$$

where q is the volumetric flow rate, C_{inf} is the infusate concentration, and r_0 is the radius of the cannula.

In general, the mathematical solution to Equation 9.20 is numerical. However, in the special case of nonendogenous macromolecules (MW > 50kDa) and high flow (e.g., 3 μL/min), Equation 9.20 can be greatly simplified because diffusive contributions to transport are negligibly small. Hence it becomes just:

$$\frac{\partial C}{\partial t} = -\frac{1}{Rr^2} \frac{\partial}{\partial r} r^2 v C - kC \tag{9.22}$$

where, as above in Equation 9.3, $k = (k_m + P \cdot s)/R$. This equation has a very simple and useful solution for the concentration profile at steady state:

$$\frac{C(r)}{C_{inf}} = R \exp\left[-\frac{4\pi(k_m + P \cdot s)}{3q} \left(r^3 - r_0^3 \right) \right] \tag{9.23}$$

For nonbinding macromolecules confined principally to the extracellular space, $R = \varphi_e$ (~ 0.2 in brain) and the interstitial concentration C_e equals C/R (c.f. Equation 9.2).

Very simple estimators of the penetration depths that can be achieved by high-flow infusion of macromolecules can be derived from Equation 9.23. The penetration depth at steady state (r_p) and the time required to reach this steady state (t_p) are:

$$r_p = \sqrt[3]{2q / [4\pi(k_m + P \cdot s)]}$$

$$\text{and} \quad t_p = 2R \big/ \left[3\left(k_m + P \cdot s \right) \right] \tag{9.24}$$

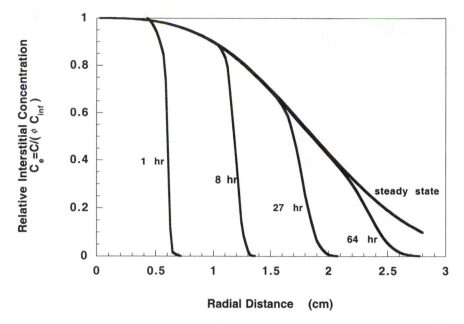

FIGURE 9.10 Simulated interstitial concentration profiles of a 180-kDa macromolecule in non-binding brain tissue at various times during high-flow microinfusion at 3 μL/min. Model parameters were taken from Table 9.1.

When the characteristic time for degradation of a macromolecule is 33 hours [i.e., $k = \ln 2/(33\text{ hr})$] and the flow rate q is 3 μL/min, Equation 9.24 predicts that a penetration depth of 1.8 cm will be achieved. This is far in excess of the penetration depth that can be achieved by simple diffusive transport, and is the theoretical result that indicates that high-flow microinfusion can achieve brain tissue penetrations that intraventricular infusion can not. Equation 9.24 also predicts that the time required to achieve this depth is 1.2 days, so that long-term infusion into the brain parenchyma is necessary.

Simulated concentration profiles for nonbinding macromolecules in brain tissue (e.g., albumin or non-binding antibodies) are presented in Figure 9.10 for $k = \ln 2/(33\text{ hr})$ and $q = 3$ μL/min. Other parameters representative of 180-kDa proteins are given in Table 9.1. The curve labeled "steady state" and forming an envelope over the other curves from top left to lower right corner is the relative concentration profile, $C_e/C_{inf} = C/(RC_{inf}) = C/(\varphi_e\, C_{inf})$, given by Equation 9.23. The curves at 1, 8, 27, and 64 hours are numerical results showing the kinetics of approach to the steady state. Note the characteristic shape of these curves. Up to

TABLE 9.1 Representative Macromolecular Parameters[a]

Parameter	Symbol	Value	Ref.
Tissue hydraulic conductivity (cm⁴/dyne/sec)	κ	0.34×10^{-8}	Morrison et al. (17)
Capillary permeability (cm/sec)	P	1.1×10^{-9}	Blasberg et al. (20)
Capillary area/tissue volume (cm²/cm³)	s	100	Bradbury (21)
Extracellular fraction	φ_e	0.2	Patlak et al. (14)
Catheter radius (cm)	r_0	0.0114	32 gauge
Diffusion coefficient (cm²/sec)	D_e	0.7×10^{-7}	Tao & Nicholson (13)[b]
Volumetric infusion rate (cm³/sec)	q	5.0×10^{-5}	Typical high-flow infusion rate (3 μL/min)
Metabolic rate constant (sec⁻¹)	k_m	5.7×10^{-6}	Arbitrary value[c]

[a] Typical of a 180 kDa protein.
[b] The value of D_e for gray matter obtained by these authors was scaled to 180 kDa molecular weight.
[c] This corresponds to a half-life of 33 hr and is roughly five times the average turnover rate of brain protein.

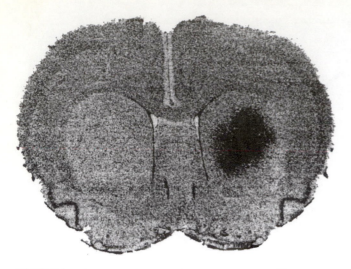

FIGURE 9.11 Autoradiogram of the distribution of ^{14}C-albumin in rat caudate following a 4 μL infusion at 0.5 μL/min. (Reproduced from Chen MY, et al. J Neurosurg 1999;90:315–20.)

the top and bottom of the leading edge. Hence, over much of the infused tissue volume, the interstitial concentration remains relatively close to the infusate concentration and provides for relatively uniform tissue dosing.

The steep concentration profiles and large penetration distances predicted for nonbinding macromolecules have been confirmed by experiment. Figure 9.11 presents an autoradiogram obtained from rat brain following a 4-μL infusion of ^{14}C-albumin at 0.5 μL/min into the gray matter of the caudate through a 32-gauge cannula (22). The image shows a relatively uniform concentration (density) over an approximately spherical infusion volume, the symmetry resulting from the isotropic structure of the gray matter on the spatial scale of these observations. Figure 9.12 is an autoradiogram obtained after infusing 75 μL of ^{111}In-transferrin (MW 80 kDa) at 1.15 μL/min into the white matter tracts of the corona radiata of the cat (18). Two findings are immediately apparent. First, with this much larger volume of infusion, delivery distances of at least a centimeter have been achieved in accordance with theoretical prediction. Second, the anisotropy of the white matter tracts is evident, indicating that the models of Equations 9.17 and 9.20 must be modified to account for such anisotropy before they are predictive of any details of white matter spread. Figure 9.13 presents both an autoradiogram and a single photon emission

well beyond 8 hours of infusion, the initial portion of the curve (nearest the cannula tip) follows the steady state profile and then drops off dramatically, approximating a step function. This concentration front moves radially outward over time with a small degree of diffusion superimposed on the advancing front, giving rise to the small curvatures observable in Figure 9.10 at

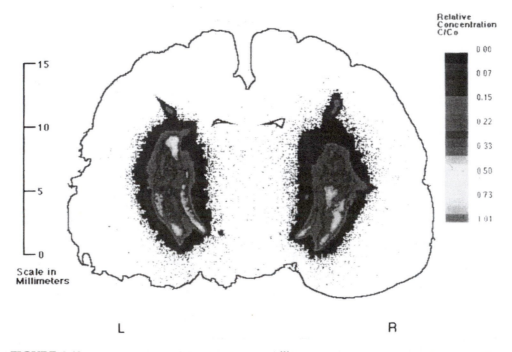

FIGURE 9.12 Autoradiogram of the distribution of ^{111}In-transferrin in cat brain following a 75-μL infusion at 1.15 μL/min into the corona radiata.

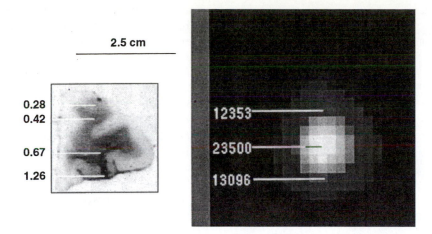

FIGURE 9.13   *Left:* Autoradiogram of a coronal section of the frontal lobe of a rhesus monkey 13 hours after completing a 10-mL infusion of ^{111}In-DTPA-transferrin into the centrum semiovale at 1.9 µL/min. Numerical values represent local tissue concentrations relative to the infusate concentration. *Right:* SPECT image corresponding to the autoradiogram. Numerical values are pixel counts used to assess spread in the dorsal-ventral and medial-lateral directions. (Reproduced from Laske DW, et al. J Neurosurg 1997;87:586–94.)

computed tomographic (SPECT) image of ^{111}In-DTPA-transferrin (81 kDa) following a 10-mL continuous infusion at 1.9 µL/min into the centrum semiovale (white matter) of a primate (23). In this case, the infused protein filled over one-third of the infused hemisphere before finding avenues of exit (10 mL exceeds the capacity of the primate hemisphere). The concentration was relatively uniform across the white matter, dropping off to only about 28% of the infusate concentration at a point over a centimeter from the cannula tip. The larger numbers reflect the presence of edema as well as tissue damage and fluid pockets in the vicinity of the cannula tip near the bottom of the section. The spread as determined from SPECT measurements was similar in the anterior-posterior, medial-lateral, and dorsal-ventral directions, ranging from 2 to 3 cm in each direction.

The high-flow distributed model of Equations 9.17, 9.20, and 9.23 describes the concentration profile that is generated in isotropic tissue at the very end of infusion. However, if these profiles are ultimately to be used to predict tissue response to a drug, these are not sufficient since they do not describe the entire history of tissue exposure to the drug. Once the pumps are turned off, there is *a post-infusion phase* during which further transport through the tissue occurs by diffusion before clearance mechanisms finally reduce the agent's concentration to a negligible value. This phase is critical in dose-response estimation since it may last a long time relative to the duration of the infusion and may broaden the sharp

concentration fronts often present at the termination of infusion. Hence, the distributed model is now extended to include a description of this phase and used in its entirety to assess likely treatment volumes as a function of degradation rate.

For isotropic tissue, the spherical distribution about the cannula tip at the end of infusion may be imagined as composed of a collection of concentric concentration shells. The post-infusion phase can then be described as the superimposed diffusion of the material from each one of these shells acting independently. Mathematically, at the start of the post-infusion period, the concentration of each shell at distance r from the cannula tip is the value of $C(r, t_{inf})$ obtained from Equation 9.20 (or 9.23 if applicable). Each of these shell concentrations can be multiplied by a function that accounts for its diffusional broadening in the post-infusion phase (24) and integration over all such shells leads to the formula for the post-infusion concentration profile, $C(r, \hat{t})$, that is:

$$C(r, \hat{t}) = \frac{e^{-k\hat{t}}}{2r\,(\pi D \hat{t})^{1/2}} \qquad (9.25)$$

$$\int_0^\infty C(r', t_{inf}) \left[e^{-(r-r')^2/(4D\hat{t})} - e^{-(r+r')^2/(4D\hat{t})} \right] r'\,dr'$$

for $\hat{t} > 0$ where $\hat{t} = t - t_{inf}$ is the time after the end of infusion (17). When this formula is applied to our macromolecule that has a 33-hour degradation time in brain, the example in Figure 9.10, the concentration

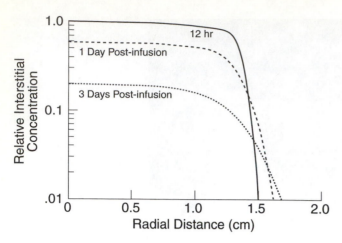

FIGURE 9.14 Simulated interstitial concentration profiles of a 180-kDa macromolecule in nonbinding brain tissue at the end of a 12-hour high-flow infusion at 3 µL/min and at 1 and 3 days post-infusion. Model parameters were taken from Table 9.1. (Reproduced from Morrison PF, et al. Am J Physiol 1994;266:R292–305.)

profiles of Figure 9.14 are generated. The solid line represents the concentration profile (the $C(r',t_{inf})$ in Equation 9.25) at 12 hours ($=t_{inf}$) after the initiation of a 3-µL/min infusion. The dotted lines show the profile at 1 and 3 days post-infusion. In the interior of the infused volume, the profile drops in value as the degradative processes exert their effect. However, beyond the initial 12-hour line, concentrations rise to appreciable values (after 1 day, to around 10% of the infusate concentration at 1.5 cm) and then fall as degradation continues. Although not immediately apparent in this figure, this outward shift could easily account for a 20% increase in dosage volume if the drug remained biologically active at 1% of its infusate concentration.

For comparison with low-flow infusion (pure diffusion) behavior, the same type of plot as Figure 9.14 is shown in Figure 9.15. In this case, computations based on Equation 9.14 were performed in which the same mass of macromolecule is infused over 12 hours but at a much lower flow rate of 0.05 µL/hr (0.00083 µL/min) to assure pure diffusive transport. Because the same infusion time is employed in both the low and high-flow simulations, the constraint of identical delivered mass at low flow requires that the infusate concentration be raised by several logs. Hence the upper end of the concentration scale in Figure 9.15 is greatly expanded relative to that of Figure 9.14. The more highly sloped lines show the movement of the concentration profile into the tissue by diffusion with the 12-hour line being the profile at end of the infusion. At this time, all regions interior to 0.3 cm are exposed to concentrations that are one to several thou-

sand-fold of that seen in the high-flow profile of Figure 9.14 and the penetration depth at 0.01 relative concentration is only 0.4 cm for low-infusion versus 1.5 cm for high-infusion. However, it is apparent in Figure 9.15 that the steep concentration profiles at the end of 12 hours of low-flow infusion lead to considerable additional penetration in the post-infusion phase, and the penetration depth at 0.01 relative concentration increases to nearly 0.9 cm by 3 days post-infusion. This raises the question of how much dose-response difference actually exists between the two delivery modes when total exposure time is considered.

Figure 9.16 answers this question for one particular dose-response metric. As discussed previously, the response of a tissue to a drug is often correlated with an area-under-the-concentration-curve *(AUC)* value in which the integrated concentration is the tissue concentration. In our example of nonbinding macromolecular infusion, the tissue concentration is a strong function of the distance from the cannula tip. Hence, the relevant *AUC* is distance-dependent and must be computed from an integral of the form presented in Equation 9.7 (with r replacing the x variable). Figure 9.16 shows this $AUC(r)$ function computed for both the low and high-flow modes of infusion and plotted, not against r, but against the corresponding spherical volume $(4/3)\pi r^3$. All cells contained within this volume will have a response equal to or greater than the response at the surface of the volume corresponding to $AUC(r)$. From independent biological information, a particular response in the target (e.g., a certain percentage of cell kill) is assumed to be identifiable with a

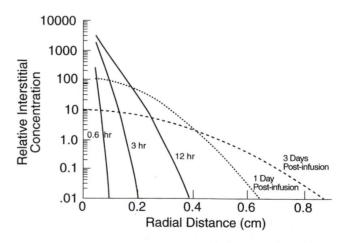

FIGURE 9.15 Simulated interstitial concentration profiles of a 180-kDa macromolecule in nonbinding brain tissue at various times during a 12-hour low-flow infusion at 0.05 µL/hr and at 1 and 3 days post-infusion. Model parameters were taken from Table 9.1. (Reproduced from Morrison PF, et al. Am J Physiol 1994;266:R292–305.)

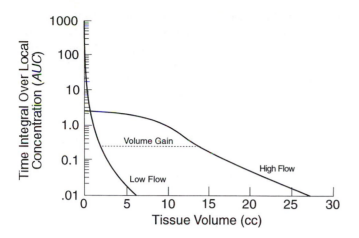

FIGURE 9.16 Simulated area-under-the-curve [$AUC(r)$] as a function of the tissue volume [$4/3\,\pi r^3$] corresponding to radial position (r). *Curves* correspond to the high- and low-flow infusion rates of Figures 9.14 and 9.15. The *dotted line* denotes a particular value of AUC corresponding to a particular response level (AUC_0). (Reproduced from Morrison PF, et al. Am J Physiol 1994;266:R292–305.)

particular AUC value, AUC_o, shown as the dotted line in Figure 9.16. The infusate concentration would be selected so that the AUC_o would lie sufficiently far below the uppermost value of the high-flow line to just assure response at a maximum desired target distance from the tip of the cannula. The difference in spherical volumes between the intersection of the AUC_o line with the low- and high-flow lines may be interpreted as the gain in treatment volume of high-flow over low-flow infusion. This gain is 14 cc for the AUC_o shown, and ranges only between 9 and 20 cc for AUC_o selections over the two logs from 1 to .01. The conclusion from this analysis is that the post-infusional spreading seen with low-flow infusion is not sufficient to compensate for the large delivery volume advantage gained during the infusion phase of high-flow microinfusion.

Tissue treatment volumes of the substance being infused are a strong function of the tissue elimination half-life that reflects the sum of both metabolic and microvascular tissue clearances. Table 9.2 summarizes how this treatment volume and associated penetration distance varies with the characteristic tissue elimination half-life of the infused species. Various elimination half-lives were used for these simulations and an infusion rate of 3 µL/min into brain for 12 hours was assumed. For the extreme case of a macromolecule undergoing no metabolism, the treatment volume is 27 cc with a penetration distance of 1.9 cm. For a more realistic tissue elimination half-life, as might be encountered with weakly binding monoclonal antibodies or stabilized analogs of somatostatin or enkephalin peptides, this

volume and distance decline only to 14 cc and 1.5 cm. When the elimination half-life drops to 1 hour, as characteristic of the rates encountered with nerve growth factor or stabilized analogs of substance P peptide or glucocerebrosidase enzyme, the treatment volume drops to 2.7 cc with a penetration distance of 0.9 cm. In a rapid metabolism situation when the elimination half-life drops to just 10 minutes, as expected for substances such as native somatostatin, enkephalin, and substance P, the treatment volume diminishes to only 0.5 cc. However, the penetration distance is still 0.5 cm and still in excess of the penetration distances encountered with modes of delivery depending on diffusional transport across tissue interfaces. Finally, it should be noted that these penetration distances, computed here for a volumetric infusion rate of 3 µL/min, will drop with decreases in the flow rate only as the cube root of the reduction factor (cf. Equation 9.24). For example, there will be only a 30% decrease in penetration distance for a three-fold drop in flow rate to 1 µL/min.

Direct interstitial infusion has been applied to the treatment of patients with advanced Parkinson's disease, and the design of the protocol is instructive (25). Motor control is severely compromised in these patients because degradation of the substantia nigra ultimately results in massive overinhibition of the motor cortex by the globus pallidus interna (Gpi). One therapeutic approach is to thermally ablate a portion of the Gpi to reduce this inhibition and restore freedom of movement. However, thermal ablation also frequently results in destruction of the optic nerve that forms the floor of the Gpi structure. Hence, a chemical means of destruction of the Gpi has been evaluated as a potentially more selective alternative.

Controlled chemical destruction of the Gpi is possible using direct interstitial infusion of the excitotoxin quinolinic acid (pyridine dicarboxylate, MW 167 Da). The property of quinolinic acid that makes it attractive for this purpose is its ability to selectively bind to and kill neurons that express the NMDA receptor but not the myelinated receptor-free fibers forming the optic nerve. Use of this compound does, however, pose a potential toxic risk to other basal ganglia surrounding the Gpi since these other structures are populated with NMDA-expressing cells. Thus, the goal is to devise a

TABLE 9.2 Tissue Treatment Volume as a Function of Tissue Elimination Half-life

Tissue elimination half-life[a]	Infinity	33.5 hr	1.0 hr	0.17 hr
Treatment volume (cm³)	27	14	2.7	0.49
Penetration distance (cm)	1.9	1.5	0.9	0.49

[a] Equal to $(\ln 2)/k$.

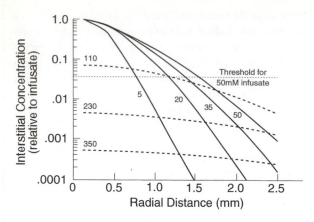

FIGURE 9.17 Relative interstitial concentration of quinolinic acid computed for a 5-μL infusion at 0.1 μL/min of a 50-mM solution in CSF into the globus pallidus interna of a primate (50-min infusion time). The threshold concentration in relative units appears as the *horizonal broken line. Other solid lines* denote profiles generated at the indicated times (minutes) during the infusion; *dashed lines* denote the profiles during the post-infusion period when the numbers are minutes after the initiation of infusion. (Reproduced from Lonser RR, et al. J Neurosurg 1999;91:294–302.)

quinolinic acid delivery procedure that targets just the Gpi while sparing its nearest neighbor, the globus pallidus externa (GPe), and other nearby ganglia.

Development of an administration protocol began with identifying the toxic threshold concentration for quinolinic acid as 1.8 mM. This was based on literature data describing neuronal cell kill in the hippocampus (26) and the assumption that an excitotoxin's toxic response is more determined by whether its concentration exceeds a threshold concentration than by an *AUC* measure. The target volume was taken as the largest inscribed sphere that would fit inside the Gpi. A conservative inflow rate of 0.1μL/min was chosen to avoid any possibility of infusate leak back along the infusion cannula. A 50-min infusion time was chosen, partly on the basis of its being the longest time easily maintained in surgery and partly because the associated delivery volume of 5 μL would suffice to initially fill the interstitial fluid volume of the inscribed sphere. The infusate concentration was then determined from theory using published transport parameters (25, 27). The complete diffusion-convection model of Equation 9.20 was solved numerically for various infusion times. This theoretical analysis was necessary to account for both convection and the substantial diffusion that results from the small molecular weight of this agent and the relatively low infusion rate. The results are expressed as the solid lines in Figure 9.17 which show tissue concentration relative to the infusate concentration. Post-infusional changes were computed using Equation 9.25, and these results are

shown in the figure as the dashed lines. In this example, it is apparent that diffusion occurring after termination of infusion has little effect on extending the volume of distribution, principally because so much diffusive transport is involved even during the infusion. The horizontal line at 0.036 is the relative concentration that is just met at any point in time at the radius of the inscribed sphere ($r = 1.5$ mm), and is equivalent to the relative toxic threshold concentration—that is, $0.036 = C_{threshold}/C_{inf}$. Using the $C_{threshold}$ of 1.8 mM, the infusate concentration C_{inf} is found to be 50 mM.

Figure 9.18 shows that the 5 μL infusion volume indeed provided localized dosing of the Gpi alone when biotinylated albumin was infused. The results in the Gpi of fully parkinsonized primates of the 5 μL infusion of 50 mM quinolinic acid are shown in Figure 9.19. Panel A presents the histology of the Gpi tissue on the infused side of the brain while Panel B presents it for the non-infused, control side. It is apparent that virtually none of the large neuronal nuclei seen in the control section is observable in the section from the infused side. The selectivity of Gpi targeting was confirmed by quantifying the number of nuclei in nearby gray matter structures. It was found that 87% of the neurons within the Gpi were destroyed, while less than 10% in the Gpe, 4% in the thalamus, 1% in the subthalamus, and 0% in the hippocampus were destroyed. In addition, no toxic changes were observed in the optic tract. Clinically, the treatment

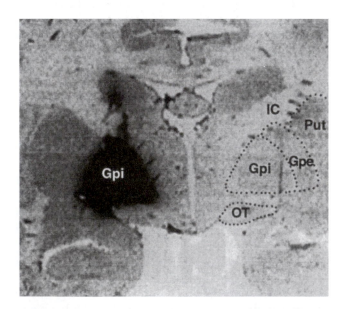

FIGURE 9.18 Coronal section of monkey brain stained for biotinylated albumin immediately after infusion of 5μL at 0.1 μL/min. Gpi = globus pallidus interna, Gpe = globus pallidus externa, OT = optic tract, Put = putamen, IC = internal capsule. (Reproduced from Lonser RR, et al. J Neurosurg 1999;91:294–302.)

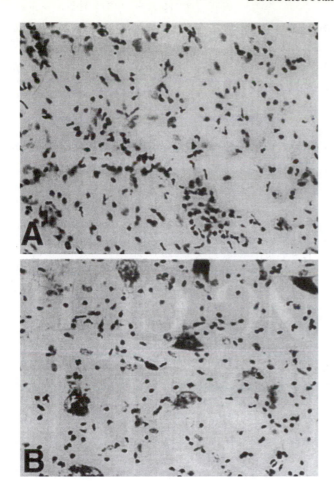

FIGURE 9.19 Photomicrographs of tissue obtained from the globus pallidus interna (Gpi) of a parkinsonian primate. There is complete neuronal ablation and minimal gliosis in the infused Gpi *(Panel A)* relative to the unlesioned control side *(Panel B)*. (Reproduced from Lonser RR, et al. J Neurosurg 1999;91:294–302.)

resulted in a stable and pronounced improvement in the principal measures of parkinsonism, including rigidity, tremor, bradykinesia, and gross motor skills.

SUMMARY

The general principles underlying distributed kinetic models of drug delivery by transfer across tissue interfaces (intraperitoneal and intraventricular delivery) and by direct interstitial infusion (low- and high-flow microinfusion) have been presented and exemplified for both small and large molecular weight substances. Formulas have been provided to assess the concentration profiles that are likely to be obtained in tissue with these delivery methods, including rough estimators of penetration depth and

time to achieve steady state penetration. Rules for obtaining needed parameters by scaling from reference values have also been provided.

Many other applications of distributed drug kinetics exist, including the spatial and time dependence of drug delivery by microdialysis (2, 27, 28, 29, 30), by the two-step delivery of targeting toxic moieties to tumors (31, 32), by the percolation of tightly binding antibodies into intervascular spaces of tissue (1, 33, 34), and by direct interstitial infusion into the spinal cord (35, 36) and peripheral nerves (37). In addition there are both mechanical and distribution issues involved in models describing potential back flow along the cannula tract during microinfusion (38). The formulations of the biological and physical phenomena involved in these cases are necessarily somewhat different from those presented in our examples. Nonetheless, the general concepts of drug delivery presented in this chapter still apply and serve as a starting point for analysis of these systems as well.

References

1. Fujimori K, Covell DG, Fletcher JE, Weinstein JN. A modeling analysis of monoclonal antibody percolation through tumors; a binding site barrier. J Nucl Med 1990;31:1191–8.
2. Morrison PF, Bungay PM, Hsiao JK, Mefford IN, Dykstra KH, Dedrick RL. Quantitative microdialysis. In: TE Robinson, JB Justice Jr, editors. Microdialysis in the neurosciences. Amsterdam: Elsevier; 1991. p. 47–80.
3. Crank J. The mathematics of diffusion. 2nd ed.. Oxford: Oxford University Press; 1975. p. 414 (see p. 334).
4. Rapaport SI, Ohno K, Pettigrew KD. Drug entry into the brain. Brain Res 1979;172:354–9.
5. Dedrick RL, Flessner MF. Pharmacokinetic considerations on monoclonal antibodies. In: Mitchell MS, editor. Progress in clinical and biological research, vol. 288. New York: Alan Liss; 1989. p. 429–38.
6. Alberts DS, Liu PY, Hannigan EV, O'Toole R, Williams SD, Young JA, Franklin EW, Clarke-Pearson DL, Malviya VK, DuBeshter B, Adelson MD, Hoskins WJ. Intraperitoneal cisplatin plus intravenous cyclophosphamide versus intravenous cisplatin plus intravenous cyclophosphamide for stage III ovarian cancer. N Engl J Med 1996;335:1950–5.
7. Dedrick RL, Myers CE, Bungay PM, DeVita VT. Pharmacokinetic rationale for peritoneal drug administration in the treatment of ovarian cancer. Cancer Treat Rep 1978;62:1–11.
8. Flessner MF, Fenstermacher JD, Dedrick RL, Blasberg RG. A distributed model of peritoneal-plasma transport: Tissue concentration gradients. Am J Physiol 1985;248:F425–35.
9. Los G, Mutsaers PHA, van der Vijgh WJF, Baldew GS, de Graaf PW, McVie JG. Direct diffusion of cis-diamminedichloroplatinum(II) in intraperitoneal rat tumors after intraperitoneal chemotherapy: A comparison with systemic chemotherapy. Cancer Res 1989;49:3380–4.
10. Pardridge WM, Oldendorf WH, Cancilla P, Frank HJ. Blood-brain barrier: interface between internal medicine and the brain. Ann Intern Med 1986;105:82–95.
11. Groothuis DR, Ward S, Itskovich AC, Dobrescu C, Allen CV, Dills C, Levy RM. Comparison of ^{14}C-sucrose delivery to the

brain by intravenous, intraventricular, and convection-enhanced intracerebral infusion. J Neurosurg 1999;90:321–31.

12. Fenstermacher JD. Pharmacology of the blood-brain barrier. In: Neuwelt EA, editor. Implications of the blood-brain-barrier and its manipulation, vol. 1. New York: Plenum Press; 1989. p. 137–55.

13. Tao L, Nicholson C. Diffusion of albumins in rat cortical slices and relevance to volume transmission. Neuroscience 1996;75:839–47.

14. Patlak CS, Fenstermacher JD. Measurements of dog blood-brain transfer constants by ventriculocisternal perfusion. Am J Physiol 1975;229:877–84.

15. Yan Q, Matheson C, Sun J, Radeke MJ, Feinstein SC, Miller JA. Distribution of intracerebral ventricularly administered neurotrophins in rat brain and its correlation with trk receptor expression. Exp Neurol 1994;27:23–36.

16. Krewson CE, Klarman ML, Saltzman WM. Distribution of nerve growth factor following direct delivery to brain interstitium. Brain Res 1995;680:196–206.

17. Morrison PF, Laske DW, Bobo RH, Oldfield EH, Dedrick RL. High-flow microinfusion: Tissue penetration and pharmacodynamics. Am J Physiol 1994;266:R292–305.

18. Bobo RH, Laske DW, Akbasak A, Morrison PF, Dedrick RL, Oldfield EH. Convection-enhanced delivery of macromolecules in the brain. Proc Natl Acad Sci USA 1994;91:2076–80.

19. Morrison PF, Dedrick RL. Transport of cisplatin in rat brain following microinfusion: An analysis. J Pharm Sci 1986;75:120–9.

20. Blasberg, RG, Nakagawa H, Bourdon MA, Groothuis DR, Patlak CS, Bigner DD. Regional localization of a glioma-associated antigen defined by monoclonal antibody 81C6 in vivo: Kinetics and implications for diagnosis and therapy. Cancer Res 1987;47:4432–43.

21. Bradbury M, The concept of a blood-brain barrier. New York: John Wiley; 1979. p. 465.

22. Chen MY, Lonser RR, Morrison PF, Governale LS, Oldfield EH. Variables affecting convection-enhanced delivery to the striatum: A systematic examination of rate of infusion, cannula size, infusate concentration, and tissue-cannula sealing time. J Neurosurg 1999;90:315–20.

23. Laske DW, Morrison PF, Lieberman DM, Corthesy ME, Reynolds JC, Stewart-Henney PA, Cummins A, Paik CH, Oldfield EH. Chronic interstitial infusion of protein to primate brain: Determination of drug distribution and clearance with SPECT imaging. J Neurosurg 1997;87:586–94.

24. Carslaw HS, Jaeger JC. Conduction of heat in solids. 2nd ed. Oxford: Oxford University Press; 1959. p. 510.

25. Lonser RR, Corthesy ME, Morrison PF, Gogate N, Oldfield EH. Convective-enhanced selective excitotoxic ablation of the neurons of the globus pallidus interna for treatment of primate parkinsonism. J Neurosurg 1999;91:294–302.

26. Vezzani A, Forloni GL, Serafini R, Rizzi M, Samanin R. Neurodegenerative effects induced by chronic infusion of quinolinic acid in rat striatum and hippocampus. Eur J Neurosci 1991;3:40–6.

27. Beagles KE, Morrison PF, Heyes MP. Quinolinic acid in vivo synthesis rates, extracellular concentrations, and intercompartmental distributions in normal and immune activated brain as determined by multiple isotope microdialysis. J Neurochem 1998;70:281–91.

28. Bungay PM, Morrison PF, Dedrick RL. Steady-state theory for quantitative microdialysis of solutes and water in vivo and in vitro. Life Sci 1990;46:105–19.

29. Morrison PF, Bungay PM, Hsiao JK, Ball BA, Mefford IN, Dedrick RL. Quantitative microdialysis: Analysis of transients and application to pharmacokinetics in brain. J Neurochem 1991;57:103–19.

30. Morrison PF, Morishige GM, Beagles KE, Heyes MP. Quinolinic acid is extruded from the brain by a probenecid-sensitive carrier system. J Neurochem 1999;72:2135–44.

31. van Osdol WW, Sung CS, Dedrick RL, Weinstein JN. A distributed pharmacokinetic model of two-step imaging and treatment protocols: Application to streptavidin conjugated monoclonal antibodies and radiolabeled biotin. J Nucl Med 1993;34:1552–64.

32. Sung CS, van Osdol WW, Saga T, Neumann RD, Dedrick RL, Weinstein JN. Streptavidin distribution in metastatic tumors pretargeted with a biotinylated monoclonal antibody: Theoretical and experimental pharmacokinetics. Cancer Res 1994;54:2166–75.

33. Juweid M, Neumann R, Paik C, Perez-Bacete J, Sato J, van Osdol WW, Weinstein JN. Micropharmacology of monoclonal antibodies in solid tumors: direct experimental evidence for a binding site barrier. Cancer Res 1992;54:5144–53.

34. Baxter LT, Yuan F, Jain RK. Pharmacokinetic analysis of the perivascular distribution of bifunctional antibodies and haptens: Comparison with experimental data. Cancer Res 1992;52:5838–44.

35. Lonser RR, Gogate N, Wood JD, Morrison PF, Oldfield EH. Direct convective delivery of macromolecules to the spinal cord. J Neurosurg 1998;9:616–22.

36. Wood JD, Lonser RR, Gogate N, Morrison PF, Oldfield EH. Convective delivery of macromolecules in to the naïve and traumatized spinal cords of rats. J Neurosurg 1999;90:115–20.

37. Lonser RR, Weil RJ, Morrison PF, Governale LS, Oldfield EH. Direct convective delivery of macromolecules to peripheral nerves. J Neurosurg 1998;89:610–15.

38. Morrison PF, Chen MY, Chadwick RS, Lonser RR, Oldfield EH. Focal delivery during direct infusion to brain: Role of flow rate, catheter diameter, and tissue mechanics. Am J Physiol 1999;277:R1218–29.

10

Population Pharmacokinetics

RAYMOND MILLER
Pfizer Global Research and Development

INTRODUCTION

Pharmacokinetic studies in patients have led to the appreciation of the large degree of variability in pharmacokinetic parameter estimates that exists across patients. Many studies have quantified the effects of such factors as age, gender, disease states, and concomitant drug therapy on the pharmacokinetics of drugs, with the purpose of accounting for interindividual variability. Finding a population model that adequately describes the data may have important clinical benefits in that the dose regimen for a specific patient may need to be individualized based on relevant physiological information. This is particularly important for drugs with a narrow therapeutic range.

The development of a successful pharmacokinetic model allows one to summarize large amounts of data into a few values that describe the whole data set. The general procedure used to develop a pharmacokinetic model is outlined in Table 10.1. Certain aspects of this procedure have been described previously in Chapters 3 and 8. For example, the technique of curve peeling frequently is used to indicate the number of compartments that are included in a compartmental model. In any event, the eventual outcome should be a model that can be used to interpolate or extrapolate to other conditions.

Population pharmacokinetic analysis is an extension of this modeling procedure. The purpose of population pharmacokinetic analysis is summarized in Table 10.2.

ANALYSIS OF PHARMACOKINETIC DATA

Structure of Pharmacokinetic Models

As discussed in Chapters 3 and 8, it is often found that the relationship between drug concentrations and time may be described by a sum of exponential terms. This lends itself to compartmental pharmacokinetic analysis in which the pharmacokinetics of a drug are characterized by representing the body as a system of well-stirred compartments with the rates of transfer between compartments following first-order kinetics. The required number of compartments is equal to the number of exponents in the sum of exponentials equation that best fits the data. In the case of a drug that seems to be distributed homogeneously in the body, a one-compartment model is appropriate and this relationship can be described in a single individual by the following monoexponential equation:

$$A = \text{Dose} \cdot e^{-kt} \qquad (10.1)$$

This equation describes the typical time course of amount of drug in the body (*A*) as a function of initial dose, time (*t*), and the first-order elimination rate constant (*k*). As described in Equation 2.14, this rate constant equals the ratio of the elimination clearance (CL_E) relative to the distribution volume of the drug (V_d), so that Equation 10.1 can then be expressed in terms of concentration in plasma (C_p).

$$C_p = \frac{\text{Dose}}{V_d} \cdot e^{-\frac{CL_E}{V_d} \cdot t} \qquad (10.2)$$

TABLE 10.1 Steps in Developing a Pharmacokinetic Model

Step	Activity
1	Design an experiment.
2	Collect the data.
3	Develop a model based on the observed characteristics of the data.
4	Express the model mathematically.
5	Analyze the model in terms of the data.
6	Evaluate the fit of the data to the model.
7	If necessary, revise the model in Step 3 to eliminate inconsistencies in the data fit and repeat the process until the model provides a satisfactory description of the data.

Therefore, if one has an estimate of clearance and volume of distribution, the plasma concentration can be predicted at different times after administration of any selected dose. The quantities that are known because they are either measured or controlled, such as dose and time, are called "fixed effects" in contrast to effects that are not known and are regarded as random. The parameters CL_E and V_d are called fixed effect parameters because they quantify the influence of the fixed effects on the dependent variable, C_p.

Fitting Individual Data

Assuming that we have measured a series of concentrations over time, we can define a model structure and obtain initial estimates of the model parameters. The objective is to determine an estimate of the parameters (CL_E, V_d) such that the differences between the observed and predicted concentrations are comparatively small. Three of the most commonly used criteria for obtaining a best fit of the model to the data are ordinary least squares (OLS), weighted least squares (WLS), and extended least squares (ELS), which is a maximum likelihood pro-

TABLE 10.2 The Purpose of Population Pharmacokinetic Analysis

Estimate the population mean of parameters of interest.

Identify and investigate sources of variability that influence drug pharmacokinetics.

Estimate the magnitude of intersubject variability.

Estimate the random residual variability.

cedure. These criteria are achieved by minimizing the following quantities, which are often called the objective function *(O)*.

Ordinary least squares (OLS) (where $\hat{C}_i$ denotes the predicted value of C_i based on the model):

$$O_{OLS} = \sum_{i=1}^{n}(C_i - \hat{C}_i)^2 \tag{10.3}$$

Weighted least squares (WLS) (where W is typically $1/$ the observed concentration):

$$O_{WLS} = \sum_{i=1}^{n}W_i(C_i - \hat{C}_i)^2 \tag{10.4}$$

Extended least squares (ELS):

$$O_{ELS} = \sum_{i=1}^{n}[W_i(C_i - \hat{C}_i)^2 + \ln \text{var}(\hat{C}_i)] \tag{10.5}$$

The correct criterion for best fit depends on the assumption underlying the functional form of the variances (var) of the dependent variable C. The model that fits the data from an individual minimizes the differences between the observed and the model predicted concentrations (Figure 10.1).

What one observes is a measured value that differs from the model-predicted value by some amount called a residual error (also called intrasubject error or within-subject error). There are many reasons why the actual observation may not correspond to the predicted value. The structural model may only be approximate, or the plasma concentrations may have been measured with error. It is too difficult to model all the sources of error separately so the simplifying assumption is made that each difference between an observation and its prediction is random. When the data are from an individual, and the error model is the additive error model, the error is denoted by ε.

$$C = \frac{\text{Dose}}{V_d} \cdot e^{-\frac{CL_E}{V_d} \cdot t} + \varepsilon \tag{10.6}$$

POPULATION PHARMACOKINETICS

Population pharmacokinetic parameters quantify population mean kinetics, between-subject variability (intersubject variability), and residual variability. Residual variability includes within-subject variability, model misspecification, and measurement error. This information is necessary to design a dosage regimen for a drug. If all patients were identical, the same dose would be appropriate for all. However, since patients

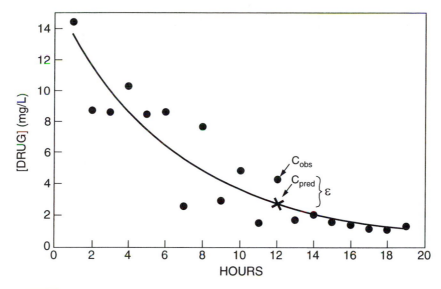

FIGURE 10.1   Fit obtained using a one-compartment model (see Equation 10.6) to fit plasma-concentration-vs.-time data observed following intravenous bolus administration of a drug. The C_{obs} designates the actual measured concentrations and C_{pred} represents the concentrations predicted by the pharmacokinetic model. (Adapted from Grasela TH Jr, Sheiner LB. J Pharmacokinet Biopharm 1991;19(suppl):25S–36S.)

vary, it may be necessary to individualize a dose depending on how large the between-subject variation is. For example, to choose an initial dose, one needs to know the relationship between the dose given and the concentration achieved and thus pharmacological response anticipated in a patient. This is the same as knowing the typical pharmacokinetics of individuals of similar sex, age, weight, and function of elimination organs. This information is available if one knows the fixed effect pharmacokinetic parameters governing the relationship of the pharmacokinetics to sex, age, weight, renal function, liver function, and so on. Large unexplained variability in pharmacokinetics in an apparently homogeneous population can lead to an investigation as to the reason for the discrepancy, which in turn may lead to an understanding of fundamental principals.

Population Analysis Methods

Assume an experiment in which a group of subjects selected to represent a spectrum of severity of some condition (e.g., renal insufficiency) are given a dose of drug and drug concentrations are measured in blood samples collected at intervals after dosing. The structural kinetic models used when performing a population analysis do not differ at all from those used for analysis of data from an individual patient. One still needs a model for the relationship of concentration to

dose and time, and this relationship does not depend on whether the fixed effect parameter changes from individual to individual or with time within an individual. The population pharmacokinetic parameters can be determined in a number of ways of which only a few will be described.

The Naive Pooled Data Method

If interest focuses entirely on the estimation of population parameters, then the simplest approach is to combine all the data as if they came from a single individual (1). The doses may need to be normalized so that the data are comparable. Equation 10.6 would be applicable if an intravenous bolus dose were administered. The minimization procedure is similar to that described in Figure 10.1.

The advantages of this method are its simplicity, familiarity, and the fact that it can be used with sparse data and differing numbers of data points per individual. The disadvantages are that it is not possible to determine the fixed effect sources of variability for the drug—for example, creatinine clearance (CL_{CR}); it cannot distinguish between variability within and between individuals, and an imbalance between individuals results in biased parameter estimates.

Pooling has the risk of masking individual behavior, but might still serve as a general guide to the mean pharmacokinetic parameters. If this method is used, it is recommended that a spaghetti plot be made to visu-

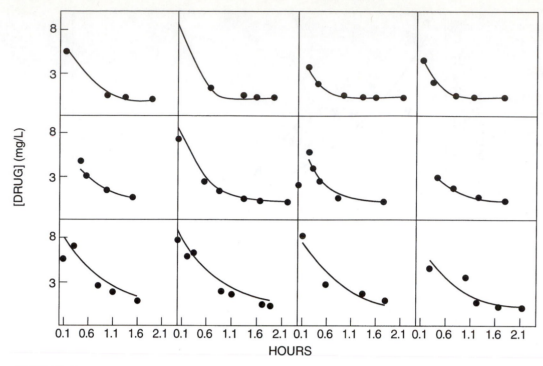

FIGURE 10.2 Fit obtained using a one-compartment model to fit plasma-concentration-vs.-time data observed following intravenous bolus administration of a drug. Each panel represents an individual subject.

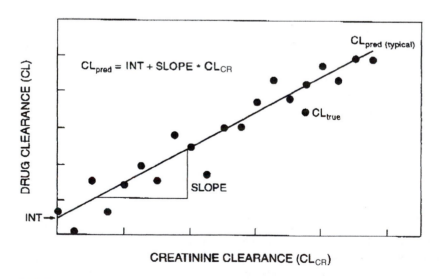

FIGURE 10.3 Linear regression analysis of drug clearance *(CL)* vs. creatinine clearance *(CL_CR)*. Typical values of drug clearance are generated for an individual or group of individuals with a given creatinine clearance. The discrepancy between the true value for drug clearance *(CL_true)* and the typical value *(CL_pred)* necessitates the use of a statistical model for interindividual variability. INT denotes the intercept of the regression line. (Adapted from Grasela TH Jr, Sheiner LB. J Pharmacokinet Biopharm 1991;19(suppl):25S–36S.)

ally determine if any individual or group of individuals deviates from the central tendency with respect to absorption, distribution, or elimination.

The Two-Stage Method

The two-stage method is so called because it proceeds in two steps (1). The first step is to use OLS to estimate each individual patient's parameters assuming a model such as Equation 10.6. The minimization procedure described in Figure 10.1 is repeated for each individual independently (Figure 10.2).

The next step is to estimate the population parameters across the subjects by calculating the mean of each parameter, its variance and covariance. The relationship between fixed effect parameters and covariates of interest can be investigated by regression techniques. To investigate the relationship between drug clearance (CL) and creatinine clearance (CL_{CR}) one could try a variety of models depending on the shape of the relationship. As described in Chapter 5, a linear relationship often is applicable, such as that given by Equation 10.7 (Figure 10.3):

$$CL = \text{INT} + \text{SLOPE} \cdot CL_{CR} \qquad (10.7)$$

The intercept in this equation provides an estimate of nonrenal clearance.

The advantages of this method are that it is easy and most investigators are familiar with it. Because parameters are estimated for each individual, these estimates have little or no bias. Pharmacokinetic/ pharmacodynamic models can be applied since individual differences can be considered. Covariates can be included in the model. Disadvantages of the method are that variance-covariance of parameters across subjects is biased and contains elements of interindividual variability, intraindividual variability, assay error, time error, model misspecification, and variability from the individual parameter estimation process. In addition, the same structural model is required for all subjects, and numerous blood samples must be obtained at appropriate times to obtain accurate estimates for Step 1.

Nonlinear Mixed Effects Modeling Method

This method is depicted in Figure 10.4 and will be described using the conventions of the NONMEM software (2, 3) and the description by Vozeh et al. (3). It is based on the principle that the individual pharmacokinetic parameters of a patient population arise from a distribution that can be described by the population mean and the interindividual variance. Each individual pharmacokinetic parameter can be expressed as a population mean and a deviation typical for that individual. The deviation is the difference between the population mean

and the individual parameter and is assumed to be a random variable with an expected mean of zero and variance ω^2. This variance describes the biological variability of the population. The clearance and volume of distribution for subject j using the structural pharmacokinetic model described in Equation 10.6 are represented by the following equations.

$$C_{ij} = \frac{\text{Dose}}{V_{dj}} \cdot e^{\frac{CL_j}{V_{dj}} \cdot t_{ij}} + \varepsilon_{ij}$$

where,

$$CL_j = \overline{CL} + \eta_j^{CL}$$

and,

$$V_{dj} = \overline{V_d} + \eta_j^{V_d}$$

where $\overline{CL}$ and $\overline{V_d}$ are the population mean of the elimination clearance and volume of distribution respectively and η_j^{CL} and $\eta_j^{V_d}$ are the differences between the population mean and the clearance (CL_j) and volume of distribution (V_{dj}) of subject j. These equations can be applied to subject k by substituting a k for j in the equations, and so on for each subject. There are, however, two levels of random effects. The first level, described previously, is needed in the parameter model to help model unexplained interindividual differences in the parameters. The second level represents a random error (ε_{ij}), familiar from classical pharmacokinetic analysis, which expresses the deviation of the expected plasma concentration in subject j from the measured value. Each ε variable is assumed to have a mean zero and a variance denoted by σ^2. Each pair of elements in η has a covariance that can be estimated. A covariance between two elements of η is a measure of statistical association between these two random variables.

NONMEM is a one-stage analysis that simultaneously estimates mean parameters, fixed effect parameters, interindividual variability, and residual random effects. The fitting routine makes use of the ELS method. A global measure of goodness of fit is provided by the objective function value based on the final parameter estimates, which, in the case of NONMEM, is minus twice the log likelihood of the data (1). Any improvement in the model would be reflected by a decrease in the objective function. The purpose of adding independent variables to the model, such as CL_{CR} in Equation 10.7, is usually to explain kinetic differences between individuals. This means that such differences were not explained by the model prior to adding the variable and were part of random interindividual variability. Therefore, inclusion of

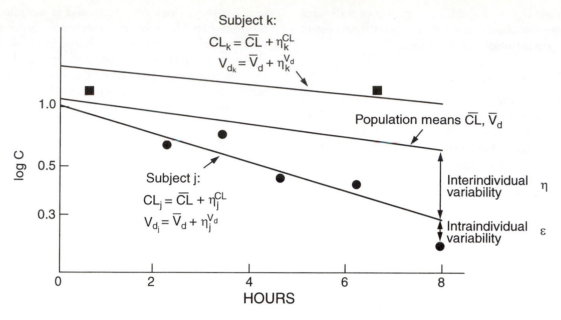

FIGURE 10.4 Graphical illustration of the statistical model used in NONMEM for the special case of a one-compartment model following intravenous bolus administration of a drug. Subject $j = \bullet$, Subject $k = \blacksquare$. (Adapted from Vozeh S, et al. Eur J Clin Pharmacol 1982;23:445–51.)

additional variables in the model is warranted only if it is accompanied by a decrease in the estimates of the intersubject variance, and under certain circumstances intrasubject variance.

The advantages of the one-stage analysis are that interindividual variability of the parameters can be estimated, random residual error can be estimated, covariates can be included in the model, parameters for individuals can be estimated, and pharmacokinetic/pharmacodynamic models can be used. Since allowance can be made for individual differences, this method can be used with routine data, sparse data, and unbalanced number of data points per patient (4, 5). The models are also much more flexible. For example, a number of studies can be pooled into one analysis while accounting for differences between study sites, and all fixed effect covariate relationships and any interindividual or residual error structure can be investigated.

Disadvantages arise mainly from the complexity of the statistical algorithms and the fact that fitting models to data is time consuming. The first-order method (FO) used in NONMEM also results in biased estimates of parameters, especially when the distribution of interindividual variability is specified incorrectly. The first-order conditional estimation procedure (FOCE) is more accurate but is even more time consuming. The objective function and adequacy of the model are based in part on the residuals, which for NONMEM are determined based on the predicted concentrations for the mean pharmacokinetic parameters rather than the predicted concentrations for each subject. Therefore, the residuals are confounded by intraindividual, interindividual, and linearization errors.

CONCLUSIONS

Population pharmacokinetics describes the typical relationships between physiology and pharmacokinetics, the interindividual variability in these relationships, and their residual intraindividual variability. Knowledge of population kinetics can help one choose initial drug dosage, modify dosage appropriately in response to observed drug levels, make rational decisions regarding certain aspects of drug regulation, and elucidate certain research questions in pharmacokinetics. Patients with the disease for which the drug is intended are probably a better source of pharmacokinetic data than healthy subjects. However, this type of data is contaminated by varying quality, accuracy, and precision, as well as by the fact that generally only sparse data is collected from each patient.

Although population pharmacokinetic parameters have been estimated either by fitting all individuals' data together as if there were no kinetic differences, or by fitting each individual's data separately and then combining the individual parameter estimates, these methods have certain theoretical problems that can only be aggravated when the deficiencies of typical clinical data are present. The nonlinear mixed effect analysis avoids many of these deficiencies and provides a flexible means of estimating population pharmacokinetic parameters.

References

1. Sheiner LB. The population approach to pharmacokinetic data analysis: Rationale and standard data analysis methods. Drug Met Rev 1984;15:153–71.
2. Beal SL, Sheiner LB. NONMEM user's guides, NONMEM Project Group, San Francisco: University of California; 1989.
3. Vozeh S, Katz G, Steiner V, Follath F. Population pharmacokinetic parameters in patients treated with oral mexiletine. Eur J Clin Pharmacol 1982;23:445–51.
4. Sheiner LB, Rosenberg B, Marathe VV. Estimation of population characteristics of pharmacokinetic parameters from routine clinical data. J Pharmacokinet Biopharm 1997;5:445–79.
5. Grasela TH Jr, Sheiner LB. Pharmacostatistical modeling for observational data. J Pharmacokin Biopharm 1991;19(suppl):25S–36S.

Suggested Additional Reading

Beal SL, Sheiner LB. Estimating population kinetics. CRC Crit Rev Biomed Eng 1982;8:195–222.

Whiting B, Kelman AW, Grevel J. Population pharmacokinetics: Theory and clinical application. Clin Pharmacokinet 1986;11:387–401.

Ludden TM. Population pharmacokinetics. J Clin Pharmacol 1988;28:1059–63.

Sheiner LB, Ludden TM. Population pharmacokinetics/dynamics. Annu Rev Pharmacol Toxicol 1992;32:185–209.

Yuh L, Beal SL, Davidian M, Harrison F, Hester A, Kowalski K, Vonesh E, Wolfinger R. Population pharmacokinetic/pharmacodynamic methodology and applications. A bibliography. Biometrics 1994;50:566–75.

Samara E, Grannenman R. Role of population pharmacokinetics in drug development. Clin Pharmacokinet 1997;32:294–312.

DRUG METABOLISM AND TRANSPORT

11

Pathways of Drug Metabolism

SANFORD P. MARKEY

Laboratory of Neurotoxicology, National Institutes of Health, Bethesda, Maryland

INTRODUCTION

Most drugs are chemically modified or metabolized in the body. The biochemical processes governing drug metabolism largely determine the duration of a drug's action, elimination, and toxicity. The degree to which these processes can be controlled to produce beneficial medical results relies on multiple variables that have been the subject of considerable study, best illustrated by examining several representative drugs. Drug metabolism may render an administered active compound inactive, or activate an inactive precursor, or produce a toxic by-product.

Phenobarbital typifies drugs that are active when administered and then converted to inactive and more polar metabolites in the liver as shown in Scheme 11.1. When phenobarbital is hydroxylated, it becomes more water- and less lipid-membrane soluble. Para-hydroxyphenobarbital is pharmacologically inactive and is either excreted directly or conjugated with glucuronide and then excreted.

Phenobarbital metabolism exemplifies the principles propounded by Richard Tecwyn Williams, a pioneering British pharmacologist active in the mid-twentieth century (1). Williams introduced the concepts of Phase I and Phase II drug metabolism. He described *Phase I* biotransformations as primary covalent chemical modifications to the administered drug (oxidation, reduction, hydrolysis, etc.), such as the hydroxylation of phenobarbital. *Phase II* reactions then synthesized or conjugated an endogenous polar species to either the parent drug or the Phase I modified drug, as exemplified by the glucuronidation of para-hydroxyphenobarbital in Scheme 11.1.

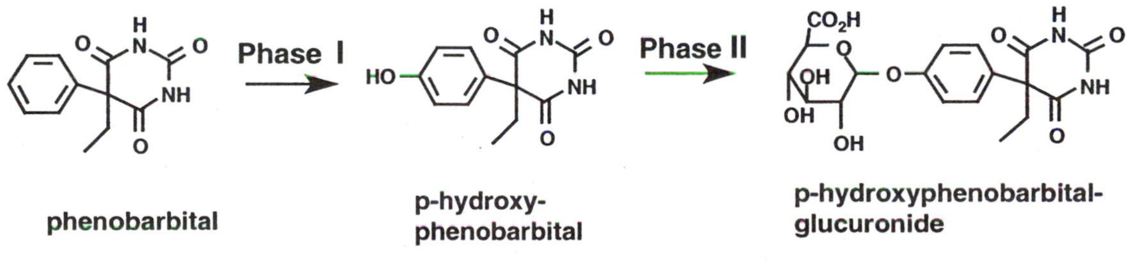

SCHEME 11.1 Metabolism of phenobarbital.

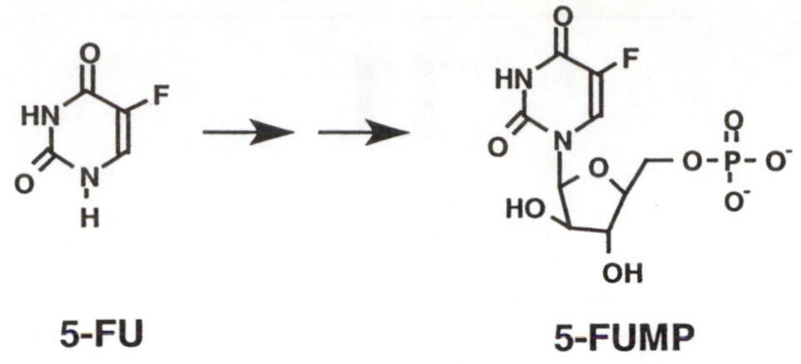

SCHEME 11.2 Metabolism of 5-FU is required to produce the active agent 5-FUMP.

These concepts have been useful to catalog and categorize newly described chemical biotransformations, especially as the field of drug metabolism developed.

Pyrimidine nucleotides exemplify a class of pharmaceuticals designed to be biotransformed in the body from inactive compounds to active cancer chemotherapeutic agents. In order to effectively interfere with thymidine synthetase, 5-fluorouracil (5-FU) must be biotransformed to 5-fluorouracil-monophosphate (5-FUMP) as shown in Scheme 11.2. The base 5-FU is not well absorbed as a drug and consequently is administered parenterally. The polar monophosphate is formed within the targeted, more rapidly dividing cancer cells, enhancing the specificity of its action.

Sometimes an active pharmaceutical produces another active agent after biotransformation. A recent example of a commercially popular drug with an active metabolite is terfenadine (Seldane™), as shown in Scheme 11.3. As discussed in Chapter 1, the terfenadine oxidative metabolite, fexofenadine (Alle-gra™), is now marketed as a safer alternative that avoids potentially fatal cardiac terfenadine side effects.

An example of a popular pharmaceutical with a toxic metabolite is acetaminophen (2,3). A portion of the acetaminophen metabolized in the liver is converted to a reactive intermediate, NAPQI, which is an excellent substrate for nucleophilic attack by free sulfhydryl groups in proteins as shown in Scheme 11.4. By substituting a high concentration of an alternative thiol for the –SH group in cysteine in liver proteins and removing the reactive NAPQI from contact with liver proteins, N-acetylcysteine (NAcCys) is an effective antidote for acetaminophen overdose (4). The N-acetyl cysteine adduct is inactive and is excreted in the urine.

Knowledge of basic principles of drug metabolism may lead to rational development of more effective pharmaceuticals, as illustrated in Scheme 11.5 by the progression from procaine to procainamide and N-acetylprocainamide. Procaine was observed in 1936

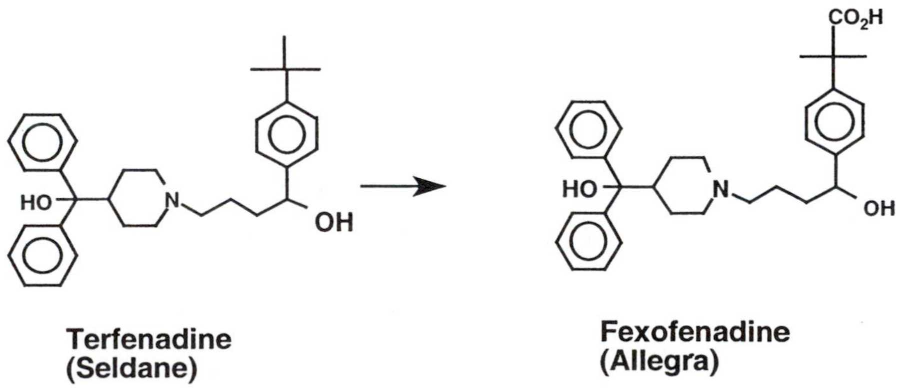

Terfenadine (Seldane)

Fexofenadine (Allegra)

SCHEME 11.3 The active agent terfenadine is converted to another active agent, fexofenadine.

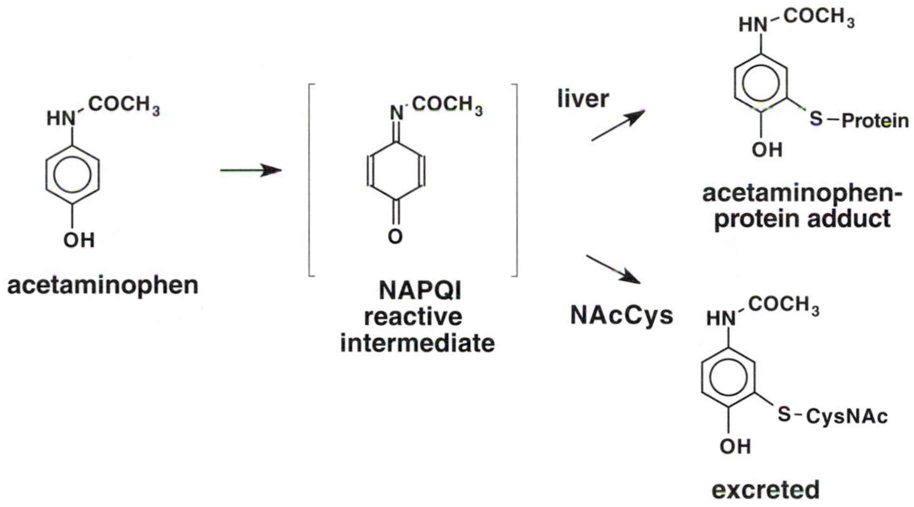

SCHEME 11.4   Acetaminophen is metabolized to a reactive and potentially toxic intermediate NAPQI that reacts with liver proteins.

to elevate the threshold of ventricular muscle to electrical stimulation, making it a promising antiarrhythymic agent (5). However, it was too rapidly hydrolyzed by esterases to be used *in vivo,* and its amide analog procainamide was evaluated (6). Procainamide had similar effects as procaine and is used clinically as an antiarrhythymic drug. It is relatively resistant to hydrolysis; about 60 to 70% of the dose is excreted as unchanged drug and 20% acetylated to *N*-acetylprocainamide (NAPA), which also has antiarrhythmic activity. NAPA has been investigated as a candidate to replace procainamide because it has a longer elimination half-life than procainamide (2.5 times) and fewer toxic side effects, representing a third generation of procaine development (7).

These examples indicate the relevance of understanding drug metabolism in the context of patient care and drug development. Presenting an overview of drug metabolism in a single chapter is challenging because the field has developed markedly in the past century with many important scientific contributions. Recent books summarize advances in understanding fundamental mechanisms of metabolic processes (8) and the encyclopedic information available regarding the metabolism of specific drugs (9). The broad concepts outlined by R. T. Williams of Phase I and Phase II metabolism are still a convenient framework for introducing the reader to metabolic processes, but these designations do not apply readily to all biotransformations. For example, the metabolic activation of 5-FU and the toxic protein binding of acetaminophen are more usefully described with regard to the specific type of chemical transformation, the enzymes involved, and the tissue site of transformation. Because the liver is a major site of drug metabolism, this chapter introduces first the hepatic Phase I enzymes and the biotransformations they effect.

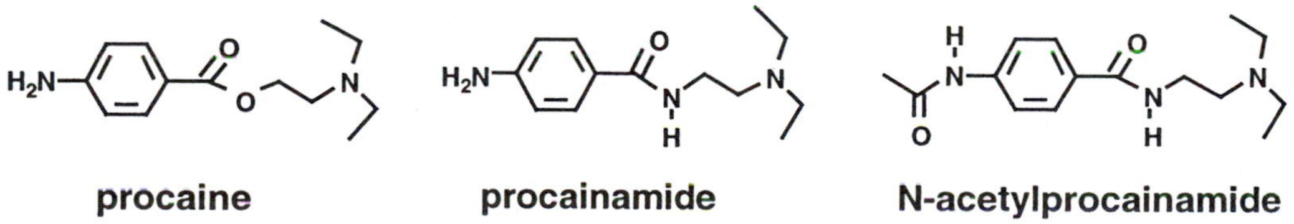

SCHEME 11.5   The structures of procaine, procainamide, and *N*-acetylprocainamide exemplify drug development based upon understanding principles of drug metabolism.

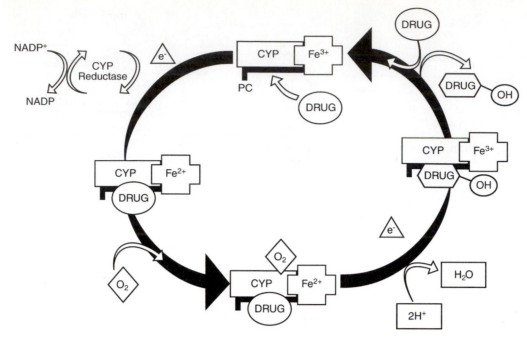

FIGURE 11.1 Free drug enters the cycle *(upper right)* and is complexed to the ferric oxidation state of the heme protein cytochrome P (CYP) in the presence of phosphatidylcholine (PC). The Fe^{3+} is reduced to Fe^{2+} by an electron generated by the conversion of NADPH to $NADP^+$ by the enzyme cytochrome P reductase *(upper left)*. The reduced complex absorbs molecular oxygen *(lower middle)*. Addition of a second electron from cytochrome P reductase results in the generation of one molecule of water, hydroxylation of one molecule of drug, and the oxidation of iron to Fe^{3+}. When hydroxylated drug is released from the enzyme complex *(upper right)*, the cycle repeats.

PHASE I BIOTRANSFORMATIONS

Liver Microsomal Cytochrome P450 Monooxygenases

Among the major enzyme systems effecting drug metabolism, the cytochrome P450 monooxygenases[1] are dominant. In humans, there are 12 gene families of functionally related proteins comprising this group of enzymes. The cytochrome P450 enzymes, abbreviated CYPs (for <u>c</u>ytochrome <u>P</u>s), catalyze drug and endogenous compound oxidations in the liver, and also in the kidneys, gastrointestinal tract, skin, and lungs. Chemically, the process of drug oxidation can be written as:

$$\text{Drug} + \text{NADPH} + \text{H}^+ + \text{O}_2 \rightarrow \text{Oxidized Drug} +$$
$$\text{NADP}^+ + \text{H}_2\text{O}$$

The requirement for NADPH as an energy and electron source necessitates the close association within the endoplasmic reticulum of the cell of CYPs with NADPH-cytochrome P reductase in a 10:1 ratio. To reconstitute the enzyme activity *in vitro*, it is necessary to include the CYP heme protein, the reductase, NADPH, molecular oxygen, and phosphatidylcholine, a lipid surfactant. The electron flow in the CYP microsomal drug oxidizing system is illustrated in Figure 11.1.

[1] In a recent historical review, R. Synder details the history of discovery of cytochrome P450 (Toxicol Sci 2000;58:3–4). Briefly, David Keilin (1887–1963) of Cambridge University named the cytochromes, pigments that absorbed light that he isolated from dipterous flies. He labeled the oxygen activating enzyme cytochrome oxidase. Otto Warburg (1833–1970) in Berlin studied cytochrome oxidase and measured its inhibition by carbon monoxide. He reported that the inhibitory effects of carbon monoxide were reversed by light and the degree of reversal was wavelength dependent. Otto Rosenthal learned these spectroscopic techniques in Warburg's lab and brought them to the University of Pennsylvania when he fled Germany in the 1930s. There, with David Cooper and Ronald Estabrook, the mechanism of steroid hydroxylation was investigated. Using the Yang-Chance spectrophotometer, they determined the characteristic spectroscopic signature of the cytochrome P450-CO complex and recognized in 1963 that it was the same as that of pig and rat liver microsomal pigments reported in 1958 independently by both M. Klingenberg and D. Garfield. These spectroscopic characteristics were used in 1964 by T. Omura and R. Sato to identify cytochrome P450 as a heme protein. Rosenthal, Cooper, and Estabrook studied the metabolism of codeine and acetanilide, and demonstrated in 1965 that cytochrome P450 is the oxygen-activating enzyme in xenobiotic metabolism as well as steroid hydroxylation.

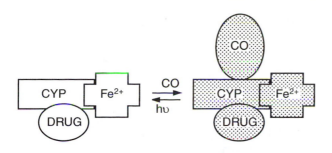

FIGURE 11.2 Cytochrome P450 has a high affinity for carbon monoxide when drugs are bound to the reduced complex, as observed spectroscopically at 450 nm.

The name cytochrome P450 derives from the spectroscopic observation that when drug is bound to the reduced heme enzyme (Fe^{+2}), carbon monoxide can bind to the complex and absorb light at a characteristic and distinctive 450 nm. The CO complex can be dissociated with light and the complex can then absorb oxygen as illustrated in Figure 11.2. The spectroscopic properties of the CYP enzyme complex were of significant utility to investigators who characterized this family of enzymes with respect to their substrate specificity, kinetics, induction, and inhibition.

Of the 12 CYP gene families, most of the drug metabolizing enzymes are in the CYP 1, 2, and 3 families. All have molecular weights of 45–60 kDa. Their naming and classification relate to their degree of amino acid sequence homology. Subfamilies have been assigned to isoenzymes with significant sequence homology to the family (e.g., CYP1A). An additional numerical identifier is added when more than one subfamily has been identified (e.g., CYP1A2). Frequently, two or more enzymes can catalyze the same type of oxidation, indicating redundant and broad substrate specificity. Thus, early efforts to categorize CYPs on the basis of biochemical transformations that they catalyzed led to confusing reports from different investigators that have now been resolved with gene sequences. Some of the principle drug metabolizing CYPs are listed in Table 11.1 (10). Three of the CYP families, 1A2, 2C, and 3A4, are shown in boldface in the table because they account for >50% of the metabolism of most drugs. Their levels can vary considerably, requiring further clinical evaluation when patient response suggests that either too much or too little of a prescribed drug is present.

It is instructive to examine which drugs are substrates for various isoforms of CYP enzymes. Table 11.2 lists some of the substrates for different CYP isoforms (10). There are examples of a single drug that is metabolized by multiple CYP enzymes (acetaminophen, diazepam), and CYP enzymes that metabolize

bioactive endogenous molecules (prostaglandins, steroids) as well as drugs.

The activity of various CYP enzymes is influenced by a variety of factors that have been identified to date. For example, genetic polymorphisms are most significant in the CYP1A, 2A6, 2C9, 2C19, 2D6, and 2E1 families. Nutrition effects have been documented in CYP1A1, 1A2, 2E1, 3A3, and 3A4,5 families; smoking influences the CYP1A1 and 1A2 families; alcohol, the CYP2E1 family; drugs, the CYP1A1, 1A2, 2A6, 2B6; 2C, 2D6, 3A3, 3A4,5 families; and environmental xenobiotics, the CYP1A1, 1A2, 2A6, 1B, 2E1, 3A3, 3A4,5 families.

The diverse nature of these effects is illustrated by recounting the experience of clinical pharmacologists who studied the pharmacokinetics of felodipine, a dihydropyridine calcium channel antagonist (11). They designed a study to test the effects of ethanol on felodipine metabolism. To mask the flavor of ethanol from the subjects, they tested a variety of fruit juices, selecting double-strength frozen grapefruit juice from concentrate as most effective. The resulting plasma felodipine concentrations did not differ between the ethanol/felodipine and felodipine groups, but the plasma concentrations in both groups were considerably higher than those seen in any previous study. The effects of repeated grapefruit juice doses are cumulative and, as shown in Figure 11.3, may increase felodipine concentrations as much as five-fold.

Upon further investigation, it was determined that grapefruit juice administration for 6 consecutive days causes a 62% reduction in small bowel enterocyte CYP3A4 protein, thereby inhibiting the first-pass metabolism of felodipine to oxidized felodipine shown in Scheme 11.6 (12). The effects of grapefruit juice are

TABLE 11.1   Human CYP Enzymes Important in Liver Metabolism of Drugs[a]

CYP enzyme	Percent total CYP content	Extent of variability
1A2	~13	~40-fold
1B1	<1	
2A6	~4	~30–100-fold
2B6	<1	~50-fold
2C	~18	**25–100-fold**
2D6	Up to 2.5	>1000-fold
2E1	Up to 7	~20-fold
2F1		
2J2		
3A4	**Up to 28**	**~20-fold**
4A, 4B		

[a] Data from Rendic S, Di Carlo FJ. Drug Metab Rev 1997;29: 413–580.

TABLE 11.2 Participation of the CYP Enzymes in Metabolism of Some Clinically Important Drugs[a]

CYP enzyme	Participation in drug metabolism (%)	Examples of substrates
1B1		17β-Estradiol
2F1	~ 1.3	Ipomeanol
4A		Prostaglandins
1A1	2.5	R-Warfarin
2A6	2.5	Cyclophosphamide, Halothane, Zidovudine
2B6	3.4	Cyclophosphamide, Testosterone
2E1	4.1	Acetaminophen, Chlorzoxazone, Dapsone, Halothane
1A2	8.2	Acetaminophen, Caffeine, Phenacetin, (R)-Warfarin
2C8,9	15.8	Tolbutamide, Diclofenac, (S)-Warfarin, Phenytoin, Hexobarbital
2C18, 19	8.3	Diazepam, Omeprazole, (S)-Mephenytoin
2D6	18.8	Codeine, Debrisoquine, Dextromethorphan, Bufuralol, Sparteine
3A4,5	34.1	Carbamazepine, Cortisol, Dapsone, Diazepam Erythromycin, Midazolam, Nifedipine, Omeprazole Testosterone

[a] Data from Rendic S, Di Carlo FJ. Drug Metab Rev 1997;29:413–580.

highly variable among individuals depending on their basal levels of small bowel CYP3A4, but grapefruit juice does not affect the pharmacokinetics of intravenously administered felodipine because the active constituents of the juice apparently are not absorbed and do not affect liver CYPs. More recent studies have shown that the degradation half-life of CYP3A4 normally is 8 hours and that at least 3 days are required to regain normal CYP3A4 function after exposure to grapefruit juice (13).

The effect of grapefruit juice on felodipine kinetics illustrates several of the difficulties and pitfalls that not only confound clinical studies of new drug products, but are a source of concern in clinical medicine. The topic of drug–drug interactions is discussed in greater detail in Chapter 14. However, pharmacologically active CYP inducers or inhibitors may derive from dietary or environmental origin (e.g., insecticides or perfumes) and can

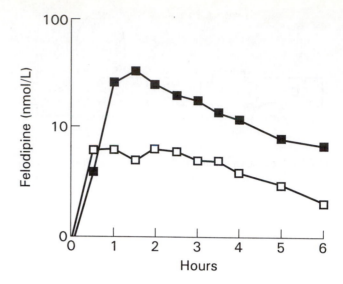

FIGURE 11.3   Plasma felodipine concentrations after oral administration to an individual of a 5 mg dose with (■) and without (□) grapefruit juice. (Reproduced with permission from Bailey DG, et al. Br J Clin Pharmacol 1998;46;101–10.)

only be recognized when appropriate *in vitro* or *in vivo* kinetic studies have been performed. Because patients have access to many new diet and food supplements, it is likely that other, currently unknown metabolic interactions will be discovered.

The example of felodipine also demonstrates that CYPs outside of the liver may have significant effects on drug concentrations. In addition to the dominant CYP3A family, the GI tract contains CYPs 2D6, 2C, 2B6, and 1A1. Similarly, CYPs are found in lung (CYP1A1, 2A6, 2B6, 2C, 2E, 2F, and 4B1), kidney (CYP1A1, 1B1, 3A, and 4A11), skin, placenta, prostate, and other tissues where their inhibition or activation may be of clinical relevance to the efficacy or toxicity of a therapeutic agent.

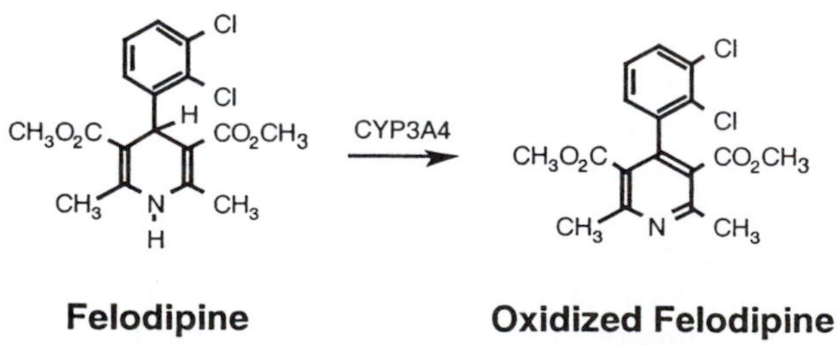

Felodipine   **Oxidized Felodipine**

SCHEME 11.6   Oxidation of felodipine is due to CYP3A4 in the small bowel.

CYP Mediated Chemical Transformations

Most drugs are relatively small organic compounds with molecular weights below 500 Da. The action of various CYP isoforms is predictable in that there are several organic structural elements that are principal targets for metabolic transformations. However, the metabolism of any specific drug is not entirely predictable in that a specific site of metabolism may be favored for one compound and a different site for another, but structurally related, compound. The following examples are chosen to reflect some of the dominant pathways for a specific drug and illustrate the selectivity of the metabolic enzymes.

Aliphatic Hydroxylation

Hydroxylation occurs at aliphatic carbon atoms, frequently at secondary or tertiary sites in preference to primary carbon atoms as shown in Scheme 11.7. Ibuprofen as shown in Scheme 11.8 is an example of aliphatic hydroxylation. Other drugs similarly metabolized include terfenadine, pentobarbital, and cyclosporin.

Aromatic Hydroxylation

Many aromatic drugs are hydroxylated either directly through asymmetrical oxygen transfer, or through an unstable arene oxide intermediate as shown in Scheme 11.9.

Because the half-life of the epoxide intermediate is short, immediate rearrangement or reaction may lead to a variety of substituted metabolites. The intermediacy of an epoxide intermediate can be inferred by the identification of para- and meta-hydroxylated and dihydrodiol metabolites, although

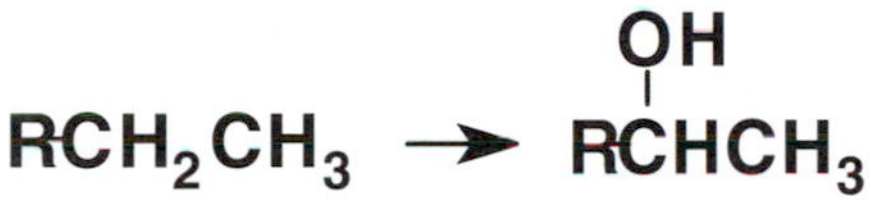

SCHEME 11.7   Aliphatic hydroxylation generally decreases lipid solubility, increases water solubility.

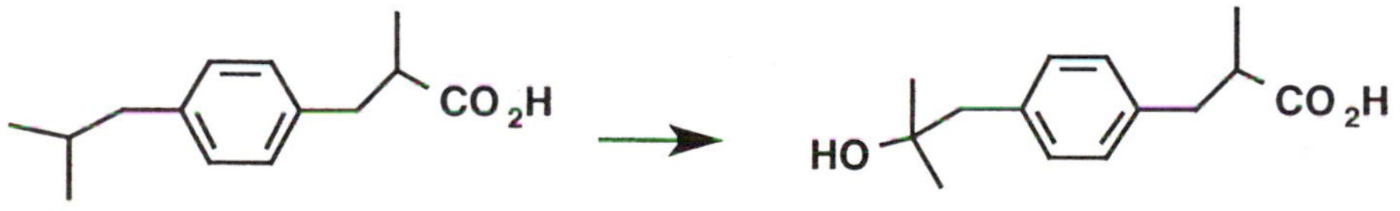

ibuprofen

SCHEME 11.8   Aliphatic hydroxylation of ibuprofen.

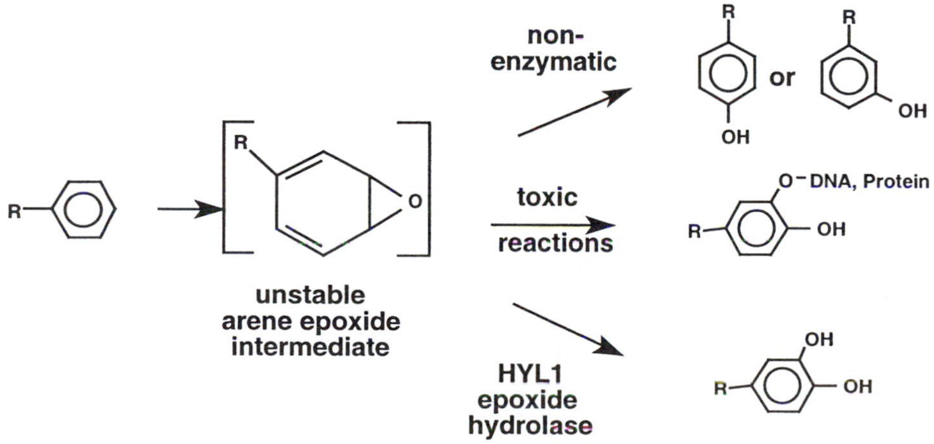

SCHEME 11.9   Hydroxylation of aromatic carbon atoms often proceeds through a reactive and unstable arene epoxide intermediate.

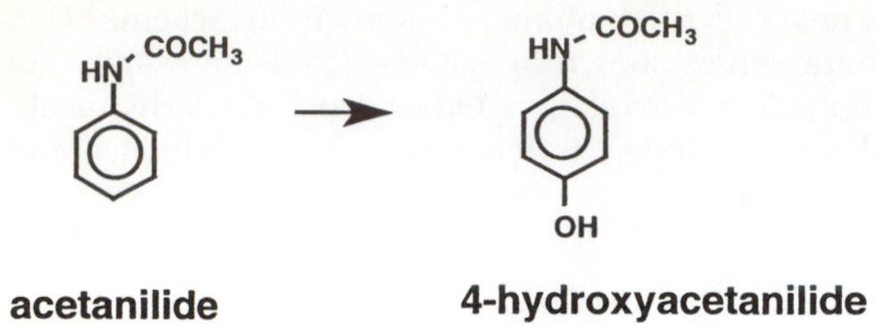

acetanilide   **4-hydroxyacetanilide**

SCHEME 11.10 Metabolism of acetanilide results in para-hydroxylation.

their relative abundances will vary with substitution and steric considerations. Acetanilide, like phenobarbital discussed previously, exemplifies the aromatic compounds that rearrange rapidly following CYP mediated arene epoxide formation leading to a single metabolite as shown in Scheme 11.10.

The major metabolite of phenytoin is para-hydroxyphenytoin, formed through an arene epoxide intermediate as shown in Scheme 11.11. Microsomal epoxide hydrolase (HYL1) is widely distributed in tissues and serves a protective role in converting longer lasting arene oxide intermediates to diols. The arene epoxide of phenytoin is detoxified through HYL1 to form the dihydrodiol (14).

Phenytoin administration during pregnancy may produce a constellation of congenital abnormalities including cleft palate. This has been ascribed to

phenytoin-arene oxide reactivity with cellular DNA in tissues lacking the protective effects of HYL1 (15, 16). Gaedigk et al. have demonstrated that there is tissue-specific expression of microsomal HYL1 and not a single HYL1 transcript and promoter region (14). They suggest that there is a post-translational regulatory pathway determining constitutive levels of enzyme in various tissues.

N-Dealkylation (O-Dealkylation, S-Dealkylation)

The mechanism of CYP catalyzed N-dealkylation has received considerable study (16). N-dealkyation appears to involve radical cation intermediates and molecular oxygen (not water). Formally, O- and S-dealkylation are related to N-dealkylation, although the mechanisms may differ. N-Demethylation is a frequent route of metabolism of drugs containing methylamine functionalities as shown in Scheme 11.12. Ethylmorphine is an example of drugs metabolized by N-dealkylation as shown in Scheme 11.13; other drugs similarly metabolized include lidocaine, aminopyrine, acetophenetedine, 6-methylthiopurine.

Drugs containing multiple functional groups are substrates for multiple drug metabolizing enzymes and pathways. The N-demethylation vs. O-dealkylation of ethylmorphine (Scheme 11.13) demonstrates that one reaction pathway may predominate. Propranolol is an example of a compound where multiple

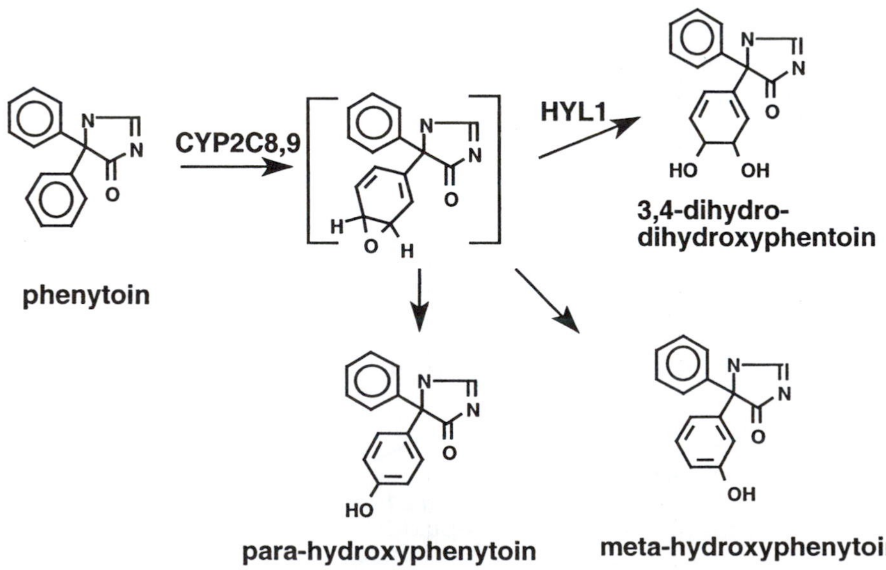

phenytoin → CYP2C8,9 → [intermediate] → HYL1 → **3,4-dihydro-dihydroxyphentoin**

para-hydroxyphenytoin   **meta-hydroxyphenytoin**

SCHEME 11.11 The metabolism of phenytoin through an arene epoxide results in a triad of oxidized metabolites that is characteristic for this intermediate.

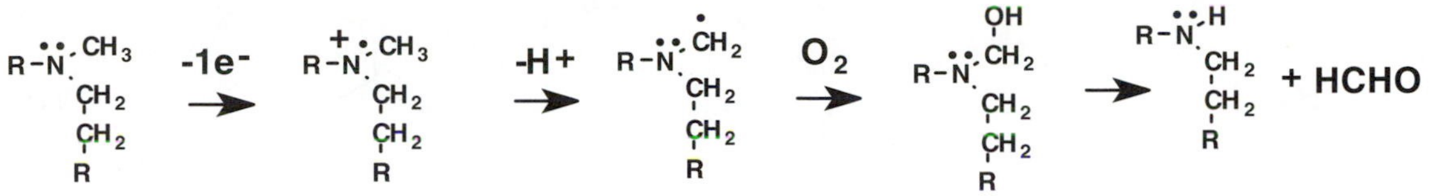

SCHEME 11.12 *N*-demethylation generates formaldehyde as a by-product.

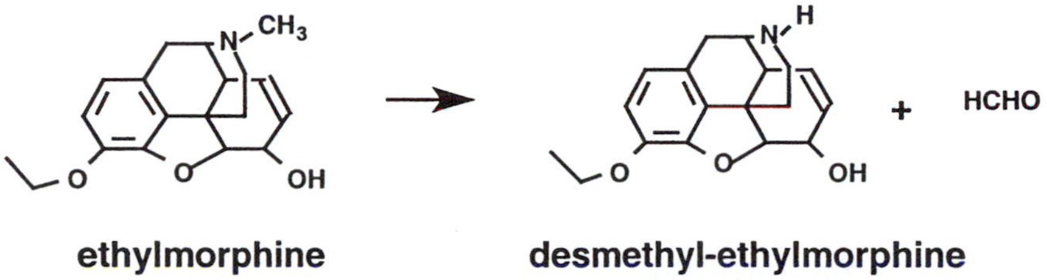

ethylmorphine   **desmethyl-ethylmorphine**

SCHEME 11.13 *N*-demethylation of ethylmorphine is favored over *O*-dealkylation.

alternative metabolites are formed as shown in Scheme 11.14.

Oxidative Deamination

Oxidative deamination proceeds through an unstable carbinolamine intermediate as shown in Scheme 11.15. Amphetamine is an example of a drug metabolized through oxidative deamination as shown in Scheme 11.16.

Dehalogenation

As discussed in Chapter 15, dehalogenation of a number of inhalation anesthetics (halothane, methoxyflurane) and halogenated solvents by liver enzymes yields chemically reactive free radicals that play an important role in the hepatotoxicity of these compounds. Dehalogenation produces a free radical intermediate that may be detected by its interaction with cellular lipids as shown in general form in

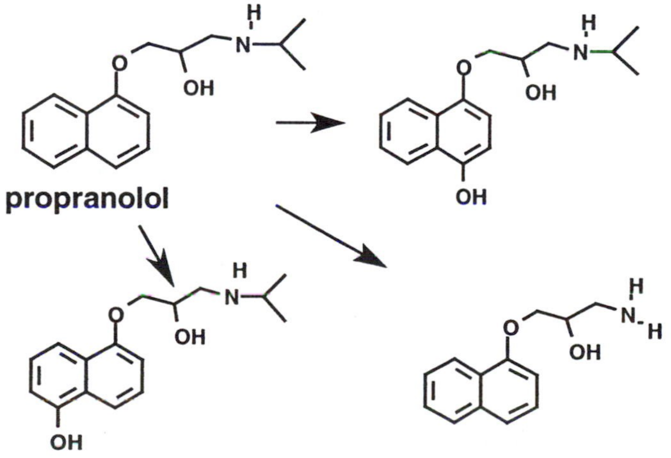

propranolol

SCHEME 11.14 Two different aromatic ring hydroxylated metabolites and the *N*-dealkylated metabolite of propranolol are excreted in urine.

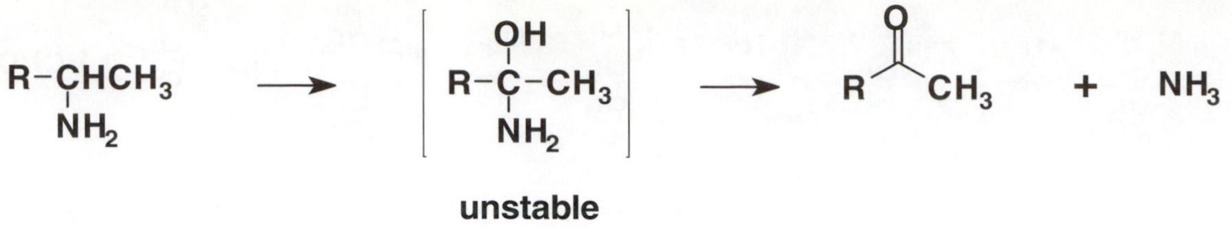

unstable

SCHEME 11.15   A general mechanism for oxidative deamination.

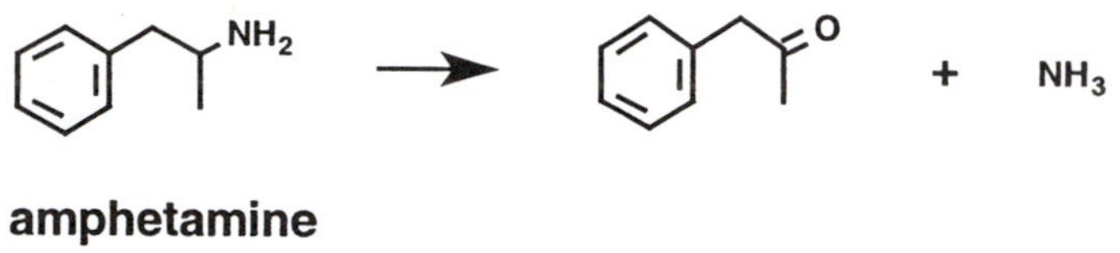

amphetamine

SCHEME 11.16   Amphetamine is metabolized to an inactive ketone.

Scheme 11.17. Dehalogenation of carbon tetrachloride is illustrated in Scheme 11.18.

N-Oxidation

Amines are readily oxidized by CYP enzymes. Aliphatic amines are converted to hydroxylamines as shown in Scheme 11.19; hydroxylamines are less basic than the parent amines. Aromatic amines are converted to products that are more toxic than their parent amines, frequently producing hypersensitivity or carcinogenicity.

Dapsone is oxidized by CYP2E1 with high affinity both *in vitro* and *in vivo*, and also by CYP3A4 as shown in Scheme 11.20. The major side effects of dapsone (methemoglobinemia, agranulocytosis) are linked to its N-oxidation (18, 19).

Other N-oxidized substrates include mianserin and clozapine, both catalyzed by CYP1A2 and 3A4. Because the products are identical to those produced by flavin monooxygenases (FMOs), *in vitro* enzymatic studies are required to identify which enzyme system is active during *in vivo* metabolism.

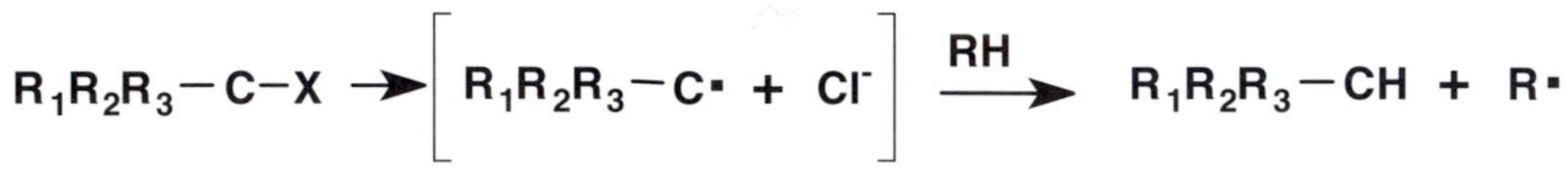

$$R_1R_2R_3-C-X \rightarrow \left[R_1R_2R_3-C\cdot + Cl^- \right] \xrightarrow{RH} R_1R_2R_3-CH + R\cdot$$

SCHEME 11.17   The mechanism for dehalogenation produces reactive free radicals.

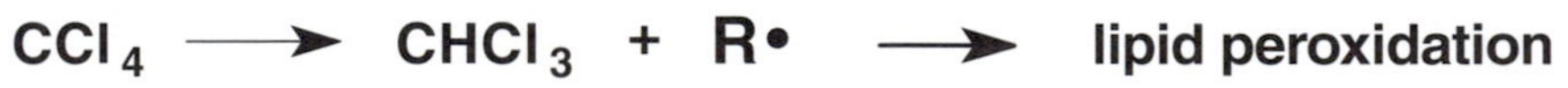

$$CCl_4 \longrightarrow CHCl_3 + R\bullet \longrightarrow \text{lipid peroxidation}$$

SCHEME 11.18   The metabolism of carbon tetrachloride can be measured by the formation of oxidized lipids.

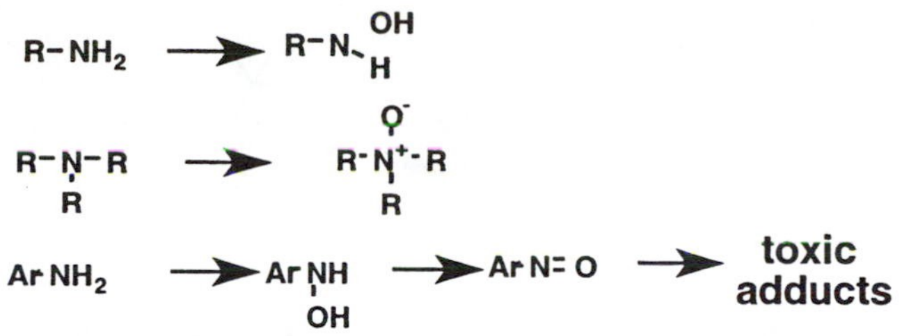

SCHEME 11.19   The nitrogen atom is a site for oxidation, potentially leading to toxic by-products.

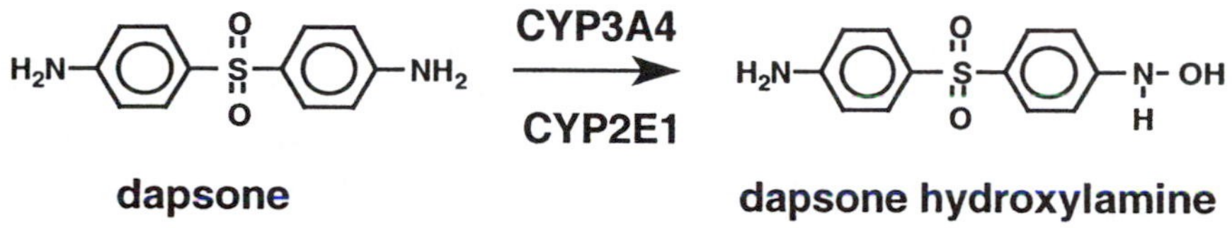

dapsone   **dapsone hydroxylamine**

SCHEME 11.20   Dapsone is a substrate for *N*-oxidation.

S-Oxidation

Sulfur is readily oxidized, non-enzymatically as well as enzymatically as shown in Scheme 11.21. Chlorpromazine is an example of *S*-oxidation by CYP3A as shown in Scheme 11.22. Chlorpromazine is also metabolized by *N*-oxidation and *N*-dealkylation pathways resulting in a multiplicity of excreted products.

There are cases of drug substrates metabolized preferentially by CYP3A and not by FMOs. Tazofelone, an experimental agent for treating patients with inflammatory bowel disease, is a sulfur and nitrogen heterocyclic compound that is sulfoxidized by human microsomal CYP3A and not FMO as shown in Scheme 11.23 (21).

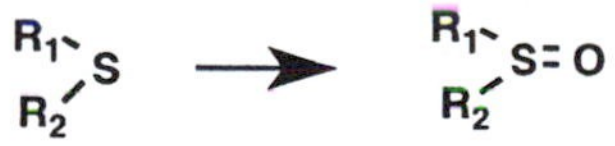

SCHEME 11.21   General formula for sulfur oxidation.

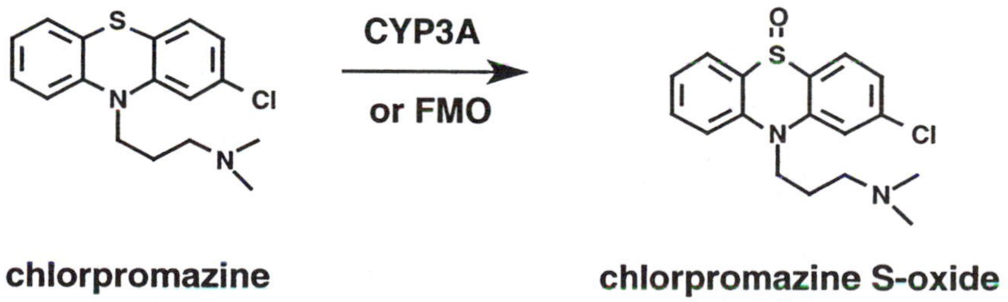

chlorpromazine   **chlorpromazine S-oxide**

SCHEME 11.22   CYP3A and FMO sulfur oxidation produce the same chlorpromazine metabolite as described in the following section (20).

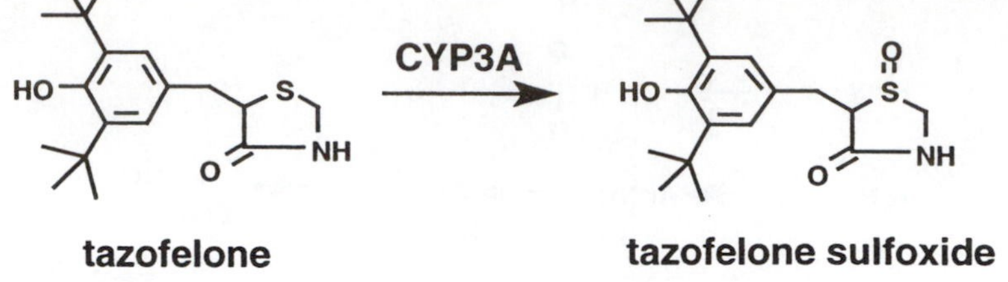

tazofelone →(CYP3A) **tazofelone sulfoxide**

SCHEME 11.23 *S-oxidation is a major route of metabolism for tazofelone.*

Non-CYP Biotransformations

Hydrolysis

Hydrolyses of esters or amides are common reactions catalyzed by ubiquitous esterases, amidases, and proteases found in every tissue and physiological fluid. These enzymes exhibit widely differing substrate specificities. The hydrolytic reactions shown in Scheme 11.24 are the reverse of Phase II conjugation reactions, especially for the acetylation reaction discussed later in this chapter.

Aspirin (acetylsalicylic acid) is an example of a compound that is hydrolyzed readily in plasma as shown in Scheme 11.25. Aspirin has a plasma half-life of 15 minutes in plasma. Salicylic acid, the active metabolite of

aspirin has a much longer half-life (12 hours for anti-inflammatory activity). However, salicylic acid irritates the gastric mucosa, leading to the use of acetylsalicylic acid or sodium salicylate in clinical practice.

Reduction

Although most drugs are metabolized by oxidative processes, reduction may be a clinically important pathway of drug metabolism. In most cases these reduction may be a clinically important pathway of drug metabolism. In most cases these metabolic transformations are carried out by reductase enzymes in intestinal anaerobic bacteria. In the case of prontosil, an aromatic azo-function ($Ar_1 - N = N - Ar_2$) is reduced to anilines ($Ar_1 - NH_2$, $Ar_2 - NH_2$). One of the reduced metabolites is sul-

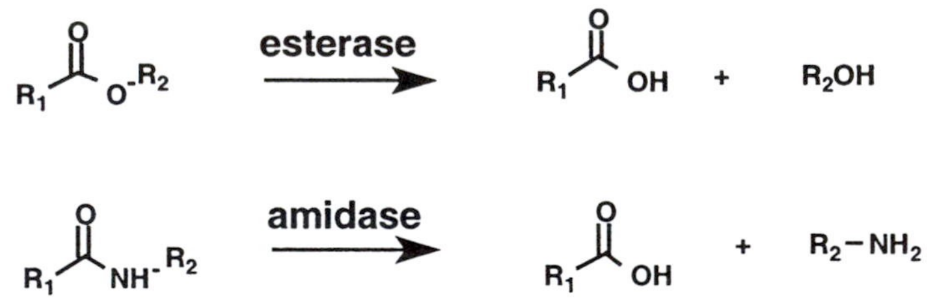

SCHEME 11.24 Hydrolytic enzymes are involved in the metabolism of many endogenous compounds.

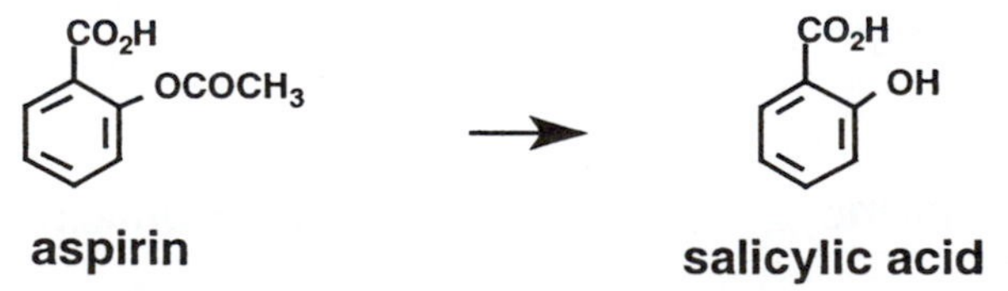

aspirin → **salicylic acid**

SCHEME 11.25 Structures of aspirin and its active metabolite salicylic acid.

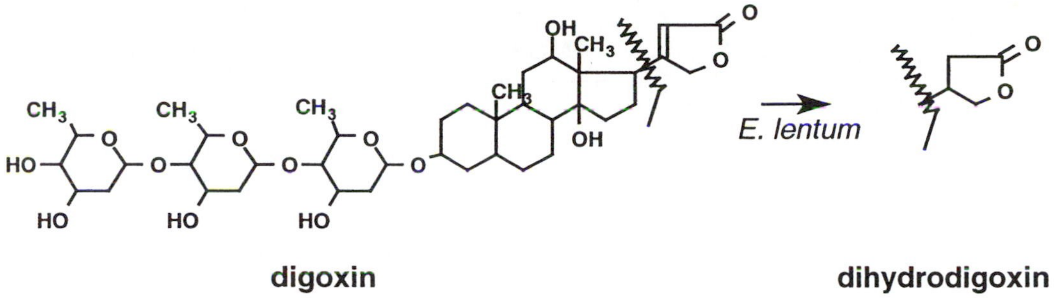

digoxin   **dihydrodigoxin**

SCHEME 11.26 Reduction of the side-chain of digoxin eliminates pharmacologic activity.

fanilamide, the active antibacterial agent, first recognized in 1935 (22). Since biotransformation is required for antibacterial activity, prontosil is referred to as a *prodrug*.

A second example is the metabolic inactivation of digoxin by *Eubacterium lentum* in the intestine (23) as shown in Scheme 11.26. Approximately 10% of patients taking digoxin excrete large quantities of the inactive reduction product dihydrodigoxin (24). As discussed in Chapter 4, the enteric metabolism of digoxin reduces digoxin bioavailability significantly in some patients. Conversely, when such patients require antibiotic therapy, the resulting blood levels of digoxin may reach toxic levels because the antibiotic halts the previously robust inactivation by *E. lentum* and digoxin bioavailability is thereby increased.

Oxidations

Flavine Monooxygenases

Flavine monooxygenases (FMOs) are microsomal enzymes that catalyze the oxygenation of nucleophilic heteroatom-containing (nitrogen, sulfur, phosphorus, selenium) compounds producing structurally similar metabolities to those produced by CYPs previously discussed. Unlike CYPs, the FMOs do not require tight substrate binding to the enzyme, but only a single point contact with the very reactive hydroperoxyflavin monooxygenating agent. FMOs are also unlike CYPs in that they do not contain metal and are very heat labile. The quantitative role of FMOs vs. CYPs in the metabolism of any specific drug cannot be predicted from an examination of the drug structure; in fact, many compounds are substrates of both enzymes. Five different mammalian FMO gene subfamilies have been identified and polyclonal antibodies have permitted identification of FMO isoforms in liver and lung from different species (human, pig, rabbit). FMOs exhibit a very broad ability to oxidize structurally different substrates, suggesting that they

contribute significantly to the metabolism of a number of drugs. FMOs require molecular oxygen, NADPH, flavin adenosine dinucleotide. Factors affecting FMOs (diet, drugs, sex) have not been as highly studied as CYPs, but it is clear that FMOs are prominent metabolizing enzymes for common drugs such as nicotine and cimetidine.

Nicotine is an example of a compound that undergoes FMO3 catalyzed N-oxidation as shown in Scheme 11.27. About 4% of a nicotine dose is stereoselectively metabolized to trans-(S)-(–)-nicotine N-1'oxide in humans by FMO3, whereas 30% of an administered dose appears as cotinine, a CYP2A6 product (20, 25). Other examples of FMO N-oxidation include trimethylamine, amphetamine, and the phenothiazines (20). As described previously, FMO3 catalyzes S-oxidation of substrates such as cimetidine, shown in Scheme 11.28, and chlorpromazine, also a CYP3A substrate (Scheme 11.22).

Monoamine Oxidases

Monoamine oxidases (MAO-A and -B) are mitochondrial enzymes that oxidatively deaminate endogenous biogenic amine neurotransmitters such as dopamine, serotonin, norepinephrine, and epinephrine. MAOs are like FMOs in that they catalyze the oxidation of drugs to produce drug metabolites that are similar in chemical structures to those formed by CYPs. Because the resulting structures are identical, oxidative deamination by

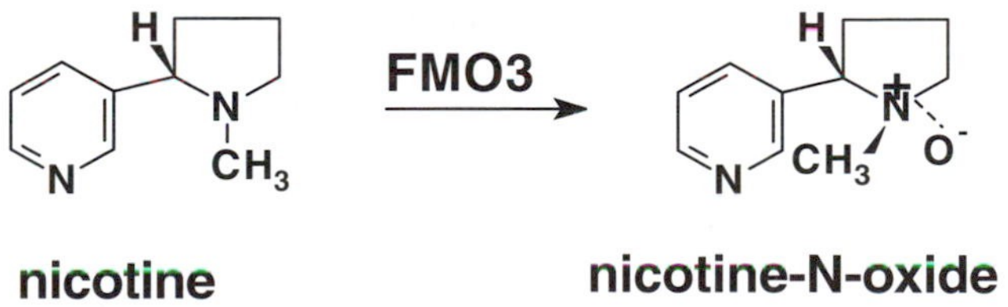

nicotine   **nicotine-N-oxide**

SCHEME 11.27 Nicotine is oxidized in a stereospecific manner to an *N*-oxide by FMO3.

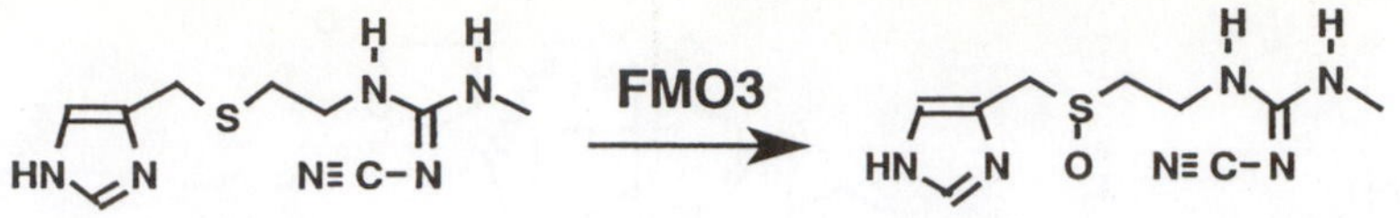

cimetidine   **cimeditine S-oxide**

SCHEME 11.28 Cimetidine is an example of a drug metabolized by FMO3 catalyzed S-oxidation; other FMO3 substrates include chlorpromazine, also a CYP3A substrate.

MAO can only be distinguished from CYP oxidative deamination by drug and enzyme characterization, not by metabolite structure. MAOs are found in liver, kidney, intestine, and brain. Some drugs (tranylcypromine, selegiline) have been designed as irreversible "suicide" substrates to inhibit MAO in order to alter the balance of CNS neurotransmitters, and the response to these inhibitors, and the study of *in vitro* enzyme preparations is used to distinguish this enzymatic process. Similarly, diamine oxidase catalyzes oxidative deamination of endogenous amines such as histamine and the polyamines putrescine and cadaverine, and can contribute to the oxidative deamination of drugs. Diamine oxidase is found in high levels in liver, intestine, and placenta, and converts amines to aldehydes in the presence of oxygen, similar to the action of CYPs.

Alcohol and Aldehyde Dehydrogenases

Alcohols and aldehydes are metabolized by nonmicrosomal liver dehydrogenases and by nonspecific liver enzymes that are important in the catabolism of endogenous compounds. Ethanol is a special example of a compound whose metabolism is clinically relevant in that ethanol may interact with prescribed pharmaceuticals either metabolically or pharmacodynamically. Ethanol is metabolized first to acetaldehyde by alcohol dehydrogenase and then to acetic acid by aldehyde dehydrogenase as shown in Scheme 11.29. These enzymes are important both for ethanol and for drugs containing alcohol functional groups.

There are also CYP-dependent microsomal ethanol oxidizing enzymes that provide metabolic redundancy, but alcohol and aldehyde dehydrogenases are the major enzymes involved in ethanol metabolism under normal physiological conditions.

PHASE II BIOTRANSFORMATIONS (CONJUGATIONS)

Drugs are frequently metabolized by covalent addition of an endogenous species such as a sugar or an amino acid. This addition, or conjugation, usually converts a lipophilic drug into a more polar product, as noted in the example of phenobarbital metabolism to hydroxyphenobarbital-glucuronide (Scheme 11.1). There are multiple conjugation reactions—glucuronidation, sulfation, acetylation, methylation, and amino acid conjugation (glycine, taurine, glutathione). Taken together, these Phase II biotransformations are analogous and comparable. However, their catalytic enzyme systems differ greatly from each other, as do the properties of resulting metabolites. Not all of these metabolites are pharmacologically inactive; some have therapeutic activity whereas others are reactive and toxic intermediates. As a consequence, it is more useful to separately present and discuss each of the three major conjugation reactions. In humans, glucuronidation is a high-capacity pathway, sulfation is a low-capacity

Alcohol Dehydrogenase

$$CH_3CH_2OH + NAD^+ \longrightarrow CH_3CHO + NADH + H^+$$

Aldehyde Dehydrogenase

$$CH_3CHO + NAD^+ + H_2O \longrightarrow CH_3CO_2H + NADH + H^+$$

SCHEME 11.29 The products of alcohol dehydrogenase are substrates for aldehyde dehydrogenase.

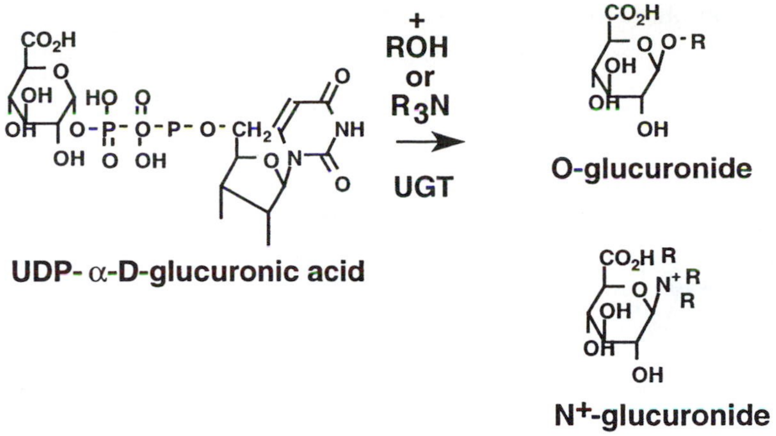

SCHEME 11.30 Nitrogen and oxygen linked glucuronide formation markedly enhances the polarity and water solubility of drugs.

pathway, and acetylation capacity exhibits high interindividual variability.

Glucuronidation

The glucuronidation pathway often accounts for a major portion of the metabolites of a drug that are found excreted in urine. Glucuronides are formed by a family of soluble microsomal enzymes, the uridine diphosphate(UDP)-glucuronosyltransferases (UGTs). Although glucuronide formation occurs predominantly in the liver, it also takes place in the kidneys and brain. There are two subfamilies comprising multiple (at least 14) isoforms with very different primary amino acid structures. The UGT1 subfamily glucuronidates phenols and bilirubin; the substrates for UGT2 include steroids and bile acids. The subfamilies that have been cloned and expressed exhibit limited substrate specificity. The high capacity of human liver for glucuronida-

tion may be due to the broad substrate redundancy in this family. UGTs catalyze the transfer of glucuronic acid from UDP-glucuronic acid to an oxygen or nitrogen atom in a drug substrate as shown in Scheme 11.30. There is considerable variation allowed in the substrates for glucuronidation, and phenols, alcohols, aromatic or aliphatic amines, and carboxylic acids are suitable functional groups for glucuronidation.

Regarding the glucuronidation of morphine shown in Scheme 11.31, morphine-3-glucuronide is the major morphine metabolite (45–55%); morphine-6-glucuronide is 20 to 30% of that level. Importantly, morphine-6-glucuronide is a more potent analgesic than its parent compound in humans. On the other hand, morphine-3-glucuronide lacks analgesic activity, but antagonizes the respiratory depression induced by morphine and morphine-6-glucuronide. Recognition of the potency of morphine-6-glucuronide has led to its evaluation as a drug for intravenous administration (26, 27).

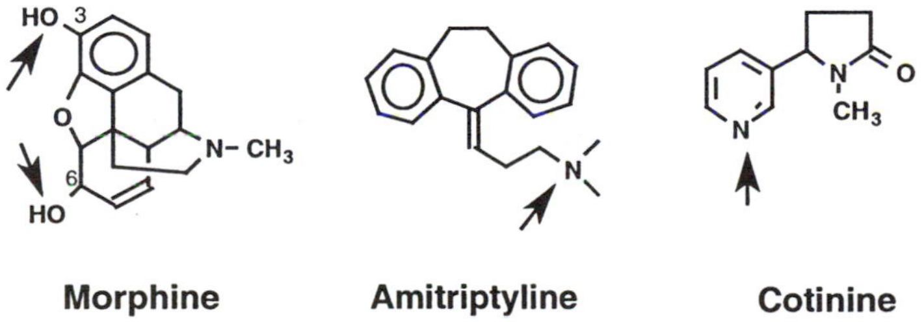

Morphine   **Amitriptyline**   **Cotinine**

SCHEME 11.31 O-glucuronides (ethers) can form from phenols such as morphine (3-phenol), p-hydroxy phenobarbital (Scheme 11.1), p-hydroxyphenytoin (Chapter 2); alcohols like morphine (6-hydroxyl). N^+-glucuronides can be formed from aliphatic amines like amitriptyline, or aromatic amines like the nicotine metabolite continine.

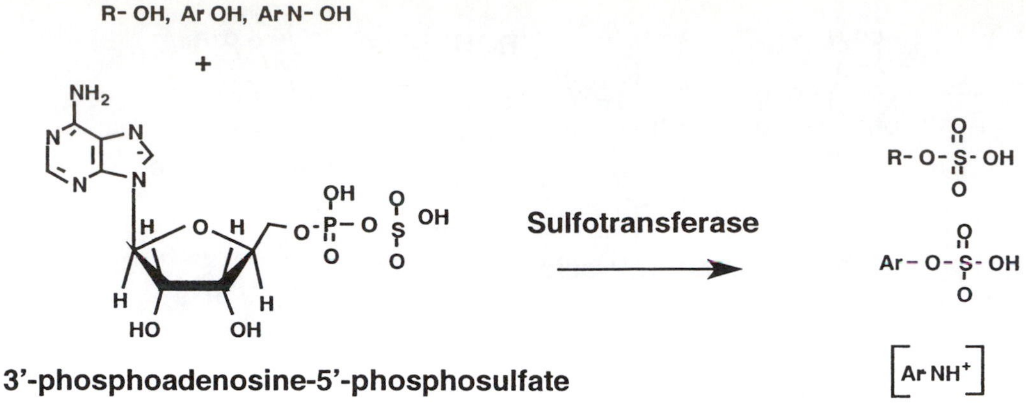

R- OH, Ar OH, Ar N- OH

+

3'-phosphoadenosine-5'-phosphosulfate

Sulfotransferase

$$R-O-\overset{O}{\underset{O}{\overset{\parallel}{S}}}-OH$$

$$Ar-O-\overset{O}{\underset{O}{\overset{\parallel}{S}}}-OH$$

$$\left[Ar\,NH^{+} \right]$$

SCHEME 11.32   General pathway for enzymatic sulfation.

Drug N^{+}-glucuronides, the quaternary ammonium products from glucuronidation of tertiary amines, have only recently been recovered as major metabolites in urine because appropriate analytical methods were not available previously (28). The percentage of the administered dose of amitryptiline excreted in human urine as amitryptiline-N^{+}-glucuronide is ~ 8%; and 17% of a nicotine dose is recovered as continine-N_1-glucuronide. The pharmacological properties of most drug N^{+}-glucuronides have not yet been determined, but the N-glucuronides of arylamines have carcinogenic properties. In particular, N-glucuronides formed in the liver can be hydrolyzed in acidic urine to a reactive electrophilic intermediate that attacks bladder epithelium.

Sulfation

Sulfation (or sulfonation) metabolizes phenols, hydroxylamines or alcohols to sulfate esters as shown in Scheme 11.32, converting somewhat polar to very polar functionalities, fully ionized at neutral pH. Like glucuronidation, sulfation is carried out by at least two subfamilies of enzyme isoforms, the sulfotransferases (STs). One subfamily is cytosolic and associated with drug metabolism and the other is membrane-bound, localized in the Golgi apparatus, and associated with sulfation of glycoproteins, proteins, and glycosaminoglycans. The STs are widely distributed in human tissues. Five cytosolic ST isoforms have been identified and characterized in human tissue; four catalyze sulfation of phenols, one the sulfation of hydroxy steroids.

Also by analogy to glucuronidation, sulfated metabolites may be pharmacologically more active than their respective parent drugs. For example, minoxidil (shown in Scheme 11.33), when applied to the scalp to promote

hair growth, requires bioactivation by STs present in hair follicles (29, 30). Minoxidil sulfate is a potent vasodilator, apparently because it is a potassium channel agonist.

A second example of sulfate bioactivation derives from the observed carcinogenicity of aromatic amines, such as those derived from coal tar (31). The polycyclic aromatic amines are N-hydroxylated by CYPs and then sulfated to form unstable N-O-sulfates that decompose and produce reactive nitrenium ion intermediates that form DNA and protein adducts. One environmental/genetic hypothesis of colon cancer etiology proposes an interaction between dietary aromatic amines and the polymorphic expression of the appropriate STs for their activation to procarcinogenic reactive intermediates (31, 32).

Acetylation

The acetyl transferase enzymes are cytosolic and found in many tissues, including liver, small intestine, blood, and kidney. Acetylation substrates are aromatic or aliphatic amines, hydroxyl or sulfhydryl groups as shown in Scheme 11.34.

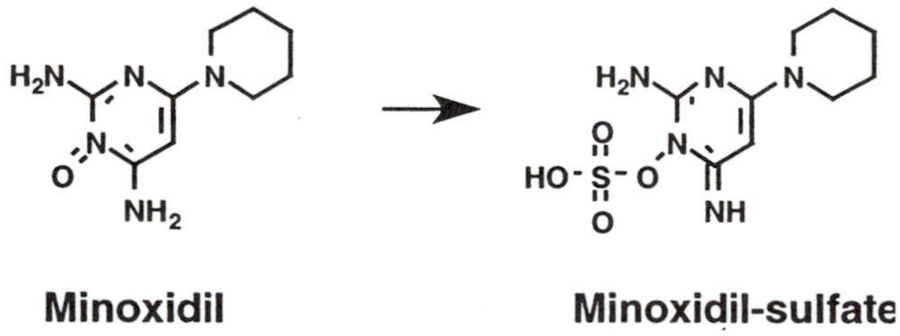

Minoxidil   **Minoxidil-sulfate**

SCHEME 11.33   Minoxidil requires sulfation for bioactivation.

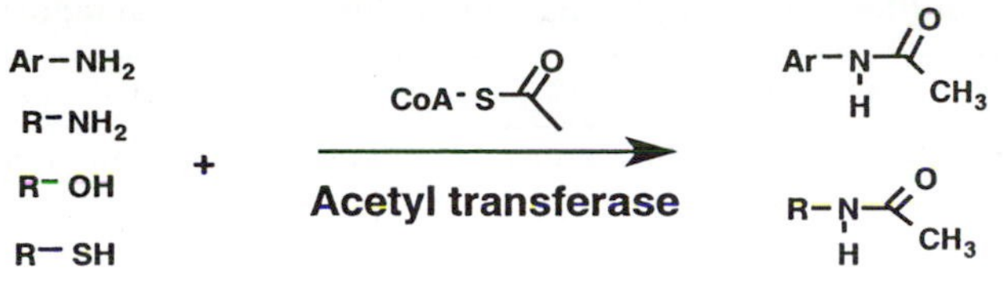

SCHEME 11.34 Acetyl transferase donates the acyl group from Coenzyme A to drug substrates.

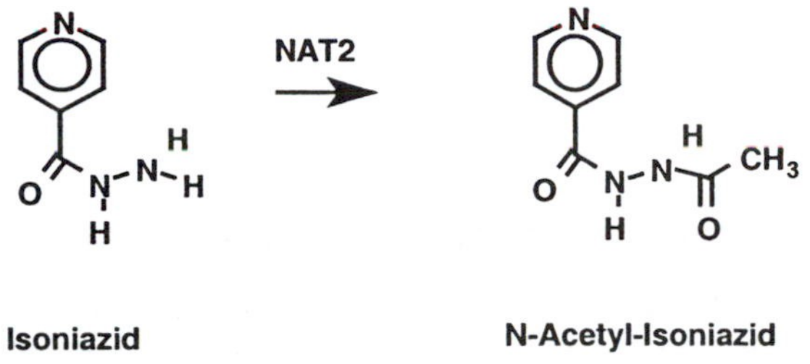

Isoniazid   **N-Acetyl-Isoniazid**

SCHEME 11.35 Isoniazid is metabolically inactivated by acetylation.

The *N*-acetyl transferase (NAT) enzymes have been most highly characterized in humans for the historical reason that isoniazid, an NAT substrate, has played a pivotal role in treating patients with tuberculosis. The major route of metabolism of isoniazid is shown in Scheme 11.35.

In treating Caucasian and black patients with isoniazid, it was noted that the half-life of the parent drug was 70 minutes in about one-half of the patients (*rapid acetylators*) and 3 hours in the other half (*slow acetylators*). There are two NAT families of enzymes, NAT1 and NAT2, that are distinguished by their preferential

acetylation of *p*-aminosalicylic acid (NAT1) or sulfamethazine (NAT2). As discussed in Chapter 13, isoniazid is a substrate for NAT2, a highly polymorphic enzyme, resulting from at least 20 different NAT2 alleles. Slow acetylators are homozygous for the NAT2 slow acetylator allele(s); rapid acetylators are homozygous or heterozygous for the fast NAT2 acetylator allele. There are clinical consequences of fast and slow acetylation from the different blood levels of isoniazid that result from patient differences in metabolism. Side effects from high levels of isoniazid, such as peripheral neuropathy (33) and hepatitis (34), are more frequent in slow acetylators.

The Phase II acetylation of aromatic hydroxylamines, the products of Phase I metabolism of aromatic amines, contitutes a toxic metabolic pathway that has been implicated in carcinogenesis as illustrated in Scheme 11.36. Rapid acetylators (with respect to NAT2) have been shown to have an increased risk of colon cancer. The mechanism of this toxicity appears to involve the reactive nitrenium ion that is formed spontaneously from unstable acetylated aromatic hydroxylamines (35).

ADDITIONAL EFFECTS ON DRUG METABOLISM

Species

Drug metabolism in different species has long been recognized as varying with regard to percentages of metabolite formed: A vs. B. vs. C, and so on. It is now recognized that there is considerable genetic variability between species in the CYPs present in liver as well as in their complement of other drug-metabolizing enzymes. As a consequence, metabolism studies con-

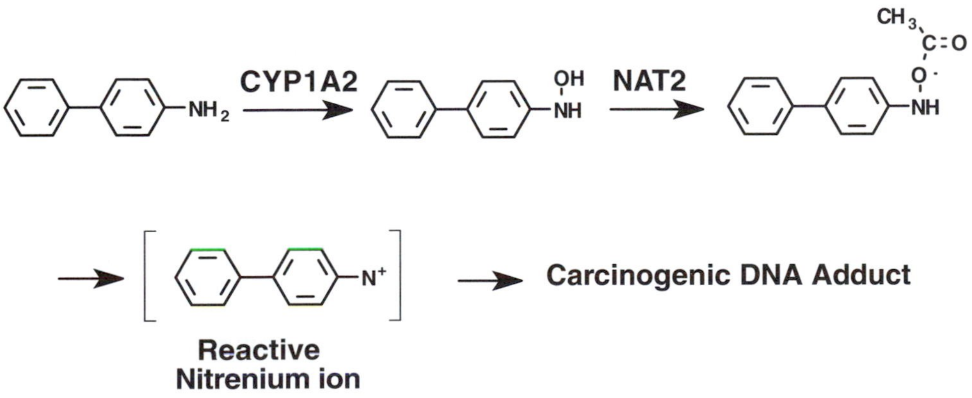

SCHEME 11.36 Reactive nitrenium ions may be produced in the metabolism of aromatic amines through hydroxylation and acetylation.

TABLE 11.3   Renal Elimination of Ciramadol and Its Major Metabolites Following a Single Oral Dose of ^{14}C-ciramadol[a]

Species	Percentage of dose in urine			
	Total radioactivity	Unchanged ciramadol	Aryl-O-glucuronide	Alicyclic-O-glucuronide
Rat	64	33	3	5
Dog	—	3	12	—
Rhesus monkey	88	<1	21	32
Man	94	44	38	2

[a] Data from Ruelius HW, Xenobiotica 1987;17:255–65.

ducted in rodents, dogs, monkeys, and other species may be useful to establish guidelines for likely drug effects in humans, but rarely can be used for predictive interspecies pharmacokinetic scaling, a topic discussed in Chapter 30.

Ruelius (36) has reviewed several examples of species differences in drug metabolism. For example, radiolabeled ciramidol, an orally active analgesic, was administered to rats, dogs, rhesus monkeys, and human. The interspecies comparison of the resulting urinary recovery of parent drug and metabolites in this study (Table 11.3) exemplifies the experience of investigators with other drugs.

Guengerich (37) has reviewed several studies of interspecies activities of CYP isoforms. For example, CYP1A2 has been purified and structurally characterized from rats, rabbits, mice, and humans. The different CYP1A2 isoforms catalyze most of the same biotransformations, but there are cases in which the rat and human isoforms differ in substrate activation. Considering that rat and human CYP1A2 are only 75% homologous in amino acid sequence, it is not surprising that their activities differ. Even single amino acid mutation in rat CYP1A2 results in significant changes in catalytic activity. Further, the concentrations of CYP 1A2 vary 25-fold in humans (10–245 pmol/mg protein) and differ from rat (4–35 pmol/mg protein in untreated vs. 830–1600 pmol/mg protein in polychlorinated biphenyl treated). Monkeys lack CYP1A2, a critical issue in the choice of this animal for cancer bioassays. Interspecies variation in the CYP3A subfamilies provides an especially important example because CYP3A4 is involved in the oxidation of 50% of the drugs used today. Humans express CYPs 3A4, 3A5, and 3A7 (fetal tissue, placenta); rats express CYPs 3A1, 3A2, 3A9, 3A18, and 3A6; rabbits express only CYP3A6. Such genetically determined enzyme differences are reflected in other drug-metabolizing enzymes and in their responses to inducers and inhibitors, further complicating extrapolation of drug metabolism between species.

Enzyme Induction and Inhibition

The effect of repeated doses of a drug, or of one drug or dietary or environmental constituent on that drug, may be to enhance or inhibit the metabolism of the drug. Both enzyme induction and inhibition are important causes of drug interactions (Chapter 14). Phenobarbital is typical of one general type of inducer; polycyclic aromatic hydrocarbons are representative of another class that affects different CYPs. With the characterization of specific human CYP isoforms, more recent studies have targeted isoforms that are induced by specific agents in an effort to understand the genetic mechanisms associated with induction.

Because of the importance of CYP3A4 in drug and steroid metabolism, the mechanism of its induction by numerous endogenous and xenobiotic compounds has received considerable attention. Rifampicin, a macrocylic antibiotic, is one of the most potent inducers of CYP3A4 activity. However, as detailed in Table 14.1, CYP3A4 activity can also be induced by phenobarbital, phenytoin, and a variety of other xenobiotics and endogenous hormones. Goodwin et al. (38) provided evidence that there is a potent enhancer gene module, 8 kb distal to the transcription start point, that mediates the transcriptional induction of the *CYP3A4* gene by rifampicin.

The opposite of the phenomenon of enzyme induction is enzyme inhibition. As previously described, there are numerous cases of dietary inhibitors of the CYPs, such as grapefruit juice, and drug inhibitors such as amphetamine, cimetidine, SKF525A (a useful tool for pharmacological research), methadone, and sulfanilimide. Because there are so many inducers and inhibitors of CYPs to which patients are likely to be exposed, clinical pharmacokinetic studies require interpretations consistent with the expected variability in CYP activity.

Sex

The effects of sex on drug disposition and pharmacokinetics may be significant, but the contribution of sex differences is sometimes difficult to separate from the major complicating effects of dietary and environmental inducers and inhibitors on drug-metabolizing enzymes. Sex differences in drug metabolism are considered in detail in Chapter 21.

Age

The effects of age on drug metabolism are discussed in specific chapters dealing with pediatric (Chapter 23) and geriatric (Chapter 24) clinical pharmacology. The most significant age differences in drug metabolism are expressed developmentally in that drug-metabolizing enzyme systems frequently are immature in neonates. An important example of this is provided by UDP-glucuronosyltransferase. Particularly in premature infants, hepatic UDP-glucuronosyltransferase activity is markedly decreased and does not reach adult levels until 14 weeks after birth (39). This results in increased serum levels of unconjugated bilirubin and a greater risk of potentially fatal kernicterus, which is likely when serum bilirubin levels exceed 30 mg/dL. This situation can be exacerbated by concurrent therapy with sulfonamides, which compete with bilirubin for albumin binding, and can be ameliorated either by prenatal therapy of the mother or postnatal therapy of the infant with phenobarbital (40). However, phenobarbital therapy is no longer favored as a pharmacologic approach to this problem because prenatal therapy with phenobarbital results in a significant decrease in prothrombin levels and because postnatal phototherapy is much more effective.

References

1. Williams RT. Detoxication mechanisms. London: Chapman and Hall Ltd.; 1959. p. 796.
2. Holtzman JL. The role of covalent binding to microsomal proteins in the hepatotoxicity of acetaminophen. Drug Metab Rev 1995;27:277–97.
3. Nelson SD. Mechanisms of the formation and disposition of reactive metabolites that can cause acute liver injury. Drug Metab Rev 1995;27:147–77.
4. Rumack BH. Acetaminophen overdose. Am J Med 1983;75:104–12.
5. Mautz FR. Reduction of cardiac irritability by the epicardial and systemic administration of drugs as a protection in cardiac surgery. J Thoracic Surg 1936;5:612–18.
6. Mark LC, Kayden HJ, Steele JM, Cooper JR, Berlin I, Rovenstine EA, et al. The physiological disposition and cardiac effects of procaine amide. J Pharmacol Exp Ther 1951;102:5–15.
7. Atkinson AJ Jr, Ruo TI, Piergies AA. Comparison of the pharmacokinetic and pharmacodynamic properties of procainamide and N-acetylprocainamide. Angiology 1988;39:655–67.
8. Woolf TF, editor. Handbook of drug metabolism. New York: Marcel-Dekker, Inc.; 1999. p. 596.
9. Baselt RC. Disposition of toxic drugs and chemicals in man. Foster City, CA: Chemical Toxicology Institute; 2000. p. 919.
10. Rendic S, Di Carlo FJ. Human cytochrome P450 enzymes: A status report summarizing their reactions, substrates, inducers, and inhibitors. Drug Metab Rev 1997;29:413–580.
11. Bailey DG, Malcolm J, Arnold O, Spence JD. Grapefruit juice-drug interactions. Br J Clin Pharmacol 1998;46:101–10.
12. Lown KS, Bailey DG, Fontana RJ, Janardan SK, Adair CH, Fortlage LA, et al. J Clin Invest 1997;99:2545–53.
13. Takanaga H, Ohnishi A, Murakami H, Matsuo H, Higuchi S, Urae A, et al. Relationship between time after intake of grapefruit juice and the effect on pharmacokinetics and pharmacodynamics of nisoldipine in healthy subjects. Clin Pharmacol Ther 2000;67:201–14.
14. Gaedigk A, Leeder JS, Grant DM. Tissue-specific expression and alternative splicing of human microsomal epoxide hydrolase. DNA Cell Biol 1997;16:1257–66.
15. Martz F, Failinger Cd, Blake DA. Phenytoin teratogenesis: Correlation between embryopathic effect and covalent binding of putative arene oxide metabolite in gestational tissue. J Pharmacol Exp Ther 1977;203:231–9.
16. Buehler BA, Rao V, Finnell RH. Biochemical and molecular teratology of fetal hydantoin syndrome. Neurol Clin 1994;12:741–8.
17. Guengerich FP, Okazaki O, Seto Y, Macdonald TL. Radical cation intermediates in N-dealkylation reactions. Xenobiotica 1995;25:689–709.
18. Coleman MD. Dapsone toxicity: some current perspectives. Gen Pharmacol 1995;26:1461–7.
19. Uetrecht J. Drug metabolism by leukocytes and its role in drug-induced lupus and other idiosyncratic drug reactions. Crit Rev Toxicol 1990;20:213–35.
20. Cashman JR. Structural and catalytic properties of the mammalian flavin-containing monooxygenase. Chem Res Toxicol 1995;8:166–81.
21. Surapaneni SS, Clay MP, Spangle LA, Paschal JW, Lindstrom TD. In vitro biotransformation and identification of human cytochrome P450 isozyme-dependent metabolism of tazofelone. Drug Metab Dispos 1997;25:1383–8.
22. Tréfouël J, Tréfouël J, Nitti F, Bouvet D. Activité du p-aminophénylsulfanilamide sur les infections streptococciques expérimentales de la souris et du lapin. Compt Rend Soc Biol (Paris) 1935;120:227–31.
23. Saha JR, Butler VP, Jr., Neu HC, Lindenbaum J. Digoxin-inactivating bacteria: identification in human gut flora. Science 1983;220:325–7.
24. Bizjak ED, Mauro VF. Digoxin-macrolide drug interaction. Ann Pharmacother 1997;31:1077–9.
25. Park SB, Jacob Pd, Benowitz NL, Cashman JR. Stereoselective metabolism of (S)-(–)-nicotine in humans: formation of trans-(S)-(–)-nicotine N-1′-oxide. Chem Res Toxicol 1993;6:880–8.
26. Christrup LL, Sjögren P, Jensen NH, Banning AM, Elbaek K, Ersboll AK. Steady-state kinetics and dynamics of morphine in can-

cer patients: Is sedation related to the absorption rate of morphine? J Pain Symptom Manage 1999;18:164–73.

27. Christrup LL. Morphine metabolites. Acta Anaesthesiol Scand 1997;41:116–22.

28. Hawes EM. N$^+$-glucuronidation, a common pathway in human metabolism of drugs with a tertiary amine group. Drug Metab Dispos 1998;26:830–7.

29. Baker CA, Uno H, Johnson GA. Minoxidil sulfation in the hair follicle. Skin Pharmacol 1994;7:335–9.

30. Buhl AE, Waldon DJ, Baker CA, Johnson GA. Minoxidil sulfate is the active metabolite that stimulates hair follicles. J Invest Dermatol 1990;95:553–7.

31. Burchell B, Coughtrie MW. Genetic and environmental factors associated with variation of human xenobiotic glucuronidation and sulfation. Environ Health Perspect 1997;105 Suppl 4:739–47.

32. Falany CN. Enzymology of human cytosolic sulfotransferases. FASEB J 1997;11:206–16.

33. Holdiness MR. Neurological manifestations and toxicities of the antituberculosis drugs. A review. Med Toxicol 1987;2:33–51.

34. Dickinson DS, Bailey WC, Hirschowitz BI, Soong S-J, Eidus L, Hodgkin MM. Risk factors for isoniazid (INH)-induced liver dysfunction. J Clin Gastroenterol 1981;3:271–9.

35. Hengstler JG, Arand M, Herrero ME, Oesch F. Polymorphisms of N-acetyltransferases, glutathione S-transferases, microsomal epoxide hydrolase and sulfotransferases: influence on cancer susceptibility. Recent Results Cancer Res 1998;154:47–85.

36. Ruelius HW. Extrapolation from animals to man: Predictions, pitfalls and perspectives. Xenobiotica 1987;17:255–65.

37. Guengerich FP. Comparisons of catalytic selectivity of cytochrome P450 subfamily enzymes from different species. Chem Biol Interact 1997;106:161–82.

38. Goodwin B, Hodgson E, Liddle C. The orphan human pregnane X receptor mediates the transcriptional activation of CYP3A4 by rifampicin through a distal enhancer module. Mol Pharmacol 1999;56:1329–39.

39. Gourley GR. Bilirubin metabolism and kernicterus. Adv Pediatr 1997;44:173–229.

40. Rubaltelli FF, Griffith PF. Management of neonatal hyperbilirubinaemia and prevention of kernicterus. Drugs 1992;43:864–72.

12

Methods of Analysis of Drugs and Drug Metabolites

SANFORD P. MARKEY

Laboratory of Neurotoxicology, National Institutes of Health, Bethesda, Maryland

INTRODUCTION

Pharmacokinetics requires the determination of a concentration of a drug, its metabolite(s), or an endogenous targeted substance in physiological fluids or tissues with respect to time. These analytical tasks have stimulated the field of analytical chemistry to devise technologies that are appropriately sensitive, precise, accurate, and matched to the demands for speed and automation, important factors in research and clinical chemistry. During the past decade, the principle determinant influencing the choice of competing analytical technologies has been speed—the coupled need to reduce both the time required for assay development and the assay cycle time for large numbers of samples. As a result, instrumentation that can measure drug concentrations in blood, tissue, and urine with minimal chemical treatment has emerged and will be discussed in this chapter using recently published examples.

Several terms used frequently in analytical laboratories have significant and specific definitions, important in the discussion of analytical assays. The *limit of detection* is the minimum mass or concentration that can be detected at a defined signal-to-noise ratio (usually 3:1). The *limit of quantification* is the analyte mass or concentration required to give an acceptable level of confidence in the measured analyte quantity, usually three-fold the limit of detection, or 10-fold background noise. *Sensitivity* of a measurement is the minimum detectable change that can be observed in a specified range. For example, a 1-pg sensitivity may be measured for a pure chemical standard, but in the presence of 1000 pg, the assay sensitivity is the ability to distinguish between 999, 1000, or 1001 pg. *Selectivity* of an assay is the ability of the technique to maintain a limit of detection independent of the sample's matrix. A highly selective assay methodology will not be affected by the presence or type of physiological fluid. *Accuracy* of a method is the ability to measure the true concentration of an analyte; *precision* is the ability to repeat the measurement of the same sample with low variance. *Reproducibility* differs from precision, connoting variability in single measurements of a series of identical samples as compared to repeated measurements of the same sample.

CHOICE OF ANALYTICAL METHODOLOGY

The types of information required largely determine the choices of analytical methodology available. Pharmacokinetic studies for new chemical entities require determinations of the administered drug and its metabolites. Selective techniques capable of distinguishing between parent drug and metabolites are necessary. For some marketed drugs, good medical practice requires measurements to determine whether patient blood concentrations are within the desired therapeutic range. Instrumentation and immunoassay kits are commercially available for highly prescribed medications with narrow therapeutic indices as well as for drugs of abuse.

The scale of a planned pharmacokinetic study further determines the assay methodologies to be considered. For a typical pharmacokinetic study of a new chemical entity, the analyst must choose methods suitable for analyzing at least 30 to 50 samples/patient plus 10 to 15 standards and procedural blanks. Quality control measures may require an additional 10 to 15 samples containing pooled and previously analyzed samples that permit assessment of run-to-run reproducibility. To maximize instrumental efficiency, analysts commonly choose to process more than a single patient's samples at one time, resulting in runs usually containing >100 patient samples plus standards and quality control samples. Standard curves are determinations of instrument response to different known concentrations of analyte, and are required to precede and follow each group of patient samples to assess quality control. Highly automated, rugged, and dependable instrumentation is critical because analyses must continue without interruption until the entire sample set has been analyzed. If the assay cycle time is short (few seconds/sample), the instrumentation requires stability of operation over only 5–10 minutes. However, when assays involve multiple procedural steps, such as derivatization and chromatographic separation, assay cycle time is more typically 5–30 minutes/sample. The resulting requirement for more than 3 days of instrumental operation may introduce conditions and costs that then serve to limit and define the study protocol. When possible, methods that are selective and sensitive and that do not require separation or chemical reactions are chosen because clearly time and cost are critical factors. Early in the drug discovery process, any conceivable and accessible analytical method may be chosen. After demonstration of the potential for commercial development, time and effort can be directed toward simpler and more cost-effective analytical methods that can be marketed as kits for therapeutic drug monitoring.

In the past ten years, pharmaceutical industry research laboratories involved in evaluating new agents have shifted their emphasis from predominantly using ultraviolet (UV) to mass spectrometric (MS) detectors with liquid chromatography (LC) separations. The driving force for the utilization of more expensive instrumentation has been the decreasing time allotted for quantitative assay method development. Improvements in mass spectrometric instrumentation have now made LC/MS routine and widely available. The required assay limit of quantification has remained relatively constant for some classes of drugs, typically in the ng-to-μg/mL range, but newer

drugs are designed to be more selective to minimize side effects, dropping therapeutic concentrations to pg/mL. Once new drugs have passed through the initial stages of development, then the market for therapeutic drug monitoring dictates that more robust and less expensive technologies be utilized, amenable to instrumentation accessible to hospital clinical chemistry laboratories. Consequently, analytical kits sold for drug monitoring are likely to be based on immunoassay methodologies. The emerging development of chip-based microanalytical methods suggests that instrumentation for therapeutic drug development and monitoring will continue to evolve while using many of the same separation and spectroscopic principles. This chapter is written to provide an introduction to the principles of some of the most commonly used analytical methodologies in clinical pharmacology.

CHROMATOGRAPHIC SEPARATIONS

Chromatography refers to the separation of materials using their relative solubility and absorption differences in two immiscible phases, one stationary and the other mobile. The defining work of M. Tswett in 1903 demonstrated the separation of colored plant pigments on a carbohydrate powder through which hydrocarbon solvents were passed. The same principles apply to the rainbow-like dispersion of colors seen when ink soaks through a shirt pocket.

Modern chromatographic science has refined these basic principles in *high-performance liquid chromatography* (HPLC). A schematic outline of an HPLC instrument is shown in Figure 12.1. Modern HPLC systems are designed to make separations rapid, reproducible, and sensitive. Particulate adsorption material that is packed in a chromatographic column is engineered to have small and uniform particle size (typically 3 or 5 microns). Columns of 1–5 mm diameter and 5–15 cm length exhibit sufficient resolution to effect useful separations. Columns packed with small particles of such lengths require high pressure (typically, 6 to 8 mega Pascals) to force solvent flow at 0.1 to 1.0 mL/min, requiring inert, precision-machined, high-pressure fittings and materials. Pumps are designed to deliver precisely metered, pulse-less flow of a mobile phase composed of either organic and/or aqueous solutions. Pumps are controlled electronically so that a gradient of the mobile phase solvents from the pumps can be continuously programmed. During an analytical run, the mobile phase can be varied so that materials in mixture partition with respect to solubility in the mobile phase and adsorption on the stationary phase.

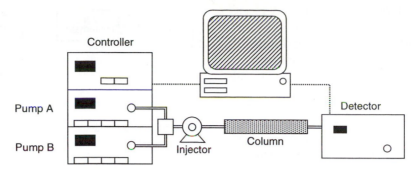

FIGURE 12.1   Schematic of HPLC system showing component modules.

The polarity, pH, or ionic concentration differs in the solutions in solvent reservoirs that are pumped into a mixing chamber and then directed into the column. When a component is more soluble in the mobile phase than in the film on the particle, it will elute from the column and be detected with respect to a characteristic chemical property, such as UV absorption (Figure 12.1).

The popularity and acceptance of HPLC in clinical assays is due to the versatility and wide applicability of the methodology. Most pharmaceuticals are small molecules (< 1000 Da) with some lipid solubility. They commonly share the property that they adsorb to silica particles coated with stable organic hydrocarbon films and can then be eluted when organic content of the mobile phase is increased. Consequently, a single analytical system can be used for many types of analyses, tailored to each by changing the solvents and gradients. The reproducibility of HPLC separations can be rigorously controlled due to extensive engineering of all the components in these systems. Reproducibility is especially dependent on consistent gradient elution and establishing equilibrium conditions before each run. The most reproducible HPLC separations are *isocratic*, using a single solvent during the analysis. In practice, the complexity of most biological fluids necessitates mobile phase gradient programming to accomplish the desired separations and cleanse the column of adsorbed components from each injected sample.

ABSORPTION AND EMISSION SPECTROSCOPY

Spectroscopy is the measurement of electromagnetic radiation absorbed, scattered or emitted by chemical species. Because different chemical species and electromagnetic radiation interact in characteristic ways, it is possible to tailor instrumentation to detect these interactions specifically and quantitatively. A simple absorption spectrophotometer contains compo-

nents that are common to many spectroscopic devices and illustrates many of the basic principles of instrumentation found in analytical biochemistry as illustrated schematically in Figure 12.2.

A light source produces radiation over the wavelength region where absorption is to be studied. For the visible spectrum, a source producing radiation between 380 and 780 nm is required; for ultraviolet radiation, 160–400 nm radiation is required. Both can be supplied by hydrogen or deuterium discharge lamps combined with incandescent lamps. A high-quality light source combines brightness with stability to produce a constant source of radiant energy. The monochromator is a wavelength selector (prism or grating), separating the discrete component energies of the light source. The quality of a monochromator is related to its ability to resolve radiation in defined wavelengths without loss of intensity. An inexpensive substitute for a monochromator is a filter, passing a fixed, discrete band of energy. When a discrete wavelength is passed through a solvent or through solvent containing dissolved sample, some of the radiant energy is absorbed, depending on the chemical structure of the sample. The absorption characteristics of each chemical structure can be predicted based on the presence or absence of component functional groups, such as aromatic, unsaturated, and conjugated groups. Colored substances, like hemoglobin, absorb in the visible region. Colorless proteins containing aromatic amino acids absorb UV light at 280 nm; all proteins absorb UV light at 214 nm due to the amide function. Many carbo-

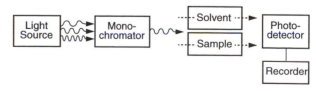

FIGURE 12.2   Schematic layout of components of an absorption spectrophotometer.

hydrates and lipids do not absorb light in the UV or visible region and are consequently transparent.

The quantity of absorbed energy is proportional to the concentration of the sample, the molar absorptivity of the sample and its solvent, and the distance or path length of the sample container or cell. Molar absorptivity is an expression of the intensity of absorbance of a compound at a given wavelength relative to its molar concentration. The light transmitted through the sample or solvent cell is directed onto a photosensitive detector, converted to an electronic signal, and sent through amplifiers to a recorder or computer. Most spectrophotometers contain optics designed so that the signal from light absorbed by the solvent is compared and subtracted from the signal from the light absorbed by the sample in an equal quantity of solvent.

The data resulting from a spectrophotometric analysis of a sample in a solvent is termed *optical density*. The measurement of the optical density of a sample at varying wavelengths is the *absorbance spectrum*. The absorbance spectrum of a drug may not be very different from absorbance spectra of many of the common metabolic intermediates in cellular metabolism. Because endogenous cellular intermediates are present typically in 10^3–10^6 greater concentrations than drugs (typically nanomolar to micromolar), it is usually not possible to use absorbance spectrophotometry alone to detect differences between drug-treated and untreated fluids. However, absorbance spectrophotometers are popular detectors for HPLC, particularly in the ultraviolet range. For many drugs, the separation power of HPLC can provide sufficient discrimination for quantifying parent drug and metabolites, as illustrated later in this chapter.

Some compounds emit light at characteristic frequencies when radiation of a particular energy is absorbed. The resulting *emission spectrum* is significantly more unique than an absorbance spectrum. Consequently, the measurement of emitted (fluorescent or phosphorescent) light can frequently be used for sensitive measurements of trace amounts of naturally luminescent compounds. The instrumentation for emission spectrophotometry is similar to absorbance instrumentation in the selection of monochromatic radiation to pass through the sample. Subsequently, a second monochromator or filter is used to collect and separate the radiation emitted prior to detection as illustrated in Figure 12.3. Drugs that are naturally fluorescent may be candidates for direct fluorescent assay, but frequently a specific separation, such as HPLC, precedes fluorescent detection in order to lower interference from background. A further way to enhance selectivity is to measure the absorption and emission of polarized light. This technique is relevant

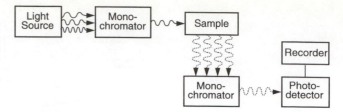

FIGURE 12.3 Schematic layout of components of an emission spectrophotometer.

to large molecules with restricted rotational movements, such as antigen-antibody complexes. An antigen, such as a drug, can be labeled with a fluorescent tag, and the florescent emission of polarized light measured in a competitive antibody binding assay, as described for cyclosporine later in this chapter.

IMMUNOAFFINITY ASSAYS

Antibodies can be powerful analytical reagents exhibiting unique specificity for molecular recognition. The analytical use of antibodies is predicated on their specificity and high affinity with regard to binding a targeted analyte in the presence of a complex mixture such as serum. This affinity interaction contrasts with chromatographic media, which bind and release components with respect to general physicochemical parameters, such as acidity, size, lipid solubility, and so on. The antibody-antigen interaction is analogous to the selectivity of a molecular lock-and-key, in contrast to the general nonspecific interactions of chromatography. The epitope (or key-like) region of an antigen that binds to an antibody can be exquisitely specific. Monoclonal antibodies recognize a single epitope; polyclonal antibodies recognize multiple epitopes. Both types of antibodies are likely to recognize or *cross-react* with metabolites or congeners of an antigen with unpredictable (but reproducible) affinity.

Antibody-based assays for drugs are developed by using the drug as a hapten and covalently linking it with proteins to form an antigen. The antibody reagent is then harvested from either an animal (polyclonal antibodies) or cell culture system (monoclonal antibodies). The specificity of the antibodies depends on the functional groups of the drug that remain exposed when the drug is coupled to the carrier protein. For example, if the hydroxyl group of *p*-HPPH (Figure 2.7) is linked to a protein carrier, the antibodies formed to this antigen will be unable to distinguish phenytoin from its *p*-HPPH metabolite.

An expanding library of antibodies is commercially available. Additionally, there are commercial services that will generate custom poly-or monoclonal antibodies to any drug or protein. The mass production and purification of mono- and polyclonal antibodies as reagents affords materials that are used routinely to recognize and separate targeted analytes. Antibodies can be bound to films, papers, surfaces, or chromatographic supports. There are inherent variations in the affinities and properties of antibodies. Consequently, cost and availability of antibody materials are directly related to the degree to which they have been pretested and characterized.

Quantification requires measurement of the extent of antibody-antigen interaction, the assessment of the amount of bound vs. free antigen. Immunoaffinity assays must be coupled with colorimetric, spectroscopic, or radiometric detection in order to create an output signal. An assay may incorporate a step to separate the antibody-ligand complex (heterogeneous assay) or may entail direct detection of the extent of antigen-antibody complex formation (homogeneous assay). Homogeneous immunoassays may use a marker-labeled antigen, for example a fluorescent-tag on a target analyte drug, to indicate whether binding has decreased or increased, directly reflecting the bound/free ratio. These assays are particularly popular in clinical chemistry because of their inherent simplicity. Examples of immunoaffinity based assays are discussed later in this chapter using cyclosporine as a target analyte.

Immunoaffinity-based assays are routinely developed for biologicals and products of the biotechnology industry as part of their characterization as new agents. In contrast, pharmacokinetic assays of new chemical entities are less likely to be immunoaffinity based because analysts are required to measure accurately the concentration of the administered parent drug. As in the case of phenytoin, metabolism of the parent drug can result in metabolites that exhibit different pharmacological activity but are structurally similar enough to the parent drug to be immunologically cross-reactive. For this reason, determination of the structures of these metabolites and, commonly, the measurement of their concentrations is a key part of the analytical requirement associated with drug development. As a general rule, immunoaffinity assays cannot be developed without prior knowledge of the metabolic fate of a drug, found by using an assay that is drug and metabolite specific.

MASS SPECTROMETRY

The analysis of the mass of an organic compound provides information on component elements and their arrangement. For example, the mass spectrum of water,

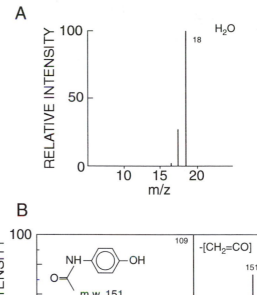

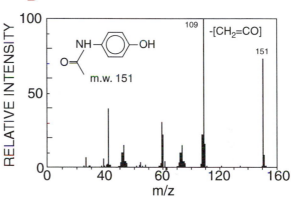

FIGURE 12.4 Electron impact ionization mass spectra of water *(Panel A)* and acetaminophen *(Panel B)*. The intensities of the fragment ions are normalized against those of the predominant ion (base peak), which, in the case of water, is also the molecular ion with mass/charge ratio (m/z) = 18.

H_2O, in Figure 12.4A illustrates several characteristics of such data. The bar graph plots mass-to-charge ratio (m/z) on the x-axis, and relative ion intensity on the y-axis. Water, composed only of one atom of oxygen (16 Da) and two atoms of hydrogen (1 Da), has a molecular weight of 18 Da. In this mass spectrum, m/z 18 is not only the *molecular ion* but also the strongest signal or *base peak*. There are signals seen for fragment ions containing the components O^+ at m/z 16, and OH^+ at m/z 17, as well as HOH^+. There are no signals at other m/z, such as 12, 13, 14, or 20, 21, because elements with those masses are not present. To generalize, mass spectra can be interpreted by a simple arithmetic accounting of elemental constituents.

The same principles of analysis can be applied to the mass spectra of more complex organic molecules. For example, the mass spectrum of acetaminophen is shown in Figure 12.4B. A molecular ion is seen for the total assembly of all of the elements $C_8H_9NO_2$ at m/z 151. The strongest signal at m/z 109 derives from the loss of ketene ($CH_2C=O$) as a stable neutral fragment

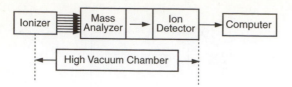

FIGURE 12.5 Schematic overview of components of a mass spectrometer.

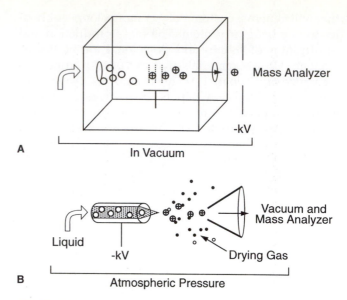

FIGURE 12.6 Schematic representations of electron impact *(Panel A)* and electrospray *(Panel B)* mass spectrometer ionization sources.

from the ionized molecule. The fragmentation pattern reveals characteristics of a molecule's architecture, such as the presence of an acetyl function. The interpretation of electron ionization mass spectra can provide rich substructural information.

How mass spectra are produced largely determines the kind of information in the spectra (1, 2). Mass spectrometry differs from absorbance or emission spectroscopy in that it is a destructive technique, consuming sample used during the measurement process. Mass spectrometry is also a very sensitive technique, consuming as little as a few attomoles in the best cases, more typically requiring ~10 pmoles for the routine quantitative analyses common in the pharmaceutical industry. From the overview outline in Figure 12.5, there are several integral components that constitute every mass spectrometer. First, all substances must be ionized in order to be mass analyzed. The physical principles focusing and separating molecules require that the molecules be positively or negatively charged so that electric and magnetic fields affect the motion of the resulting ions. Second, the ions must enter a mass analyzer in a vacuum chamber maintained at a pressure sufficiently low as to permit ions to travel without interacting with other molecules or ions. Third, there must be an ion detector capable of converting the impinging ion beam into an electronic signal. Fourth, there must be controlling electronics, usually integrated with a computer, to regulate the ionization, mass analysis, ion detection, and vacuum systems and to record and process ion signals. There are efficient ionization methods for producing ions *in vacuo* of organic compounds of any size or complexity from gases, liquids, or solids. Figures 12.6A and B picture two of the most common ionization mechanisms, electron and electrospray, widely used by investigators in clinical pharmacology.

Electron ionization of neutral organic molecules in the vapor phase occurs when electrons emitted from a heated filament remove an electron from the molecule. The resulted odd-electron ions are focused and accelerated into a mass analyzer by electric fields. Electron ionization and a closely related method, chemical ionization, were the principal methods used in clinical

pharmacology until around 1990. Electrospray ionization of neutral organic molecules in liquid solutions occurs when liquids flow through a conductive needle bearing a charge of several thousand volts at atmospheric pressure. The emerging liquid forms a sharp cone, with microdroplets of ion clusters bearing multiple charges and attached solvent molecules. A gas stream dries the clusters and the resulting desolvated singly and multiply charged ions are guided into the vacuum system of the mass analyzer. Because of its compatibility with liquid samples, electrospray is currently the principal method of ionization used in clinical pharmacology assays.

Following ionization, the charged molecular, cluster, or fragment ions are accelerated and focused into a mass analyzer. The type of mass analyzer influences the range and quality of the mass spectrum. Some analyzers have a limited mass range, for example, m/z 0 to 1000, or 0 to 20,000. Others have limited resolution of m/z, for example the ability to resolve the difference between m/z 1000 and 1001, or 1001.000 and 1001.010. The first work applying mass analysis to pharmacology used magnetic sector mass analyzers in the identification of metabolites of chlorpromazine (3). This work introduced the concept of *selected ion monitoring* or mass fragmentography, a technique of alternating between pre-selected ions of interest, thereby enhancing sensitivity and making the mass spectrometer a sophisticated gas chromatographic detector. The principles of online chromatography and selected ion monitoring are integral in all modern mass spectrometric instrumentation. Currently, however the most commonly used mass analyzers in pharmacology include time-of-flight, quadrupole, and ion traps, which are illustrated in the panels in Figure 12.7 and discussed below.

The time-of-flight (TOF) mass analyzer separates ions by accelerating a pulse of ions in vacuum and then measuring their time of arrival at a detector. Because all ions are given the same initial kinetic energy, lighter ions arrive at the detector faster than heavier ions. All ions from a single pulse are analyzed, so there is no upper mass limit on TOF analyzers. Resolution is a function of flight path length and initial position in the beam of pulsed ions. The inherent simplicity, speed, and mass range of TOF analyzers has resulted in low-cost, higher performance instrumentation for routine analyses.

A quadrupole mass analyzer filters ions using radio-frequency alternating voltages at a constant dc potential on paired cylindrical rods. A continuous beam of ions enters the alternating field region at low energy. Resonant positive ions of a particular m/z ratio traverse the field region through to the detector, attracted first to poles of negative charge and then, when the field alternates, they are drawn toward to the opposite pair of rods. Nonresonant ions collide with the surface of the rods. Quadrupole mass filters are designed to filter limited mass ranges, typically m/z 10 to 2000 for organic ion analysis. Quadrupole analyzers are widely used in clinical pharmacology, especially with electrospray ionization.

A quadrupole ion trap mass analyzer collects ions in stable trajectories using a radio-frequency oscillating voltage on a central ring electrode. A gated electron beam ionizes neutral molecules within the trap or ions may be injected into the trap from external ion sources. A second radio-frequency field between the end caps causes ions of a particular m/z to go into an unstable trajectory and pass through the holes in one end cap to the ion detector. Several millisecond trapping and ejection cycles are performed over defined m/z ranges. The capability of ion traps to store and accumulate selected ions, and subsequently to fragment and analyze the fragments, has made these a popular low-cost alternative to tandem mass spectrometers.

Alternative permutations of ionization and mass analyzer alternatives present many instrument configurations to prospective users, and there continues to be significant instrumentation development leading to new capabilities with different configurations. Consequently, no single ionizer/mass analyzer dominates the clinical pharmacology market. For example, the option of tandem mass analysis may be the deciding factor in instrument selection. Tandem mass analysis is the separation of a mass-resolved ion beam, and its subsequent frag-

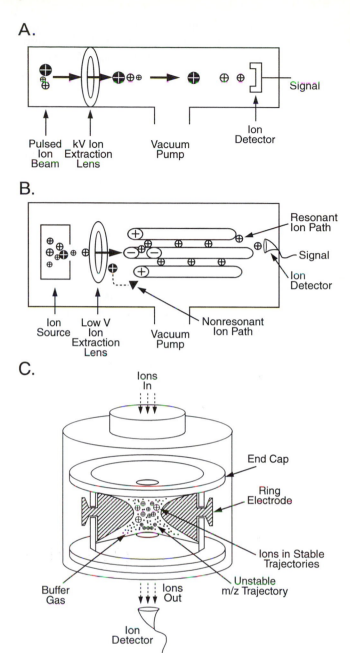

FIGURE 12.7 Schematic representations of three mass analyzers. *Panel A:* Time-of-flight; *Panel B:* Quadrupole; *Panel C:* Quadrupole ion trap

mentation and further mass analysis, that is, the mass spectrum of ions in a mass spectrum, or MS/MS analysis. Some of the most common tandem mass analyzer configurations are quadrupole-quadrupole-quadrupole (qqq), quadrupole-quadrupole-TOF (qqTOF), and ion trap. MS/MS analysis significantly increases the selectivity of analytical mass spectrometry by requiring not only that a specific mass is characteristic of a compound, but that specific mass fragments be present in a characteristic pattern to yield a second product ion. For example, in Figure 12.4B, the primary mass spectrum of acetaminophen is characterized by m/z 151 as a base peak with a significant fragment ion at m/z 109 that derived from that molecular species. Thus, in a chromatography-MS/MS analysis, an instrument could be set to pass m/z 151 in a first stage of analysis and m/z 109 in the second stage. The result would be a time-varying signal representing only ions of m/z 109 that derived from m/z 151, a very stringent criteria for mass detection. Thus, this particular signal would result only when acetaminophen eluted from the chromatograph.

Ion traps have a further advantage of allowing serial experiments, by trapping an ion, fragmenting it, trapping a specific fragment, and then fragmenting and mass analyzing the secondary fragment, and so on (e.g., MS^3 or MS^n). MS/MS analysis is possible with high sensitivity because the transmission and storage of mass resolved ions is efficient. Frequently, sensitivity and selectivity are enhanced by MS/MS analyses because chemical background is reduced when compared to MS analyses.

EXAMPLES OF CURRENT ASSAY METHODS

There are many possible permutations for coupling one of the chromatographic or immunoaffinity separations with one or another of the spectrometric detection technologies. HPLC coupled with UV or fluorescence spectrometry and HPLC interfaced with MS are among the most widely used quantitative analytical methods for new chemical entities because of their general applicability and sensitivities relevant to clinical pharmacology. Homogeneous immunoaffinity assays are frequently a first choice for protein or other biotechnology products. Immunoaffinity with fluorescence polarization or enzyme reaction monitoring are popular commercialized methods for marketed chemical entities. A discussion contrasting alternative combined methods of analysis for nucleoside drugs and cyclosporine follows because these analyses illustrate the variety and respective merits of combined analytical methods widely used in pharmacological research.

HPLC/UV and HPLC/MS Assay of New Chemical Entities—Nucleoside Drugs

Examples of the use of HPLC/UV and HPLC/MS/MS are provided by the analyses of fluoro-dideoxyadenosine (F-ddA, Figure 12.8), a synthetic dideoxynucleoside inhibitor of HIV reverse transcrip-

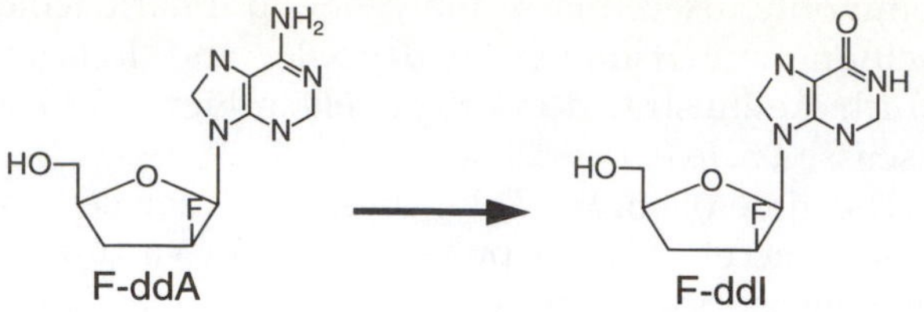

FIGURE 12.8   Chemical structures of F-ddA and F-ddI.

tase under investigation in the Laboratory of Medicinal Chemistry of the National Cancer Institute. F-ddA is metabolized to fluoro-dideoxyinosine (F-ddI), also a reverse transcriptase inhibitor.

Selection of a suitable assay method began with consideration of chemical characteristics of the drug and the determination of the likely range of blood and tissue concentrations required for pharmacological effect (4). F-ddA and F-ddI absorb UV at 260 nm, making them logical candidates for an HPLC/UV assay. The analytical conditions reported for the previously marketed analogue didanosine (ddI) were useful for reference, but fluorine substitution makes F-ddA more lipophilic and acid stable than ddI.

The analyst facing the challenge of designing an assay begins by characterizing the chromatography of analytes, choosing column materials and eluents either recommended for structurally similar compounds or broadly applicable in pharmacology. Conditions are required that provide retention and elution of F-ddA and F-ddI with symmetrical peak shape and adequate separation. Choice of any specific chromatographic column and mobile phase buffer and elution program results from incremental trials, with the objective of improving chromatographic separation and peak shape sufficiently to enable quantitative measurement in the biological fluid being sampled. In this case, the investigators used a phenylsilicon reverse phase column with a mobile phase linear gradient ranging in composition from 2 to 36% methanol in 0.01 M phosphate buffer.

Direct injection of biological fluids into chromatographic columns is possible, but, to preserve the life of the column, some type of solvent extraction or pre-filtration is recommended to remove cellular debris, proteins, and particulate material. After obtaining satisfactory chromatograms of pure analyte, the analyst adds the same quantity of analyte to a blank biological fluid sample to determine the chromatography and background in the presence of just the biological matrix. The chromatographic profile of the biological fluid with and without added analyte standards will determine the necessity for alternative chromatographic conditions, column selection, and sample cleanup.

Often filtration can be combined with sample enrichment using cartridges containing chromatographic packings. Solid phase extraction cartridges contain any of a wide variety of chromatographic media, such as normal or reverse phase coated silica or ion exchange polymers. They are like mini-columns, but are optimized for sample cleanup prior to chromatography and not for analytical separations. A cartridge is chosen that will trap target analytes from the biological fluid, permit rinses to remove salts, and allow efficient elution of the analytes in a convenient quantity of organic solvent. The eluent is concentrated either under a nitrogen stream in a chemical fume hood or in a centrifugal rotary evaporator, and the final sample re-dissolved for injection into the analytical column. In many cases, the process of solid phase extraction cleanup has been adapted to robotic systems, enabling analysts to scale procedures from single samples to automated 96- or 384-well formats. For this F-ddA and F-ddI analysis, patient plasma was diluted with water and applied to an octadecylsilyl reverse phase cartridge, washed with phosphate buffer, and the analytes eluted with methanol/water.

Contemporary quantitative assays require the analyst to select appropriate compounds to serve as internal standards. A fixed quantity of an internal standard is added to each sample so that the intensity of the signals from the analyte from each sample can be normalized to those from the internal standard and compared to samples analyzed during the same run or from another analytical set on another date. Internal standards must have similar chemical properties to the target analyte, be available in pure form, and be separable on chromatography. Like the target analyte, it is critical that the internal standards are well separated from endogenous components. For F-ddA and F-ddI analyses, the investigators selected the structurally related chloro-analogs as internal standards.

An aliquot of the mixture of the internal standards is precisely added to every tube in an analysis set. One set of six to eight different concentrations of the analyte is prepared to construct a *standard curve* that covers the sample concentration range of measurement. Appropriately chosen internal standards will result in the generation of linear standard curves, with proportional increases in the ratio of analyte to internal standard with increasing mass of analyte. Data from the resulting standard curve is used to convert relative signal response to absolute concentration data.

Biological sample processing may require additional considerations prior to actual implementation. For example, the expected presence of HIV in the blood samples for F-ddA analysis required the analysts to test methods to inactivate this virus without altering the quantification of drug or metabolite. Several procedures were tested and it was determined that the addition of a small quantity of Triton X-100 detergent eliminated virus without affecting sample integrity or chromatography. Many drugs are stable in biological fluids when stored frozen, but chemical stability, reactive intermediary metabolites, and effects of storage need to be evaluated in developing assays of drugs and their metabolites. The addition of chemical preservatives, protein denaturants, or detergents may be required, and these issues are best reviewed at the outset of assay development.

A *chromatogram* is the plot or graph of detector signal (e.g., UV absorbance) vs. time that results when a sample is eluted from the chromatographic column and passed through the detector. Typical analytical HPLC chromatographic analysis of many drugs requires 15 to 35 minutes. Following each chromatographic run, the mobile phase gradient must be returned to the starting condition, requiring an additional 5–15 minutes for column stabilization.

The HPLC/UV chromatograms of pre-dose and F-ddA patient plasma with added 5'-Cl-deoxyadenosine internal standard are shown in Figure 12.9. The dotted line on the chromatogram indicates the composition of the programmed linear elution gradient throughout the run. The pre-dose plasma analysis contains peaks for endogenous plasma components absorbing at 260 nm. These background peaks will vary from individual to individual because dietary substances, other drugs, and intermediary metabolites may all contribute to the recorded signal. However, it was important to design the assay so that there were no interfering signals for endogenous components eluting at the expected retention times of F-ddI, F-ddA, or the internal standard (5'-Cl-dA).

The HPLC/UV F-ddA method was used to generate preclinical pharmacokinetic data in monkeys (5). The limits of quantification for both F-ddA and F-ddI were 50 ng/mL using this assay. However, for clinical pharmacokinetic studies, the NCI investigators required a more sensitive assay. Due to the number of clinical samples, an assay time faster than 45–50/min/sample was also desirable. For these reasons, an HPLC/MS/MS assay was developed. Conversion from an HPLC/UV assay to MS detection conditions required the substitution of volatile buffers compatible with electrospray ionization. The analysts defined fast isocratic conditions for the HPLC/MS chromatography, eliminating the need for gradient programming. Because of enhanced detection selectivity, background interference is significantly less than with UV detection, thereby eliminating the need for gradient programming. Therefore, the analysts were

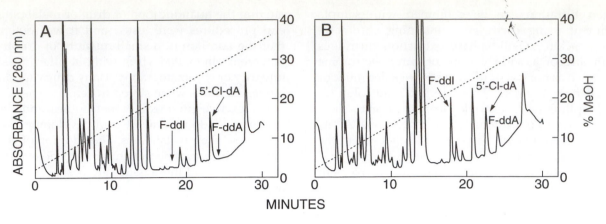

FIGURE 12.9 HPLC/UV analysis of plasma from a patient before *(Panel A)* and after *(Panel B)* receiving an F-ddA dose with 5'-Cl-dA added as internal standard. The plasma analyzed in Panel B was drawn 85 min after beginning a 100-min i.v. infusion. *Arrows* indicate the elution time for each component. The *dotted line* indicates the methanol concentration gradient.

able to reduce assay time by employing fast isocratic conditions for the HPLC/MS/MS assay. For F-ddA HPLC/MS/MS, analyses were completed in 10-min cycles using a 25% methanol/0.25% acetic acid eluent, about four to five times faster and at 10-fold greater sensitivity than for HPLC/UV gradient analyses.

The electrospray ionization mass spectra of F-ddA and F-ddI are similar to other nucleosides and typical of many drugs in that they exhibit intense MH^+ protonated molecular ions. By recording the signal from a single characteristic ion, *selected ion monitoring*, a chromatogram is produced that is considerably more specific than a UV absorbance chromatogram. However, MS/MS offers even greater stringency by recording the signal characteristic of a fragment formed from a selected ion, a process known as *selected reaction monitoring* (2). Using MS/MS, the F-ddA-MH^+ ion at m/z 254 is further fragmented in the second mass spectrometer stage to produce an intense adenine ion (BH_2^+) at m/z 136 and a weak F-dideoxy fragment at m/z 119. Using these unique characteristics, signals are monitored from compounds eluting from LC producing ions at m/z 254 *and* fragmenting to mz/136. Selected reaction monitoring reduces background without sacrificing signal strength. There is no background signal in pre-dose patient plasma at the retention value for F-ddA. Likewise, there are no interfering signals for F-ddI (m/z 255 to 137).

Like HPLC/UV, quantitative mass spectrometric assays require internal standards to be added to every sample to compensate for fluctuations in sample handling and instrument performance. Commonly, structural analogs of the target analytes are the most readily available internal standards, although for highest precision and accuracy, nonradioactive, stable isotope analogs (deuterium, ^{13}C, ^{15}N) are preferred. For the HPLC/MS/MS analysis of F-ddA, the chloro-analog internal standards 2-Cl-A (m/z 302 to 170) and 2-Cl-I (m/z 303 to 171) were chosen, and the limit of quantification (LOQ) was 4 ng/mL (16 nM) for F-ddA and 8 ng/mL (32 nM) for F-ddI.

The pharmacokinetic results obtained with HPLC/UV and HPLC/MS/MS are compared in Figure 12.10. Dotted lines indicate the limits of quantification for F-ddA by both assay methods. Data for F-ddI obtained by either method shows good agreement, being well above the LOQ for both techniques. On the other hand, all the F-ddA data points are below the LOQ for HPLC/UV. Nonetheless, measurements reported below LOQs can be useful in that they help define what additional assay sensitivity must be achieved to generate data suitable for pharmacokinetic analysis.

This description of F-ddA quantification provides a specific example from which some general observations about HPLC/UV and LC/MS assays may be drawn. Liquid chromatographic separations are well suited to pharmacokinetic requirements, because the same physicochemical characteristics that determine drug bioavailability (solubility, polarity, chemical stability) can be translated to liquid chromatography. The selectivity of detection (UV absorbance, fluorescence, mass, or mass-to-mass fragment), and not the detector sensitivity, frequently defines assay LOQ. The general applicability of LC/MS/MS recommends its acceptance as a preferred assay method. This preference is reinforced by simpler and more facile assay development using LC/MS/MS than HPLC/UV. Chromatographic separation is critical in HPLC/UV because there is an unavoidable UV background arising from biological matrix components with similar physico-

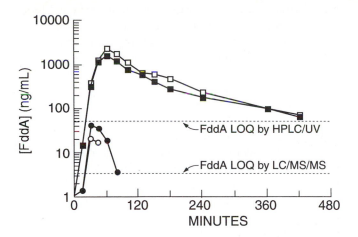

FIGURE 12.10 Plasma concentration vs. time profiles for F-ddA and F-ddI after oral administration of 4.5-mg/kg F-ddA to a patient. The levels of F-ddA measured by HPLC/MS/MS are shown as ●, by HPLC/UC as ○. The levels of F-ddI measured by HPLC/MS/MS are shown as ■; by HPLC/UV, as □.

chemical characteristics to drugs. Consequently, analysts developing HPLC/UV (or fluorescence) methods must test and refine chromatographic columns, solvents, and gradients in order to establish the required selectivity for any target analyte. That process may require days or weeks of research time. Even after chromatographic conditions have been optimized, the analysis of each sample is likely to require 15 to 30 minutes of chromatography, followed by another 5 to 30 minutes to accommodate column flushing and reequilibration to initial conditions. In contrast, LC/MS/MS assays can be developed rapidly by choosing generic chromatographic separation conditions. LC is required mostly to separate analytes from the physiological fluid matrix, with most of the separation selectivity provided by the MS/MS selected reaction monitoring. Analysis cycle times can be reduced to 5 to 10 minutes or less because fast, isocratic separation conditions are generally acceptable. Finally, LC/MS/MS procedures can be easily modified to include drug metabolites in the analyses, simply by adding another target mass and mass fragment.

The capability of mass spectrometry to analyze multiple drugs in physiological fluids and the demand of high-throughput screening (see Chapter 28) has led some pharmaceutical companies to test the concept of "cassette dosing," the analysis of pharmacological data generated by administering several drugs to a single animal, cell preparation, or enzyme incubation (6, 7). Although LC/MS is compatible with the determination of multiple drugs in a mixture, the drugs are not independent variables when co-administered *in vivo* because of their interactions with metabolic

enzymes. Consequently, cassette dosing has not been generally adopted as a means of short-cutting either the *in vitro* or *in vivo* study of drug metabolism.

HPLC/UV and Immunoassays of Cyclosporine: Assays for Therapeutic Drug Monitoring

Cyclosporine (cyclosporine A) is a potent and widely used immunosuppressive agent with a narrow therapeutic index. As a consequence, there is ongoing competition to develop rapid and accurate assays for therapeutic monitoring of cyclosporine blood concentrations in transplant patients treated with this drug. This competition produced refinement and automation of the reference HPLC/UV methods initially developed for cyclosporine as well as the development of faster, automated immunoassays suitable for routine use in hospital clinical laboratories. Consideration of the chromatographic and immunoassay methods developed for cyclosporine offers an opportunity to review the usual process of clinical assay development and maturation. When developing new chemical entities, pharmaceutical researchers pay a premium for the speed of assay development and an assurance of assay selectivity. However, for marketed drugs, clinical laboratories require reliable and accurate assays that are less expensive and less demanding of sophisticated equipment and operator skill.

Cyclosporine is a hydrophobic cyclic peptide of fungal origin that is composed of 11 amino acid residues. The structure of cyclosporine shows that all of the constituent amino acids are aliphatic (Figure 12.11). UV absorbance at 210 nm is due to the amide bonds in the molecule and is consequently not as intense or distinctive as that of many drugs containing aromatic rings. Development of cyclosporine as a pharmaceutical occurred in the 1970s, a period when HPLC/UV, but not LC/MS methods were available. Consequently,

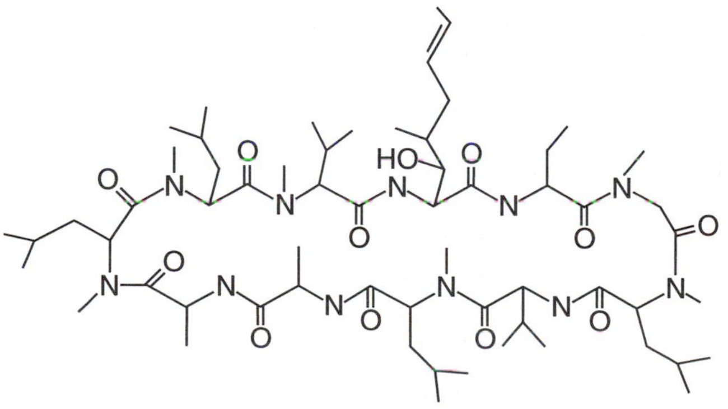

FIGURE 12.11 Chemical structure of cyclosporine.

HPLC/UV was the initial benchmark clinical chemical assay method for cylcosporine, verified recently by comparison with LC/MS/MS methods (8, 9).

HPLC/UV methods for cyclosporine analyses use whole blood samples with cyclosporine D added as an internal standard (10, 11). Patient blood samples are diluted with a solution of the internal standard in organic solvents to effect cell lysis, dissociation, and solubilization of the cyclosporine. After centrifugation, the analytes in the supernatant are adsorbed on a solid phase extraction cartridge, washed, and eluted. Interfering lipids are removed from the eluent by extraction with a hydrocarbon solvent, and the sample is separated on a reverse phase column at 70° C under isocratic conditions, monitoring UV absorbance at 210 nm. Isocratic elution conditions facilitate faster analytical runs because, as previously noted, no time is required for resetting gradients and stabilizing chromatographic conditions. As a result, one sample requires only 5 to 15 minutes chromatography time. The LOQ of the HPLC/UV method is ~20–45 μg/L, which is acceptable because the therapeutic range is 80 to 300 μg/L. Cyclosporine HPLC/UV assay methods have been optimized in a variety of research and commercial laboratories. It is possible for future improvements to be made in sample processing, but this assay represents the state-of-the-art for HPLC/UV analyses in the mid-1990s (10, 11).

There are several widely used commercial immunoassays for cyclosporine measurement. Fluorescence polarization immunoassay (FPIA) is one popular technique, typical of a homogeneous immunoassay, and instructive with regard to its principles and limitations. FPIA depends on the difference in fluorescence characteristics of bound and free fluorescent antigen (12, 13). FPIA instrumentation uses a polarized light source to excite emission by the fluorescein-tagged-cyclosporine. Cyclosporine is not fluorescent so competition of fluorescein-tagged-cyclosporine and cyclosporine in blood for binding to a monoclonal antibody is used as the basis of quantitation of cyclosporine in patient blood samples. In the absence of available antibody, the fluorescein-tagged-cyclosporine is randomly oriented in solution. Polarized light preferentially excites those molecules with the fluorescein oriented relative to the plane of the incident light. The degree of polarization of the emitted light depends on the percentage of molecules that are fixed or highly oriented. Binding to a macromolecule has the effect of slowing random molecular motion in solutions, and thus bound fluorescein-tagged-cyclosporine-antibody complexes emit polarized light more efficiently than free fluorescein-tagged-cyclosporine. By competing with free fluorescein-tagged-cyclosporine for antibody com-

plex formation, cyclosporine present in patient blood reduces emission of polarized light and enables the FPIA assay to measure the bound/free ratio of fluorescein-tagged-cyclosporine directly and, by reference to a standard curve, the cylosporine concentration in the blood sample. FPIA is not affected by background light interference, but is affected by cyclosporine metabolites that cross-react with the antibody. FPIA instrumentation can, in principle, be adapted to quantify any drug for which a fluorescein-tagged analog and specific antibodies can be prepared. The instrumentation is highly automated and designed for routine use in hospital clinical laboratories. Unattended assay of a single sample requires 14 minutes; but most of the time is required for incubation, so analysis of a full carousel of 20 samples requires only 19 minutes. The LOQ for FPIA assay of cyclosporine in 25 μg/L.

Several enzyme immunoassays (EIAs) are also popular commercial clinical assays with cyclosporine measurement capability [e.g., Enzyme Monitored (Multiplied) Immunoassay Technique (EMIT™), Cloned Enzyme Donor Immunoassay (CEDIA™)]. All homogeneous EIAs are competitive immunoassays in which enzyme-labeled antigen competes with sample antigen for a limited quantity of antibody binding sites. The resulting enzyme-labeled antigen-antibody bound complex exhibits a change in its rate of enzymatic action in comparison with free enzyme-labeled antigen. A kinetic measurement of the rate of reaction corresponds to determination of bound/free antigen ratio and consequently permits the drug concentration in the sample to be measured. The reagents for cyclosporine EMIT use cyclosporine-linked to recombinant glucose-6-phosphate-dehydrogenase. The active enzyme converts bacterial coenzyme NAD^+ to NADH resulting in a change of UV absorbance. Enzyme activity is decreased when added monoclonal antibody binds to the cyclosporine-linked enzyme. Highest enzyme activity corresponds to occupation of all antibody sites by high levels of cyclosporine in the blood sample.

The reagents for CEDIA detect the reassociation of two cloned fragments of β-galactosidase, an enzyme that catalyzes the hydrolysis of a chlorophenol-β-galactopyranoside to generate a product detected by UV absorbance at 570 nm. One cloned fragment of the β-galactosidase is linked to cyclosporine. When a monoclonal antibody to cyclosporine is added, competition is established between the cyclosporine in the blood sample and cyclosporine-linked to the fragment of β-galactosidase. Higher enzyme activity correlates with higher concentrations of cyclosporine in patient blood. Both EMIT and CEDIA assays are kinetic measurements that are performed in clinical autoanalyzers much like the FPIA assay previously described.

In addition to the FPIA, EMIT and CEDIA methods, several other commercial homogeneous immunoassays have been developed for cyclosporine quantification. Each manufacturer develops and controls the distribution of their antibodies and labeled cyclosporine antigen reagents that define the quantitative response characteristics of an assay kit. Although both polyclonal and monoclonal antibody reagents have been developed, more than 30 cyclosporine metabolites have been characterized and many of them exhibit cross-reactivity (i.e., high affinity) toward both these antibody types. As a consequence, most of the immunoassays report values that are elevated in comparison to the HPLC/UV or LC/MS/MS reference data. This has led to considerable debate and discussion in the clinical chemistry community with regard to methods for the analysis of cyclosporine and interpretation of the resulting data (8–11, 14–29).

Summary of F-ddA and Cyclosporine Analyses

The choice of assay technologies illustrated in the discussions of methods for F-ddA and cyclosporine demonstrates that there are many chemical, enzymatic, and instrumental options in devising quantitative measurements of drugs and drug metabolites. When new chemical entities are being studied, it is likely that a premium will be paid for the versatility and power of mass spectrometry and the requisite trained scientists required to obtain and interpret data. However, after drugs with narrow therapeutic indices are marketed and widely distributed, commercial considerations will drive the development of techniques that can be applied using general clinical laboratory instrumentation and less highly trained technical staff.

References

1. Johnston RAW, Rose ME. Mass spectrometry for chemists and biochemists. Cambridge: Cambridge University Press; 1996. p. 501.
2. Watson JT. Introduction to mass spectrometry. Philadelphia: Lippincott-Raven; 1997. p. 496.
3. Hammer CG, Holmstedt B, Ryhage R. Mass fragmentography. Identification of chlorpromazine and its metabolites in human blood by a new method. Anal Biochem 1968;25:532–48.
4. Roth JS, Ford H, Jr., Tanaka M, Mitsuya H, Kelley JA. Determination of 2'-beta-fluoro-2',3'-dideoxyadenosine, an experimental anti-AIDS drug, in human plasma by high-performance liquid chromatography. J Chromatogr B Biomed Sci Appl 1998;712:199–210.
5. Roth JS, McCully CM, Balis FM, Poplack DG, Kelley JA. 2'-beta-fluoro-2',3'-dideoxyadenosine, lodenosine, in rhesus monkeys: plasma and cerebrospinal fluid pharmacokinetics and urinary disposition. Drug Metab Dispos 1999;27:1128–32.
6. Bu HZ, Magis L, Knuth K, Teitelbaum P. High-throughput cytochrome P450 (CYP) inhibition screening via cassette probe-dosing strategy. I. Development of direct injection/on-line guard cartridge extraction/tandem mass spectrometry for the simultaneous detection of CYP probe substrates and their metabolites. Rapid Commun Mass Spectrom 2000;14:1619–24.
7. Floyd CD, Leblanc C, Whittaker M. Combinatorial chemistry as a tool for drug discovery. Prog Med Chem 1999;36:91–168.
8. Oellerich M, Armstrong VW, Schutz E, Shaw LM. Therapeutic drug monitoring of cyclosporine and tacrolimus. Update on Lake Louise Consensus Conference on cyclosporine and tacrolimus. Clin Biochem 1998;31:309–16.
9. Simpson J, Zhang Q, Ozaeta P, Aboleneen H. A specific method for the measurement of cyclosporin A in human whole blood by liquid chromatography-tandem mass spectrometry. Ther Drug Monit 1998;20:294–300.
10. McBride JH, Kim SS, Rodgerson DO, Reyes AF, Ota MK. Measurement of cyclosporine by liquid chromatography and three immunoassays in blood from liver, cardiac, and renal transplant recipients. Clin Chem 1992;38:2300–6.
11. Salm P, Norris RL, Taylor PJ, Davis DE, Ravenscroft PJ. A reliable high-performance liquid chromatography assay for high-throughput routine cyclosporin A monitoring in whole blood. Ther Drug Monit 1993;15:65–9.
12. Diamandis EP, Christopoulos TK, editors. Immunoassay. San Diego: Academic Press; 1996. p. 579.
13. Price CP, Newman DJ, editors. Principles and practice of immunoassay. London: Macmillan; 1997. p. 667.
14. Aspeslet LJ, LeGatt DF, Murphy G, Yatscoff RW. Effect of assay methodology on pharmacokinetic differences between cyclosporine Neoral and Sandimmune formulations. Clin Chem 1997;43:104–8.
15. Dusci LJ, Hackett LP, Chiswell GM, Ilett KF. Comparison of cyclosporine measurement in whole blood by high-performance liquid chromatography, monoclonal fluorescence polarization immunoassay, and monoclonal enzyme-multiplied immunoassay. Ther Drug Monit 1992;14:327–32.
16. Gulbis B, Van der Heijden J, van As H, Thiry P. Whole blood cyclosporin monitoring in liver and heart transplant patients: evaluation of the specificity of a fluorescence polarization immunoassay and an enzyme-multiplied immunoassay technique. J Pharm Biomed Anal 1997;15:951–63.
17. Hamwi A, Veitl M, Manner G, Ruzicka K, Schweiger C, Szekeres T. Evaluation of four automated methods for determination of whole blood cyclosporine concentrations. Am J Clin Pathol 1999;112:358–65.
18. Holt DW, Johnston A, Kahan BD, Morris RG, Oellerich M, Shaw LM. New approaches to cyclosporine monitoring raise further concerns about analytical techniques. Clin Chem 2000;46:872–4.
19. Kivisto KT. A review of assay methods for cyclosporin. Clinical implications. Clin Pharmacokinet 1992;23:173–90.
20. McBride JH, Kim S, Rodgerson DO, Reyes A. Conversion of cardiac and liver transplant recipients from HPLC and FPIA (polyclonal) to an FPIA (monoclonal) technique for measurement of blood cyclosporin A. J Clin Lab Anal 1998;12:337–42.
21. McGuire TR, Yee GC, Emerson S, Gmur DJ, Carlin J. Pharmacodynamic studies of cyclosporine in marrow transplant recipients. A comparison of three assay methods. Transplantation 1992;53:1272–5.
22. Morris RG. Cyclosporin assays, metabolite cross-reactivity, and pharmacokinetic monitoring. Ther Drug Monit 2000;22:160–2.
23. Murthy JN, Yatscoff RW, Soldin SJ. Cyclosporine metabolite cross-reactivity in different cyclosporine assays. Clin Biochem 1998;31:159–63.
24. Oellerich M, Armstrong VW, Kahan B, Shaw L, Holt DW, Yatscoff R, Lindholm A, Halloran P, Gallicano K, Wonigeit K and

others. Lake Louise Consensus Conference on cyclosporin monitoring in organ transplantation: report of the consensus panel. Ther Drug Monit 1995;17:642–54.

25. Schutz E, Svinarov D, Shipkova M, Niedmann PD, Armstrong VW, Wieland E, Oellerich M. Cyclosporin whole blood immunoassays (AxSYM, CEDIA, and Emit): A critical overview of performance characteristics and comparison with HPLC. Clin Chem 1998;44:2158–64.

26. Shaw LM, Holt DW, Keown P, Venkataramanan R, Yatscoff RW. Current opinions on therapeutic drug monitoring of immunosuppressive drugs. Clin Ther 1999;21:1632–52; discussion 1631.

27. Steimer W. Performance and specificity of monoclonal immunoassays for cyclosporine monitoring: How specific is specific? Clin Chem 1999;45:371–81.

28. Takagi H, Uchida K, Takahara S, Takahashi K. 12th quality assessment of cyclosporin blood monitoring by 56 Japanese laboratories. Transplant Proc 1998;30:1706–8.

29. Taylor PJ, Salm P, Norris RL, Ravenscroft PJ, Pond SM. Comparison of high-performance liquid chromatography and monoclonal fluorescence polarization immunoassay for the determination of whole-blood cyclosporin A in liver and heart transplant patients. Ther Drug Monit 1994;16:526–30.

CHAPTER

13

Clinical Pharmacogenetics

DAVID A. FLOCKHART

Division of Clinical Pharmacology, Georgetown University Medical Center, Washington, D.C.

INTRODUCTION

The juxtaposition in time of the sequencing of the entire human genome and the realization that medication errors constitute one of the leading causes of death in the United States (1) has led many to believe that pharmacogenetics may be able to improve pharmacotherapy. As a result, a fairly uncritical series of hopes and predictions have led not only physicians and scientists, but also venture capitalists and Wall Street to believe that genomics will lead to a new era of personalized medications. If this is to occur, it will require a series of accurate and reliable genetic tests that allow physicians to predict clinically relevant outcomes with confidence. This short summary of the state of pharmacogenetics as we enter the new millennium is intended as an introduction to the field, using pertinent examples to emphasize the important principles of the discipline, which I hope will transcend the moment and serve as a useful group of principles with which to evaluate and follow this rapidly evolving field.

One of the most important principles in this particular discipline at this particular time is that the huge amount of media, Internet, and device marketing hyperbole should be greeted with a healthy dose of scientific skepticism. First, we must note that pharmacogenetics is *not* a new discipline. The coalition of the science of genetics, founded by the work of an Austrian monk Gregor Mendel with peas, and the ancient science of pharmacology did not occur until the twen-

tieth century, but it was early in that century. After the rediscovery of the Mendelian laws of genetics at the turn of the century, some connection with the ancient science of pharmacology would seem inevitable, and indeed a series of investigators contributed important observations that named and then laid the foundations of the field (Table 13.1) (2). These rested in part in genetics and in part in pharmacology.

In the area of genetics, the separate observations of Hardy and Weinberg that resulted in the Hardy-Weinberg Law are particularly pertinent to modern pharmacogenetics. This law states that when an allele with a single change in it is distributed at equilibrium in a population, the incidences p and q of the two resulting alleles will result in a genotype incidence that can be represented by the following equation:

$$p^2 + 2\,pq + q^2 = 1$$

Two important predictions follow: 1) The incidence of heterozygotes ($2pq$) and of the homozygous q genotype (q^2) can be predicted if the incidence of the p genotype (p^2) is known. 2) If this equation accurately predicts the incidence of genotypes and alleles, then we are dealing with a single change that results in two alleles and two resultant phenotypes. If genotypes are present in a population in dysequilibrium with this law, the influence of population concentrating factors or environment must be invoked and a pure genetic etiology is inadequate.

In the area of pharmacology, the identification of the series of proteins in the familiar pharmacologic

TABLE 13.1   The Early History of Pharmacogenetics

1932	First inherited difference in a response to a chemical—inability to taste phenythiourea.
World War II	Hemolysis in African-American soldiers treated with primaquine highlights importance of genetic deficiency of glucose-6-phosphate dehydrogenase (G6PD).
1957	Motulsky proposes that "inheritance might explain many individual differences in the efficacy of drugs and in the occurrence of adverse drug reactions."
1959	Vogel publishes "pharmacogenetics: the role of genetics in drug response."
1959	Genetic polymorphism found to influence isoniazid blood concentrations.
1964	Genetic differences found in ethanol metabolism.
1977	CYP2D6 polymorphism identified by Mahgoub et al.

cascade essentially identified not only a series of targets for drugs but also a series of genetic "targets" that might contribute to interindividual variability in drug response. The proteins involved turned out to be diverse in structure, function, and location, ranging from those that control and facilitate drug absorption, through the enzymes in the gastrointestinal tract and liver that influence drug elimination, to molecules involved in the complex series of events that occur during and after the interaction between drugs and cellular receptor molecules. Along the way, the complexity of human response to exogenous xenobiotics was constantly reemphasized. The complexity was then exploited to the benefit of patients, as demonstrated by the early work on propranolol, the first β-adrenoreceptor blocker, and cimetidine, the first H_2-receptor blocker. Subsequent work demonstrated the involvement of multiple intracellular proteins in the second messenger response proposed by Earl Sutherland, and in the responses to steroids and other exogenous molecules that have intranuclear sites of action. The twentieth century in pharmacology therefore laid the ground for work in the twenty-first, which will involve the study of genetic changes in this cascade of important proteins, even as genetic information itself leads to the identification of a large number of new protein and genetic drug targets.

THE HIERARCHY OF PHARMACOGENETIC INFORMATION

An important second principle of modern pharmacogenetics is illustrated in Figure 13.1 in which the

hierarchy of useful information from pharmacogenetic studies is illustrated. Although this figure illustrates an information hierarchy for single nucleotide polymorphisms (SNPs), it could equally well be used for deletions, insertions, duplications, splice variants, or genetic variants in general. There is a large amount of activity at the base of this pyramid at the moment, and available information about the presence, incidence, and validity of individual SNPs is large and rapidly expanding as the result of the work of the SNP consortium, the Human Genome Project, and a large number of individual scientists. As we ascend the pyramid toward increasingly functional data, the pyramid becomes dramatically thinner as the databases containing data about nonsynonymous SNPs, nonconservative amino acid changes, and SNPs that change activity *in vitro*, clinical pharmacokinetics, drug response, or finally clinically important outcomes are progressively smaller. The number of SNPs that have been clearly shown to bring about clinically important outcomes is indeed small, and this is reflected in the fact that, as of this writing, no pharmacogenetic test is routinely available to physicians.

This figure also makes clear the long scientific route from the discovery of an individual SNP to the actual demonstration of a clinically important outcome. This is particularly pertinent in view of the simple fact that the vast majority of individual polymorphisms in human DNA likely have no dynamic consequence. A lot of work in the laboratories of molecular biologists and geneticists can therefore be expended to little avail. As a result, a number of clinical pharmacologists, i.e. scientists with expertise in genetics, pharmacology, and medicine have elected to start at the other end, the top of the pyramid. By searching for outliers in populations that demonstrate aberrant clinical responses and by focusing on these polymorphisms, they intend to elicit valuable genetic, mechanistic, and clinical lessons. This approach has already born considerable fruit, as illustrated later in this chapter. It is important to note that the most successful of these approaches have occurred when collaborative groups of physicians, pharmacologists, and geneticists have been able to form translational teams to carry research from the clinic to the laboratory and back.

It is possible for scientists who study specific drug responses to place the phenomena that they study at individual points in time within this hierarchy of information. For example, the cytochrome P450 enzymes present in the human liver and gastrointestinal tract have a long pharmacogenetic history and variants in some of these, notably those designated CYP2C9, CYP2C19, and CYP2D6, could reasonably be placed at present in the top two rows of the hierarchy. Of course,

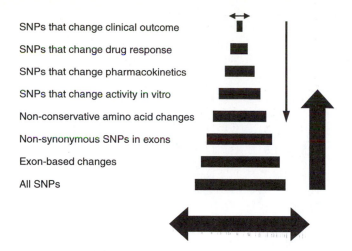

SNPs that change clinical outcome

SNPs that change drug response

SNPs that change pharmacokinetics

SNPs that change activity in vitro

Non-conservative amino acid changes

Non-synonymous SNPs in exons

Exon-based changes

All SNPs

FIGURE 13.1 The hierarchy of pharmacogenetic information from single nucleotide polymorphisms (SNPs). The size of the bar at each level of the pyramid represents an approximation of the number of SNPs in each category. At the base is the total number of SNPs, estimated to be somewhere between 20 and 80 million. Most of these are not in exons, the expressed sequences that code for proteins, and so the second level is much smaller, in the 300,000 range. Exon-based changes are more likely to result in a clinical effect, but there are good examples of intronic changes and promoter variants that result in important, expressed changes. Non-synonymous SNPs are those that result in a change in amino acid, and the number of these that are nonconservative and therefore have a greater chance of changing the structure or activity of the protein domain they code for is even smaller. Through a wide range of techniques, laboratory scientists are expressing these variants and testing whether they change activity *in vitro,* and it is clear that most do not, so the number of SNPs at this level of the hierarchy shrinks further. SNPs that result in statistically significant changes in pharmacokinetics due to changes in receptors, transporters, or drug-metabolizing enzymes that are rate limiting are well described, but few and far between. Very few of these result in clinically significant changes in drug response, and even fewer could be measured by the epidemiologists and managers that measure aggregate clinical outcomes.

there are many individual SNPs in these enzymes that have no functional consequence, and remain in the bottom row. In contrast, the majority of pharmacogenetic information available at present about drug receptors, transporters or ketoreductases occupies the lower few rows of the pyramid, although this is starting to change.

For obvious reasons, we have more information about drug responses that are easy to measure. Genetic variants that result in changes in plasma concentrations of drugs that can be measured easily are relatively amenable to study by analytical chemists and clinical pharmacokineticists, whereas genetic polymorphisms in receptors that might influence drug response require careful clinical pharmacologic studies. These simple observations emphasize the need for a qualified cadre of clinical pharmacologists in the

field of pharmacogenetics to effectively exploit the huge amount of information made available by the sequencing of the human genome. They perhaps explain also the already apparent concentration of contributions from clinical pharmacologists to the field.

IDENTIFICATION AND SELECTION OF OUTLIERS IN A POPULATION

Figure 13.2 illustrates one useful means of identifying population outliers that allows investigators to focus on these individuals, to take information from the top of the hierarchy of information presented in Figure 13.1, and to apply it fairly quickly to questions of clinical relevance. Figure 13.2 contains both histograms and Normit plots from a population with a range of metabolic capacities for CYP2C19. A Normit plot is essentially a means of describing the population as a cumulative distribution in units of standard deviation from the mean. The cumulative plot of a pure normal distribution will be a straight line, the slope of which is determined by the variance of the distribution. In other words, the steeper the slope, the more tightly the group would be distributed around the mean, whereas a more shallow line would indicate a more broadly distributed group. The value of this analysis to pharmacogeneticists is that changes in the slope of the line indicate a *new* distribution, and if this different population represents more than 1% of the total, it can reasonably be expected to be genetically stable and be termed a polymorphism. In the case illustrated, the six subjects on the right of each histogram were all shown to possess a SNP in both the alleles coding for CYP2C19 that was subsequently shown to render the enzyme inactive (3). Figure 13.2 also illustrates the point that a number of probes can be developed to determine the *phenotype* that results from the expression of such a *genotype.* In this case, the study was carried out to demonstrate the utility of a single dose of the proton pump inhibitor omeprazole as a probe for the genetic polymorphism in CYP2C19. As summarized in Table 13.2, ideal characteristics of probes for phenotyping include specificity for the trait in question, sensitivity and ease of available assays, and, most important, the requirement that they be clinically benign. The absence of some of these characteristics in many probes and the difficulty in finding ideal probes are some of the most significant impediments to progress in developing clinically useful pharmacogenetic tests, and are key issues that critical scientific evaluators should address.

Upon the identification of an outlier phenotype such as this, the logical next step is a valid demonstration that it can be explained by a genetic change. Family and twin studies are a valuable means of confirming this, and

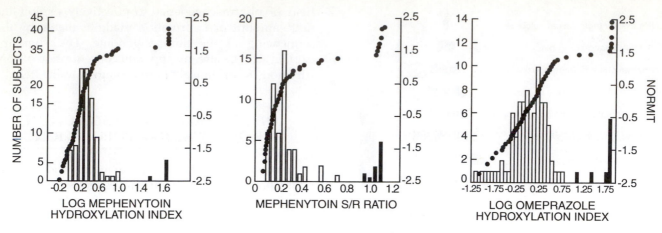

FIGURE 13.2   Normit plots (•) of CYP2C19 activity as indicated by the metabolism of mephenytoin and omeprazole as probe drugs. Comparisons for a population of 142 subjects are shown based on log hydroxylation indices for mephenytoin [$\log_{10}$ (µmole S-phenytoin given/µmole 4'-hydroxymephenytoin recovered in urine)] and omeprazole [$\log_{10}$(omeprazole/5'-hydroxyomeprazole)], and ratio of S-mephenytoin/R-mephenytoin recovered in urine. In the histograms, rapid metabolizers are represented by open bars and slow metabolizers by solid bars. The same seven individuals were identified by all three methods as poor CYP2C19 metabolizers. (Reproduced with permission from Balian JD, et al. Clin Pharmacol Ther 1998;57:662–9.)

have been the standard in the field since the days of Mendel. These remain an important part of any genetic association study, but they are now being replaced in a few cases, such as this, by genetic tests that are able to define changes at specific loci and test for their presence in broad, unrelated groups of people.

The clinical relevance of CYP2C19 polymorphism, primarily present in Asian populations (4), has been studied by a number of investigators, in whom it has been shown that the cure rate for *Helicobacter pylori* infection is greater in patients who are genetic poor metabolizers (5). When given omeprazole doses of 20 mg per day for 4 weeks, these individuals have plasma *AUCs* that are 5- to 10-fold higher than those of extensive metabolizers (6). The resultant decreases in gastric acid exposure are associated with a clinically important difference in the response of *H. pylori* infection (7). As illustrated in Figure 13.3, patients with duodenal ulcers who were poor metabolizers had a 100% cure rate, but extensive metabolizers with both alleles active had only a 25% cure rate when given an omeprazole dose of 20 mg per day. Despite the apparent importance of these data, it might reasonably be argued that therapy of all patients with 40 or 60 mg of omeprazole might result a uniformly beneficial outcome without the need for pharmacogenetic testing.

EXAMPLES OF IMPORTANT GENETIC POLYMORPHISMS

Pharmacologically significant genetic variants have been described at every point of the cascade leading from the pharmacokinetics of drug absorption to the pharmacodynamics of drug effect (Figure 2.1), including proteins involved in the absorption, distribution, elimination, and direct cellular action of drugs.

Drug Absorption

One of the most well-known polymorphisms relevant to pharmacodynamic response is in the aldehyde dehydrogenase gene *(ALDH2)* (8). There are 10 human *ALDH* genes and 13 different alleles that result in an autosomal dominant trait that lacks catalytic activity if one subunit of the tetramer is inactive. *ALDH2* deficiency occurs in up to 45% of Chinese, but rarely in Caucasians or Africans, and results in buildup of toxic acetaldehyde and alcohol-related flushing in Asians. Although the genetics of this enzyme and of alcohol metabolism are generally well characterized, a genetic diagnostic test would have little clinical utility because the carriers of the defective alleles are usually acutely aware of it. This illustrates a more widely relevant

TABLE 13.2   Properties of an Ideal Probe for Phenotyping

Specific for the pharmacogenetic trait in question

Sensitive

Simple to administer

Inexpensive

Easy to assay

Clinically benign

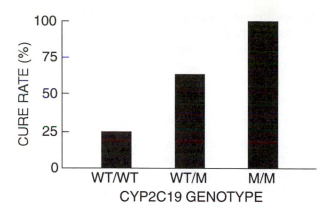

FIGURE 13.3 Effectiveness of omeprazole and amoxacillin in eradicating *Helicobacter pylori* infection in duodenal ulcer patients with CYP2C19 genotypes (WT = wild type allele, M = mutant allele). (Data from Furuta T, et al. Ann Intern Med 1998;129:1027–30.)

point in that the *availability of genetic testing methodology does not necessarily mean that it is clinically useful.*

Drug Distribution

P-glycoprotein (P-gp)

As discussed in Chapter 16, studies in mice that have the MDR-1 gene that codes for P-gp knocked out have clearly demonstrated an important role for this multidrug transporter in the absorption and disposition of a large number of clinically important medicines (9–11). The first significant polymorphism in this protein was recently shown to change the pharmacokinetics of digoxin in a marked and likely clinically significant manner. Figure 13.4 diagrams the action of P-gp and illustrates the point that plasma digoxin concentration changes in P-gp knockout mice are accompanied by a proportionately greater change in its concentration in the brain. Many other transporters have been identified recently, but the contribution of mutations in them to clinical response remains unclear at present.

Drug Elimination

P450 CYP2D6

No protein involved in drug metabolism or response has a pharmacogenetic component that has been more studied than this enzyme. CYP2D6 is now known to be the principal catalyst for the metabolism of more than 40 drugs and has been the subject of extensive and excellent reviews (8, 12–14). The original reports of population outliers by Mahgoub et al. (15) and Eichelbaum et al. (16) were the result of observations of sensitivity to debrisoquine, or sparteine by these astute clinical investigators. These

reports were followed by the first identification of genetic changes responsible for altered activity in the metabolism of CYP2D6 substrates (17). Eventually, a legion of genetic changes were identified by a large number of groups such that there are now 38 identified alleles containing more than 50 mutations; progress in this area can be accessed on the Internet at http://www.imm.ki.se/CYPAlleles. This remarkable story contains within it a large number of important lessons and illustrates a number of key pharmacogenetic principles. First among these is that genetic variants can result in both decreases and increases in activity.

The incidence of the poor metabolizer phenotype for CYP2D6 is now known to vary considerably in different human populations, from an average of 7% in Caucasians to about 2% in the African and Asian populations that have been studied. However, it is clear that extensive metabolizers from China or Africa do have mean rates of metabolism that are slower than Caucasian extensive metabolizers, and that this is likely the result of the presence of the *10 allele in Asians (18–20) and of the *17 allele in Africans (21, 22). Relatively subtle genetic effects may therefore contribute to differences in interindividual response.

Ultrarapid metabolizers who carry multiple copies of the *CYP2D6* gene have also been identified (23). This phenotype appears to be present in approximately 10% of a Spanish population (24), 1–2% of a Swedish population (25), and notably in up to 30% of Ethiopians (26). This trait may result in treatment failures when standard doses of a large number of medications are prescribed, and forms the basis for

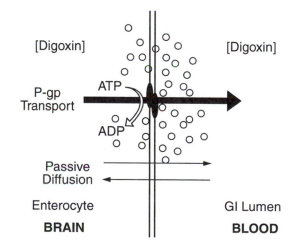

FIGURE 13.4 Schematic drawing of P-glycoprotein (P-pg) efflux pumping in enterocytes and at the blood-brain barrier. Because P-gp efflux pump action is absent, knockout mice lacking the *P-gp* gene have increased digoxin bioavailability and an increased brain/plasma digoxin concentration ratio.

what has been described as "rational megaprescribing" (27).

Although CYP2D6 represents a relatively small proportion of the immunoblotable CYP450 protein in human livers (28), it is clear that it is responsible for the metabolism of a relatively large number of important medicines. These include all the β-adrenoreceptor blockers that are known to be metabolized, including propranolol (29), metoprolol (30), carvedilol (31) and timolol (32). Although few studies of patient response are available, an elegant clinical pharmacologic study has demonstrated lower resting heart rates in poor metabolizers who were administered the CYP2D6 substrate timolol (32). On the other hand, a key principle is illustrated by studies demonstrating that increased propranolol plasma concentrations in Chinese poor metabolizers were *not* accompanied by the expected increase in cardiac slowing, so that *the alterations in pharmacokinetics in poor metabolizers apparently were offset by changes in pharmacodynamic responsiveness* (33).

While it is often held that genetic polymorphisms are most important when they affect drugs of narrow therapeutic range for which dangerous toxicity may result or perilous lack of effect may ensue, this need not be the case. For example, CYP2D6 converts codeine, likely the most widely prescribed opiate in the world and the mainstay of pain control for a large number of patients, to its active metabolite morphine. It follows that patients who have deficient CYP2D6 are unable to make morphine, and pharmacodynamic studies have shown that this results in decreased pain control (34), as well as decreased codeine effects on pupillary and respiratory function (35).

A large number of studies have demonstrated the effects of the CYP2D6 polymorphism on the pharmacokinetics of tricyclic antidepressants and antipsychotic drugs (3). Although both drugs have a narrow therapeutic range and the clinical consequences of this polymorphism have been documented for tricyclic antidepressants (36), it has been surprisingly difficult to demonstrate that CYP2D6 polymorphism has clinically significant consequences for patients treated with antipsychotic drugs.

Lastly, an important lesson that has been learned from research on CYP2D6 is that many, but not all, *genetic polymorphisms can be mimicked by drug interactions.* Not only is CYP2D6 metabolism of codeine potently inhibited by quinidine (35), but the inhibition of this enzyme by commonly prescribed drugs such as fluoxetine (37), paroxetine (38, 39), and the majority of antipsychotic drugs (40), including haloperidol (41) is well described. These interactions are likely clinically relevant and more prevalent in many circumstances than the poor metabolizer phenotype (42). Of note, the ultrarapid metabolizer phenotype of CYP2D6 has not at present been shown to be mimicked by a drug interaction, and the rare reports of effects of metabolic inducers on CYP2D6 activity are not well substantiated, and appear modest at best (43).

Genetic Variants in Thiopurine Methyltransferase

A number of rare mutations in this Phase II conjugative enzyme, which is responsible for critical steps in the metabolism of azathioprine and 6-mercaptopurine, demonstrate the principal that a *low incidence of a genetic change in the population does not obviate its clinical importance.* Although the genetic variants responsible for deficient thiopurine methyltransferase activity are present in less than 0.5% of studied populations (44, 45), it is clear that they can have fatal consequences in children treated with 6-mercaptopurine for acute lymphocytic leukemia. They also can bring about clinically important intolerance to azathioprine that results in decreased ability to continue taking effective doses of this drug (46). These dramatic changes allowed investigators from the groups of Weinshilboum (47) and Evans (45) to identify outlier individuals in clinical populations early on, and enabled these investigators to adopt a "phenotype to genotype" approach that relatively quickly identified the mutations responsible for the polymorphism. As a result, the genetic variants that contribute to these dangerous toxicities can be firmly placed at the top of the pyramid of pharmacogenetic data and are among the few that have important clinical consequences for pharmacotherapy. Despite its clinical importance, pharmacogenetic testing for this polymorphism remains problematic, since a large number of alleles must be tested, genetic haplotype identification is difficult, and phenotypic measurements that quantify the enzyme in platelets remain more useful than genetic tests.

N-Acetyltransferase 2 (NAT-2)

In marked contrast to the data on genetic changes in thiopurine methyltransferase, genetic variants in this enzyme are very common, but have little clinical significance (8). NAT-2 can therefore be placed on the pyramid of genetic information at a point where clear pharmacokinetic changes have been noted, but important pharmacodynamic consequences have not yet been demonstrated. In addition, as with CYP2D6, it is clear that a large number of mutations and at least 17 different alleles contribute to this change in activity (48). The slow acetylator phenotype is present in roughly 50% of Caucasian and African populations studied, but in as few 10% of Japanese, and as many as 80% of Egyptians

(49, 50). Woosley et al. (51) demonstrated that slow acetylators develop positive antinuclear antibody (ANA) titers and procainamide-induced lupus more quickly than rapid acetylators. However, this finding did not lead to widespread phenotypic or genetic testing because all patients will develop positive ANA titers after one year of procainamide therapy and almost a third will have developed arthralgias and/or a skin rash (52). Although a number of studies have attempted to associate this polymorphism with the risk for xenobiotic-induced bladder, colorectal (53) or breast cancer (54), there are at present no compelling data that warrant phenotypic testing for this polymorphism in order to improve treatment with any medicine, much less a genetic test that would have to accurately identify such a large number of alleles.

Genetic Variants in Drug Receptors

β-*Adrenoreceptor (beta2AR) Mutations in Asthma*

Since the first descriptions of genetic polymorphisms in beta2AR that may play a pathogenic role in the development of asthma (55, 56), a number of investigators have shown an association between these mutations and patient response to treatment for this disease. A number of missense mutations within the coding region of the type 2 β-receptor gene on chromosome 5q31 have been identified in humans. In studies utilizing site-directed mutagenesis and recombinant expression, three loci at amino acid positions 16, 27, and 164 have been found to significantly alter *in vitro* receptor function. The Thr164Ile mutation displays altered coupling to adenylyl cyclase, the Arg16Gly mutation displays enhanced agonist-promoted downregulation, and the Gln27Glu form is resistant to downregulation (56). The frequencies of these various beta2AR mutations are not different in asthmatic than in normal populations, but Lima et al. (53) have shown that albuterol-evoked FEV1 was higher and the bronchodilatory response was more rapid in Arg 16 homozygotes than in a cohort of carriers of the Gly 16 variant. In addition, an association has been demonstrated between the same beta2AR polymorphism and susceptibility to bronchodilator desensitization in moderately severe stable asthmatics. Although these data are compelling, careful studies have concluded that the beta2AR genotype is not a major determinant of fatal or near-fatal asthma (58), and widespread testing of asthmatic patients for the presence of genetic polymorphisms in the beta2AR is not yet routinely carried out. Nevertheless, a number of other potential target proteins may alter the susceptibility and response of asthmatic patients, including histamine N-

methyltransferase (59), and the lipoxygenase system and further developments in the genetics of asthma pharmacotherapy seem likely.

Mutations in Endothelial Nitric Oxide Synthase (e-NOS)

An association has been made between cardiovascular disease and specific mutations in e-NOS, the enzyme that creates nitric oxide via the conversion of citrulline to arginine in endothelial cells and in platelets (60). A firmer understanding of the mechanism of this effect has been provided by a series of careful studies of forearm vascular vasodilation conducted by Abernethy and Babaoglu (61), who showed that acetylcholine, but not nitroprusside-mediated vasodilation, was compromised by the Glu298Asp mutation in this enzyme. These results demonstrate the value of careful clinical pharmacologic studies in confirming a pharmacological consequence of a polymorphism that otherwise would only have had an association with cardiovascular disease. The implications of these findings for patients with hypertension, congestive heart failure, and a variety of other disorders are clear issues for future investigation.

CONCLUSIONS AND FUTURE DIRECTIONS

There are many potential pitfalls that lie in the way of researchers on the route from the discovery of a mutation in human DNA that codes for a pharmacologically important protein to the development of a clinically useful pharmacogenetic test. Very few such tests have been developed as yet, but a considerable number seem likely to be found useful over the next decade in guiding the treatment of patients with cancer, asthma, hypertension, and pain.

In the development of new pharmacogenetic tests, as for any other clinically applied test, assay sensitivity, specificity, and positive predictive value will have to be scrutinized rigorously. In addition, the reliability of DNA testing in terms of intra- and interday variability and the rigor of assays when applied to multiple DNA samples will have to be demonstrated almost more carefully than it would be for routine assays for serum chemistries or hematology. This is because there are significant societal pressures that insist on the accuracy of a diagnostic test that informs a physician and a patient about an individual's genetic makeup. The requirement for robust tests has not prevented any other technology from entering clinical practice though, and I think it likely that a number of array-based genetic tests will soon be available that are able to diagnose genotypes simultaneously at a relatively large number of loci.

When the technical barriers of sensitivity, specificity, and reproducibility are overcome, it seems very likely that the practice of medicine will enable individual patients to be treated for a variety of different drug targets with different doses of medicines, or indeed different medicines, based on their genotype or phenotype.

References

1. Lesar TS, Lomaestro BM, Pohl H. Medication-prescribing errors in a teaching hospital. Arch Intern Med 1997;157:1569–76.

2. Nebert DW. Pharmacogenetics: 65 candles on the cake. Pharmacogenetics 1997;7:435–40.

3. Balian JD, Sukhova N, Harris JW, Hewett J, Pickle L, Goldstein JA, Woosley RL, Flockhart DA. The hydroxylation of omeprazole correlates with S-mephenytoin metabolism: A population study. Clin Pharmacol Ther 1995;57:662–9.

4. Flockhart DA. Drug Interactions and the cytochrome P450 system: The role of cytochrome P450 2C19. Clin Pharmacokinet 1995;29:45–52.

5. Furuta T, Ohashi K, Kamata T, Takashiima M, Kosuge K, Kawasaki T, et al. Effect of genetic differences in omeprazole metabolism on cure rates for *Helicobacter pylori* infection and peptic ulcer. Ann Intern Med 1998;129:1027–30.

6. Andersson T, Regardh CG, Lou YC, Zhang Y, Dahl ML, Bertilsson L. Polymorphic hydroxylation of S-mephenytoin and omeprazole metabolism in Caucasian and Chinese subjects. Pharmacogenetics 1992;2:25–31.

7. Furuta T, Ohashi K, Kosuge K, Zhao XJ, Takashima M, Kimura M, et al. CYP2C19 genotype status and effect of omeprazole on intragastric pH in humans Clin Pharmacol Ther 1999;65:552–61.

8. Kalow W, Bertilsson L. Interethnic factors affecting drug metabolism. Adv Drug Res 1994;25:1–53.

9. Schinkel AH, Smit JJ, van Tellingen O, Beijnen JH, Wagenaar E, van Deemter L et al. Disruption of the mouse mdr1 a p-glycoprotein gene leads to a deficiency in the blood-brain barrier and to increase sensitivity to drugs. Cell 1994;77:491–502.

10. Schinkel AH, Wagenaar E, Mol CA, van Deemter L. P-glycoprotein in the blood-brain barrier of mice influences the brain penetration and pharmacological activity of many drugs. J Clin Invest 1996;97:2517–24.

11. van Asperen J, Schinkel AH, Beijnen JH, Nooijen WJ, Borst P, van Telligen O. Altered pharmacokinetics of vinblastine in Mdr1a P-glycoprotein-deficient mice. J Natl Cancer Inst 1996;88:994–9.

12. Bertilsson L., Dahl M-L. Polymorphic drug oxidation—Relevance to the treatment of psychiatric disorders. CNS Drugs 1996;5:200–23.

13. Dahl ML, Bertilsson L. Genetically variable metabolism of antidepressants and neuroleptic drugs in man. Pharmacogenetics 1993;3:61–70.

14. Jick H, Jick SS, Gurewich V, Myers MW, Vasilakis C. Risk of idiopathic cardiovascular death and nonfatal venous thromboembolism in women using oral contraceptives with differing progestagen components. Lancet 1995;346:1589–92.

15. Mahgoub A, Idle JR, Dring LG, Lancaster R, Smith RL. Polymorphic hydroxylation of debrisoquine in man. Lancet 1977;2:584–6.

16. Eichelbaum M, Spannbrucker N, Steincke B, Dengler HJ. Defective N-oxidation of sparteine in man: A new pharmacogenetic defect. Eur J Clin Pharmacol 1979;16:183–7.

17. Kimura S, Umeno M, Skoda RC, Meyer UA, Gonzalez FJ. The human debrisoquine 4-hydroxylase (CYP2D) locus: Sequence and identification of the polymorphic CYP2D6 gene, a related gene, and a pseudogene. Am J Hum Genet 1989;45:889–904.

18. Johansson I, Oscarson M, Yue QY, Bertilsson L, Sjöqvist F, Ingelman-Sundberg M. Genetic analysis of the Chinese chromosome P4502D locus: Characterization of variant *CYP2D6* genes present in subjects with diminished capacity for debrisoquine hydroxylation. Mol Pharmacol 1994;46:452–9.

19. Mihara K, Suzuki A, Kondo T, Yasui N, Furukori H, Nagashima U, et al. Effects of the *CYP2D6*10* allele on the steady-state plasma concentrations of haloperidol and reduced haloperidol in Japanese patients with schizophrenia. Clin Pharmacol Ther 1999;65:291–4.

20 Yue QY, Zhong ZH, Tybring G, Dalen P, Dahl ML, Bertilsson L, et al. Pharmacokinetics of nortriptyline and its 10-hydroxy metabolite in Chinese subjects of different CYP2D6 genotypes. Clin Pharmacol Ther 1998;64:384–90.

21. Masimirembwa C, Persson I, Bertilsson L, Hasler JA, Ingelman-Sundberg M. A novel mutant variant of the *CYP2D6* gene (*CYP2D6*17*) common in a black African population: Association with diminished debrisoquine hydroxylase activity. Br J Clin Pharmacol 1996;42:713–19.

22. Oscarson M, Hidestrand M, Johansson I, Ingelman-Sundberg M. A combination of mutations in the *CYP2D6*17 (CYP2D6Z)* allele causes alterations in enzyme function. Mol Pharmacol 1997;52:1034–40.

23. Johansson I, Lundqvist E, Bertilsson L, Dahl ML, Sjöqvist F, Ingelman-Sundberg M. Inherited amplification of an active gene in the cytochrom P450 CYP2D6 locus as a cause of ultrarapid metabolism of debrisoquine. Genetics 1993;90:11825–9.

24. Bernal ML, Sinues B, Johansson I, McLellan RA, Wennerholm A, Dahl ML, et al. Ten percent of North Spanish individuals carry duplicated or triplicated *CYP2D6* genes associated with ultrarapid metabolism of debrisoquine. Pharmacogenetics 1999;9:657–60.

25. Dahl ML, Johansson I, Bertilsson L, Ingelman-Sundberg M, Sjöqvist F. Ultrarapid hydroxylation of debrisoquine in a Swedish population: Analysis of the molecular genetic basis. J Pharmacol Exp Ther 1995;274:516–20.

26. Aklillu E, Persson I, Bertilsson L, Johansson I, Rodrigues F, Ingelman-Sundberg M. Frequent distribution of ultrarapid metabolizers of debrisoquine in an Ethiopian population carrying duplicated and multiduplicated functional *CYP2D6* alleles. J Pharmacol Exp Ther 1996;278:441–6.

27. Bertilsson L, Dahl ML, Sjöqvist F, Aberg-Wistedt A, Humble M, Johansson I, et al. Molecular basis for rational megaprescribing in ultrarapid hydroxylators of debrisoquine [letter]. Lancet 1993;341:63.

28. Shimada T, Yamazaki H, Mimura M, Inui Y, Guengerich FP. Interindividual variations in human liver Cytochrome P-450 enzymes involved in the oxidation of drugs, carcinogens and toxic chemicals: Studies with liver microsomes of 30 Japanese and 30 Caucasians. J Pharmacol Exp Ther 1994;270:414–23.

29. Ward SA, Walle T, Walle UK, Wilkinson GR, Branch RA. Propanolol's metabolism is determined by both mephenytoin and debrisoquin hydroxylase activities. Clin Pharmacol Ther 1989;45:72–9.

30. Johnson JA, Burlew BS. Metoprolol metabolism via cytochrome P4502D6 in ethnic populations. Drug Metab Dispos 1996;24:350–5.

31. Zhou HH, Wood AJ. Stereoselective disposition of carvedilol is determined by CYP2D6. Clin Pharmacol Ther 1995;57:518–24.

32. McGourty JC, Silas JH, Fleming JJ, McBurney A, Ward JW. Pharmacokinetics and beta-blocking effects of timolol in poor and extensive metabolizers of debrisoquine. Clin Pharmacol Ther 1985;38:409–13.

33. Zhou HH, Koshakji RP, Silberstein DJ, Wilkinson GR, Wood AJ. Racial differences in drug response: Altered sensitivity to and clearance of propanolol in men of Chinese descent as compared with American whites. N Engl J Med 1989;320:565–70.

34. Poulsen L, Brosen K, Arendt-Nielsen L, Gram LF, Elbaek K, Sindrup SH. Codeine and morphine in extensive and poor metabolizers of sparteine: pharmacokinetics, analgesic effect and side effects. Eur J Clin Pharmacol 1996;51:289–95.

35. Caraco Y, Sheller J, Wood AJ. Impact of ethnic origin and quinidine coadministration on codeine's disposition and pharmacodynamic effects. J Pharmacol Exp.Ther 1999;290:413–22.

36. Sjöqvist F. Towards optimal use of tricyclic antidepressants: The new pharmacogenetics. In: Costa E, editor. Neurochemical pharmacology—A tribute to B. B. Brodie. New York: Raven Press; 1989.p.303–18.

37. Otton SV, Wu D, Joffe RT, Cheung SW, Sellers EM. Inhibition by fluoxetine of cytochrome P450 2D6 activity. Clin Pharmacol Ther 1993;53:401–9.

38. Sindrup SH, Brøsen K, Gram LF, Hallas J, Skjelbo E, Allen A, et al. The relationship between paroxetine and the sparteine oxidation polymorphism. Clin Pharmacol Ther 1992;51(1)1:278–87.

39. Alderman J, Preskorn SH, Greenblatt DJ, Harrison W, Penenberg D, Allison J, et al. Desipramine pharmacokinetics when coadministered with paroxetine or sertraline in extensive metabolizers. J. Clin Psychopharmacol. 1997;17:284–91.

40. Shin JG, Soukhova N, Flockhart DA. Effect of antipsychotic drugs on human liver cytochrome P-450 (CYP) isoforms in vitro: Preferential inhibition of CYP2D6. Drug Metab Dispos 1999;27:1078–84.

41. Ereshefsky L. Pharmacokinetics and drug interactions: Update for new antipsychotics [see comments]. J Clin Psychiatry 1996;57 (suppl 11):12–25.

42. Goff DC, Midha KK, Brotman AW, Waites M, Baldessarini RJ. Elevation of plasma concentrations of haloperidol after the addition of fluoxetine. Am J Psychiatry 1991;148:790–2.

43. Dilger K, Greiner B, Fromm MF, Hofmann U, Kroemer HK, Eichelbaum M. Consequences of rifampicin treatment on propafenone disposition in extensive and poor metabolizers of CYP2D6. Pharmacogenetics 1999;9:551–9.

44. Krynetski EY, Tai HL, Yates CR, Fessing MY, Loennechen T, Schuetz JD, et al. Genetic polymorphism of thiopurine S-methyltransferase: Clinical importance and molecular mechanisms. Pharmacogenetics 1996;6:279–90.

45. Yates CR, Krynetski EY, Loennechen T, Fessing MY, Tai HL, Pui CH, et al. Molecular diagnosis of thiopurine S-methyltransferase deficiency: genetic basis for azathioprine and mercaptopurine intolerance. Ann Intern Med 1997;126:608–14.

46. Black AJ, McLeod HL, Capell HA, Powrie RH, Matowe LK, Pritchard SC, et al. Thiopurine methyltransferase genotype predicts therapy-limiting severe toxicity from azothioprine. Ann Intern Med 1998;129:716–18.

47. Weinshilboum RM, Sladek SL. Mercaptopurine pharmacogenetics: monogenic inheritance of erythrocyte thiopurine methyltransferase activity. Am J Hum Genet 1980;32:651–62.

48. Agundez JAG, Olivera M, Martinez C, Ladero JM, Benitez J. Identification and prevalence study of 17 allelic variants of the human NAT2 gene in a white population. Pharmacogenetics 1996;6:423–8.

49. Lin HJ, Han CY, Lin BK, Hardy S. Ethnic distribution of slow acetylator mutations in the polymorphic N-acetyltransferase (NAT2) gene. Pharmacogenetics 1994;4:125–34.

50. Lin HJ, Han CY, Lin BK, Hardy S. Slow acetylator mutations in the human polymorphic N-acetyltransferase gene in 786 Asians, Blacks, Hispanics, and Whites: Application to metabolic epidemiology. Am J Hum Genet 1993;52:827–34.

51. Woosley RL, Drayer DE, Reidenberg MM, Nies AS, Carr K, Oates JA. Effect of acetylator phenotype on the rate at which procainamide induces antinuclear antibodies and the lupus syndrome. N Engl J Med 1978;298:1157–9.

52. Kosowsky BD, Taylor J, Lown B, Ritchie RF. Long-term use of procaine amide following acute myocardial infarction. Circulation 1973;47:1204–10.

53. Lee EJ, Zhao B, Seow-Choen F. Relationship between polymorphism of N-acetyltransferase gene and susceptibility to colorectal carcinoma in a Chinese population. Pharmacogenetics 1998;8:513–17.

54. Ambrosone CB, Freudenheim JL, Graham S, Marshall JR, Vena JE, Brasure JR, et al. Cigarette smoking, N-acetyltransferase 2 genetic polymorphisms, and breast cancer risk. JAMA 1996;276:1494–501.

55. Reihsaus E, Innis M, MacIntyre N, Liggett SB. Mutations in the gene encoding for the beta2-adrenergic receptor in normal and asthmatic subjects. Am J Respir Cell Mol Bio 1993;8:334–9.

56. Liggett SB. Polymorphisms of the beta2-adrenergic receptor and asthma. Am J Respir Crit Care Med 1997;156:S156–62.

57. Lima JJ, Thomason DB, Mohamed MH, Eberle LV, Self TH, Johnson JA. Impact of genetic polymorphisms of the beta2-adrenergic receptor on albuterol bronchodilator pharmacodynamics. Clin Pharmacol Ther 1999;65:519–25.

58. Weir TD, Mallek N, Sandford AJ, Bai TR, Awadh N, Fitzgerald JM, et al. beta2-Adrenergic receptor haplotypes in mild, moderate and fatal/near fatal asthma. Am J Respir Crit Care Med 1998;158:787–91.

59. Preuss CV, Wood TC, Szumlanski CL, Raftogianis RB, Otterness DM, Girard B, et al. Human histamine N-methyltransferase pharmacogenetics: common genetic polymorphisms that alter activity. Mol Pharmacol 1998;53:708–17.

60. Hibi K, Ishigami T, Tamura K, Mizushima S, Nyui N, Fujita T, et al. Endothelial nitric oxide synthase gene polymorphism and acute myocardial infarction. Hypertension 1998;32:521–6.

61. Abernethy DR, Babaoglu MO. Polymorphic variant of endothelial nitric oxide synthase (eNOS) markedly impairs endothelium-dependent vascular relaxation [abstract]. Clin Pharmacol Ther 2000;67:141.

14

Drug Interactions

CARA L. ALFARO AND STEPHEN C. PISCITELLI

Clinical Center, National Institutes of Health, Bethesda, Maryland

INTRODUCTION

Pharmacologists have been studying, interpreting, and managing the interactions of drugs since concomitant medicines have been administered to patients. Literature reports of interactions have been documented as far back as 1879 when Index Medicus was first cataloged (1). Currently, thousands of drug interactions are studied each year, contributing to an enormous knowledge base that describes both simple and complex alterations that occur when drugs are used in combinations.

A *drug interaction* is defined as the pharmacologic or clinical response to the administration of a drug combination different from that anticipated from the known effects of the two agents when given alone (2). It should be noted that the term "drug interaction" usually has a negative connotation. Although drug interactions may lead to a loss of therapeutic effect or toxicity, they may also benefit the patient. The use of certain drugs in combination can lead to improved outcomes or improve a drug regimen's convenience, reduce costs, or improve the side effect profile. For example, the concomitant use of probenecid and ampicillin has been used for years to achieve high and prolonged concentrations of the antibiotic (3).

In addition to drug–drug interactions, a variety of other substances can alter the pharmacokinetics and/or effect of drugs. These include foods, nutritional supplements, cytokines, formulation excipients, and environmental factors (e.g., cigarette smoke). All these factors require consideration in the evaluation of a patient with a suspected drug interaction.

The assessment of drug interactions remains an integral component of patient management. This is especially true in elderly patients who often have various chronic diseases for which they receive multiple medications. Patients who receive their care from more than one provider and their medications from more than one pharmacy are also prone to interactions. In addition, drug interactions are common in disease states for which multidrug therapy is the standard of care, such as tuberculosis, HIV infection, and cancer. It is not uncommon for HIV-infected patients to be receiving 8 to 10 different medications, with each having its own food restrictions, dose-spacing requirements, and complex interaction profile.

In this chapter, drug interactions will be described on the basis of major mechanisms. *Pharmacokinetic interactions* are those in which the concentrations of one or more drugs may be altered by another. These interactions may occur by changes in absorption, distribution, metabolism, or excretion. However, it is important to note that multiple mechanisms may co-exist. For example, co-administration of quinidine and digoxin leads to increased digoxin levels by reducing the renal and biliary clearance of digoxin, decreasing its volume of distribution, and perhaps modulating transport proteins (4). *Pharmacodynamic interactions* refer to additive, synergistic, or antagonistic effects resulting from co-administration of two or more drugs. The synergistic actions of certain antibiotics have long been a mainstay of therapy against organisms that are difficult to eradicate such as *Pseudomonas aeruginosa* or *Mycobacterium tuberculosis*. Drugs with overlapping toxicities, such as ethanol and benzodiazepines, could lead to more serious adverse effects than when either is given alone. An understanding of interaction mechanisms is needed to optimize drug therapy.

Epidemiology

The incidence of drug interactions varies widely in the literature ranging from 2.2 to 70.3% (5–12). The incidence is increased in the elderly, especially in those patients who are confined to nursing homes. Patients with multiple organ dysfunction and those receiving polypharmacy are also at an increased risk. Recent data on HIV-infected patients estimate that drug interactions occur in up to 77% of patients receiving protease inhibitors (13). The clinical consequences of these interactions have not been well described. One study of hospitalized patients reported that the incidence of symptoms due to a drug interaction was only between 0 and 1% (11). However, many serious drug interactions have been described. In some cases, such as interactions of terfenadine or cisapride with azole antifungals, interactions may result in death (14, 15). Terfenadine, astemizole, and cisapride have been removed from the U.S. market in recent years solely because of the life-threatening potential of interactions with these drugs.

Classifications

Drug interactions can be classified based on their severity and on the probability that the interaction exists. Severity is usually classified as minor, moderate, or severe. *Minor drug interactions* usually have limited clinical consequences and require no change in therapy. For example, acetaminophen may reduce the effects of furosemide. However, this interaction is unlikely to cause any clinical effects or warrant a change in dose (16). A *moderate interaction* would be the increased incidence in hepatitis resulting from combined therapy with rifampin and isoniazid. Although the increased toxicity of this combination is clearly known, it would still be used along with frequent monitoring of liver enzymes. A *severe drug interaction* would involve potentially serious toxicity and require a change in dose, drug, or dosing schedule. The classic example of a severe interaction that is discussed in Chapter 1 is the life-threatening cardiac arrhythmia that may occur when terfenadine is combined with

ketoconazole (14). Severe interactions require the discontinuation of one of the co-administered agents.

The likelihood that an interaction is caused by a drug is usually classified as established, probable, suspected, possible, or unlikely. This is determined by documentation of similar interactions in published clinical and *in vitro* studies, case reports, pre-clinical studies, and anecdotes. Interactions may further be classified on the basis of the time course of the interaction. Certain interactions occur immediately with concomitant administration such as the chelation of fluoroquinolone antibiotics and antacids, which results in an immediate decrease in fluoroquinolone absorption. Other interactions require several hours or days to develop such as the reduction in the effects of warfarin by co-administration of vitamin K.

MECHANISMS OF DRUG INTERACTIONS

Interactions Affecting Drug Absorption

Interactions that affect drug absorption can be dramatic. A number of mechanisms can affect drug absorption including a change in gastric pH, chelation, ion exchange, change in gastric motility, alteration in gut flora, modulation of transport proteins, or inhibition of intestinal enzymes.

Certain drugs, such as ketoconazole and itraconazole, require an acidic gastric pH for optimal dissolution so they can be absorbed in the small intestine. The addition of agents, such as proton pump inhibitors, H_2 receptor antagonists, and antacids, that raise the gastric pH will markedly reduce the absorption and plasma concentrations of these antifungal drugs (17, 18). For example, the combination of ranitidine and ketoconazole led to a reduction in the area under the plasma level-vs.-time curve (AUC) of ketoconazole by over 50% (17). Decreases in ketoconazole absorption by pH-raising agents have led to therapeutic failure (19). In these situations, fluconazole can be used as an alternative since its absorption is not pH-dependent (20).

Chelation is the irreversible binding of drugs in the gastrointestinal tract. Tetracyclines have long been reported to bind with antacids, leading to inactivation of these antibiotics (21). Quinolone antibiotics also chelate with di- and tri-valent cations such as the aluminum or magnesium in antacids, calcium in dairy products, and ferrous sulfate in iron replacement agents (22). In general, these interactions reduce the AUC of the quinolone by over 75%. Although these interactions are clearly clinically relevant, they are also easy to avoid by administering the antibiotic two hours before the antacid is given. A change in dose or drug is unnecessary. Chelation interactions represent a severe interaction in which a simple change in dose scheduling is all that is required to avoid the loss of antibiotic activity.

A large number of drugs have been reported to interact with the anionic exchange resins such as cholestyramine (23). These exchange resins form insoluble complexes with warfarin, digoxin, beta-blockers, nonsteroidal anti-inflammatory drugs, and other drugs, thereby decreasing their absorption and leading to low plasma concentrations. A separation between doses is often the only intervention required. However, exchange resins need to be administered frequently during the day and staggered dosing may be very inconvenient for the patient.

As discussed in Chapter 4, enteric bacteria can metabolize digoxin within the intestine and reduce its bioavailability. Conversely, administration of antibiotics that alter gut flora has been reported to increase digoxin absorption in some patients (24). Antibiotics may also inhibit the growth of gut flora that hydrolyze steroid conjugates. This inhibition decreases enterohepatic recirculation of oral contraceptives and may lower their plasma concentration. Although reports of unplanned pregnancies have been attributed to this interaction, several other clinical studies have found that contraceptive blood concentrations are unchanged by concomitant antibiotic therapy (25, 26).

Interactions Affecting Protein Binding

The extent to which protein binding displacement interactions result in clinically significant drug interactions has been largely overstated (27). Very few drug interactions have been identified based on this mechanism, and many that were previously thought to be protein-binding interactions have been identified as being metabolically based. The extent and significance of protein binding displacement interactions are to some extent dependent on whether the displaced drug is restrictively or nonrestrictively eliminated (see Chapters 5 and 7).

Restrictively Metabolized Drugs

For restrictively metabolized drugs, only unbound drug in plasma can be cleared. An increase in the unbound fraction in plasma will result in a proportional increase in total (bound + unbound) drug elimination clearance and a decrease in total drug concentration in plasma. An increase in the unbound concentration of drug in plasma occurs immediately after addition of the displacing drug. However, as shown in Figure 7.2, it will gradually return to pre-displacement concentrations as long as intrinsic clearance remains unchanged (27–29). For most drugs, this transient increase in unbound concentration will not be clinically significant. However, this transient increase may be clinically significant for drugs with a small volume of distribution, a long elimination half-life, and a narrow therapeutic index. A clinically significant interaction that occurs solely by plasma protein displacement is the displacement of warfarin from serum albumin by a metabolite of chloral hydrate (trichloroacetic acid), which transiently increases the unbound concentration of warfarin (29).

Nonrestrictively Metabolized Drugs

For nonrestrictively metabolized drugs, elimination clearance is dependent on hepatic blood flow and increases in unbound drug concentrations in plasma will not lead to an increase in clearance. Therefore, in contrast to the situation with restrictively metabolized drugs, an increase in the unbound fraction will lead to an immediate and sustained increase in unbound concentration (27, 29). However, no examples of clinically significant plasma protein displacement interactions involving nonrestrictively metabolized drugs have been identified (29, 30). Some reasons for the lack of clinically significant interactions are that many nonrestrictively cleared drugs have a relatively wide therapeutic index and the relationships between drug concentration and response are not well defined (30).

Interactions Affecting Drug Metabolism

As described in Chapter 11, most drugs undergo biotransformation via Phase I and/or Phase II metabolic reactions in the liver. Many Phase I reactions, such as dealkylation, deamination, and hydroxylation, involve the cytochrome P-450 (CYP450) monooxygenases. Research on CYP450 isoenzymes has grown exponentially in the past decade. Advances in the application of scientific methods to identify the amino acid sequences of specific CYP450 isoenzymes has furthered research in this area as well as the identification of specific genetic polymorphisms for these isoenzymes (see Chapter 13). Additionally, the ability to fully characterize the CYP450 metabolism of drugs and their interaction with CYP450 isoenzymes, largely through in vitro methods using drug probes and cDNA expressed isoenzymes in human liver microsomes, has furthered understanding of this area of drug metabolism.

Phase II conjugation reactions, such as glucuronidation and sulfation, involve the microsomal uridine diphosphate (UDP) glucuronosyltransferases and the cytosolic sulfotransferases, respectively. Although drug interactions involving Phase II enzymes can occur, much less research has been completed in this area. Therefore, this chapter will focus on drug metabolism interactions involving the CYP450 enzyme system. Thus far, 14 families of CYP450 enzymes common to all mammals have been identified (31). However, only three of these families (CYP1, CYP2, and CYP3) are thought to be important in the metabolism of drugs. Isoenzymes within these families that have been identified as important in drug metabolism include CYP1A2, CYP2B6, CYP2C9, CYP2C19, CYP2D6, CYP2E1, and CYP3A4. Of these isoenzymes, CYP3A4 is the most abundant, constituting 25% of total hepatic CYP450 (32). This isoenzyme is responsible for the metabolism of a vast array of structurally diverse drugs and, coupled with its expression in gut wall, may be responsible for the metabolism of the majority of xenobiotics.

Table 14.1 lists drugs as substrates, inhibitors, and/or inducers of various isoenzymes. Although this table can be used as a basic guide to predict drug–drug interactions involving CYP450 isoenzymes, many variables are not included that would assist in interpreting the clinical significance of these interactions (e.g., potency of inhibition). In simplistic terms, a drug that is a substrate for an isoenzyme may be considered an inhibitor of that isoenzyme, although the potency of the inhibition will depend on many factors. However, the converse is not necessarily true. Quinidine, for example, is the most potent inhibitor thus far identified for CYP2D6, but it is metabolized by CYP3A4 (33).

Until recently, the pathways of drug metabolism and the inhibiting or inducing effects of drugs on various CYP450 isoenzymes were not fully determined. However, a new emphasis on characterizing the metabolism of drugs and their effects on CYP450 isoenzymes occurred secondary to identification of the potentially fatal metabolic drug interaction between terfenadine, a prodrug that is metabolized by CYP3A4 to an active metabolite, and ketoconazole and macrolide antibiotics that inhibit the activity of CYP3A4 (see Chapter 1) (14, 34). Due to the life-threatening risk of *torsades de pointes* when terfenadine is used with CYP3A4 inhibiting drugs and the non-life-threatening indications for which this drug was developed, it was deemed that the risk/benefit ratio did not merit its continued availability. Therefore, this drug is no longer marketed in the United States.

As a result of this experience, the Food and Drug Administration now requires characterization of the metabolic pathways of a new drug and its inducing and inhibiting effect on specific isoenzymes (35). In addition, pharmaceutical companies are beginning to base product development decisions on the information generated from these studies. For example, knowledge of the drug interaction involving terfenadine led to the development of the active metabolite, fexofenadine, which is a nonsedating antihistamine without QT-interval prolonging effects. Norastemizole and (+) norcisapride are also being evaluated as improved chemical entities that are thought not to have the QT-interval prolonging properties of their respective parent compounds (36). However, the overall benefit of a specific drug is another factor that must be considered in making risk/benefit decisions. For example, the protease inhibitors are potent inhibitors of CYP3A4 but, in the absence of other more effective therapies, their utility in treating HIV warrants their continued availability. Conversely, the calcium channel blocker mibefradil was withdrawn from the U.S. market because of its potent CYP3A4 inhibitory effects and the availability of equally effective therapeutic alternatives.

Inhibition of CYP450 Enzymes

Inhibition can be characterized as reversible, quasi-irreversible, and irreversible (32, 37). The type of inhibition most commonly involved in drug interactions is reversible upon discontinuation of the inhibitor, and isoenzyme function is regained generally over one elimination half-life of the inhibitor. Distinguishing between quasi-irreversible and irreversible inhibition from a clinical standpoint is less important since the differentiation is the reversibility of the inhibition in an *in vitro* environment. The mechanism of both of these irreversible inhibitions involves formation of a stable complex with the inhibitor and the prosthetic heme group of CYP450 such that the CYP450 is sequestered in a functionally inactive state. Enzyme activity can only be restored by generating new CYP450. Examples of inhibitors that form complexes with CYP450 enzymes include the macrolide antibiotics, erythromycin and troleandomycin.

Reversible inhibition can be described as having a competitive, noncompetitive, or uncompetitive mechanism. *Competitive inhibition*, the most common type implicated in drug–drug interactions, occurs when the inhibitor binds to the active site of the free enzyme, thus preventing substrate binding. The onset and time course of competitive inhibition follow the half-life and time to steady state of the inhibitor drug. The time to maximal drug interaction will also depend on the time required for the substrate to reach a new steady state. For *noncompetitive inhibition*, substrate binds to one site on the enzyme while the inhibitor binds to another site, thereby making the enzyme-substrate-inhibitor complex nonfunctional. *Uncompetitive inhibi-*

TABLE 14.1 Selected CYP450 Substrates, Inhibitors and, Inducers (Adapted from 68, 69)

Substrates

CYP1A2	CYP2B6	CYP2C9 (polymorphic)	CYP2C19 (polymorphic)	CYP2D6 (polymorphic)	CYP2E1	CYP3A4		
Amitriptyline	Amitriptyline	Amitriptyline	Amitriptyline	Bufuralol	Acetaminophen	Alfentanyl	Erythromycin	Progesterone
Caffeine	Bupropion	Celecoxib	Citalopram	Codeine	Chlorzoxazone	Alprazolam	Estradiol	Quetiapine
Clomipramine	Cyclophosphamide	Fluoxetine	Clomipramine	Desipramine	Enflurane	Astemizole	Felodipine	Quinidine
Clozapine	Diazepam	Fluvastatin	Cyclophosphamide	Dexfenfluramine	Ethanol	Atorvastatin	Fentanyl	Ritonavir
Cyclobenzaprine	Lidocaine	Diclofenac	Imipramine	Dextromethorphan	Halothane	Buspirone	Finasteride	Salmeterol
Estradiol	Midazolam	Fluoxetine	Indomethacin	Donepezil	Isoflurane	Caffeine	Haloperidol	Saquinavir
Fluvoxamine	Nevirapine	Glipizide	Lansoprazole	Encainide	Methoxyflurane	Carbamazepine	Hydrocortisone	Sertraline
Imipramine	Procainamide	Ibuprofen	Nelfinavir	Fluoxetine	Sevoflurane	Cerivastatin	Indinavir	Sildenafil
Melatonin	Promethazine	Irbesartan	Nilutamide	Fluvoxamine	Theophylline	Chlorpheniramine	Lidocaine	Simvastatin
Mexiletine	Tamoxifen	Losartan	Omeprazole	Haloperidol		Cisapride[a]	Loratadine	Tacrolimus
Olanzapine	Temazepam	Phenytoin	Pantoprazole	Lidocaine		Citalopram	Lovastatin	Tamoxifen
Propranolol	Testosterone	Piroxicam	Phenytoin	Mexiletine		Clarithromycin	Methadone	Taxol
Riluzole	Valproic acid	Sertraline	Progesterone	Nortriptyline		Clozapine	Midazolam	Testosterone
Ropivacaine	Verapamil	Sulfamethoxazole	Propranolol	Ondansetron		Codeine	Nefazodone	Terfenadine[a]
Tacrine		Suprofen	Teniposide	Propranolol		Cyclosporine	Nelfinavir	Trazodone
Theophylline		Tamoxifen	R-warfarin	Risperidone		Dapsone	Nifedipine	Triazolam
Verapamil		Tolbutamide		Tamoxifen		Dextromethorphan	Nisoldipine	Verapamil
R-warfarin		Torsemide		Thioridazine		Diazepam	Nitrendipine	Vincristine
Zileuton		S-warfarin		Tramadol		Diltiazem	Ondansetron	Zaleplon
Zolmitriptan				Venlafaxine			Pimozide	Zolpidem

(continued)

171

TABLE 14.1 Continued

Inhibitors

CYP1A2	CYP2B6	CYP2C9 (polymorphic)	CYP2C19 (polymorphic)	CYP2D6 (polymorphic)	CYP2E1	CYP3A4
Amiodarone	Amiodarone	Amiodarone	Cimetidine	Amiodarone	Disulfiram	Amiodarone
Cimetidine	Ketoconazole	Fluconazole	Felbamate	Celecoxib		Cimetidine
Ciprofloxacin	Orphenadrine	Fluoxetine	Fluoxetine	Chlorpheniramine		Ciprofloxacin
Enoxacin	Tranylcypromine	Fluvastatin	Fluvoxamine	Cimetidine		Clarithromycin
Fluvoxamine	Troglitazone	Fluvoxamine	Indomethacin	Clomipramine		Delaviridine
Furafylline	Troleandomycin	Isoniazid	Ketoconazole	Fluoxetine		Diltiazem
Methoxsalen		Lovastatin	Lansoprazole	Methadone		Erythromycin
Mibefradil[a]		Paroxetine	Modafinil	Mibefradil[a]		Fluconazole
Norfloxacin		Phenylbutazone	Omeprazole	Paroxetine		Fluoxetine
Ticlopidine		Sertraline	Oxcarbazepine	Quinidine		Fluvoxamine
		Teniposide	Paroxetine	Ritonavir		Gestodene
		Zafirlukast	Ticlopidine	Terbinafine		Grapefruit juice
			Topiramate			Indinavir
						Itraconazole
						Ketoconazole
						Mibefradil[a]
						Mifepristone
						Nefazodone
						Nelfinavir
						Norfloxacin
						Ritonavir
						Saquinavir
						Troleandomycin

Inducers

CYP1A2	CYP2B6	CYP2C9 (polymorphic)	CYP2C19 (polymorphic)	CYP2D6 (polymorphic)	CYP2E1	CYP3A4
Cruciferous vegetables	Dexamethasone	Rifampin	Norethindrone	None identified	Ethanol	Barbiturates
Char-grilled meat	Phenobarbital	Secobarbital	Prednisone		Isoniazid	Carbamazepine
Insulin	Rifampin		Rifampin			Efavirenz
Omeprazole	Sodium valproate					Glucocorticoids
Tobacco						Modafinil
						Nevirapine
						Oxcarbazepine
						Phenobarbital
						Phenytoin
						Rifampin
						St. John's wort
						Troglitazone

[a] Withdrawn from U.S. market.

172

tion occurs when the inhibitor binds to the enzyme-substrate complex, rendering it nonfunctional. These inhibition mechanisms have different kinetics that can be described by the following equations:

Competitive inhibition:

$$\% \text{ inhibition} = \frac{\dfrac{[I]}{K_i}}{1 + \dfrac{[I]}{K_i} + \dfrac{[S]}{K_m}}$$

Noncompetitive inhibition:

$$\% \text{ inhibition} = \frac{\dfrac{[I]}{K_i}}{1 + \dfrac{[I]}{K_i}}$$

Uncompetitive inhibition:

$$\% \text{ inhibition} = \frac{\dfrac{[I]}{K_i}}{1 + \dfrac{[I]}{K_i} + \dfrac{K_m}{[S]}}$$

Where $[I]$ is the concentration of the inhibitor, $[S]$ is the concentration of the substrate, K_i is the inhibition constant of the inhibitor, and K_m is the Michaelis–Menten constant of the enzyme metabolizing the substrate.

Although inhibition of CYP450 enzymes leads to increased concentrations of the substrate drug, the following questions need to be considered to assess the clinical relevance of these interactions.

1. *What is the toxic potential and therapeutic index of the substrate?* When evaluating the clinical relevance of a drug interaction, it is important to consider the therapeutic index of the substrate drug. For example, inhibition of terfenadine metabolism may result in QT prolongation and *torsades de pointes* while inhibition of sertraline metabolism is not associated with such serious cardiovascular sequelae. However, it should be kept in mind that inhibition of sertraline metabolism could lead to an increased incidence of other side effects.

2. *What are the other pathways involved in the metabolism of the substrate?* If the substrate drug is metabolized by multiple CYP450 pathways and is combined with an inhibitor that is specific for one pathway, the drug will be less affected than if it is only metabolized by the inhibited pathway. For example, *in vitro* studies have estimated that zolpidem is metabolized by CYP3A4 (61%), CYP2C9 (22%), CYP1A2 (14%), CYP2D6 (<3%), and CYP2C19 (<3%), whereas triazolam is almost exclusively metabolized by CYP3A4 (38,

39). Addition of ketoconazole to zolpidem will increase zolpidem AUC by 67% compared to a 1200% increase in triazolam AUC (40, 41).

3. *What is the role of active metabolites of the substrate?* If active metabolites are required for therapeutic efficacy, an inhibitor may decrease formation of the metabolites with resultant loss of therapeutic efficacy. As discussed in Chapter 13, codeine is metabolized to its active analgesic metabolite, morphine, via CYP2D6. Inhibition of this isoenzyme is likely to reduce the analgesic effect of codeine and codeine derivatives (42).

4. *What are the consequences of metabolic inhibition of metabolites?* For many metabolites, especially ones that are devoid of desired pharmacologic effects, the metabolic pathways may not be well understood. However, one should be aware of possible clinical consequences of this type of inhibition. For example, nefazodone is a CYP3A4 substrate while one of its main metabolites, meta-chlorophenylpiperazine (mCPP) is a substrate of CYP2D6. Inhibition of CYP2D6 will result in increases in mCPP concentration and side effects such as anxiety (43).

5. *Does the inhibitor inhibit multiple CYP450 isoenzymes?* One should consider if the inhibitor inhibits multiple CYP450 isoenzymes. Drugs that inhibit multiple pathways will be more likely to inhibit the metabolism of drugs that are metabolized by multiple pathways. For example, cimetidine is a well-known inhibitor of multiple CYP450 isoenzymes.

6. *Is the patient a poor metabolizer of an isoenzyme for which the inhibitor is specific?* At the current time, patients are not generally genotyped or phenotyped for polymorphic CYP450 isoenzymes (CYP2C9, CYP2C19, and CYP2D6). However, if a patient is a poor metabolizer of a specific isoenzyme, addition of an inhibitor will not affect the metabolism of the substrate drug because the isoenzyme already contributes relatively little to that drug's metabolism. For example, a CYP2D6 poor metabolizer receiving desipramine (a CYP2D6 substrate) would not be expected to exhibit elevated desipramine concentrations with co-administration of a specific CYP2D6 inhibitor (42, 44). However, the therapeutically effective dose of desipramine for this individual would be lower than a standard dose due to the absence of functional CYP2D6 and the lack of full metabolic compensation by other CYP isoenzymes.

7. *Do otherwise pharmacologically inert metabolites of the inhibitor inhibit CYP450 isoenzymes?* In most cases, this information will not be known. However, otherwise inert drug metabolites can affect the activity of CYP450 isoenzymes. Paroxetine is a well-documented potent CYP2D6 inhibitor, and it appears that one of its glucuronidated metabolites (M-II) also contributes to this inhibition (45).

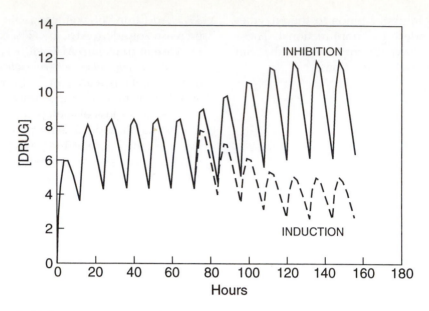

FIGURE 14.1 Theoretical plasma concentration–time profiles of a drug in the presence of a CYP enzyme inducer *(broken line)* and inhibitor *(solid line)*

8. *Is the inhibition potentially harmful or helpful?* Although one usually considers inhibition of drug metabolism as potentially harmful, these interactions can be exploited to enhance therapeutic effect. Combinations of ketoconazole and cyclosporine have been used as a way to save drug costs and doses of this expensive immunosuppressant (46). Ritonavir, an inhibitor of CYP3A4, also increases the bioavailability of saquinavir by 20-fold, allowing for a reduced saquinavir dosage and a lower pill burden (47).

Induction of CYP450

The net effect of induction is increased DNA transcription and synthesis of CYP450 enzymes. With the exception of CYP2D6, all of the CYP450 isoenzymes are inducible. The time course of induction depends on the elimination half-life of the inducer as well as the time required for enzyme degradation and new enzyme production (48). As with CYP450 inhibition, there are multiple clinical consequences of CYP450 induction. Addition of an inducer will decrease the substrate concentration and therapeutic failure may result. (Figure 14.1). Similarly, discontinuation of an inducer will increase the substrate concentration in a time-dependent fashion, and toxicity may result. CYP450 inducers may also accelerate formation of reactive metabolites which may be harmful. For example, alcohol induces CYP2E1 with a resultant increase in formation of acetaminophen toxic metabolites, thus predisposing patients to hepatotoxicity. At the current time, at least five mechanisms of enzyme induction have been identified: induction by the aryl hydrocarbon receptor, ethanol, peroxisome proliferators, the constitutive androstane receptor (CAR), and the pregnane X receptor (PXR) (49). Two additional nuclear receptors, liver X receptors and farnesoid X receptors, may also be involved in enzyme induction (48, 50).

The CAR and PXR orphan nuclear receptors are primarily affected by drugs and there appears to be considerable overlap of drugs affecting these receptors (48). Induction involving PXR is most pronounced on CYP3A4, while induction involving the CAR receptor is most pronounced on CYP2B6. The orphan nuclear receptor, CAR, appears to be the target of phenobarbital-type induction (48). Data regarding specific isoenzymes linked to CAR-mediated induction come largely from drug interaction studies with phenobarbital-type inducers. The most pronounced inductive effect involves CYP2B6 with some effects also noted for CYP2C9, CYP3A4, CYP1A2, and some UDP-glucuronosyltransferases. Induction involving PXR was formerly termed rifampicin/glucocorticoid-type induction. It has recently been determined that the human PXR (hPXR) binds to the rifampicin/dexamethasone response element in the CYP3A4 promotor region as a heterodimer with the 9-cis-retinoic acid receptor (RXR). The hPXR/RXR complex is activated by a number of drugs, including rifampin, dexamethasone, phenobarbital, clotrimazole, and spironolactone, which have been shown to modulate *CYP3A4* expression. Additionally, the CYP3A4-inducing herbal preparation, St. John's wort, has been shown to activate PXR (51). The identification of this receptor is important in that PXR binding and activation assays can be used to predict which com-

TABLE 14.2   P-glycoprotein Substrates and Inhibitors (53, 70, 71)

Substrates		Inhibitors	
Actinomycin	Mitoxantrone	Amiodarone	Mefloquine
Amprenavir	Morphine	Bepridil	Nicardipine
Colchicine	Nelfinavir	Cefoperazone	Nifedipine
Cortisol	Nicardipine	Ceftriaxone	Nitrendipine
Cyclosporine	Nifedipine	Clarithromycin	Progesterone
Daunorubicin	Paclitaxel	Cortisol	Propranolol
Dexamethasone	Progesterone	Cyclosporine	Quercetin
Digoxin	Rifampin	Diltiazem	Quinine
Diltiazem	Ritonavir	Dipyridamole	Quinidine
Docetaxel	Saquinavir	Erythromycin	Reserpine
Doxorubicin	Tacrolimus	Felodipine	Tacrolimus
Erythromycin	Taxol	Fluphenazine	Tamoxifen
Etoposide	Teniposide	Hydrocortisone	Terfenadine[a]
Fexofenadine	Terfenadine[a]	Itraconazole	Testosterone
Hydrocortisone	Topotecan	Ketoconazole	Trifluoperazine
Indinavir	Verapamil	Lidocaine	Verapamil
Ivermectin	Vinblastine		
Loperamide	Vincristine		
Mitomycin C			

[a] Withdrawn from U.S. market.

pounds are likely to induce CYP3A4 rather than relying on *in vitro* assay methodology using human liver slices.

Induction of P-glycoprotein and Intestinal CYP450

As discussed in Chapter 4, CYP450 is expressed in large concentrations on the intestinal epithelium and can be involved in presystemic drug metabolism. Levels of CYP450 in the gut wall are generally 20 to 50% of those in the liver, but there is considerable variability (52). Substances that inhibit gastrointestinal CYP3A4 can markedly increase the bioavailability of CYP3A4 substrates. The enterocytes in the intestinal mucosa are also a site of expression of transporter proteins that also play a critical role in drug metabolism and disposition (see Chapter 16). Many drug transporters have thus far been identified including organic anion-transporting polypeptide (OATP), organic cation transporters (OCTs), and P-glycoprotein (P-gp). Although all these transporters are likely important in drug disposition, P-gp has been the most studied of the drug transporters.

P-gp is the product of the human multidrug resistance gene (*mdr1*) that has been recognized as a contributor to resistance for a variety of chemotherapeutic agents by decreasing the intracellular accumulation of anticancer drugs (53). P-gp is an efflux transporter present in the gastrointestinal epithelium, liver, kidney, and endothelial cells making up the blood-brain barrier. This transporter is thought to be important in the absorption, distribution, and elimination of many drugs. P-gp restricts drug entry into and through the intestinal epithelium by transporting drugs back into the intestinal lumen, thereby decreasing drug bioavailability. Because P-gp transports drugs back into the lumen, it may also increase their exposure time to CYP3A4 present in the gut wall. Thus, intestinal expression of CYP3A4 and P-gp may serve complementary roles in limiting drug absorption.

In addition to tissue distribution, there appears to be a significant overlap with regard to CYP3A4 substrates and inhibitors and P-gp substrates and inhibitors (Tables 14.1 and 14.2). This overlap obscures the specific contribution of inhibition of CYP3A4 and modulation of P-gp function to gastrointestinal site interactions. One exception is the P-gp substrate digoxin, a metabolite of the CYP3A4 substrate digitoxin, but not itself a substrate of this isoenzyme. However, not all drugs listed as CYP3A4 substrates or inhibitors have been evaluated with regard to their role as substrates or inhibitors of P-gp. In addition, drugs that inhibit both CYP3A4 and P-gp may have very different inhibitory potencies—that is, a drug may be more selective for P-gp inhibition compared to CYP3A4 inhibition (54).

Some substances, such as grapefruit juice, affect CYP3A4 only in the gut wall and not the liver. Grapefruit juice contains various flavinoids that have been well documented to be inhibitors of gastrointestinal CYP3A4. Large increases in bioavailability have been reported when grapefruit juice has been administered concomitantly with drugs that have extensive intestinal wall metabolism (55, 56). For example, saquinavir exposure increases by 50 to 200% when co-administered with grapefruit juice (57). Other drugs noted to have increased bioavailability with grapefruit juice include beta-blockers, calcium channel blockers, benzodiazepines, and HMG CoA-reductase inhibitors (55).

Grapefruit juice also appears to have inhibitory effects on P-gp-mediated enterocyte transport. For example, P-gp inhibition may mediate the large increase in cyclosporine bioavailability that occurs when this drug is co-administered with grapefruit juice. However, P-gp and CYP3A4 may have opposing effects. Co-administration of the protease inhibitor indinavir and grapefruit juice leads to either a decrease in indinavir levels or no effect, suggesting that activation of P-gp may negate any increased bioavailability from CYP3A4 inhibition (57, 58). Regardless, inhibition of CY3PA4 or modulation of P-gp in the gut wall can have a major impact on drug absorption and drug interactions. Since grapefruit juice is a natural product, there is wide variability that makes these interactions very unpredictable in individual patients. The severity of the interaction may depend on how much and how often the grapefruit juice was consumed, the timing of the grapefruit juice and the medication dose, the specific brand of juice, and whether it was double or single strength.

The use of P-gp inhibitors to increase intracellular concentrations of chemotherapeutic agents in tumor cells is being evaluated in patients with multidrug resistant tumors. Such compounds also may be very useful to target drug delivery to the central nervous system. Studies in *mdr 1* knockout mice have suggested that P-gp inhibition may result in higher cerebrospinal fluid concentrations of P-gp substrates (59). Ketoconazole, an inhibitor of both CYP3A4 and P-gp, was shown to cause a larger increase in CSF levels of saquinavir and ritonavir relative to unbound plasma levels (60). Unfortunately, potent P-gp inhibitors often have limited utility since they have pharmacologic effects that set dose limits below those needed for P-gp inhibition. Currently, specific P-gp inhibitors are being developed that lack undesired pharmacologic effects. However, the strategy of administering a P-gp inhibitor to increase drug exposures must be considered in light of the consequences of inhibiting a drug transporter with wide distribution in the body. General inhibition of P-gp function in various tissues may be met with significant central nervous system and other adverse effects.

PREDICTION AND CLINICAL MANAGEMENT OF DRUG INTERACTIONS

In Vitro Screening Methods

It is impossible to study every possible combination of drugs that may be used clinically. Although nonhuman mammalian species are often used for *in vivo* screens for drug interactions, well-documented differences in enzyme expression and regulation between these species and humans weaken clinical extrapolation of these results. For these reasons, a variety of *in vitro* systems are being relied on to screen for and assess CYP450-mediated drug interactions (61). Microsomes, hepatocytes, liver slices, purified P450 enzymes, and recombinant human P450 enzymes have all been used to assess if a drug candidate will affect concomitantly administered agents. For new drug development, the ability to predict *in vivo* drug interactions from *in vitro* studies has become a useful tool in the decision to develop a drug candidate (62). *In vitro* methods have been shown to predict *in vivo* interactions with some drugs such as paclitaxel (63).

Although these *in vitro* systems can certainly be useful, numerous limitations and caveats warrant consideration. In general, many systems can only evaluate enzyme inhibition, and are not useful to assess induction. Also, *in vitro* results cannot necessarily be extrapolated to clinical studies for drugs with multiple metabolic pathways. *In vitro* studies predicted that methadone concentrations would be markedly increased by concomitant use of ritonavir (64). However, a study in healthy volunteers demonstrated that methadone concentrations actually decreased (65). These discordant results were due to a variety of factors not evaluable *in vitro*, including protein binding, disposition of isomers, and involvement of multiple CYP isoenzymes. Additionally, it is important that concentrations of inhibitors are used for *in vitro* testing that are not several-fold higher than expected *in vivo*. Finally, all *in vitro* screening studies should include positive controls for inhibition (e.g., ketoconazole for CYP3A4, quinidine for CYP2D6) and induction (e.g., rifampin for CYP3A4).

Predicting Drug Interactions in Individual Patients

An understanding of basic interaction mechanisms is essential to identifying and managing drug interactions. Interactions involving drug metabolism are of greatest clinical significance and a working knowledge of the major classes of drugs that affect CYP450 metab-

TABLE 14.3   Drug Interaction Resources

Anderson GD. A mechanistic approach to antiepileptic drug interactions. Ann Pharmacother 1998;32:554–63.

Fugh-Berman A. Herb-drug interactions. Lancet. 2000;355:134–8.

Flockhart D. CYP450 Interaction table. Internet at http://www.georgetown.edu/departments/pharmacology/davetab.html

Hansten PD, Horn JR. Drug interactions analysis and management. St. Louis, MO: Facts and Comparisons; 1999.

Levy RH, Thummel KE, Trager WF, Hansten PD, Eichelbaum M, editors. Metabolic drug interactions. Philadelphia: Lippincott Williams & Wilkins; 2000.

Michalets EL. Update: clinically significant cytochrome P-450 drug interactions. Pharmacotherapy 1998;18:84–112.

Piscitelli SC, Rodvold KA. Drug interactions in infectious diseases. Totowa, NJ: Humana Press; 2000.

Tatro DS. Drug interaction facts. St. Louis, MO: Facts and Comparisons; 2000.

Zucchero FJ, Hogan MJ, Schultz CD. Evaluations of drug interactions, St. Louis, MO: First DataBank; 1999.

olism combined with a review of medication profiles can prevent serious interactions from occurring. However, a variety of additional factors may be responsible for the occurrence and severity of an interaction in an individual patient. Genetics, environmental factors (e.g., cigarette smoke), foods, concomitant diseases, impaired organ function, and age may all play a role in determining if an interaction will occur and what clinical effects will result. These factors make it difficult to predict the magnitude or clinical significance of a drug interaction for an individual patient.

As discussed in Chapter 13, it is possible to genotype individuals to identify mutant genes that cause patients to be poor metabolizers or extensive metabolizers of some drugs. Another approach involves phenotyping patients using various probe drugs for specific CYP450 isoenzymes (44). After patients receive a probe drug that is almost exclusively metabolized by one CYP450 isoenzyme, the effect of a putative inhibitor or inducer can be evaluated by examining the formation of metabolites from the probe drug in the presence of the inhibitor or inducer. Some examples of probe drugs include caffeine (CYP1A2), tolbutamide (CYP2C9), S-mephenytoin (CYP2C19), chlorzoxazone (CYP2E1), debrisoquine (CYP2D6), sparteine (CYP2D6), dextromethorphan (CYP2D6), erythromycin (CYP3A4), and midazolam (CYP3A4). As discussed in Chapter 7, "cocktails" of probe drugs can be given in combination to evaluate various metabolic pathways simultaneously.

After administration of a probe drug, urine or blood is collected for a period of time and the ratio of a metabolite and the parent drug is calculated. These ratios serve as a biomarker of enzyme activity. For drug interaction studies, these tests can be especially useful when performed prior to, and then after administration of a suspected interacting drug. For example, if an investigator wanted to evaluate the effect of fluoxetine on CYP2D6, subjects might be given a dose of dextromethorphan. Urine would be collected and the ratio of metabolite (dextrorphan) to parent drug (dextromethorphan) would be measured. Subjects would then receive either a single dose or steady-state dosing of fluoxetine, after which the dextromethorphan phenotyping would be repeated. The dextromethorphan/dextrorphan ratios before and after fluoxetine would be compared to assess the effect of fluoxetine on CYP2D6 (66). Phenotyping is not widely used in clinical practice due to the need for extensive analytical capability and expert interpretation, and the invasiveness and expense of the procedures. Despite these limitations, phenotyping remains a useful research tool for characterizing the inhibiting or inducing effects of a drug on a specific isoenzyme.

Clinical Approach to Drug Interactions

Some general principles for recognizing and managing drug interactions are:

1. At each outpatient visit or hospital admission, a thorough drug history should be recorded that includes over-the-counter medications, investigational drugs, and alternative therapies.

2. Because patients may often seek treatment from more than one provider, they should be advised to have all their medications dispensed at one pharmacy.

3. Maintain a high index of suspicion for a drug interaction when assessing cases of exaggerated toxicity or treatment failure. Consider concomitant diseases and toxicities of current drugs in the patient's regimen, and use the clinical approach for diagnosing adverse drug reactions that is discussed in Chapter 25. The resources listed in Table 14.3 will be helpful in identifying drug interactions that have been documented previously.

4. If warranted by the clinical circumstances, select drugs with fewer potential interactions. For example, azithromycin is not metabolized by CYP450 and does not possess the inhibition properties associated with other macrolide antibiotics. Similarly, low doses of fluconazole are associated with fewer drug interactions than ketoconazole or itraconazole.

5. Drugs that can be administered once or twice daily may reduce food-related interactions or dosing separation problems.

6. Patient counseling is especially important when proper separation of drug doses is necessary to avoid an interaction (e.g., didanosine and indinavir).

7. The successful management of drug interactions often requires only minimal modifications in dosage or dose scheduling. In some cases, blood level monitoring is available and changes in drug dosing can be guided by pharmacokinetic principles.

8. In some instances pharmacokinetic interactions may be used to simplify complex regimens and reduce pill burden.

Drug interactions remain a major cause of patient morbidity, but can also be used to optimize patient care. The ever-increasing numbers of new agents in development will only make management of medication regimens more complex. An understanding of the basic concepts and mechanisms of drug interactions will be a valuable tool in designing safe and effective multidrug regimens.

Available Resources That List Drug Interactions

It is easy to be overwhelmed by the sheer numbers of documented and theoretical drug interactions. Table 14.3 lists various drug interaction resources. While most adequately describe the mechanism and likely effects, there are inherent limitations. Since textbooks cannot be updated as often as new information becomes available, Internet websites may offer the most up-to-date information. However, sites that do not charge a fee for their use may not be regularly updated and may not have supportive documentation and bibliographies. It is also important to remember that these resources can only provide information. They are no substitute for clinical judgment and common sense.

To facilitate research in the area of drug interactions, the Food and Drug Administration has issued a guidance on conducting drug interaction studies (67). This document is available online and reviews the current state of the art in the design and analysis of such studies.

References

1. Davis WB. A consideration of the alleged antagonism of opium and belladonna. Cincin Lancet & Clinic 1879;ii (n.s.):141–3.
2. Tatro DS. Drug interaction facts. St. Louis, MO: Facts and Comparisons; 2000.
3. Karney WW, Turck M, Holmes KK. Comparative therapeutic and pharmacological evaluation of amoxicillin and ampicillin plus probenecid for the treatment of gonorrhea. Antimicrob Agents Chemother 1974;5:114–8.
4. Fromm MF, Kim RB, Stein CM, Wilkinson GR, Roden DM. Inhibition of P-glycoprotein-mediated drug transport: A unifying mechanism to explain the interaction between digoxin and quinidine. Circulation 1999;99:552–7.
5. Fichtl B, Doering W. The quinidine-digoxin interaction in perspective. Clin Pharmacokinet 1983;8:137–54.
6. Cooper JW, Wellins I, Fish KH, et al. Frequency of potential drug-drug interactions. J Am Pharm Assoc. 1975;15:24–31.
7. Mitchell GW, Stanaszek WF, Nichols NB. Documenting drug-drug interactions in ambulatory patients. Am J Hosp Pharm 1979;36:653–7.
8. Jinks MJ, Hansten PD, Hirschman JL. Drug interaction exposures in an ambulatory Medicaid population. Am J Hosp Pharm 1979;36:923–7.
9. Jankel CA, Fitterman LK. Epidemiology of drug-drug interactions as a cause of hospital admissions. Drug Safety 1993;9:51–9.
10. Gosney M, Tallis R. Prescription of contraindicated and interacting drugs in elderly patients admitted to hospital. Lancet 1984;1:564–7.
11. Puckett WH, Visconti JA. An epidemiologic study of the clinical significance of drug-drug interactions in a private community hospital. Am J Hosp Pharm 1971;28:247–53.
12. Durrence CW, DiPiro JT, May JR, et al. Potential drug interactions in surgical patients. Am J Hosp Pharm 1985;42:1553–6.
13. Van Cleef GF, Fisher EJ, Polk RE. Drug interaction potential with inhibitors of HIV protease. Pharmacotherapy 1997;17:774–8.
14. Honig PK, Wortham DC, Zamani K, et al. Terfenadine-ketoconazole interaction. JAMA 1993;269:1513–8.
15. Pohjola-Sintonen S, Viitasalo M, Toivonen L, Neuvonen P. Torsades de pointes after terfenadine-itraconazole interaction. Br Med J 1993;306:186.
16. Martin U, Prescott LF. The interaction of paracetamol with frusemide. Br J Clin Pharmacol 1994;37:464–7.
17. Piscitelli SC, Goss TF, Wilton JH, D' Andrea DT, Goldstein H, Schentag JJ. Effects of ranitidine and sucralfate on ketoconazole bioavailability. Antimicrob Agents Chemother 1991;35:1765–71.
18. Kanda Y, Kami M, Matsuyama T, Mitani K, Chiba S, Yazaki Y, Hirai H. Plasma concentration of itraconazole in patients receiving chemotherapy for hematological malignancies: The effect of famotidine on the absorption of itraconazole. Hematol Oncol 1998;16:33–7.
19. Van Der Meer JWM, Keuning JJ, Scheijgrond HW, Heykants J, Van Cutsem J, Brugmans J. The influence of gastric acidity on the bioavailability of ketoconazole. J Antimicrob Chemother 1980;6:552–4.
20. Blum RA, D'Andrea DT, Florentino BM, et al. Increased gastric pH and the bioavailability of fluconazole and ketoconazole. Ann Intern Med 1991;114:755–7.
21. D'Arcy PF, McElnay JC. Drug-antacid interactions: assessment of clinical importance. Drug Intell Clin Pharm 1987;21:607–17.
22. Polk RE. Drug-drug interactions with ciprofloxacin and other fluoroquinolones. Am J Med 1989;87(suppl 5A):76S–81S.
23. Farmer JA, Gotto AM Jr. Antihyperlipidaemic agents. Drug interactions of clinical significance. Drug Safety 1994;11:301–9.
24. Midoneck SR, Etingin OR. Clarithromycin-related toxic effects of digoxin. N Engl J Med 1995;333:1505.

25. Weisberg E. Interactions between oral contraceptives and anti-fungals/antibacterials. Is contraceptive failure the result? Clin Pharmacokinet 1999;36:309–13.

26. Weaver K, Glasier A. Interaction between broad-spectrum antibiotics and the combined oral contraceptive pill. A literature review. Contraception 1999;59:71–8.

27. Rolan PE. Plasma protein binding displacement interactions—Why are they still regarded as clinically important? Br J Clin Pharmacol 1994;37:125–8.

28. Sansom LN, Evans AM. What is the true clinical significance of plasma protein binding displacement interactions? Drug Safety 1995;12:227–33.

29. MacKichan JJ. Influence of protein binding and use of unbound (free) drug concentrations. In: Evans WE, Schentag JJ, Jusko WJ, editors. Applied pharmacokinetics: Principles of therapeutic drug monitoring. 3rd ed. Vancouver: Applied Therapeutics; 1992. p. 5-1–48.

30. MacKichan JJ. Protein binding drug displacement interactions: Fact or fiction? Clin Phamacokinet 1989;16:65–73.

31. Nelson DR, Koymans L, Kamataki T, Stegeman JJ, Feyereisen R, Waxman DJ, et al. P450 superfamily: Update on new sequences, gene mapping, accession numbers and nomenclature. Pharmacogenetics 1996;6:1–42.

32. Lin JH, Lu AWH. Inhibition and induction of cytochrome P450 and the clinical implications. Clin Pharmacokinet 1998;35:361–90.

33. Guengerich FP, Muller-Enoch D, Blair IA. Oxidation of quinidine by human liver cytochrome P-450. Mol Pharmacol 1986;30:287–95.

34. Yun C, Okerholm RA, Guengerich FP. Oxidation of the antihistaminic drug terfenadine in human liver microsomes: Role of cytochrome P-450 3A(4) in N-dealkylation and C-hydroxylation. Drug Metab Dispos 1992;21:403–9.

35. Collins JM. Regulatory viewpoint: Prediction of drug interactions from in vitro studies. In: Levy RH, Thummel KE, Trager WF, Hansten PD, Eichelbaum M, editors. Metabolic drug interactions. Philadelphia: Lippincott Williams & Wilkins; 2000. p. 41–7.

36. Tucker GT. Chiral switches. Lancet 2000;355:1085–7.

37. Thummel KE, Kunze KL, Shen DD. Metabolically-based drug-drug interactions: Principles and mechanisms. In: Levy RH, Thummel KE, Trager WF, Hansten PD, Eichelbaum M, editors. Metabolic drug interactions. Philadelphia: Lippincott Williams & Wilkins; 2000. p. 3–19.

38. von Moltke LL, Greenblatt DJ, Granda BW, Duan SW, Grassi JM, Venkatakrishnan K, et al. Zolpidem metabolism in vitro: Responsible cytochromes, chemical inhibitors and in vivo correlations. Br J Clin Pharmacol 1999;48:89–97.

39. von Moltke LL, Greenblatt DJ, Harmatz JS, Duan SX, Harrel LM, Cotreau-Bibbo MM, et al. Triazolam biotransformation by human liver microsomes in vitro: Effects of metabolic inhibitors and clinical confirmation of a predicted interaction with ketoconazole. J Pharmacol Exp Ther. 1996;276:370–9.

40. Greenblatt DJ, von Moltke LL, Harmatz JS, Mertzanis P, Graf JA, Durol ALB, et al. Kinetic and dynamic interaction study of zolpidem with ketoconazole, itraconazole, itraconazole, and fluconazole. Clin Pharmacol Ther 1998;64:661–71.

41. Greenblatt DJ, Wright CE, von Moltke LL, Harmatz JS, Ehrenberg BL, Harrel LM, et al. Ketoconazole inhibition of triazolam and alprazolam clearance: differential kinetic and dynamic consequences. Clin Pharmacol Ther 1998;64:237–47.

42. Sindrup SH, Brøsen K, Gram LF, et al. The relationship between paroxetine and the sparteine oxidation polymorphism. Clin Pharmacol Ther 1992;51:278–87.

43. Rotzinger S, Fang J, Coutts, RT, Baker GB. Human CYP2D6 and metabolism of m-chlorophenylpiperazine. Biol Psychiatry 1998;44:1185–91.

44. Brøsen K. Recent developments in hepatic drug oxidation: Implications for clinical pharmacokinetics. Clin Pharmacokinet 1990;18:220–39.

45. Crewe HK, Lennard MS, Tucker GT, Woods FR, Haddock RE. The effect of selective serotonin re-uptake inhibitors on cytochrome P4502D6 (CYP2D6) activity in human liver microsomes. Br J Clin Pharmacol 1992;34:262–5.

46. Jones TE. The use of other drugs to allow a lower dosage of cyclosporin to be used: Therapeutic and pharmacoeconomic considerations. Clin Pharmacokinet 1997;32:357–67.

47. Hsu A, Granneman GR, Cao G, Carothers L, El-Shourbagy T, Baroldi, P, et al. Pharmacokinetic interactions between two human immunodeficiency virus protease inhibitors, ritonavir and saquinavir. Clin Pharmacol Ther 1998;63:453–64.

48. Fuhr U. Induction of drug metabolizing enzymes: Pharmacokinetic and toxicological consequences in humans. Clin Pharmacokinet 2000;38:493–504.

49. Lehmann JM, McKee DD, Watson MA, Willson TM, Moore JT, Kliewer SA. The human orphan nuclear receptor PXR is activated by compounds that regulate CYP3A4 gene expression and cause drug interactions. J Clin Invest 1998;102:1016–23.

50. Kliewer SA, Lehmann JM, Milburn MV, Willson TM. The PPARs and PXRs: Nuclear xenobiotic receptors that define novel hormone signaling pathways. Recent Prog Horm Res 1999;54:345–67.

51. Moore LB, Goodwin B, Jones SA, Wisely GB, Serabjit-Singh CJ, Willson TM, Collins JL, Kliewer SA. St. John's wort induces hepatic drug metabolism through activation of the pregnane X receptor. Proc Natl Acad Sci USA 2000;97:7500–2.

52. Wacher VJ, Silverman JA, Zhang Y, Benet LZ. Role of P-glycoprotein and cytochrome P450 3A in limiting oral absorption of peptides and peptidomimetics. J Pharm Sci 1998;87:1322–30.

53. Silverman, JA. P-glycoprotein. In: Levy RH, Thummel KE, Trager WF, Hansten PD, Eichelbaum M, editors. Metabolic drug interactions. Philadelphia: Lippincott Williams & Wilkins; 2000. p. 135–44.

54. Wandel C, Kim RB, Kajiji S, Guengerich FP, Wilkinson GR, Wood AJJ. P-glycoprotein and cytochrome P-450 3A inhibition: Dissociation of inhibitory potencies. Cancer Res 1999;59:3944–8.

55. Bailey DG, Malcolm J, Arnold O, Spence JD. Grapefruit juice-drug interactions. Br J Clin Pharmacol 1998;46:101–10.

56. Fuhr U. Drug interactions with grapefruit juice. Extent, probable mechanism and clinical relevance. Drug Safety 1998;18:251–72.

57. Shelton MJ, Wynn HE, Hewitt RG, DiFrancesco R. Effects of grapefruit juice on the parmacokinetic exposure to indinavir in HIV-positive subjects. J Clin Pharmacol 2001;41:435–42.

58. Crixivan (indinavir) product information. West Point, PA: Merck & Co; 1998.

59. Kim RB, Fromm MF, Wandel C, et al. The drug transporter P-glycoprotein limits oral absorption and brain entry of HIV-1 protease inhibitors. J Clin Invest 1998;101:289–94.

60. Khaliq Y, Gallicano K, Venance S, Kravcik S, Cameron DW. Effect of ketoconazole on ritonavir and saquinavir concentrations in plasma and cerebrospinal fluid from patients infected with human immunodeficiency virus. Clin Pharmacol Ther 2000;68:637–46.

61. Ring BJ, Wrighton SA. Industrial viewpoint: Application of in vitro drug metabolism in various phases of drug development. In: Levy RH, Thummel KE, Trager WF, Hansten PD, Eichelbaum M, editors. Metabolic drug interactions. Philadelphia: Lippincott Williams & Wilkins; 2000. p. 29–39.

62. Yuan R, Parmelee T, Balian JD, Uppoor RS, Ajayi F, Burnett A, et al. In vitro metabolic interaction studies: Experience of the Food and Drug Administration. Clin Pharmacol Ther 1999;66:9–15.

63. Jamis-Dow CA, Pearl ML, Watkins PB, Blake DS, Klecker RW, Collins JM. Predicting drug interactions in vivo from experiments in vitro. Human studies with paclitaxel and ketoconazole. Am J Clin Oncol 1997;20:592–9.

64. Guibert A, Furlan V, Martino J, Taburet AM. In vitro effect of HIV protease inhibitors on methadone metabolism. Abstracts of the 37th Interscience Conference on Antimicrobial Agents and Chemotherapy, Toronto, September 28–October 1, 1997 (abstract A-58).

65. Hsu A, Granneman GR, Carothers L, et al. Ritonavir does not increase methadone exposure in healthy volunteers. Abstracts of the 5th Conference on Retroviruses and Opportunistic Infections, Chicago, February 1–5, 1998 (abstract 342).

66. Alfaro CL, Lam YW, Simpson J, Ereshefsky L. CYP2D6 inhibition by fluoxetine, paroxetine, sertraline, and venlafaxine in a crossover study: Intraindividual variability and plasma concentration correlations. J Clin Pharmacol 2000;40:58–66.

67. Guidance for Industry. In vivo drug metabolism/drug interaction studies—Study design, data analysis, and recommendations for dosing and labeling. Food and Drug Administration, US Department of Health and Human Services, November 1999. (Internet at http://www.fda.gov/cder/guidance/index.htm)

68. Flockhart D. Cytochrome P450 drug interaction table. (Internet at http://www.georgetown.edu/departments/pharmacology/davetab.html)

69. Ekins S, Wrighton SA. The role of CYP2B6 in human xenobiotic metabolism. Drug Metab Rev 1999;31:719–54.

70. Rodriguez I, Abernethy DR, Woosley RL. P-glycoprotein in clinical cardiology. Circulation 1999;99:472–74.

71. Wacher VJ, Wu CY, Benet LZ. Overlapping substrate specificities and tissue distribution of cytochrome P450 3A and P-glycoprotein: Implications for drug delivery and activity in cancer chemotherapy. Mol Carcinog 1995;13:129–34.

15

Biochemical Mechanisms of Drug Toxicity

ARTHUR J. ATKINSON, JR.* AND SANFORD P. MARKEY†

*Clinical Center, National Institutes of Health, Bethesda Maryland, †Laboratory of Neurotoxicology,
National Institute of Mental Health, Bethesda, Maryland

INTRODUCTION

Several attempts have been made to classify different types of adverse drug reactions, and different classifications actually may be appropriate for different purposes. The approach taken in Chapter 25 is that proposed by Rawlins and Thomas (1). According to this classification, Type A reactions consist of augmented but qualitatively normal pharmacological responses, whereas Type B reactions are those that are qualitatively bizarre. Some Type B reactions represent drug allergy or hypersensitivity and others were initially labeled idiosyncratic. However, progressively fewer adverse drug reactions are still regarded as simply idiosyncratic as more is learned about their mechanistic basis.

Approximately 70 to 80% of the adverse drug reactions that occur in clinical practice can be classified as Type A (2). This category consists of reactions that generally are mediated through pharmacologic receptors and have a pharmacokinetic basis with an obvious dose-response relationship. Hepatotoxic reactions to acetaminophen have also been assigned to this category. However, this and a number of other adverse reactions are mediated by chemically reactive cytotoxic metabolites and deserve separate consideration from a mechanistic standpoint. Allergic or hypersensitivity reactions constitute an additional 6 to 10% of the adverse drug reactions that are encountered clinically (3), and most of them also entail initial covalent bind-

ing of a chemically reactive drug metabolite to an endogenous macromolecule.

This chapter will focus on some representative adverse drug reactions that reflect the chemical reactivity of drugs and metabolites rather than their binding to specific pharmacologic receptors. Although these reactions are commonly thought of as not being dose related, they occur in many cases only after the dose-dependent formation of chemically reactive compounds exceeds a critical threshold that overcomes host detoxification and repair mechanisms. Therefore, it may be possible to minimize the severity or even occurrence of these reactions by prescribing the lowest therapeutically effective drug dose or by co-administering an agent that blocks reactive metabolite formation or bolsters endogenous detoxification mechanisms.

Drug-Induced Methemoglobinemia

Drug-induced methemoglobinemia is an adverse reaction that has been studied for over 50 years and serves as a paradigm for our understanding of the biochemical mechanism underlying a number of toxic reactions to drugs. Pioneering investigations by Brodie and Axelrod (4) on the metabolism of acetanilide demonstrated that methemoglobin levels following administration of this drug paralleled plasma levels of aniline, suggesting that phenylhydroxylamine was involved in methemoglobin formation (Figure 15.1). These investigators also found that when another metabolite of

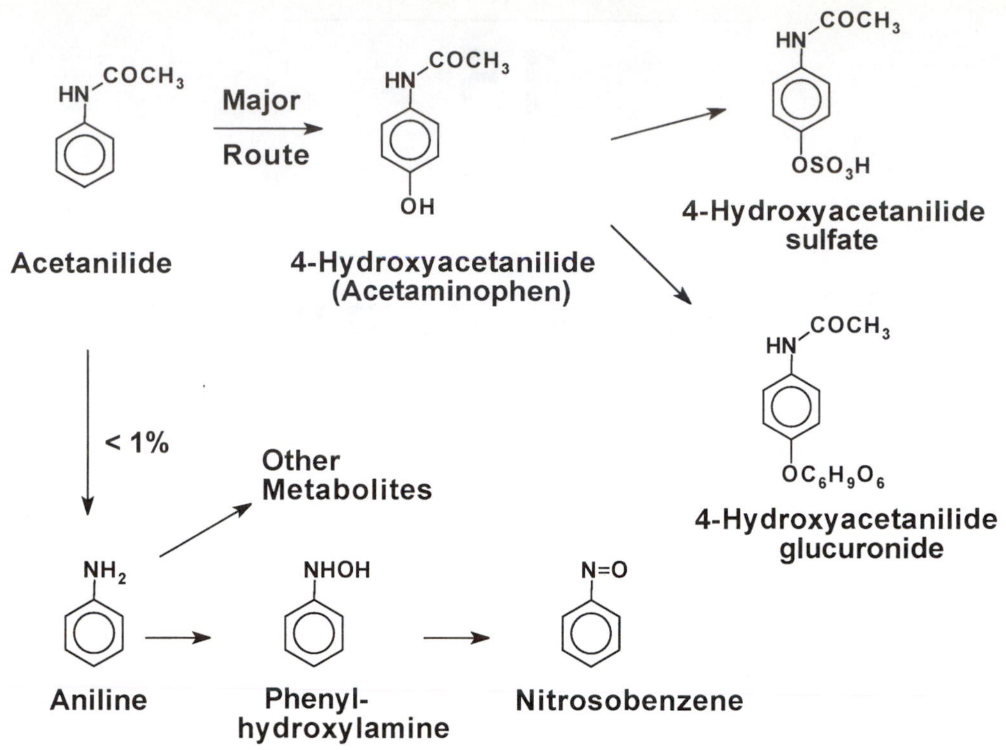

FIGURE 15.1 Metabolism of acetanilide. The major route of metabolism is via hydroxylation to form *p*-hydroxyacetanilide (acetaminophen). Less than 1% is deacetylated to form aniline.

acetanilide, *N*-acetyl *p*-aminophenol, was administered to humans it had analgesic activity that was equal to that of acetanilide, yet did not cause an increase in methemoglobin levels. These findings provided the impetus for the subsequent introduction of this metabolite as the analgesic drug acetaminophen.

In fact, methemoglobin is being formed constantly in normal erythrocytes. In the process of binding oxygen, oxyhemoglobin is converted to a superoxo-ferriheme ($Fe^{+++}O_2^{\bullet-}$) complex (5, 6). Although tissue release of oxygen restores heme iron to its ferrous state, some oxygen is dissociated from hemoglobin as superoxide ($O_2^{\bullet-}$), resulting in oxidation of hemoglobin to ferric methemoglobin. The spontaneous formation of methemoglobin is counteracted by the enzymatic reduction of heme iron to the ferrous form so that less than 1% of total hemoglobin normally is present as methemoglobin. However, higher levels of methemoglobinemia are present in individuals with hemoglobin M or other genetically rare hemoglobins that are highly vulnerable to low levels of oxidizing agents. Another rare cause of methemoglobinemia results from a deficiency in NADH-dependent cytochrome b_5 methemoglobin reductase (NADH-diaphorase) that normally reduces ferric to ferrous heme.

Drugs and other xenobiotics that cause methemoglobinemia react either stoichiometrically or in a cyclic fashion to convert heme iron from the ferrous to the ferric state. A partial list of these compounds is provided in Table 15.1. Nitrites are representative of stoichiometrically acting compounds. An account of an outbreak of methemoglobinemia that occurred in a cafeteria, whose staff had inadvertently placed sodium nitrite in a batch of oatmeal and a salt shaker, was popularized several years ago in a story entitled "Eleven Blue Men" (7). Abuse of amyl, butyl, and isobutyl nitrates continues to result in a number of fatal episodes of methemoglobinemia (5). On the other hand, most drugs that cause methemoglobinemia form metabolites that interact in a cyclic fashion to convert hemoglobin to methemoglobin, as shown for acetanilide in Figure 15.2. Because less than 1% of an administered acetanilide dose is metabolized to aniline, relatively little methemoglobin would be formed were it not for the fact that phenylhydroxylamine is regenerated from nitrosobenzene by the reducing action of cellular glutathione (6). The drugs listed in Table 15.1 also are presumably converted to hydroxylamine metabolites by *N*-oxidation, as described in Chapter 11. It is not clear why some people are more prone to develop methemoglobinemia than others. However, it is known that neonates express low levels of functional NADH-diaphorase and are particularly prone to this adverse reaction when treated with methemoglobin-forming drugs (5).

TABLE 15.1   Partial List of Compounds Producing Methemoglobinemia[a]

Stoichiometrically acting	Presumed cylical mechanism
Sodium nitrite	Aniline
Amyl nitrite	Nitrobenzene
Butyl nitrite	Acetanilinde
Isobutyl nitrite	Phenacetin
Nitric oxide	Sulfanilamide
Silver nitrate	Sulphamethoxazole
	Dapsone
	Primaquine
	Benzocaine
	Prilocaine
	Metoclopramide

[a] Data from Coleman MD, Coleman NA. Drug Saf 1996;14:394–405.

The fact that many of the drugs listed in Table 15.1 incorporate aniline or aniline analogs in their structure is a legacy that for many drugs stems from the origin of early pharmaceutical development in the German dye industry. Chloramphenicol, which actually is a natural compound that incorporates a nitrosobenzene moiety (Figure 15.3), causes aplastic anemia in 1 in 20,000 to 40,000 of individuals who are treated with this antibiotic (8). The exact mechanism by which chloramphenicol causes aplastic anemia is unknown, but also appears to involve the nitroso group, since similar toxicity has not been associated with thiamphenicol, a choloramphenicol analog in which the nitroso group is replaced with a methylsulfone group (Figure 15.3).

The Role of Covalent Binding in Drug Toxicity

With the exception of some anticancer drugs, chemicals directly toxic to tissues are eliminated in the drug

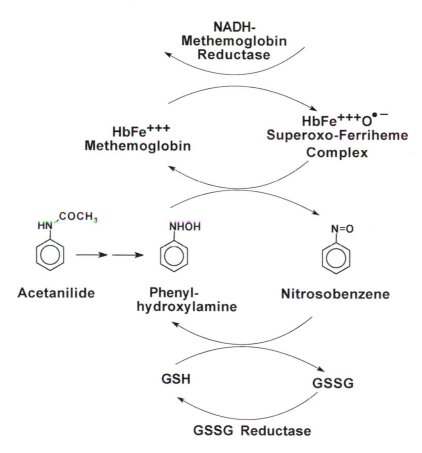

FIGURE 15.2   Cyclic mechanism by which a single molecule of phenylhdroxylamine is able to oxidize several hemoglobin molecules to methemoglobin, thereby overcoming the reductive capacity of NADH-methemoglobin reductase (NADH-diaphorase). Glutathione (GSH) maintains the cycle by reducing nitrosobenzene back to phenylhdroxylamine, and is itself regenerated from the GSSG dimer by the action of GSSG reductase (also called glutathione reductase).

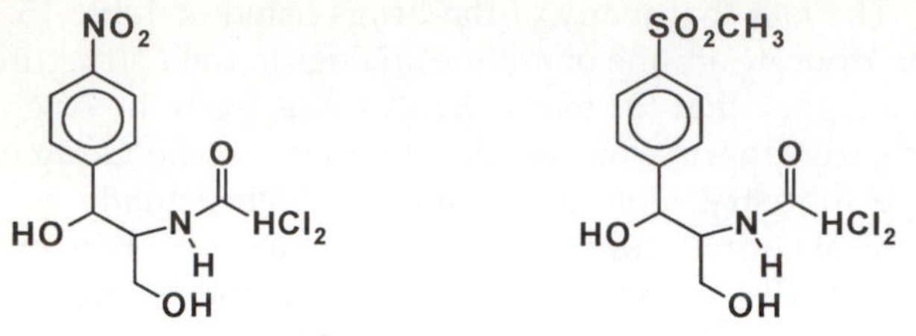

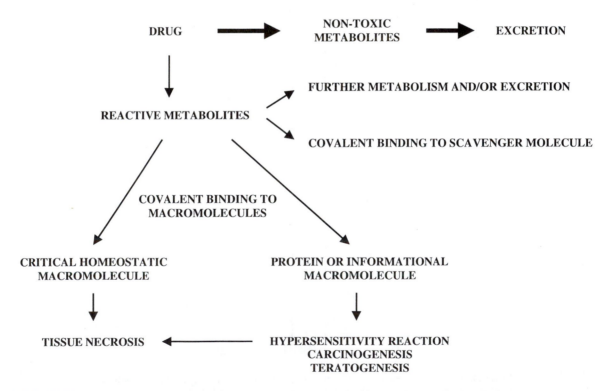

Chloramphenicol   **Thiamphenicol**

FIGURE 15.3 Chemical structures of chloramphenicol and thiamphenicol. Thiamphenicol, in which the nitroso group of chloramphenicol is replaced by a methylsulfone group, retains antibiotic activity, but does not cause the aplastic anemia that is a major concern with chloramphenicol therapy.

development process, so drug toxicity involving covalent binding usually is mediated by chemically reactive metabolites. Current mechanistic understanding of these toxic reactions usually extends to identification of the reactive metabolite and metabolic pathway involved. In some cases, protective mechanisms for scavenging reactive metabolites and metabolite-target protein adducts have also been identified. However, mechanistic information about events linking adduct formation to observed clinical toxicity is lacking in most cases.

A general scheme for adverse reaction mechanisms of this type is shown in Figure 15.4. As emphasized in Chapter 11, drug metabolizing enzymes can convert drugs into either inactive, nontoxic compounds or chemically reactive metabolites. Although these reactive metabolites can cause toxic reactions by forming covalent linkages with a variety of macromolecules, in many cases they also can be inactivated by further metabolism and excretion, or by binding to endogenous scavenger molecules such as glutathione. In these cases, there is a metabolic balance between reactive metabolite formation and elimination that may be altered by genetic factors, or perturbed by disease, environmental factors, or concomitant therapy with other drugs.

These reactions are not generally thought of as dose related. However, mass-action law considerations dictate that the extent of reactive metabolite formation, and hence adverse reaction risk, will also

FIGURE 15.4 General scheme for the role played by reactive drug metabolites in causing a variety of adverse reactions. The reactive metabolites usually account for only a small fraction of total drug metabolism and are too unstable to be chemically isolated and analyzed. In many cases, covalent binding of these metabolites to tissue macromolecules only occurs after their formation exceeds a critical threshold that overcomes host detoxification and repair mechanisms.

be a function of drug dosage. It also can be inferred from Figure 15.4 that part of the interindividual variability in incidence of these reactions reflects varying activity in the parallel pathways involved in metabolizing drugs to either nontoxic or reactive metabolites. In some cases, it has been possible to actually relate the risk of an adverse drug reaction to polymorphic drug metabolizing phenotype.

DRUG-INDUCED LIVER TOXICITY

Few areas have been as confusing to clinicians as the perplexing array of adverse drug reactions affecting the liver. Given the central role that the liver plays in drug metabolism, it is not surprising that many drugs are converted to compounds that cause liver damage. In fact, liver injury has been estimated to be the principal safety reason for terminating clinical trials during drug development and for withdrawing marketed drugs (9). Traditional classifications of drug hepatotoxicity, such as that shown in Table 15.2, have been based on descriptions of observed histopathology rather than on an understanding of the basic mechanism involved (10). We will focus our discussion on representative adverse reactions that damage the liver either through covalent binding of a reactive metabolite or through an idiosyncratic mechanism.

Hepatotoxic Reactions Resulting from Covalent Binding of Reactive Metabolites

A major advance in our understanding of the role of covalent binding of reactive metabolites in causing hepatotoxic drug reactions was provided by Brodie and his co-workers in 1971 (11). These investigators administered ^{14}C-labeled bromobenzene to rats and showed that the radioactivity was localized to centrilobular hepatocytes in the region of greatest liver damage and could not be removed from this area by washing with solvents. Binding did not occur when the bromobenzene was added directly to liver slices *in vitro*, but binding after *in vivo* administration was enhanced when rats were pre-treated with phenobarbital, and was reduced when they were pre-treated with SKF-525A, an inhibitor of drug metabolism. The conclusion was drawn that bromobenzene was being converted to an active arene oxide metabolite that was the proximate hepatotoxin (Figure 15.5). It was subsequently shown that detoxifying enzymes and glutathione played an important protective role in removing this arene oxide before it could react covalently with liver macromolecules (12).

TABLE 15.2   Classification of Drug-induced Liver Toxicity

I. Hepatocellular necrosis

   A. Zonal necrosis (CCl$_4$-type)

      CCl$_4$

      Halogenated benzenes

      Acetaminophen

   B. Viral hepatitis like (cinchophen-type)

      Isoniazid

      Iproniazid

      Halothane

II. Uncomplicated cholestasis (steroid-type)

      Anabolic steroids

      Estrogens

III. Nonspecific hepatitis with cholestasis (chlorpromazine-type)

      Phenothiazines

      Isoniazid

      Erythromycin estolate

IV. Drug-induced steatosis

      Tetracycline

Acetaminophen

A pattern of liver necrosis similar to that caused by bromobenzene is observed in patients who ingest massive doses of acetaminophen (Table 15.2). This toxic reaction also has been produced experimentally in rats and is thought to be mediated by a reactive metabolite, *N*-acetyl-*p*-benzoquinone imine (NAPQI), as shown in Scheme 11.4, (13). A number of NAPQI-hepatic protein adducts have been identified (14, 15). Although it is presumed that covalent binding of hepatic proteins with NAPQI leads to functional alterations that result in hepatotoxicity, it is not known what hepatic macromolecules are the critical targets. However, the demonstration that covalent binding only occurred after hepatic glutathione levels were depleted by more than 70% (16, 17) has provided the rationale for the clinical use of *N*-acetylcysteine to minimize toxicity following acetaminophen overdose (18).

Isoniazid

The widespread use of isoniazid prophylaxis for tuberculosis has focused attention on the liver injury caused by this drug. About 20% of patients treated with isoniazid will show elevated blood concentrations of liver enzymes and bilirubin that subside as treatment is continued (19). However, clinical hepatitis develops in some patients, and these reactions have

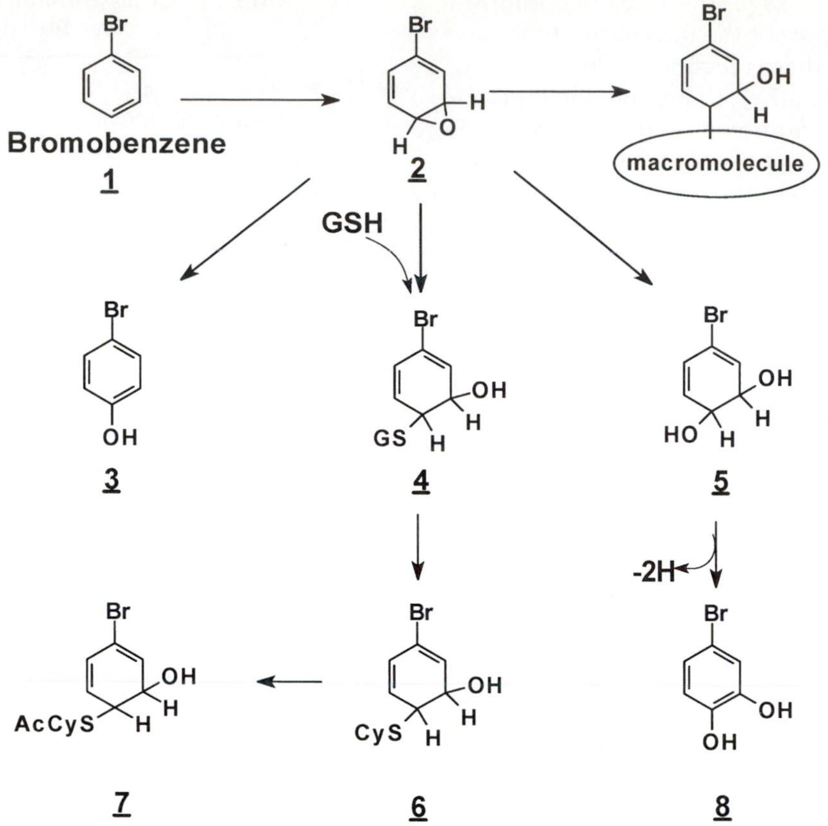

FIGURE 15.5 Metabolism of bromobenezene **1** to a chemically reactive epoxide (arene oxide) metabolite **2** that can then either bind covalently to nearby macromolecules, be scavenged by glutathione (GSH) **4** and further metabolized (**2, 6**), or be converted nonenzymatically or by expoxide hydrolase to stable hydroxylated metabolites (**3, 5, 8**).

proved fatal. Current understanding of the mechanism of isoniazid-induced hepatotoxicity is based on the metabolic pathways shown in Figure 15.6 (20, 21). It has been demonstrated in an animal model that hepatotoxicity is correlated with plasma concentration of hydrazine but not of acetyhydrazine or isoniazid (22), and that pre-treatment with an amidase inhibitor can prevent toxicity (21). However, it is postulated that hydrazine is further metabolized to a chemically reactive hepatotoxin by the cytochrome P-450 system.

A number of features of isoniazid hepatotoxicity can be interpreted by reference to the metabolic scheme shown in Figure 15.6. First, phenotypic slow acetylators are more prone to liver damage than rapid acetylators (Table 15.3) (23). Not only were hydralazine plasma concentrations higher in slow acetylators than in rapid acetylators treated with isoniazid for 14 days (24), but, in another study, urine excretion of hydrazine was higher in slow than in rapid acetylators whereas urine excretion of acetylhydrazine and diacetylhydrazine was lower (25). Second, the incidence of liver damage is increased in alcoholic patients who are treated with isoniazid to

the extent that the protective benefit of the rapid acetylator phenotype is lost (23). It has been proposed that induction of cytochrome P-450 enzymes by alcohol is responsible for an increased formation rate of the reactive metabolite that binds to hepatic macromolecules (20). Despite these advances in our understanding of the risk factors that predispose to isoniazid-induced hepatotoxicity, it remains unclear whether age, the predominant risk factor (Table 15.3), exerts its effects on either isoniazid metabolism or on protective mechanisms that

TABLE 15.3 Age and Acetylator Phenotype Affect Risk of Isoniazid-induced Hepatitis[a]

| | Acetylator phenotype | |
Age	Fast	Slow
<35 years	3.7%	13.0%
≥35 years	13.2%	37.0%

[a] Data from Dickinson DS, et al. J Clin Gastroenterol 1981;3:271–9.

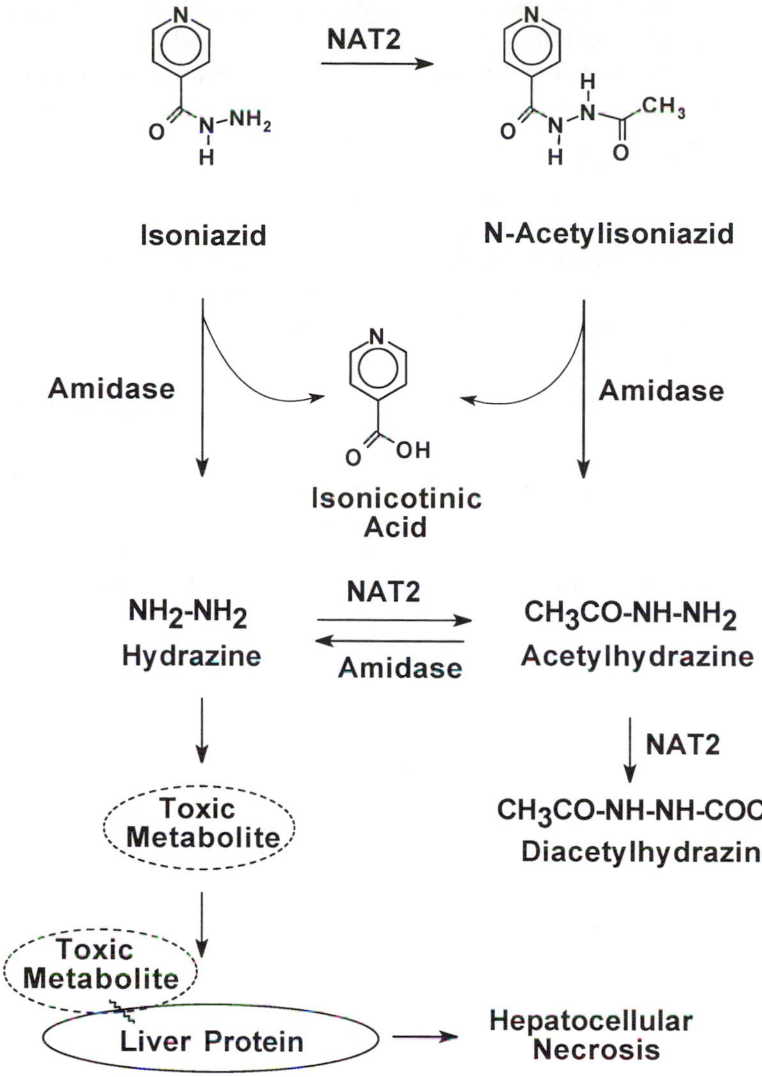

FIGURE 15.6 Metabolism of isoniazid to hydrazine that is then activated by cytochrome P-450 enzymes to a chemically reactive metabolite. *N*-Acetyltransferase (NAT2) acts at several points in this scheme to reduce hydrazine concentrations. This accounts for the fact that rapid acetylators are less likely than slow acetylators to develop isoniazid-induced hepatitis. On the other hand, chronic alcohol consumption induces cytochrome P-450 enzymes, thereby increasing the extent of toxic metabolite formation from hydrazine and the risk of hepatitis.

as yet remain undefined. The importance of understanding the biochemical basis of these risk factors stems from the important role that consideration of them plays in developing guidelines for the use of isoniazid for chemoprophylaxis of tuberculosis (26).

Immunologically Mediated Hepatotoxic Reactions

Immune mechanisms also play a prominent role in some hepatotoxic adverse drug reactions (27).

Because a minimum molecular weight of 1000 Da generally is needed for a molecule to elicit an immune response, most drugs elicit immune responses by functioning as haptens. In most cases this entails initial formation of a chemically reactive metabolite that then binds covalently to a macromolecule to form a neoantigen. As shown in Figure 15.4, the reactive metabolite may in some cases function as a direct hepatotoxin as well as an immunogen (28). The enzyme that metabolizes the drug may be among the macromolecular targets and may subsequently be inactivated by the reactive metabolite, a phenomenon referred to as *suicide inhibition*. After transport of the neoantigen to the cell membrane, humoral or cellular immune responses are triggered and result in hepatocellular damage.

Traditionally, immune-mediated toxicity has been suspected on clinical grounds, such as the presence of fever, rash, an eosinophil response, a delay between exposure to the toxin and the onset of clinical symptoms, and the accelerated recurrence of symptoms and signs of toxicity after re-administration of the drug (29). However, recent investigations are beginning to provide a framework for understanding the mechanism of these reactions.

Halothane

Halothane is a volatile general anesthetic that was introduced into the practice of clinical anesthesia in 1956. Shortly after its introduction, two forms of hepatic injury were noted to occur in patients who received halothane anesthesia. A subclinical increase in blood concentration of transaminase enzymes is observed in 20% of patients and has been attributed to the free radical metabolite shown in Figure 15.7 (30). The second form of toxicity is a hepatitis-like reaction that is characterized by severe hepatocellular necrosis that is potentially fatal (31). This adverse reaction

occurs in only 1 of 35,000 patients on initial exposure to this agent and in 1 of 3,700 patients on repeat exposure. Because the onset of halothane hepatitis is delayed but is more frequent and occurs more rapidly following multiple exposures, and because these patients usually are febrile and demonstrate eosinophilia, this reaction was suspected of having an immunologic basis. This hypothesis was strengthened by the finding that serum from patients with halothane hepatitis contained antibodies that reacted specifically with the cell membrane of hepatocytes harvested from halothane-anesthetized rabbits, rendering them susceptible to the cytotoxic effects of normal lymphocytes (29).

Satoh et al. (32) have provided further mechanistic information on this reaction by demonstrating that the reactive acyl chloride metabolite shown in Figure 15.7 binds covalently to the surface membranes of hepatocytes of rats injected with halothane. Among the macromolecular targets of this metabolite is CYP2E1, the cytochrome P-450 isoform that forms trifluoroacetyl chloride from halothane, and 45% of patients with halothane hepatitis form autoantibodies against CYP2E1 as well as antibodies against the neoantigen formed by this reaction (33). A number of other macromolecular targets are located in the endoplasmic reticulum where they appear to act as chaperones involved in protein folding (34). At present, it is not clear that

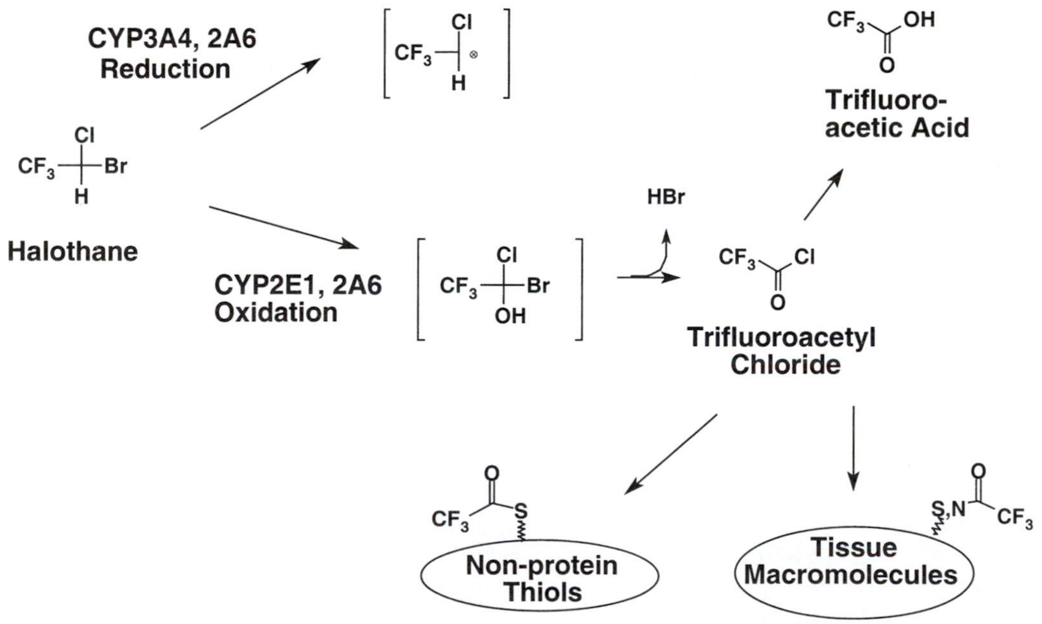

FIGURE 15.7 Oxidation of halothane by CYP2E1 leads to formation of trifluoroacetylchloride that can be nonenzymatically converted to trifluoroacetic acid, scavanged by glutathione, or bound covalently to tissue macromolecules, thereby causing liver damage. A reductive metabolic pathway generates free radicals that cause lipid peroxidation, but this pathway does not appear to be involved in the pathogenesis of halothane hepatitis.

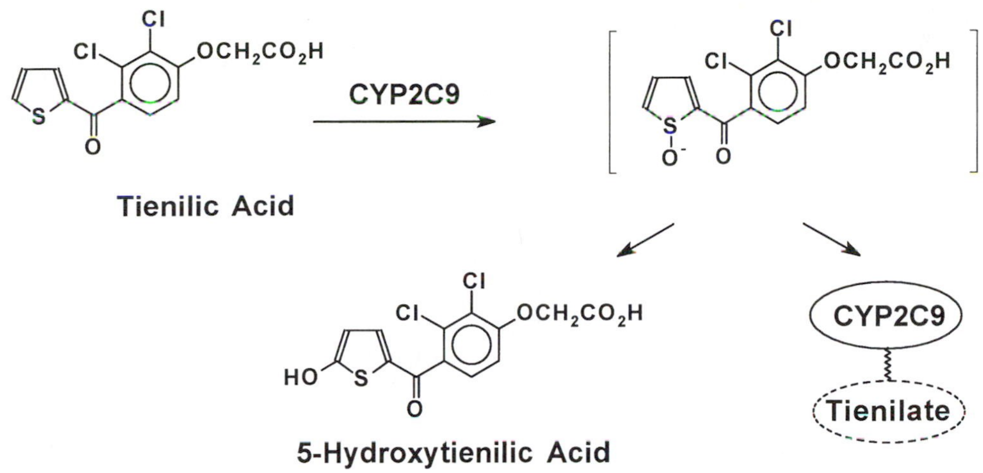

FIGURE 15.8 Oxidation of tienilic acid by CYP2C9 to an unstable electrophilic thiophene sulfoxide that binds specifically with CYP2C9 to form a haptenic conjugate or reacts with water to form 5-hydroxytienilic acid.

these antibodies play a pathogenetic role in halothane hepatitis, and it is possible that cell-mediated immune mechanisms might be of greater importance. In that regard, Furst et al. (35) have demonstrated that Kupffer cells are involved as antigen presenting cells in a guinea pig model of halothane hepatitis.

It is not clear why so few patients who receive halothane anesthesia are prone to develop hepatitis. Eliasson et al. (36) propose that patient risk reflects alterations in the balance between the activity of CYP2E1, which they found to vary by 30-fold in human liver samples, and the protective ability of glutathione and other nonprotein thiols to scavenge trifluoroacetyl chloride (Figure 15.7). This would explain the increased risk of halothane hepatitis in obese subjects, who have elevated activities of CYP2E1, and older individuals, in whom hepatic glutathione levels may be decreased. In this regard, Kharasch et al. (37) have found that patients pre-treated with disulfiram, a specific CYP2E1 inhibitor, before halothane anesthesia formed less trifluoroacetic acid than those who received no pre-treatment. These investigators proposed that a single pre-anesthetic dose of disulfiram might be effective in reducing neoantigen formation and thereby also effective in preventing halothane hepatitis.

Tienilic Acid

Tienilic acid (ticrynafen) is a uricosuric diuretic that was initially marketed in the United States in 1979. It was withdrawn a few months later because of hepatitis-like adverse reactions that developed in approximately 1 of 1000 patients treated with the drug but were fatal in 10% of the patients who developed overt

jaundice (38). The onset of overt toxicity generally occurred 1 to 6 months after starting therapy with tienilic acid, and fever, rash and eosinophilia were reported in some of the patients. These findings led investigators to suspect an immunologic basis for this adverse reaction.

Beaune et al. (39) found that the serum of patients with tienilic acid-induced hepatitis contained antimicrosomal antibodies that inhibited formation of the 5-hydroxymetabolite of tienilic acid (Figure 15.8). These antibodies are specifically directed to the CYP2C9 isoenzyme that metabolizes tienilic acid and to the neoantigen formed by covalent binding of this isoenzyme with the presumed thiophene sulfoxide reactive intermediate shown in Figure 15.8 (40, 41). This specificity of antibody formation is in contrast with the spectrum of antibodies that are formed after halothane exposure, suggesting that the reactive metabolite formed from tienilic acid is so unstable that it reacts primarily with the enzyme that forms it. In that regard, a three-site conformational epitope has recently been identified near the active site of CYP2C9 that reacts with autoantibodies in sera from patients with tienilic acid-induced hepatitis (42).

Robin et al. (40) have shown in a rat model that both unaltered CYP2C11, the analog of CYP2C9 in humans, and the CYP2C11 adduct formed after tienilic acid exposure migrate from the endoplasmic reticulum to the plasma membrane by a microtubule-dependent vesicular route. However, plasma membrane expression of the adduct is more prolonged than that of CYP2C11. These authors hypothesize that the immune reaction in tienilic acid hepatitis is directed against both CYP2C9 and alkylated CYP2C9

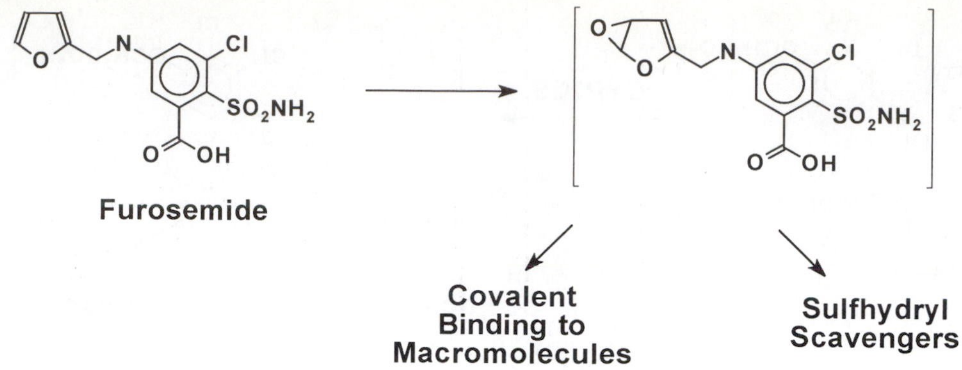

FIGURE 15.9   Proposed metabolism of furosemide to a chemically reactive furanic epoxide.

that are expressed on the plasma membrane of hepatocytes. As yet unknown are the relative roles played by antibody and cell-mediated mechanisms in mediating the hepatotoxicity that occurs subsequent to immune recognition (42).

MECHANISMS OF OTHER DRUG TOXICITIES

Although little is known about the mechanism of many drug toxic reactions, it is likely that covalent binding mediates many of them. Small alterations in chemical structure also may result in quite different patterns of organ involvement in drug toxic reactions. Mitchell et al. (43) have shown that mice treated with large doses of furosemide develop hepatocellular necrosis, presumably due to epoxidation of the furan ring (Figure 15.9). However, these investigators found that furan and several closely related furan congeners also may cause toxic reactions in the kidney and lung, as shown in Table 15.4 (44). In some cases, the site of toxicity could be shifted from one organ to another by pre-treatment with agents such as phenobarbital that altered the activity of drug metabolizing enzymes. In each case, the presumed reactive metabolite was a furan epoxide analogous to that shown for furosemide in Figure 15.9. Similarly, *in situ* metabolism of acetaminophen by kidney microsomal enzymes occurs by the same pathways shown in Scheme 11.4 and is responsible for causing acute renal tubular necrosis (45).

These observations underscore the importance of extrahepatic drug metabolism because toxic reactions targeting organs other than the liver probably reflect the formation of reactive metabolites in these tissues, rather than the peripheral effects of toxic metabolites formed in the liver. Tissue specific

differences in protective mechanisms may also underlie the organ specificity of some adverse drug reactions. Chemically reactive metabolites not only are involved in the pathogenesis of localized tissue or organ cytotoxic reactions, but play an important role in mediating adverse drug reactions that are characterized by systemic manifestations of hypersensitivity, as well as carcinogenic and teratogenic adverse reactions.

Systemic Reactions Resulting from Drug Allergy

Only recently has there been appreciation of the important role of immune mechanisms in mediating hepatotoxicity and other organ-specific damage. However, anaphylaxis and other systemic reactions traditionally associated with drug allergy also usually entail covalent binding of a drug or reactive drug metabolite to form multivalent hapten-carrier com-

TABLE 15.4   Predominant Sites of Toxicity Caused by Furan Analogs[a]

Liver	Kidney	Lung
Furan	Furan	Ipomeanol
Furosemide	2-Ethyl furan	
2-Furamide	2,3-Benzofuran	
2-Acetyl furan	2-Furoic acid	
2-Furfurol	3-Furoic acid	
2-Ethyl furoate		
2-Methoxy furan		
Dibenzofuran		

[a] Data in mice and rats from Mitchell JR, et al. Nature 1974;251:508–10.

plexes. Exceptions to this general rule are insulin, dextran and other macromolecules, and quaternary ammonium compounds that have multiple copies of a single epitope (46).

Allergic Reactions to Penicillin

Allergic reactions to penicillin are a common cause of allergic drug reactions and have been reported in various studies to occur in 0.7 to 8% of patients treated with this drug (47). As shown in Table 15.5, the spectrum of allergic reactions to penicillin spans all four categories of the Gell and Coombs classification that is described in Chapter 25. Anaphylaxis is the most serious of these reactions. It occurs in about 0.01% of patients who receive penicillin and has a fatality rate of 9% (48). Penicillin-induced cytopenias, interstitial nephritis, and serum sickness reactions occur more frequently with prolonged high-dose therapy (49). Contact dermatitis occurs primarily after cutaneous exposure to penicillin, but is infrequent in

patients since topical penicillin formulations have been discontinued; it occurs primarily in nurses, pharmacists, and others whose skin comes in repeated contact with the drug.

Penicillin is unusual in that it forms immunogenic hapten-carrier complexes by binding directly to macromolecules in plasma and on cell surfaces (Figure 15.10). But even though prior metabolic activation is not required, it has been found that hapten formation is facilitated by one or more low molecular weight serum factors (47). Conversely, the haptenation of penicillin-protein conjugates has been shown to be reversible, although the specific enzymes mediating this have not been identified (50). The penicilloyl-protein conjugate constitutes more than 90% of the haptenic products and is the major antigenic determinant for the formation of penicillin-specific immunoglobulins and T-cells (51). This antigenic determinant is involved in 75% of IgE-mediated allergic reactions and most of the other reactions shown in Table 15.5. Although the minor antigenic determinants are pres-

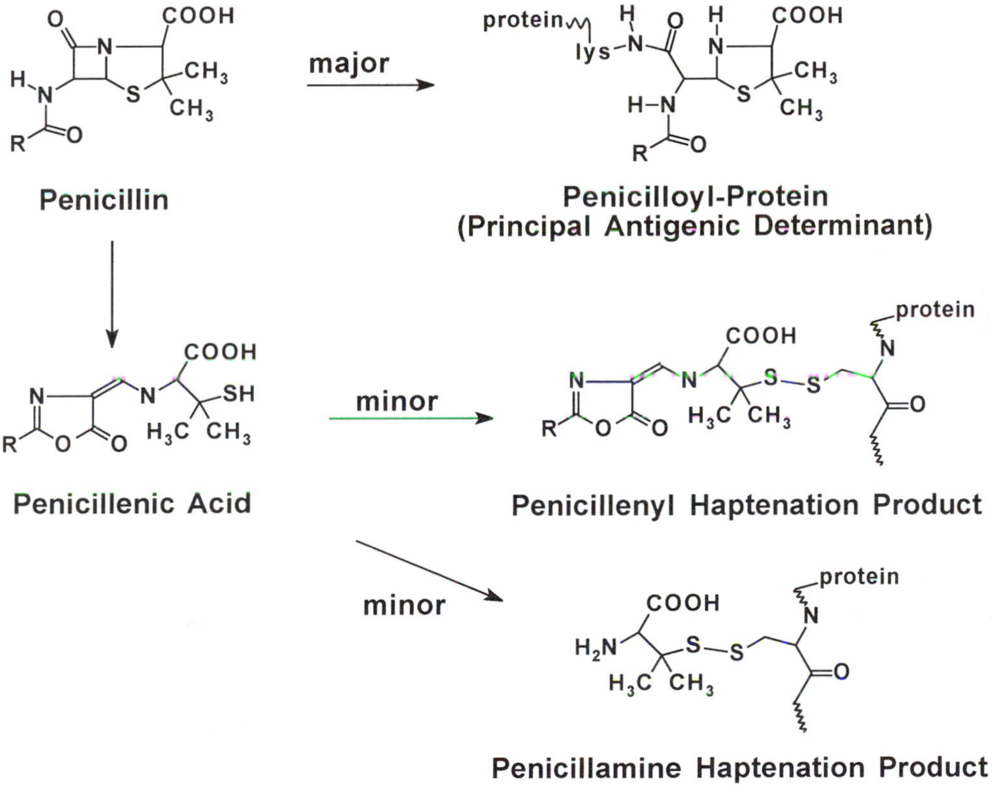

FIGURE 15.10 Hapten determinants formed by pencillins that contain a β-lactam ring linked to various side chains (R). The primary route of haptenation involves acylation of the ε-amino group of lysine residues of serum or cell surface proteins to form a penicilloyl or major antigenic determinant. Isomerization of penicillin leads to the generation of compounds that form disulfide bonds with the cysteine sulfhydryl groups of proteins. These epitopes are termed minor determinants.

TABLE 15.5   Representative Immune-mediated Reactions
to Penicillin

Gell and Coombs type[a]	Mechanism	Clinical presentation
I	IgE-mediated	Anaphylaxis Urticaria
II	IgG or IgM-mediated, complement dependent cytolysis	Hemolytic anemia Thrombocytopenia Interstitial nephritis
III	Immune complex-mediated, complement dependent	Serum sickness Drug fever Vasculitis
IV	T-cell lymphocyte-mediated	Contact dermatitis Morbilliform skin rash

[a] Gell PGH, Coombs RRA. Clinical aspects of immunology. Oxford: Blackwell; 1963.

TABLE 15.6   Comparison of Allergy History with
Penicillin Skin Test Results[a]

	Allergy history	
Skin test	Positive	Negative
Positive	18%	4%
Negative	80%	95%
Uninterpretable	3%	1%

[a] Data from Sogn DD, et al. Arch Intern Med 1992;152:1025–32.

ent only in low abundance, they play an important role in some IgE-mediated reactions. The extent of hapten formation and the probability of eliciting a penicillin-specific immune response appear to increase as a function of the cumulative penicillin dose (52). In one study, 50% of patients who received at least 2 gm of penicillin for 10 days had an IgG and/or an IgE antibody response (49).

The likelihood that haptenic products are formed in everyone who receives penicillin, and the frequency with which penicillin-specific antibody responses occur, stand in marked contrast to the infrequent occurrence of allergic reactions to this drug. The cumulative risk of penicillin allergy appears to be related to the persistence of penicillin-specific antibodies, with the half-life of pencilloyl IgE antibodies reported to range from 10 to more than 1000 days (49). In this regard, dehaptenation was noted to be slower than normal in penicillin allergic patients (50). Although it has been found that penicillin allergic reactions are less common in the young, it is not clear that youth is an independent protective factor or simply reflects the fact that the young are likely to have had less cumulative exposure to penicillin. Other constitutional or genetic factors are also likely to be important determinants of individual proclivity to develop allergic reactions to penicillin and other drugs.

In clinical practice, both a history of prior penicillin allergy and skin testing can be used to identify individuals at risk for penicillin allergic reactions. These approaches were compared in a National Institute of Allergy and Infectious Diseases-sponsored study of 1539 hospitalized patients in whom penicillin therapy was indicated (53). Patients received skin tests with both benzylpenicilloyl-octalysine to determine major determinant reactivity, and a minor determinant mixture of benzylpenicillin, benzylpenicilloate, and benzylpenicilloyl-N-propylamine. Of the positive skin test reactors, 84% had major determinant reactivity, and the remaining 16% had positive tests with only the minor determinant mixture. As shown in Table 15.6, most patients with a negative history also had negative skin tests, and none of these patients had an allergic reaction to penicillin. A substantial percentage of patients with a history of penicillin allergy were found to have negative skin tests. Penicillin therapy of patients with a positive or unknown history of penicillin allergy but negative skin tests resulted in a 1.3% incidence of immediate or accelerated IgE-mediated allergic reactions. Most patients with positive skin tests were treated with other antibiotics but two of the nine individuals who received penicillin had immediate or accelerated allergic reactions and two others developed rashes on days 3 and 9 of penicillin therapy, respectively. Because primary reliance is placed on history to identify penicillin allergic individuals, it would appear that the patients at greatest risk are the 4% of history-negative patients who nonetheless react to skin testing.

Procainamide-induced Lupus

Although a number of drugs are capable of inducing a systemic lupus erythematosus-like reaction, procainamide is the most common cause of drug-related lupus. Kosowski et al. (54) found that all patients treated with procainamide for more than a year developed antinuclear antibodies, but that procainamide-induced lupus occurred in slightly less than one-third of those who began therapy. The fact that procainamide contains an aniline moiety, similar to many drugs that cause methemoglobinemia, led to initial speculation that its N-acetylated metabolite (NAPA) might have antiarrhythmic efficacy but would be less likely to cause this adverse effect (Figure 15.11) (55).

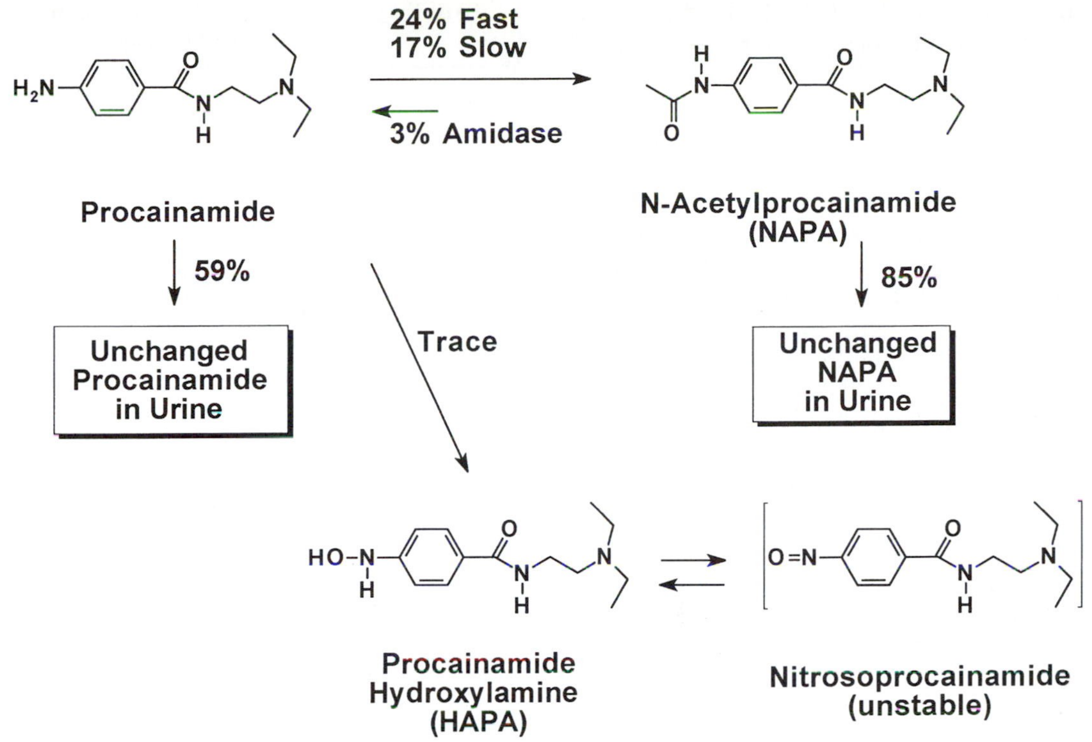

FIGURE 15.11 Simplified scheme of procainamide metabolism. In subjects with normal kidney function, renal excretion of unchanged drug accounts for more than half the elimination of a procainamide dose, whereas acetylation by NAT2 accounts for only 24% and 17% of elimination in rapid and slow acetylators, respectively. A small amount of procainamide is metabolized to a hydroxylamine that is in equilibrium with a postulated chemically unstable and reactive nitroso compound that is capable of haptenic binding to histone proteins.

This was first demonstrated by switching a patient with procainamide-induced lupus to NAPA whereupon both the arthralgic symptoms of drug-induced lupus and antinuclear antibody titers returned to normal (56). Subsequent confirmation was provided by long-term studies in which patients received effective antiarrhythmic therapy with NAPA without developing this reaction (57, 58). However, the immunologic safety of NAPA is relative rather than absolute because approximately 3% of an administered NAPA dose is converted to procainamide by deacetylation (Figure 15.11) (59). In this regard, Kluger et al. (57) described a patient who developed drug-induced lupus when treated with NAPA doses sufficient to produce plasma procainamide concentrations of 1.6 µg/mL. The fact that these symptoms subsided when the NAPA dose was reduced so that procainamide levels fell to 0.7 µg/mL suggests that there is a threshold procainamide level that must be exceeded before this toxic reaction occurs.

Uetrecht (60) provided further evidence that the aryl amine group of procainamide is implicated in the development of drug-induced lupus by demonstrating that procainamide is metabolized to a hydroxylamine (HAPA) (Figure 15.11). HAPA is in equilibrium with a chemically unstable nitroso compound that is capable of covalent binding to histones and other proteins and, by rendering them antigenic, may initiate the immune reaction leading to procainamide-induced lupus (61). Although hepatic CYP2D6 is capable of forming HAPA from procainamide (62), it is likely that the relevant reactive metabolites are generated by myeloperoxidase within activated neutrophiles or monocytes (61, 63). An alternative possibility to the immunogenic role played by direct covalent binding of the nitroso metabolite is the suggestion that this metabolite initiates the immune response of drug-induced lupus by directly activating lymphocytes through redox cycling or inhibition of DNA methylation reactions (64).

Although the exact mechanism of initial sensitization remains unclear, it was found in a group of prospectively studied patients that serum IgG, IgM, and IgA autoantibodies against histone, single-stranded DNA and the [(H2A-H2B)-DNA] complex appeared after an average of 7 months of procainamide therapy (65). The (H2A-H2B) dimer is a component of the histone octamer (66), and it is of particular interest that 16 of the 19 patients in this study who were destined to develop procaine-induced lupus developed high titers of IgG autoantibodies to the [(H2A-H2B)-DNA] complex. By contrast, only two of the nine asymptomatic patients were found to have IgG anti-[(H2A-H2B)-DNA] activity that was at most only 3% of that measured in the symptomatic patients. Similar antibodies are found in patients with systemic lupus erythematosus and it has been proposed that lupus nephritis results from IgG binding to [(H2A-H2B)-DNA] in nucleosomal material that is deposited in the glomerulus by the circulation (66). Because renal involvement is not a feature of drug-induced lupus, it appears that factors other than antibody binding to [(H2A-H2B)-DNA] are responsible for nephritis. However, the systemic symptoms of drug-induced lupus may result from inflammatory mechanisms involved in the clearance of immune complexes.

Carcinogenic Reactions to Drugs

It has been realized that chemicals can cause cancer since 1775 when Percival Potts observed a high incidence of scrotal cancer in chimney sweeps (67). Despite intensive study, much remains to be learned about the mechanistic details of chemical carcinogenesis, of which drug-induced carcinogenesis is a subcategory. Since 1969, the International Agency for Research on Cancer (IARC) has conducted an evaluation of the carcinogenic risk of pharmaceuticals, assigning them to five groups based on the strength of evidence linking compounds to carcinogenesis (68). Table 15.7 lists pharmaceuticals that are regarded as being either carcinogenic or probably carcinogenic to humans. In addition to these single compounds, combinations of the following are also regarded as carcinogenic: analgesic formulations containing phenacetin, MOPP chemotherapy (nitrogen mustard, vincristine, procarbazine, and prednisone), 8-methyoxypsoralen combined with UVA radiation, and combined or sequential oral contraceptive regimens containing estrogens and progestins.

Chemical carcinogens are generally regarded as being either genotoxic or non-genotoxic, although some carcinogens, such as estrogens, may exert a combination of these effects. Some toxic drugs, such as alkylating agents used in cancer chemotherapy, are directly genotoxic but others require prior conversion to reactive metabolites. Dioxin and some other non-genotoxic carcinogens appear to activate intracellular receptors, leading to changes in gene expression that result in cancer (69). Regardless of mechanism, chemi-

TABLE 15.7 IARC List of Carcinogenic and Probably Carcinogenic Pharmaceuticals[a]

	Carcinogenic	Probably carcinogenic
Cytotoxic drugs	Chlornaphazine	Adriamycin
	Myleran	Azacitidine
	Chlorambucil	BCNU
	Methyl-CCNU	CCNU
	Cyclophosphamide	Chlorozotocin
	Melphalan	Cisplatin
	Thiotepa	Nitrogen mustard
	Treosulfan	N-nitroso-N-methylurea
		Procarbazine
Immuno-suppressants	Azathioprine Cyclosporine	
Hormone agonists and antagonists	Diethylstilbestrol Tamoxifen	Oxymetholone Testosterone
Other	Arsenic trioxide	Phenacetin
		Chrloramphenicol
		5-Methoxypsoralen

[a] Data from Marselos M and Vainio H. Carcinogenesis 1991;12:1751–66, and White INH. Carcinogenesis 1999;20:1153–60.

cal carcinogenesis is a complex process requiring sequential stages of initiation, promotion and progression (67). As a result, there is usually a delay of several years between exposure to carcinogens and the appearance of drug-induced cancers.

Secondary Leukemia Following Cancer Chemotherapy

The success of chemotherapeutic regimens for cancer has resulted in an increasing number of patients who develop a secondary myeloid leukemia. Data collected from patients who were treated with alkylating agents for Hodgkin's disease, ovarian cancer, and other malignancies have demonstrated that following chemotherapy there is an excess risk of treatment-related myelodysplastic syndrome (MDS) that progresses to acute myeloid leukemia (70, 71). This risk is greatest in patients more than 40 years old, is greater in males than in females, and is proportionate to the dose and duration of chemotherapy. The risk reaches a peak approximately 5 years after initiating chemotherapy and persists for up to 10 years. Estimates range from less than 0.3% to 10% for the cumulative 10-year incidence of secondary acute myeloid leukemia in

INITIATION   PROMOTION   PROGRESSION

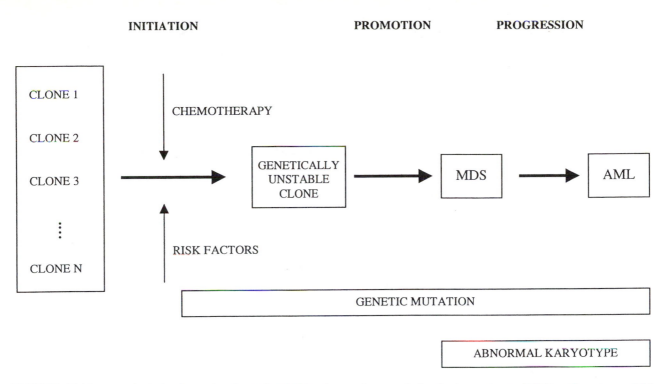

FIGURE 15.12 Hypothetical scheme for the pathogenesis of secondary myelodysplastic syndrome (MDS) and acute myeloid leukemia (AML) following cancer chemotherapy with alkylating agents.

patients who have received chemotherapy for Hodgkin's disease (71).

Alkylation of hematopoietic progenitor cell DNA during chemotherapy with alkylating agents appears to be the genotoxic event that initiates the carcinogenic process by causing genetic mutations that alter cell growth (Figure 15.12). In animal studies, this has been shown to result in a permanent loss of stem-cell reserve and the maintenance of hematopoiesis by a succession of individual stem-cell clones (70). Following this preliminary clonal restriction, it appears that a chromosomal abnormality develops in a clone that results in some selective growth advantage. Deletion or loss of chromosomes 7 and 5 are the most frequent chromosomal abnormalities that have been found in MDS secondary to therapy with alkylating agents (72). Chromosome 5 encodes a number of genes that may play an important role in the pathogenesis of secondary MDS and its further progression to leukemia (73). For example, it has been proposed by analogy with Fanconi anemia that abnormalities affecting the long arm of chromosome 5 (5q-) may lead to a structural or functional loss of interferon response factor-1 *(IRF-1)* that functions as a tumor suppressor gene (74). The product of this gene (IRF-1) is expressed constitutively in normal progenitor cells and has the biological effect of inhibiting growth and stimulating inhibition. In normal cells, IFNγ induces IRF-1 and inhibits cell growth. But IFNγ actually stimulates cell growth in cells incapable of an IRF-1 response and may provide the selection pressure that is needed for the outgrowth of a leukemogenic mutant stem-cell clone.

Secondary acute myeloid leukemia also follows chemotherapy with DNA-intercalating anthracyclines and topoisomerase II-directed epipodophyllotoxins. The onset of leukemia in these patients generally occurs only 2 to 3 years after chemotherapy and is rarely preceded by MDS (71, 73). These agents cause translocations involving the myeloid-lymphoid leukemia gene that is located at chromosome band 11q23. This gene appears to play an important role in controlling the differentiation of primitive hematopoietic stem cells.

Diethylstilbestrol-induced Vaginal Cancer

In 1971, Herbst et al. (75) reported the unusual occurrence of clear cell adenocarcinoma of the vagina in eight young women. The precipitating factor appeared to be the fact that their mothers had been treated with diethylstilbestrol (DES) in order to prevent spontaneous abortion and premature delivery in what were deemed to be high-risk pregnancies. Recent estimates place the incidence of clear cell adenocarci-

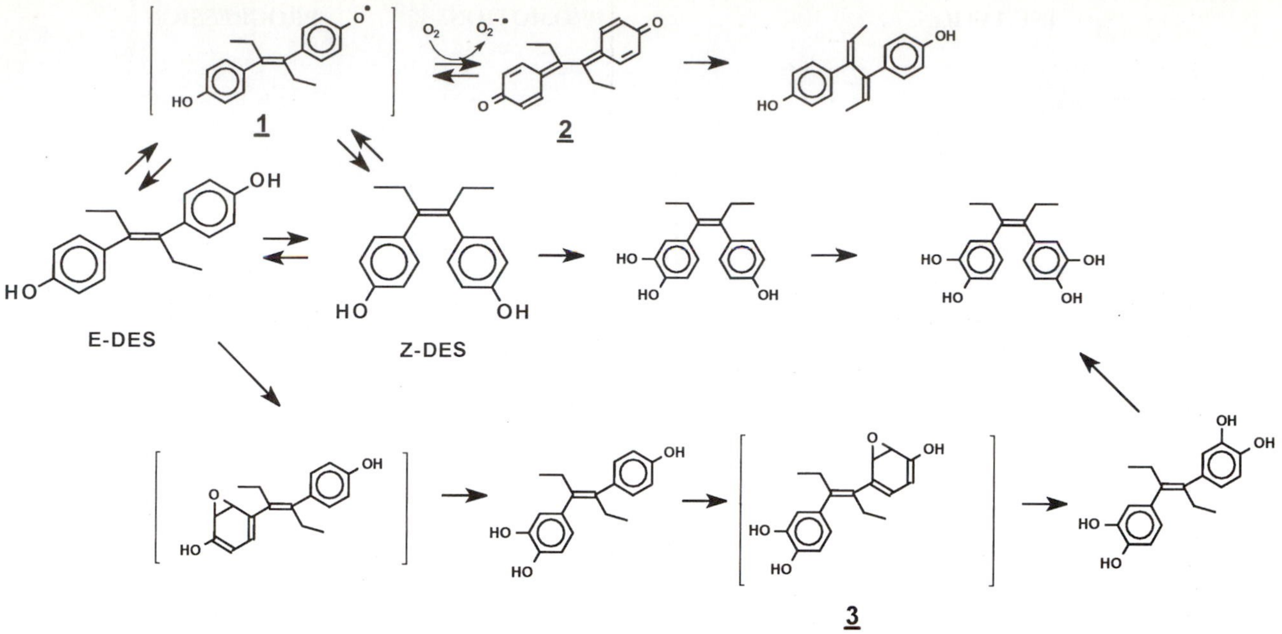

FIGURE 15.13 Partial scheme for the metabolism of diethylstilbestrol (DES). DES is administered as the trans-isomer (E-DES) that in solution is in equilibrium with the cis-isomer (Z-DES). Cytochrome P-450 enzymes oxidize E-DES and Z-DES to a postulated chemically reactive semiquinone **1** which is further oxidized to a quinone **2**, thereby generating reactive oxygen species (ROS) that oxidize cellular macromolecules. Redox cycling is perpetuated and ROS formation amplified by cytochrome P-450 or cytochrome b_5 reductase that reduce the quinone back to the semiquinone. The unstable semiquinone and diol epoxide **3** metabolites are presumably those that bind to DNA to form adducts and initiate carcinogenesis.

noma of the vagina at 1.5 per 1000 women who were exposed *in utero* to DES (76).

DES is a nonsteroidal estrogen that crosses the placenta and targets intranuclear estrogen receptors that develop in the fetal genital tract early in intrauterine life. During fetal development, Müllerian-derived columnar epithelium is replaced by a hollow core of squamous epithelium that arises from the vaginal plate (77). But neonatal DES exposure leads in mice to persistence of Müllerian-type columnar epithelium in the upper vagina and cervix and subsequent adenosis. DES exerts proliferative effects by binding to the classic estrogen receptor (ER-α), and it has been thought that increased cell proliferation might be carcinogenic by causing an increase in spontaneous errors associated with DNA replication and increasing the replication of clones of cells carrying these errors (78). Consistent with a role for ER-α in mediating DES carcinogenesis are observations following neonatal exposure to DES that the incidence of atypical uterine hyperplasia and cancer was increased in mutant mice that overexpress ER-α, and that squamous metaplasia of the vaginal epithelium was absent in ER-α knockout mice (78).

However, estrogen receptor-mediated events cannot fully explain the carcinogenic properties of estrogens, and there is mounting evidence that DES has direct genotoxic effects that result from its metabolism in target tissues (79, 80). The pathways of DES metabolism are partly depicted in Figure 15.13 (79, 81). It can be seen that redox cycling between the semiquinone and quinone metabolites generates superoxide anion radicals that may cause oxidative damage to DNA and other cellular macromolecules (79). In addition, chemically reactive semiquinone and diol epoxide metabolites are formed that are capable of forming either stable or depurinating DNA adducts (80). Stable DNA adducts are formed when reactive metabolites react with exocyclic amino groups on adenine or guanine. Depurinating adducts result when these metabolites bind to the N-3 or N-7 position of adenine or the N-7 or C-8 position of guanine. The depurinating adducts destabilize the glycosidic bond to deoxyribose, spontaneously releasing the purine base and the metabolite that is bound to it. It is believed that depurinating adducts are the primary culprits in the process of tumor initiation, and that mutations result from misrepair or misreplication of the apurinic sites (80). Stable DNA adducts could also play a role in carcinogenesis by interfering with error-free repair of the apurinic sites.

Consistent with the pathogenetic role of impaired DNA repair is the finding of mutations in DNA polymerase β that have been observed in a hamster kidney model of DES carcinogenesis (79). Although specific gene defects have not been identified in DES-induced clear cell adenomas in humans, up-regulation of the normal p53 tumor suppressor gene has been described and attributed to a normal cellular response to persistent DNA damage or genetic instability (82). Molecular genetic analysis has provided evidence of microsatellite instability in all the DES-induced and 50% of the spontaneous clear-cell adenoma tissue samples that were analyzed, again suggesting that defective DNA repair represents a critical molecular feature of this tumor type (83). Even though the genotoxic effects of DES may initiate carcinogenesis, estrogen receptor-mediated proliferative stimuli from endogenous estrogens would appear to play an important role in tumor promotion and progression, insofar as the adenocarcinomas primarily occur after the onset of menstruation (77).

Teratogenic Reactions to Drugs

Although the principles of teratogenesis are described more fully in Chapter 22, certain general concepts are central to an understanding of the way in which drugs cause teratogenic adverse reactions. First, teratogens cause a specific abnormality, or pattern of abnormalities, in the fetus, such as phocomelia resulting from maternal therapy with thalidomide (84). However, even known teratogens will not exert a teratogenic effect unless they are given during the relevant period of fetal organogenesis, generally during the first trimester of pregnancy. In addition, fetal exposure must also exceed a critical threshold for teratogenesis to occur. The level of exposure is not only determined by the rate of drug transfer across the placenta but by fetal clearance mechanisms (85). Unfortunately, the ability of the fetal liver to provide teratogenic protection is limited by the facts that the liver does not begin to form until the fourth week of pregnancy and that smooth endoplasmic reticulum is not detectable in fetal hepatocytes until the twelfth week of pregnancy (86). Finally, it is likely that genetic factors also determine the outcome of exposure to teratogens.

The Fetal Hydantoin Syndrome

Hanson et al. (87) coined the term fetal hydantoin syndrome to describe a pattern of malformations that occurs in epileptic women who are treated with phenytoin during pregnancy. The clinical features of the syndrome include craniofacial anomalies, such as cleft lip or palate, a broad, depressed nasal bridge and inner epicanthic folds, nail and digital hypoplasia, prenatal and postnatal growth retardation, and mental retardation. These authors estimated that about 11% of exposed fetuses have the syndrome with serious sequelae, but that almost three times as many have lesser degrees of impairment. The magnitude and difficulty of this problem are underscored by the estimate that hydantoin therapy is prescribed during 2 per 1,000 pregnancies, and by the fact that the risks of untreated epilepsy exceed the teratogenic risk of anticonvulsant therapy.

Phenytoin, phenobarbital, and carbamazepine are teratogenic anticonvulsant drugs that also cause hypersensitivity reactions that include skin rash, fever, and hepatitis (88). The cytochrome P-450-mediated hydroxylation of all three drugs proceeds via the formation of chemically reactive epoxide intermediates, as shown for phenytoin in Scheme 11.11. A pathogenetic role for phenytoin epoxide is suggested by the finding that the activity of epoxide hydrolase, the enzyme that converts the epoxide to a nontoxic dihydrodiol metabolite, is deficient in lymphocytes from patients with phenytoin-induced hepatotoxic reactions (89). Covalent binding of phenytoin to rat gingival proteins also suggests that metabolic activation plays a pathogenetic role in the gingival hyperplasia that occurs in 30 to 70% of patients receiving long-term phenytoin therapy (90).

Martz et al. (91) used a mouse model to provide the first evidence that the epoxide metabolite of phenytoin might be similarly implicated in mediating teratogenic reactions to this drug. Pregnant mice were treated with a single dose of phenytoin on gestational day 11. Their fetuses were subsequently found to have a 4% incidence of cleft palate and other anomalies, and inhibition of epoxide hydrolase with trichloropropene oxide resulted in at least a doubling of this incidence. Furthermore, administration of radioactive phenytoin resulted in covalent binding of the radioactivity to gestational tissue macromolecules. By assaying lymphocytes for epoxide hydrolase activity, as had been done for patients with phenytoin hepatotoxicity, Strickler et al. (92) demonstrated that the occurrence of major birth defects, including cleft lip or palate, congenital heart anomalies, and microcephaly, was correlated with subnormal epoxide hydrolase activity. Subsequently, Buehler et al. (93) obtained samples of amniocytes at amniocentesis and were able to correlate low amniocyte levels of epoxide hydrolase activity with an increased risk of developing the fetal hydantoin syndrome. More recently, Winn and Wells (94) have used a mouse model to demonstrate that peroxidase-catalyzed metabolic activation of phenytoin by fetal tissues results in the formation of reactive oxygen species that oxidize fetal macromolecules.

At present it appears that phenytoin damages fetal macromolecules either by covalent binding of its epoxide or a free radical reactive intermediate, or by free radical-initiated oxidation (95, 96). Although the relative teratologic contributions of covalent binding and free-radical oxidation have yet to be determined, it appears that DNA damage plays a critical role in much the same way as has been described for carcinogenic reactions. In this regard, it has been demonstrated that mice deficient in the *p53* tumor suppressor gene, which is necessary for DNA repair, are more susceptible to phenytoin teratogenic reactions (96).

References

1. Rawlins MD, Thomas SHL. Mechanisms of adverse drug reactions. In: Davies DM, Ferner RE, de Glanville H, editors. Davies's textbook of adverse drug reactions. 5th ed. London: Chapman & Hall Medical; 1998. p. 40–64.
2. Melmon KL. Preventable drug reactions—Causes and cures. New Engl J Med 1971;284:1361–8.
3. Goldstein RA, Patterson R. Drug allergy: prevention, diagnosis, and treatment. Ann Intern Med 1984;100:302–3.
4. Brodie BB, Axelrod J. The fate of acetanilide in man. J Pharmacol Exp Ther 1948;94:29–38.
5. Coleman MD, Coleman NA. Drug-induced methaemoglobinaemia—Treatment issues. Drug Saf 1996;14:394–405.
6. Coleman MD. Use of *in vitro* methaemoglobin generation to study antioxidant status in diabetic erythrocyte. Biochem Pharmacol 2000;60:1409–16.
7. Roueché B. The medical detectives. New York: Penguin Books;1988. p. 3–13.
8. Yunis AA. Chloramphenicol: relation of structure to activity and toxicity. Ann Rev Pharmacol Toxicol 1988;28:83–100.
9. Ballet F. Hepatotoxicity in drug development: detection, significance and solutions. J Hepatol 1997;26 (suppl 2):26–36.
10. Popper H, Rubin E, Gardiol D, Schaffer F, Paronetto F. Drug-induced liver disease: a penalty for progress. Arch Intern Med 1965;115:128–36.
11. Brodie BB, Reid WD, Cho AK, Sipes G, Krishna G, Gillette JR. Possible mechanism of liver necrosis caused by aromatic organic compounds. Proc Natl Acad Sci USA 1971;68:160–4.
12. Zampaglione N, Jollow DJ, Mitchell JR, Stripp B, Hamrick M, Gillette JR. Role of detoxifying enzymes in bromobenzene-induced liver necrosis. J Pharmacol Exp Ther 1973;187:218–27.
13. Dahlin DC, Miwa GT, Lu AYH, Nelson SD. N-Acetyl-*p*-benzoquinone imine: A cytochrome P-450 mediated oxidation product of acetaminophen. Proc Natl Acad Sci USA 1984;81:1327–31.
14. Pumford NR, Halmes NC. Protein targets of xenobiotic reactive intermediates. Annu Rev Pharmacol Toxicol 1997;37:91–117.
15. Qui Y, Benet LZ, Burlingame AL. Identification of the hepatic protein targets of reactive metabolites of acetaminophen *in vivo* in mice using two-dimensional gel electrophoresis and mass spectrometry. J Biol Chem 1998;273:17940–53.
16. Mitchell JR, Jollow DJ, Potter WZ, Gillette JR, Brodie BB. Acetaminophen-induced hepatic necrosis. IV. Protective role of glutathione. J Pharmacol Exp Ther 1973;187:211–17.
17. Mitchell JR, Thorgeirsson SS, Potter WZ, Jollow DJ, Keiser H. Acetaminophen-induced hepatic injury: Protective role of glutathione in man and rationale for therapy. Clin Pharmacol Ther 1974;16:676–84.
18. Rumack BH. Acetaminophen overdose. Am J Med 1983;75:104–12.
19. Mitchell JR, Long MW, Thorgeirsson UP, Jollow DJ. Acetylation rates and monthly liver function tests during one year of isoniazid preventive therapy. Chest 1975;68:181–90.
20. Lauterberg BH, Smith CV, Todd EL, Mitchell JR. Oxidation of hydrazine metabolites formed from isoniazid. Clin Pharmacol Ther 1985;38:566–71.
21. Sarich TC, Adams SP, Petricca G, Wright JM. Inhibition of isoniazid-induced hepatotoxicity in rabbits by pretreatment with an amidase inhibitor. J Pharmacol Exp Ther 1999;289:695–702.
22. Sarich TC, Youssefi M, Zhou T, Adams SP, Wall RA, Wright JM. Role of hydrazine in the mechanism of isoniazid hepatotoxicity in rabbits. Arch Toxicol 1996;70:835–40.
23. Dickinson DS, Bailey WC, Hirschowitz BI, Soong S-J, Eidus L, Hodgkin MM. Risk factors for isoniazid (INH)-induced liver dysfunction. J Clin Gastroenterol 1981;3:271–9.
24. Blair IA, Tinoco RM, Brodie MJ, Care RA, Dollery CT, Timbrell JA, et al. Plasma hydrazine concentrations in man after isoniazid and hydralazine administration. Human Toxicol 1985;4:105–202.
25. Peretti E, Karlaganis G, Lauterburg BH. Increased urinary excretion of toxic hydrazino metabolites of isoniazid by slow acetylators. Effect of a slow-release preparation of isoniazid. Eur J Clin Pharmacol 1987;33:283–6.
26. American Thoracic Society. Treatment of tuberculosis and tuberculosis infection in adults and children. Am Rev Respir Dis 1986;134:355–63.
27. Boelsterli UA, Zimmerman HJ, Kretz-Rommel A. Idiosyncratic liver toxicity of nonsteroidal antiinflammatory drugs: molecular mechanisms and pathology. Crit Rev Toxicol 1995;25:207–35.
28. Chen M, Gandolfi AJ. Characterization of the humoral immune response and hepatotoxicity after multiple halothane exposures in guinea pigs. Drug Metab Rev 1997;29:103–22.
29. Vergani D, Mieli-Vergani G, Alberti A, Neuberger J, Eddleston ALWF, Davis M, et al. Antibodies to the surface of halothane-altered rabbit hepatocytes in patients with severe halothane-associated hepatitis. N Engl J Med 1980;303:66–71.
30. Beaune P, Pessayre D, Dansette P, Mansuy D, Manns M. Autoantibodies against cytochromes P450: role in human diseases. Adv Pharmacol 1994;30:199–245.
31. Park BK, Pirmohamed M, Kitteringham NR. Role of drug disposition in drug hypersensitivity: a chemical, molecular, and clinical perspective. Chem Res Toxicol 1998;11:969–88.
32. Satoh H, Fukuda Y, Anderson DK, Ferrans VJ, Gillette JR, Pohl LR. Immunological studies on the mechanism of halothane-induced hepatotoxicity: immunohistochemical evidence of trifluoroacetylated hepatocytes. J Pharmacol Exp Ther 1985;233:857–62.
33. Bourdi M, Chen W, Peter RM, Martin JL, Buters JTM, Nelson SD, et al. Human cytochrome P450 2E1 is a major autoantigen associated with halothane hepatitis. Chem Res Toxicol 1996;9:1159–66.
34. Amouzadeh HR, Bourdi M, Martin JL, Martin BM, Pohl LR. UDP-glucose:glycoprotein glucosyltransferase associates with endoplasmic reticulum chaperones and its activity is decreased in vivo by the inhalation anesthetic halothane. Chem Res Toxicol 1997;10:59–63.
35. Furst SM, Luedke D, Gaw H-H, Reich R, Gandolfi AJ. Demonstration of a cellular immune response in halothane-exposed guinea pigs. Toxicol Appl Pharmacol 1997;143:245–55.
36. Eliasson E, Gardner I, Hume-Smith H, de Waziers I, Beaune P, Kenna JG. Interindividual variability in P450-dependent generation of neoantigens in halothane hepatitis. Chem Biol Interact 1998;116:123–41.

37. Kharasch ED, Hankins D, Mautz D, Thummel KE. Identification of the enzyme responsible for oxidative halothane metabolism: Implications for prevention of halothane hepatitis. Lancet 1996;347:1367–71.

38. Zimmerman HJ, Lewis JH, Ishak KG, Maddrey WC. Ticrynafen-associated hepatic injury: Analysis of 340 cases. Hepatology 1984;4:315–23.

39. Beaune P, Dansette PM, Mansuy D, Kiffel L, Finck M, Amar C, et al. Human antiendoplasmic reticulum autoantibodies appearing in a drug-induced hepatitis are directed against a human liver cytochrome P-450 that hydroxylates the drug. Proc Natl Acad Sci USA 1987;84:551–5.

40. Robin M-A, Maratrat M, Le Roy M, Le Breton F-P, Bonierbale E, Dansette P, et al. Antigenic targets in tienilic acid hepatitis. Both cytochrome P450 2C11 and 2C11-tienilic acid adducts are transported to the plasma membrane of rat hepatocytes and recognized by human sera. J Clin Invest 1996;98:1471–80.

41. López-Garcia MP, Dansette P, Mansuy D. Thiophene derivatives as new mechanism-based inhibitors of cytochromes P-450: Inactivation of yeast-expressed human liver cytochrome P-450 2C9 by tienilic acid. Biochemistry 1994;33:166–75.

42. Lecoeur S, André C, Beaune PH. Tienilic acid-induced hepatitis: anti-liver and kidney microsomal type 2 autoantibodies recognize a three-site conformational epitope on cytochrome P4502C9. Mol Pharmacol 1996;50:326–33.

43. Mitchell JR, Nelson WL, Potter WZ, Sasame HA, Jollow DJ. Metabolic activation of furosemide to a chemically reactive, hepatotoxic metabolite. J Pharmacol Exp Ther 1976;199:41–52.

44. Mitchell JR, Potter WZ, Hinson JA, Jollow DJ. Hepatic necrosis caused by furosemide. Nature 1974;251:508–10.

45. McMurtry RJ, Snodgrass WR, Mitchell JR. Renal necrosis, glutathione depletion, and covalent binding after acetaminophen. Toxicol Appl Pharmacol 1978;46:87–100.

46. Adkinson NF Jr. Drug allergy. In: Middleton E Jr, Ellis EF, Yunginger JW, Reed CE, Adkinson NF Jr, Busse WW. Allergy: principles and practice. St. Louis:Mosby;1998. p. 1212–24.

47. Dipiro JT, Adkinson NF Jr, Hamilton RG. Facilitation of penicillin haptenation to serum proteins. Antimicrob Agents Chemother 1993;37:1463–7.

48. Saxon A, Beall GN, Rohr AS, Adelman DC. Immediate hypersensitivity reactions to beta-lactam antibiotics. Ann Intern Med 1987;107:204–15.

49. Adkinson NF. Risk factors for drug allergy. J Allergy Clin Immunol 1984;74:567–72.

50. Sullivan TJ. Dehaptenation of albumin substituted with benzylpenicillin G determinants [abstract]. J Allergy Clin Immunol 1988;81:222.

51. Weltzien HU, Padovan E. Molecular features of penicillin allergy. J Invest Dermatol 1998;110:203–6.

52. Lafaye P, Lapresie C. Fixation of penicilloyl groups to albumin and appearance of anti-penicilloyl antibodies in penicillin-treated patients. J Clin Invest 1988;82:7–12.

53. Sogn DD, Evans R III, Shepherd GM, Casale TB, Condemi J, Greenberger PA, et al. Results of the National Institute of Allergy and Infections Diseases Collaborative Clinical Trial to test the predictive value of skin testing with major and minor penicillin derivatives in hospitalized adults. Arch Intern Med 1992;152:1025–32.

54. Kosowsky BD, Taylor I, Lown B, Ritchie RF. Long-term use of procainamide following acute myocardial infarction. Circulation 1973;47:1204–10.

55. Drayer DE, Reidenberg MM, Sevy RW. N-Acetylprocainamide: An active metabolite of procainamide. Proc Soc Exp Biol Med 1974;146:358–63.

56. Stec GP, Lertora JJL, Atkinson AJ Jr, Nevin MJ, Kushner W, Jones C, et al. Remission of procainamide-induce lupus erythematosus

with N-acetylprocainamide therapy. Ann Intern Med 1979;90:799–801.

57. Kluger J, Drayer DE, Reidenberg MM, Lahita R. Acetylprocainamide therapy in patients with previous procainamide-induced lupus syndrome. Ann Intern Med 1981;95:18–23.

58. Atkinson AJ Jr, Lertora JJL, Kushner W, Chao GC, Nevin MJ. Efficacy and safety of N-acetylprocainamide in the long-term treatment of patients with ventricular arrhythmias. Clin Pharmacol Ther 1983;33:565–76.

59. Stec GP, Ruo TI, Thenot J-P, Atkinson AJ Jr, Morita Y, Lertora JJL. Kinetics of N-acetylprocainamide deacetylation. Clin Pharmacol Ther 1980;28:659–66.

60. Uetrecht JP. Reactivity and possible significance of hydroxylamine and nitroso metabolites of procainamide. J Pharmacol Exp Ther 1985;232:420–5.

61. Kubicka-Muranyi M, Goebels R, Goebel C, Uetrecht J, Gleichmann E. T lymphocytes ignore procainamide, but respond to its reactive metabolites in peritoneal cells: Demonstration by the adoptive transfer popliteal lymph node assay. Toxicol Appl Pharmacol 1993;122:88–94.

62. Lessard É, Hamelin BA, Labbé L, O'Hara G, Bélanger PM, Turgeon J. Involvement of CYP2D6 activity in the N-oxidation of procainamide in man. Pharmacogenetics 1999;9:683–96.

63. Jiang X, Khursigara G, Rubin RL. Transformation of lupus-inducing drugs to cytotoxic products by activated neutrophils. Science 1994;266:810–13.

64. Rubin RL. Response to technical comment. Science 1995;268:585–6.

65. Rubin RL, Burlingame RW, Arnott JE, Totoritis MC, McNally EM, Johnson AD. IgG but not other classes of anti-[(H2A-H2B)-DNA] is an early sign of procainamide-induced lupus. J Immunol 1995;154:2483–93.

66. Burlingame RW, Rubin RL. Autoantibody to the nucleosome subunit (H2A-H2B)-DNA is an early and ubiquitous feature of lupus-like conditions. Mol Biol Rep 1996;23:159–66.

67. Graham MA, Riley RJ, Kerr DJ. Drug metabolism in carcinogenesis and cancer chemotherapy. Pharmacol Ther 1991;51:275–89.

68. Marselos M, Vainio H. Carcinogenic properties of pharmaceutical agents evaluated in the IARC Monographs programme. 1991;12:1751–66.

69. Green S. Nuclear receptors and chemical carcinogenesis. Trends Pharmacol Sci 1992;13:251–5.

70. List AF, Jacobs A. Biology and pathogenesis of the myelodysplastic syndromes. Semin Oncol 1992;19:14–24.

71. Leone G. Mele L, Pulsoni A, Equitani F, Pagano L. The incidence of the secondary leukemias. Haematologica 1999;84:937–45.

72. Levine EG, Bloomfield CD. Leukemias and myelodysplastic syndromes secondary to drug, radiation, and environmental exposure. Semin Oncol 1992;19:47–84.

73. Smith MA, McCaffrey RP, Karp JE. The secondary leukemias: challenges and research directions. J Natl Cancer Inst 1996;88:407–18.

74. Lensch MW, Rathbun RK, Olson SB, Jones GR, Bagby GC Jr., Selective pressure as an essential force in molecular evolution of myeloid leukemic clones: a view from the window of Fanconi anemia. Leukemia 1999;13:1784–9.

75. Herbst AL, Ulfelder H, Poskanzer DC. Adenocarcinoma of the vagina: association of maternal stilbestrol therapy with tumor appearance in young women. N Engl J Med 1971;284:878–81.

76. Hatch EE, Palmer JR, Titus-Ernstoff L, Noller KL, Kaufman RH, Mittendorf R, et al. Cancer risk in women exposed to diethylstilbestrol in utero. JAMA 1998;280:630–4.

77. Herbst AL. Behavior of estrogen-associated female genital tract cancer and its relation to neoplasia following intrauterine exposure to diethylstilbestrol (DES). Gynecol Oncol 2000;76:147–56.

78. Dickson RB, Stancel GM. Chapter 8: Estrogen receptor-mediated processes in normal and cancer cells. J Natl Cancer Inst Monogr 2000;27:135–45.

79. Roy D, Palangat M, Chen C-W, Thomas RD, Colerangle J, Atkinson A, Yan Z-J. Biochemical and molecular changes at the cellular level in response to exposure to environmental estrogen-like chemicals. J Toxicol Environ Health 1997;50:1–29.

80. Cavalieri E, Frenkel K, Liehr JG, Rogan E, Roy D. Chapter 4: Estrogens as endogenous genotoxic agents—DNA adducts and mutations. J Natl Cancer Inst Monogr 2000;27:75–93.

81. Haaf H, Metzler M. *In vitro* metabolism of diethylstibestrol by hepatic, renal and uterine microsomes of rats and hamsters. Effects of different inducers. Biochem Pharmacol 1985;34:3107–15.

82. Waggoner SE, Anderson SM, Luce MC, Takahashi H, Boyd J. p53 protein expression and gene analysis in clear cell adenocarcinoma of the vagina and cervix. Gynecol Oncol 1996;60:339–44.

83. Boyd J, Takahashi H, Waggoner SE, Jones LA, Hajek RA, Wharton JT, et al. Molecular genetic analysis of clear cell adenocarcinomas of the vagina and cervix associated and unassociated with diethylstibestrol exposure in utero. Cancer 1996;77:507–13.

84. Taussig HB. A study of the German outbreak of phocomelia: The thalidomide syndrome. JAMA 1962;180:1106–14.

85. Szeto HH. Maternal-fetal pharmacokinetics: summary and future directions. NIDA Res Monogr 1995;154:203–7.

86. Ring JA, Ghabrial H, Ching MS, Smallwood RA, Morgan DJ. Fetal hepatic drug elimination. Pharmacol Ther 1999;84:429–45.

87. Hanson JW, Myrianthopoulos NC, Harvey MAS, Smith DW. Risks to the offspring of women treated with hydantoin anticonvulsants, with emphasis on the fetal hydantoin syndrome. Pediatr 1976;89:662–8.

88. Shear NH, Spielberg SP. Anticonvulsant hypersensitivity syndrome. In vitro assessment of risk. J Clin Invest 1988;82:1826–32.

89. Spielberg SP, Gordan GB, Blake DA, Goldstein DA, Herlong HF. Predispostion to phenytoin hepatotoxicity assessed in vitro. N Engl J Med 1981;305:722–7.

90. Wortel JP, Hefferren JJ. Rao GS. Metabolic activation and covalent binding of phenytoin in the rat gingiva. J Periodontal Res 1979;14:178–81.

91. Martz F, Failinger C 3rd, Blake DA. Phenytoin teratogenesis: correlation between embryopathic effect and covalent binding of putative arene oxide metabolite in gestational tissue. J Pharmacol Exp Ther 1977;203:231–9.

92. Strickler SM, Dansky LV, Miller MA, Seni M-H, Andermann E, Spielberg SP. Genetic predisposition to phenytoin-induced birth defects. Lancet 1985;2:746–9.

93. Buehler BA, Delimont D, van Waes M, Finnell RH. Prenatal prediction of risk of the fetal hydantoin syndrome. N Engl J Med 1990;322:1567–72.

94. Winn LM, Wells PG. Phenytoin-initiated DNA oxidation in murine embryo culture, and embryo protection by the antioxidative enzymes superoxide dismutase and catalase: evidence for reactive oxygen species-mediated DNA oxidation in the molecular mechanism of phenytoin teratogenicity. Mol Pharmacol 1995;48:112–20.

95. Wells PG, Winn LM. Biochemical toxicology of chemical teratogenesis. Crit Rev Biochem Mol Biol 1996;31:1–40.

96. Wells PG, Kim PM, Laposa RR, Nicol CJ, Parman T, Winn LM. Oxidative damage in chemical teratogenesis. Mutat Res 1997;396:65–78.

16

Equilibrative and Concentrative Drug Transport Mechanisms

PETER C. PREUSCH

Pharmacological Sciences Training Program, National Institutes of Health, Bethesda, Maryland

INTRODUCTION

The processes of drug absorption, distribution, metabolism, and elimination have been reviewed in earlier chapters. Inherent in each of these processes are membrane transport steps that traditionally have been thought of as being mediated by passive diffusion. For example, as discussed in Chapter 3, inulin diffuses freely through interendothelial junctions of continuous capillaries and through fenestrated or discontinuous capillaries, but does not cross cell-wall membranes. Hence, it is a marker for extracellular fluid space. On the other hand, ethyl alcohol diffuses freely though both capillary and cell-wall membranes and serves as a marker for total body water. Passive diffusion also mediates the distribution of anesthetic gases and many lipophilic drugs.

In recent years, there has been increased appreciation of the role that specific membrane transport proteins play in the processes of drug absorption, distribution, and elimination by both renal and nonrenal pathways. The potential to exploit such transporters to enhance drug bioavailability and improve tissue specific delivery has been recognized. For example, the role of membrane transporters in mediating drug–drug interactions and the potential benefit of intentional co-therapy to enhance drug absorption have been described in Chapter 14. The role of membrane transport proteins as principal agents in the resistance of some tumors to chemotherapy and in the development of microbial antibiotic resistance has also become well established. Finally, it is possible that individual variations in drug transport may contribute

to individual variations in drug responses and adverse drug reactions. Interest in membrane transporters and drug therapy has lead to a number of recent meetings and books on the topic (1–3).

MECHANISMS OF TRANSPORT ACROSS BIOLOGICAL MEMBRANES

Research *in vitro* and *in vivo* (particularly in microorganisms) has defined several modes of transport across biological membranes (4–6):

1. Passive diffusion
2. Facilitated diffusion (i.e., through membrane channels)
3. Carrier-mediated transport
4. Carrier-mediated active transport

Active transport may be subdivided into primary transport, which is directly coupled to substrate oxidation or high-energy phosphate hydrolysis, or secondary transport, which is coupled to co-transport of another molecule or ion down its thermodynamic gradient. We will first consider the thermodynamics of membrane transport and then review mechanisms of both passive and active transport.

Thermodynamics of Membrane Transport

The basic principles of transport across a semipermeable membrane and the relevant thermodynamic

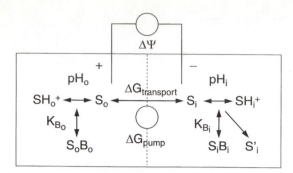

FIGURE 16.1 Model for equilibrative transport across a permeable membrane separating two compartments, arbitrarily designated outside (**o**) or inside (**i**), containing a diffusible solute **S**. The solute is shown as occurring in equilibrium with a non-membrane permeant protonated state **SH⁺** and with non-membrane permeant macromolecular bound species **SB**. The **pH** and dissociation constants (**K_B**) of the binding sites for **S** may differ in the two compartments. **S** is shown as undergoing irreversible chemical conversion to another species **S′** in the inside compartment, only. (See text for additional details.)

TABLE 16.1   Thermodynamic Factors in Drug Transport

Driving force	Example	Relevant compartments
Diffusion	Caffeine	All body compartments
Membrane potential	^{99m}Tc-sestamibi	Cardiac mitochondria
pH trapping	Phenobarbital	Renal tubule
Protein binding	Warfarin	Plasma/liver distribution
Active transport	Captopril	Small intestine
Chemical modification	Cytarabine	Leukocyte

and flux equations governing transport are well established. Books on transport appear quite regularly and often include this material in an introductory chapter. References 4, 7, and 8 give quite exhaustive treatments of the problem from the bioengineering, biophysical, and biological points of view. The following discussion with reference to Figure 16.1 and Table 16.1 is limited to the most basic thermodynamic equations and a qualitative discussion of the principles.

For a neutral solute, the thermodynamic driving force for transport across the membrane (ΔG_{transp}) is the difference in concentation of the solute across the membrane and is given by the first term of Equation 16.1.

$$\Delta G_{transp} = 2.303\, RT \log [S_i]/[S_o] + nF\Delta\psi + \Delta G_{pump} \quad (16.1)$$

where:

> $R = 1.987\ \text{cal/mol°K} = 8.314\ \text{Joules/mol°K}$
> T = absolute temperature in °K
> n = Avogadro's number
> $F = 23.06\ \text{cal/mol-mV} = 96.5\ \text{Joule/mol-mV}$
> $\Delta\psi$ = transmembrane electrical potential (mV)

This movement is entropically driven, since there are more ways to arrange molecules in the larger volume represented by the sum of the compartment volumes than by the donor volume alone. An order of magnitude difference in concentration corresponds to an energy of 1.35 kcal/mol (5.67 kJ/mol) at 23°C or 1.41 kcal/mol (5.94 kJ/mol) at 37°C. At equilibrium, the concentration on both sides of the membrane will be equal.

For a charged solute, the driving force must also include a term reflecting any transmembrane potential difference ($\Delta\psi$). This term may add to or oppose that of the initial concentration gradient. At equilibrium ($\Delta G = 0$) the concentration gradient must be in balance with the electrostatic potential difference. Thus, charged species may be concentrated (electrophoresed) into a compartment against a concentration gradient. An order of magnitude difference in concentration of a charged solute across a membrane corresponds to 58.5 mV at 23°C and 61.5 mV at 37°C for a singly charged species, and about 30 mV for a doubly charged species, and so on. Alternately, one can consider the process of transporting a charged molecule across a membrane as one which will contribute to establishing a transmembrane potential. Such transport is called electrogenic. The combined effect of the concentration gradient of an ion across the membrane and the influence of the membrane potential defines the electrochemical potential gradient for that species across the membrane. This total electrochemical potential may be expressed in kcal, joules, or, commonly, in mV. Most cells, whether microorganisms in growth medium or mammalian cells in communication with the blood stream, have a negative potential inside versus their surroundings. Therefore, the uptake of cations into cells is a thermodynamically favorable process.

In the case of active transport, the movement of the substrate is coupled to some other energetic process (ΔG_{pump}), such as co-transport of another substrate or ion according to its electrochemical potential gradient or the hydrolysis of ATP. Active transport is generally considered to involve specifically coupled reactions catalyzed by a single transmembrane protein assembly. For example, members of the ABC family of transport proteins specifically couple the energy of ATP hydrolysis to the pumping of substrate molecules across a transmembrane concentration gradient. Members of the major facilitator superfamily couple the transport of protons, sodium, potassium, or other ions (including organic ions such as α-keto-glutarate) down their electrochemical concentration gradients to transport of a host of other ions and molecules.

In real cells, multiple transmembrane pumps and channels maintain and regulate the transmembrane potential. Furthermore, those processes are at best only in a quasi steady state, not truly at equilibrium. Thus, electrophoresis of an ionic solute across a membrane may be a passive equilibrative diffusion process in itself, but is effectively an active and concentrative process when the cell is considered as a whole. Other factors that influence transport across membranes include pH gradients, differences in binding, and coupled reactions that convert the transported substrate into another chemical form. In each case, transport is governed by the concentration of free and permeable substrate available in each compartment. The effect of pH on transport will depend on whether the permeant species is the protonated form (e.g., acids) or the unprotonated form (e.g., bases), the pK_a of the compound, and on the pH in each compartment. The effects can be predicted with reference to the Henderson-Hasselbach equation (Equation 16.2), which states that the ratio of acid and base forms changes by a factor of ten for each unit change in either pH or pK_a.

$$pH = pK_a + \log \frac{[base]}{[acid]} \qquad (16.2)$$

Thus, if the unprotonated form of a base with pK_a of 9.0 is permeant (e.g., amines) and the pH outside increases from 7 to 8, the concentration of the free base increases from 1% to about 10% of the total (a large effect). If the protonated from were the permeant species of similar pK_a (e.g., phenols), the same unit pH change would yield a change in the permeant species from about 99 to 90% of the total (not a very important change). Transmembrane gradients of metal ions or other titrants that interact with drug molecules will similarly affect drug transport depending on the concentration ranges, dissociation constants, and identity of the free drug or complex as the permeant species.

Plasma protein binding is important in pharmacokinetics because it influences the concentration of free drug available for transport. As discussed in Chapter 14, this leads to interactions between compounds that compete for the same binding sites on serum albumin. However, co-administered compounds also may compete for tissue binding sites as demonstrated by the interaction between quinidine and digoxin (9). The extent of drug distribution across a membrane will depend on the relative affinity of competing compounds for both plasma and tissue binding sites.

Finally, transport can also be driven by the conversion of intracellular substrate into another chemical form. For example, in the case of nucleoside drugs, conversion to the corresponding nucleotides by appropriate kinases may be the limiting factor in cellular uptake

and activation. The same principle applies to sulfation, glucuronidation, prodrug activations, or other metabolic processes that provide a removal of the transported species from the transportable (free) internal pool. In some cases, transport is directly coupled to substrate modification as in the uptake of sugars in to bacterial cells by PEP-coupled phosphorylation systems.

Passive Diffusion

Passive diffusion is the transport of a molecule across a lipid bilayer membrane according to its electrochemical potential gradient without the assistance of additional transporter molecules. This process can be studied in pure lipid membranes, although it is acknowledged that the properties of even relatively pure lipid patches in native membranes are altered by the high density of neighboring protein molecules. The physical and functional properties of membranes can be modeled with varying levels of detail and mathematical complexity. The simplest model represents the membrane as a single semipermeable barrier separating two uniform aqueous compartments. Transport is characterized by a single reversible rate constant. A more complex model represents the membrane as an intervening third compartment of 25–30 Å thickness with properties equivalent to a bulk organic solvent. Transport is modeled as a reversible partition of molecules from the donor aqueous phase into the membrane compartment and rate-limiting release of the solute from the organic membrane phase into the receiving compartment. This model yields a rate equation of the same form as the Michaelis–Menten equation in enzyme kinetics. Although such kinetics are observed for mediated membrane transport, they are not typically observed for simple diffusive transport. A more sophisticated model adds barriers of high charge density and high dielectric constant on either side of the organic compartment to represent the phospholipid head groups. Still other models may incorporate unstirred diffusion layers extending into the aqueous compartments. These models reveal different points of view about what constitutes the most important rate determining barrier to bulk transport.

Molecular dynamics simulations (10, 11) have provided a provocative image of passive diffusion of solute molecules within the membrane bilayer (Figure 16.2). These simulations illustrate the rapid but restricted mobility of the lipid side chains, and demonstrate that the membrane hydrophobic region is not particularly well modeled by bulk solvent properties. They suggest the spontaneous formation of voids and transient channels within the membrane and the ability of small molecules and ions to diffuse within the membrane by hopping among these voids (*ca.* 8 Å

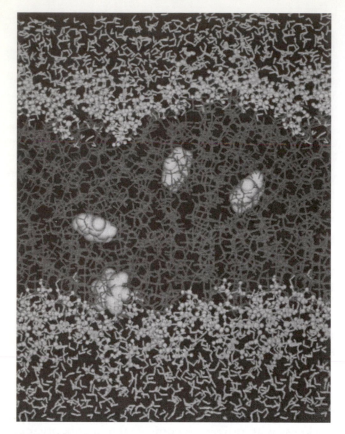

FIGURE 16.2 Molecular dynamics simulation of the diffusion of benzene within a hydrated lipid bilayer membrane. Benzene molecules are shown as CPK models; atoms in the phospholipid head groups are shown as ball and stick models; and hydrocarbon chains and water molecules as dark and light stick models, respectively. (Reproduced with permission from Bassolino-Klimas D, Alper HE, Stouch TR. Biochemistry 1993;32:12624–37.)

jumps on a 5 psec time scale). They highlight the importance of concerted large conformational motions, occurring with relatively low frequency compared to continual small motions (*ca.* 1.5 Å occurring on the 100 fsec time scale). Thus far, these methods have been used to successfully model the diffusion of water, hydrogen ions, small organics, and various drugs within the bilayer. They have provided reasonably good agreement with experimental data on intramembrane diffusion. The types of motion available to small molecules such as benzene differ qualitatively from those available to a fairly large organic drug such as nifedipine. Thus far, no one has successfully modeled the full process of transport from one aqueous compartment into the membrane and into the other aqueous compartment. The problem has been that the feasible time scale for molecular dynamics simulations is presently in the nsec range, whereas the rates of drug transport are typically in the msec range. Although diffusion within the organic phase of the

membrane appears to be facile, the steps for insertion into and exit from that phase across the polar head group region are exceedingly slow.

Extensive efforts have been made to develop Quantitative Structure/Activity Relationships (QSAR) that predict membrane transport (12, 13). Particularly extensive use has been made of log P (log solvent/water partition coefficient values) and the Hansch equation (Equation 16.3).

$$\log(1/C) = -k (\log P)^2 + k'(\log P) + \rho\sigma + k'' \qquad (16.3)$$

where:

C = substrate concentration or dose producing a given effect (ED_{50}, IC_{50}, rate of reaction or transport)

log P = partition coefficient or lipophilicity factor π

σ = Hammet electronic substituent effect constants

k, k', k'', ρ = regression coefficients

Derivation of this correlation originally was based on the expectation that passive diffusion across a lipid bilayer would be the limiting factor in drug action, but many other factors, such as enzyme inhibition and receptor binding data, often also correlate well. The octanol/water partition coefficient (log $P_{octanol/water}$) is most commonly used and is generally assumed unless otherwise noted. Reverse phase HPLC and immobilized artificial membrane methods for estimating log P have largely replaced actual liquid/liquid extraction methods for determining these values. The ability to correlate log P values with structure has become quite good, and calculated values (CLOGP) are now often used.

Table 16.2 presents a selection of drugs, transport sites, and parameters that have been studied in QSAR studies relevant to drug absorption and excretion measurements excerpted from a much larger table (13). Overall conclusions from this work are that transportability correlates with: 1) lipophilicity (log P), 2) water solubility, 3) pK_a, and 4) molecular weight. Correlations with lipophilicity are almost always good. Although different log P ranges are optimal for oral (log P = 0.5 – 2.0), buccal (log P = 4 – 4.5), and topical (log P>2.0) delivery, there is much overlap. Unfortunately, increasing drug lipophilicity may increase delivery generally throughout the body and do little to improve selective delivery to target tissues. Water solubility bears on the total concentration available for transport (e.g., in GI absorption). Solubility is more difficult to predict from structure than is log P, although calculated estimates can be made from melting point data and calculated solvation energies. Molecular weight is related to diffusivity ($D \propto 1/\sqrt{mw}$), both in the membrane and the aqueous phases. It has

TABLE 16.2 Sample of QSAR Studies on Transport[a]

Drug classes	Systems	Physical parameters correlated with activity[b]
Absorption as log (% absorbed), log permeability, or log k		
Barbiturates	Gastric	$\log P_{CHCl_3/water}$, R_m
Sulfonamides	Gastric	$\log P_{isoamyl\ alcohol/water}$
Anilines	Gastric	pK_a
Xanthines	Intestinal	$D_{pH\ 5.3}$
Cardiac glycosides	Intestinal	$\log P_{octanol/water}$, R_m
Excretion as log (% excreted), log CL, or log k		
Penicillins	Biliary	$\log P$
Sulfathiazoles	Biliary	$\log P_{octanol/water}$, pK_a
Sulfapyridines	Renal	R_m, pK_a
Sulfonamides	Renal	π, pK_a
Amphetamines	Renal	$\log P_{heptane/buffer}$

[a] Adapted from Table VI in Austel B, Kutter R. Absorption, distribution and metabolism of drugs. In: Toplis JG, editor. Quantitative structure activity relationships. Medicinal Chemistry Monographs, vol 19. New York: Academic Press, 1983. p. 437–96.

[b] k = rate constant, CL = clearance, P = partition coefficient for indicated solvents,

R_m = relative mobility under specific chromatographic conditions, $D_{pH5.3}$ = distribution coefficient (a partition coefficient corrected for fractional ionization at pH 5.3), π = substitutent lipophilicity values.

been found empirically that there is a cutoff molecular weight (< 500–650 Da) above which passive diffusion across most biological membranes is excluded.

Apart from these basic rules of thumb, the ability to predict the relationship between molecular structure and transport across biological membranes is limited outside a narrow range of compounds. Confounding factors include inaccurate, incomplete and/or noncomparable data, and the potential existence of multiple drug transport mechanisms in real biological membranes. In particular, limited QSAR data is available for the specific drug transporters that are considered next.

Carrier-Mediated Transport: Facilitated Diffusion and Active Transport

Several characteristics distinguish carrier-mediated transport from passive diffusion. Rates are generally faster than for passive diffusion, and transport is solute specific and shows a greater temperature variation (Q_{10}). Transport is saturable, resembling Michaelis–Menten enzyme kinetics. Transport rates may not be the same in both directions across the membrane at a given substrate concentration. Transport may be inhibitable by competitive transport substrates or by

noncompetitive inhibitors acting at other sites. Transport may be regulated by cell state (e.g., by phosphorylation, induction, or repression of transporter molecules), or by gene copy number. Transport is tissue specific because it depends on the expression of particular transporters that do not occur in all membranes. Active transport is a special from of carrier-mediated transport in which solute concentration is mechanistically linked to energetically favorable reactions (Equation 16.1). Distinction between primary pumps and secondary transporters may be made on the basis of cosubstrate dependence (e.g., oxidative substrate, ATP, or PEP requirement) or the effects of various ionophores, uncouplers, and inhibitors of primary pumps.

Mechanisms of drug transport *in vivo* have been better established in bacterial systems than in mammalian systems, owing the greater experimental control and access to genetic manipulations that can be achieved. Table 16.3 lists examples of drugs for which the transport in bacteria is dominated by the indicated mechanisms (6).

The distinction between facilitated diffusion through channels and carrier-mediated transport is somewhat artificial, but may be justified on the basis of specificity. For example β-lactams in general can pass through nonselective bacterial outer cell membrane channels (e.g., OmpF) via passive diffusion, whereas imipenem (and related zwitterionic carbapenems) can also utilize OprD channels, which preferentially recognize basic amino acids and dipeptides. The identification of mutants that selectively confer imipenem resistance suggests that more intimate protein-drug associations are involved in carrier-mediated transport than in facilitated diffusion, which may be limited only by pore diameter.

TABLE 16.3 Transport Mechanisms in Bacteria[a]

Transport mechanism	Example
Passive diffusion across lipid bilayer	Fluroquinolones
	Tetracyclines (hydrophobic)
Facilitated diffusion (non-selective)	Beta-lactams
	Tetracyclines (hydrophylic)
Mediated transport (selective)	Imipenem
	Catechols
Active transport	Aminoglycosides
	Cycloserine

[a] Adapted from Table 1 in Hancock REW. Bacterial transport as an import mechanism and target for antimicrobials. In: Georgopapadakou NH, editor. Drug transport in antimicrobial and anticancer chemotherapy. New York: Marcel Dekker, Inc.; 1995. p. 289–306.

The tetracyclines provide an interesting example in that bacterial uptake is passive (by both nonmediated and carrier-mediated pathways), efflux is active, and they are subject to pH, membrane potential, and metal ion gradient effects (14). Tetracycline is both a weak base (pK_{a1} = 3.3) and a weak acid (pK_{a2} = 7.7, pK_{a3} = 9.7) and is subject to pH trapping. Furthermore, the anions can chelate divalent cations such as magnesium and the metal chelates have altered solubility. Uptake across the outer membrane of gram negative bacteria is nonmediated for hydrophobic tetracyclines and carrier mediated via porins (e.g. OmpF) for hydrophilic homologs. Nonmediated diffusion via the lipopolysaccharide depends on the neutral species, whereas carrier-mediated diffusion via the porins favors the magnesium-bound anion (net positive charge) and is enhanced by the Donnan membrane potential. In contrast to most mammalian membranes, passive diffusion across the lipopolysaccharide outer membrane of *E. coli* is slower for more hydrophobic analogs and may account for their lower antimicrobial activity. Uptake across the cytoplasmic membrane is by nonmediated passive diffusion of the neutral species, and is thermodynamically driven by the pH gradient across the inner membrane (pH 7.8 inside, pH 6.1 outside, for cells grown at a nominal pH 7.0). Efflux of tetracycline, on the other hand, is due to active transport via TetA, which catalyzes antiport of the [Mg-anion chelate]$^{+1}$ (out) in exchange for a proton (in).

Uptake Mechanisms Dependent on Membrane Trafficking

Pinocytosis (cell sipping) has been thought to be a nonspecific, nonsaturable, noncarrier-mediated form of membrane transport via vesicular uptake of bulk fluid into cells from the surrounding medium (15, 16). This mechanism is most relevant to large particles and polymer conjugates. The term has fallen from favor and one suspects that many events previously ascribed to nonspecific pinocytosis are now recognized as being due to specific receptor-mediated endocytosis. *Endocytosis* is specific and intrinsic to the mechanism of action of many macromolecular drugs This process is also used to deliver small molecules as prodrugs, and mediates the distribution and clearance of many contemporary drug materials, including many biotechnology products, most peptide hormones, and cytokines (e.g., insulin, growth hormone, erythropoetin, G-CSR, and interleukins) (17). Receptor-mediated endocytosis plays an important role in the nephrotoxicity of aminoglycoside antibiotics (18). After glomerular filtration, aminoglycosides bind to charge-mediated receptor sites on the brush border of proximal renal tubule cells. They are then incorporated into apical endocytotic vac-

uoles and are translocated intracellularly where they cause lysosomal disruption and cell necrosis. *Transcytosis* is a variant that involves coupled cellular pathways for receptor-mediated uptake, transcellular vesicle migration, and exocytosis on the opposite cell surface (Figure 16.3) (19, 20).

DESCRIPTION OF SELECTED MEMBRANE PROTEIN TRANSPORTERS

A large number of transport functions in various tissues have been defined physiologically and/or pharmacologically. A substantial number can now be associated with specific gene, mRNA, and deduced protein sequences. Relatively few have been isolated and fully characterized biochemically. Lists of transport functions, transporters, and substrates can be found in various reviews (21–29). It is not always clear when the nomenclature refers to a transport activity or to specific, genetically defined transport proteins. Table 16.4 provides a partial listing of membrane transporter families.

The ATP-binding cassette (ABC) superfamily and the major facilitator (MF) superfamily account for the majority of membrane transporters. Peptide transporters of both types have been reported. Both anion and cation pumps of both types are known. Although most ABC family members catalyze active transport coupled to ATP hydrolysis, members of the MF superfamily may catalyze either mediated diffusion or active transport (coupled most often to H^+ or Na^+ co-transport). A few examples suffice to illustrate the general points.

The P-glycoprotein Efflux Pump

The most extensively studied drug transporter is undoubtedly P-glycoprotein (P-gp), the product of the *mdr1* (multidrug resistance) gene (30, 31). This transporter was discovered during the 1970s through studies of chemotherapy-resistant tumors in cancer patients. Multidrug resistance can be acquired both by patients receiving chemotherapy and by cultured cells exposed to chemotherapeutic agents *in vitro*. Cells, which become resistant to one chemotherapeutic agent, are often found to be cross-resistant to a wide range of other drugs to which they have never been exposed. Although other mechanisms can occur, the most common mechanism entails increased expression of a membrane phospho-glycoprotein of approximately 170 kDa, which is an active efflux transporter. This protein was dubbed P-glycoprotein [P for altered permeability]. Human MDR1 and MDR2 are 76% identical in sequence, but only MDR1 plays a role in drug resistance. MDR2 is most likely involved in

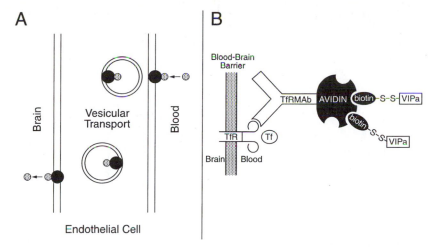

FIGURE 16.3 Mechanism of transcellular drug delivery across the blood-brain barrier. *Panel A:* Schematic representation of vesicle trafficking and topology. *Panel B:* An example of this drug transport mechanism in the delivery of a biotin-vasoactive intestinal peptide (VIPa) disulfide-linked prodrug across the blood-brain barrier via the transferrin receptor (20, 21). Binding of a monoclonal antibody (TfRMAb) to the transferrin receptor (TfR) on the blood side of brain endothelial cells results in endocytosis of the MAb-receptor complex along with attached materials (avidin-biotin-VIPa conjugate). Fusion of the vesicle on the brain interstitial side of the cell exposes the modified mAB-transferrin receptor complex to the brain side of the barrier. Reductases on the brain side cleave the disulfide linkages that attach the peptide drug to the delivery vehicle, releasing vasoactive intestinal peptide to express its pharmacological effect. (Adapted from: Bickel U, Pardridge WM. Vector-mediated delivery of opiod peptides to the brain. In: Rapaka RS, editor. Membranes and barriers: targeted drug delivery. NIDA Res Monograph 154, NIH Pub. #95–3889. p. 28–46.)

TABLE 16.4   Partial Listing of Membrane Transporters

Transporter family	Representative substrates
ABC superfamily	
ABC peptide transporter family	
P-glycoprotein (MDR) family	
MDR 1a, 1b, 2, 3	Organic cations, lipids (PC)
MRP1,2,3	Organic anions, GSX conjugates, GSH co-transporter
cMOAT	Canalicular multispecific anion transporter = MRP2
MXR	Mitoxantrone, doxorubicin, daunorubicin
cBAT	Canalicular bile acid transport
Major facilitator superfamily	
POT	Proton-coupled oligopeptide transporter
NT	Na$^+$-coupled nucleotide transporter
NTCP	Na$^+$-copuled taurocholate protein
OATP	Polyspecfic organic anion transport protein
OAT-K1	Renal methotrexate transporter
OCT	Organic cation transporter—electrogenic
RFC	Reduced folate carrier
sGSHT	Glutathione conjugate transporter

transport of phosphatidylcholine. Similar proteins occur in rodents, and knockout mice have been valuable in defining the *in vivo* roles of these proteins.

The *mdr1* gene encodes a 1280-amino acid protein and is thought to contain 12 hydrophobic transmembrane helices (two groups of six) with globular cytosolic domains inserted between TM6 and TM7 and at the end of TM12 (Figure 16.4). This motif is characteristic of the ABC superfamily of membrane transport proteins. Each of the globular domains contains one ATP hydrolysis site, that includes the canonical Walker A (nucleotide binding) and Walker B (magnesium binding) sequences, which also occur in other ATPases. In addition, both include the Walker C (linker peptide or dodecapetide) region that is a signature of the ABC superfamily. Another notable member of the class is the cystic fibrosis transmembrane conductance regulator (CFTR), which has an identical topology, but seems to function as an ATP-regulated chloride channel.

The multidrug resistance-related protein (MRP) family and the mitoxantrone-resistance (MXR) family discussed later are also ABC transporters. All members of the class include two TM domains and two cytoplasmic ATPase domains. The order of these domains within a polypeptide and their arrangements into single or multiple polypeptides include all possible variations. In some cases, the proteins are expressed as half-trans-

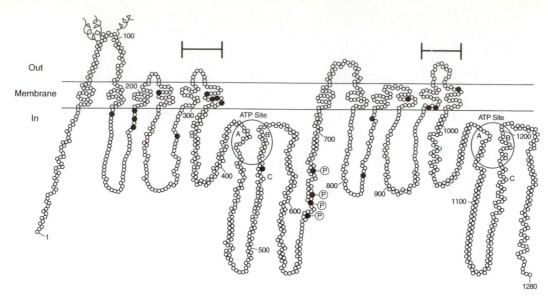

FIGURE 16.4 A hypothetical two-dimensional model of human P-glycoprotein based on hydropathy analysis of the amino acid sequence and its functional domains. Amino acid residues (o); the positions of selected mutations that alter the substrate specificity of P-gp (•); ATP sites *(large circles)*; N-linked glycosylation sites *(squiggly lines)*; phosphorylation sites *(circled P)*; and Walker A, B, and C regions are indicated. Numbers refer to specific amino acid positions, and bars above the model indicate regions labeled with photoaffinity analogs. (Reproduced with permission from Ambudkar SV, Dey S, Hrycyna CA, Ramachandra M, Pastan I, Gottesman MM. Annu Rev Pharmacol Toxicol 1999;39:361–98.)

porters containing only one TM domain and one ATPase domain. However, these appear to be functional as either homo- or heterodimers with another TM and ATPase domain. Three glycosylation sites occur within the first extracellular loop of P-gp. These are not required for transport function, but do affect the half-life of the protein, its folding within the endoplasmic reticulum, and its delivery to the cell surface. A series of phosphorylation sites occur in the linker domain between the first half-molecule and the second half. Again, these are not required for transport activity, but may play a regulatory role.

The mechanism of ATP hydrolysis by MDR1 has been examined and is not fundamentally different from that of the more familiar F1 ATPase, but the mechanism of coupling ATP hydrolysis to transmembrane transport of substrates is unclear. An X-ray crystallographic structure has been determined for the ATPase domain (RbsA) of the *E. coli* ribose transport protein (32). This structure illustrated details of the active site and demonstrated that the ABC signature sequence was far removed from the ATP binding site. It is believed that this sequence is involved in communicating conformational changes occurring at the active site to binding sites in the TM domains. Turnover of the enzyme probably involves a two-stroke sequence: 1) binding of substrate and hydrolysis at one of the ATP sites in order to load the transported molecule on one side of the membrane; and 2) hydrolysis at the second ATP site in order to expel the

substrate from the other side of the membrane. An alternate two-stroke model involves: 1) substrate binding followed by ATP hydrolysis to expel the substrate from the cell; and 2) ATP hydrolysis at the second site in order to re-cock the enzyme into a conformation that can bind substrate. These mechanisms are not distinguishable at this time. Evidence suggests that substrate binds by absorption from within the inner leaflet of the membrane bilayer, rather than from bulk solvent in the cytosol. In this sense, the action of MDR1 is like that of MDR2, which is thought to flip phosphatidylcholine from the inner leaflet to the outer leaflet of the membrane. MDR1 has been called a hydrophobic vacuum cleaner, whose evolutionary job was to clean membranes of foreign natural toxins. Expulsion of substrate into the aqueous phase outside the cell is facilitated by trapping agents such as serum albumin that prevent reentry of the hydrophobic substrate into the membrane. Intracellular auxillary proteins may also play a role in delivering hydrophobic substrates to the transporter binding site.

The most challenging mechanistic question about P-gp is the basis for its ability to transport such a wide range of molecular structures (Table 14.2). Extensive substrate structure/activity studies and transporter mutagenesis, chemical, and photolabeling studies have been used to test structure/function hypotheses for P-gp. The model that emerges is one of multiple partially overlapping binding sites with few absolutely required determinants. Most of the substrate contacting residues are located in two clusters in TM5,6 and TM11,12. It is hypothesized that these form two binding sites: one for high affinity substrate recognition inside the cell, and one for low affinity binding effectively outside the cell. There may also be an allosteric binding site, but the kinetics of membrane-bound enzymes and their substrates are difficult to interpret. Numerous drugs are known to be transported by P-gp and are competitive inhibitors of the transport of other drugs. These are commonly hydrophobic, often planar aromatic compounds, and compounds that are neutral or positively charged at physiological pH, with molecular weights in the 200–1000 Da range. However, there is very little other obvious structural similarity. Pharmacophore recognition methods only work across a small subset of closely related compounds, and the rules for one class do not carry over to another class of molecules. A few drugs are nonsubstrate competitive inhibitors that bind, but are not transported. Another class of inhibitors act through inhibition of the ATP hydrolysis steps (e.g., vanadate ion). These latter inhibitors are useful mechanistic probes; however, none have the selectivity relative to other ATP utilizing enzymes that is required for them to be developed for clinical use as MDR inhibitors.

The MRP Family of Transporters

The Multidrug-resistance Related Protein (MRP) family is closely related and structurally similar to the MDR family (26, 27). MRP1 was initially identified in lung cells, which were known not to express P-gp. It has been shown to pump anionic compounds (as opposed to the cations pumped by P-gp). Substrates for MRP1 include anionic natural products; glutathione, glucuronyl, and sulfate conjugates; and, in some cases, neutral molecules coupled to glutathione transport without conjugation. In liver, MRP1 is present on the sinusoidal surface of the hepatocyte. MRP2 is similar to MRP1, except in its tissue distribution and localization. In liver, it is expressed on the canalicular membrane, and is also known as the canalicular multispecific organic anion transporter (cMOAT). Homology searching has revealed seven MRP family members. MRP3 is similar to MRP1, but with narrower substrate specificity. MRP4 and MRP5 act as nucleotide transporters. MRP6 and MRP7 can be recognized by their sequences, but their functions are unknown at this time.

The Nucleoside Transporter Family

The nucleoside transporter (NT) family is illustrative of the multifacilitator superfamily (22, 23). Both naturally occurring nucleosides and most nucleoside drugs are very hydrophilic and do not readily cross

bilayer membranes except by mediated or active transport. The relevant transport activities have been defined functionally by their substrates, co-substrates, and inhibitor sensitivities. Currently known nucleoside transport activities are either equilibrative or concentrative. The equilibrative transporters allow the free exchange of nucleosides across membranes according to their concentration gradients. Concentrative transporters translocate nucleosides into a cell against a thermodynamic gradient by coupling transport to the electrogenic co-transport of sodium ions into the cell. Equilibrative transporters are ubiquitous. Two classes can be distinguished as nitrobenzylthioinosine sensitive (es) or insensitive (ei). Five classes of concentrative transporters (N1–N5) can be distinguished by their substrate specificities. These transporters are more selectively expressed in epithelial tissues (intestine, kidney, and choroid plexus) and in lymphoid cells and tissues.

The es transporter of erythrocytes has been identified by photoaffinity labeling, purified, and characterized as a relative of the equilibrative GLUT1 glucose transporter (a member of the 12 transmembrane spanning major facilitator superfamily). Variations in molecular weight and glycosylation state occur in various species and tissues. The N3 concentrative transporter of rabbit kidney SNST1 was cloned by hybridization to a probe for the rabbit intestine Na^+-coupled glucose transporter SGLT1 (a member of the Na^+-coupled organic co-transporter family). As in the case of the GLUT1 family, the sequence suggests a protein with 12 transmembrane spans; however, in this instance several amino acid residues are clearly implicated in the Na^+ co-transport function. An N2 transporter gene (cnt1) has been cloned from rat intestine by expression in *Xenopus* oocytes. In this case, the sequence suggests a 14 TM protein with multiple glycosylation and phosphorylation sites. Although differing in molecular detail, it is likely that all members of the equilibrative and Na^+-linked families will be similar in overall three-dimensional structure and transport mechanism. However, there is a wealth of detailed variation on which selectivity in drug transport or transporter inhibition may eventually be based.

Cells differ in their reliance on nucleoside uptake and salvage versus *de novo* biosynthetic pathways for normal growth, and hence, they differ in their sensitivity to nucleoside drugs. Table 16.5 (adapted from Tables 1–4 in reference 23) lists some nucleoside drugs, diseases for which they have been used, and the transporters that recognize them. In addition to the es, ei, and N1–N5 nucleoside transporters, some nucloside drugs also utilize nucleobase (NB) transporters.

TABLE 16.5   Nucleoside Drugs, Indications, and Transporters [a]

Nucleoside drug	Clinical indication	Transporter specificity
Cladribine (Cl-dAdo)	Leukemia	es, ei, N1, N5
Cytarabine (araC)	Leukemia	es, ei
2-Fludarabine (F-araA)	Leukemia	es, N1, N5
Pentostatin (dCF)	Leukemia	es
Floxidine (F-dURd)	Colon Cancer	es, ei
Didanosine (ddI)	HIV	es, NB
Zalcitabine (ddC)	HIV	es, N2
Zidovudine (AZT)	HIV	N2
Acyclovir (ACV)	HSV	NB
Gancyclovir (GCV)	HSV	es, NB
Vidarabine (araA)	HSV	es, ei, N1
Idoxuridine (IdUrd)	HSV	es
Trifluridine (F3-dThd)	HSV	Not Determined
Ribavirin (RBV)	RNA/DNA viruses	Not Determined

[a] Adapted from Tables 1–4 in Cass CE. Nucleoside transport. In: Georgopapadakou NH, editor. Drug transport in antimicrobial and anticancer chemotherapy. New York: Marcel Dekker, Inc.; 1995. p. 408–51.

The greatest successes with nucleoside drugs have been in the treatment of leukemias, lymphomas, HIV, and herpes virus infections. These drugs act intracellularly after conversion to nucleotide phosphates, generally by blocking DNA synthesis. Although nucleoside transport is important, the limiting step that defines the activity of nucleoside drugs is often the nucleotide kinase-mediated conversion of the nucleoside to the nucleotide. However, resistance to nucleoside therapy has been observed for cells with reduced transport activity as well as for cells with altered kinase activity or altered target sensitivity. Furthermore, these processes may be subject to coordinate regulation.

ROLE OF TRANSPORTERS IN PHARMACOKINETICS AND DRUG ACTION

There is increasing recognition of the important role played by protein transporter molecules in the processes of drug absorption, distribution, and elimination. This is particularly true with respect to the barrier and drug-eliminating functions of gastrointestinal epithelial cells, hepatocytes, and renal tubule cells (24). Figure 16.5 schematizes drug transport in the body and some of the known transport proteins. Trans-

porters also are important determinants of the response of cancers and bacteria to chemotherapy.

Role of Transporters in Drug Absorption

As described in Chapter 4, oligopeptide and monocarboxylic acid transporters facilitate the absorption of certain drugs. There have been a number of recent demonstrations that these natural transport pathways can be exploited to enhance drug action. An example demonstrating this concept is the discovery that valacyclovir is a substrate for the PEPT-1 transporter (33). Valacyclovir is an amino acid ester prodrug of the antiviral drug acyclovir. The usefulness of acyclovir is somewhat limited by its poor bioavailability. However, the oral bioavailability of valacyclovir is increased three- to five-fold in human subjects. Experiments using a rat intestinal perfusion model demonstrated a 3- to 10-fold increased intestinal permeability of valacyclovir over acyclovir. The effect was specific (i.e., exhibited structure/activity preferences among a family of amino acid ester prodrugs), stereospecific for L-valine, saturable, inhibitable by known PEPT-1 substrates (cephalexin, dipeptides), and competitive with other amino acid ester prodrugs (e.g., gly-acyclovir, val-AZT). Studies using Chinese hamster ovary (CHO) cells expressing hPEPT-1 demonstrated competition between valacyclovir and the classic PEPT-1 substrate ^{3}H-glycyl-sarcosine. Experiments in Caco-2 cells showed enhanced, saturable, and inhibitable mucosal to serosal transport, consistent with active transport via the PEPT-1 transporter. In contrast, serosal to mucosal transport was shown to be by passive diffusion. Furthermore, transport was accompanied by hydrolysis of the prodrug, such that although drug was taken up as valacyclovir, it appeared on the serosal side as acyclovir.

This example is unusual in that valacyclovir is an amino acid ester of a nucleoside that does not closely resemble the normal dipeptide substrates of the PEPT-1 transporter. A number of other drugs such as methotrexate are probably transported by proteins that normally transport the metabolites that they resemble and antagonize (e.g., folates). However, these cases represent fortuitous examples of drug transportability "natural selection" during the drug discovery and development process. With increased understanding of the specificity determinants of nutrient transport, a rational basis for designing or redesigning drugs to exploit specific transporters may emerge.

As discussed in Chapters 4 and 14, both P-gp and CYP3A4 are co-localized in intestinal epithelial cells and may limit bioavailability either by intestinal first-pass metabolism by CYP3A4 or by P-gp-mediated exsorption. Many of the substrates for CYP3A4 are

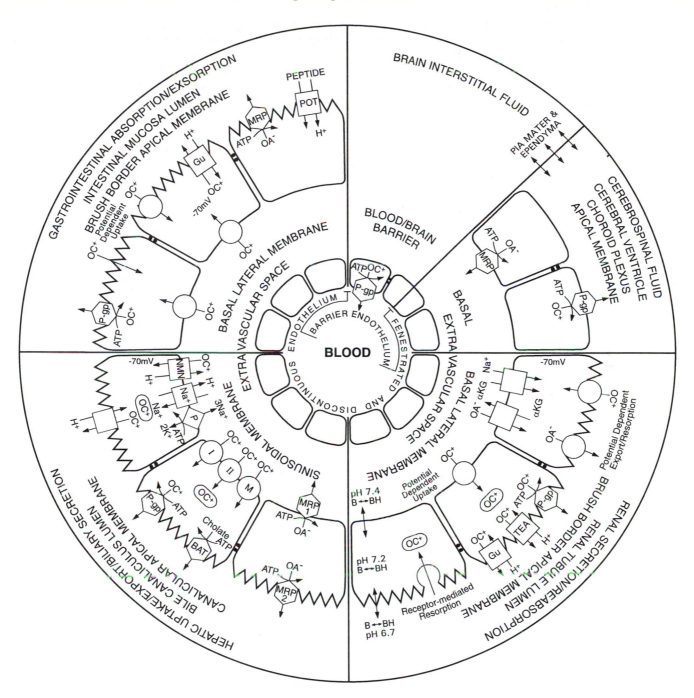

FIGURE 16.5 Schematic of drug transport in the body indicating cellular topology for selected transporters. Capillaries with tight junctions are designated by •=•, organic cations by OC$^+$, and organic anions by OA$^-$. Members of the ABC superfamily of transport proteins, designated by ⬡ include P-glycoprotein (P-gp), multidrug resistance proteins (MRP), MRP1, MRP2 or cMOAT, and the bile acid transporter (BAT). Active-transporters, designated by ☐ include the guanidium transporter (Gu), triethylammonium transporter (TEA), N-methyl nicotinamide transporter (NMN), proton-coupled oligopeptide transporter (POT). Carrier-mediated transport or facilitated diffusion, designated by ○ includes the Type I (I) and Type II (II) cation carriers and the multi-specific non-charge selective carrier (M). Na$^+$/K$^+$ P-type ATPase is designated by ⬦, and ◠ denotes intracellular sequestration.

also substrates for P-gp (see Tables 14.1 and 14.2), so that many CYP3A4 substrates may also be competing for transport by P-gp or may modify its level of expression (34). There is no sequence homology between these proteins and likely no tertiary structural homology. However, both likely have similar broadly accessible hydrophobic pockets.

Competition between substrates for limiting transporter molecules and other effects lead to drug–drug, drug–food, and drug–dietary supplement interactions very similar to those seen with CYP450s. In an explicit test of GI absorption/exsorption interactions, small intestinal secretion of intravenously infused talinolol, a β1-adrenergic receptor antagonist, has been studied in healthy volunteers using a steady-state perfusion technique (35). Perfusion of dexverapamil (R-verapamil) into the intestinal lumen lowered the intestinal secretion of talinolol 29–56%. The conclusion is that bioavailability of talinolol is in part limited by exsorption and may be subject to drug interactions during absorption. In this study R-verapamil was used because it is known to affect P-gp-mediated drug transport, but is devoid of the pharmacological effects of S-verapamil. Hence, it can be used safely as a probe in clinical studies of P-gp inhibition. P-gp can be activated as well as inhibited, as evidenced by the ability of grapefruit juice to increase P-gp activity, partially counteracting its inhibition of CYP3A4-mediated first-pass metabolism (36, 37).

Role of Transporters in Drug Distribution

Transporters are critical in the function of capillary endothelium, where they contribute to the blood-brain, blood-germinal epithelium (blood-testis and blood-ovary), and blood-placental barriers. Endothelial cells in each of these tissues express high levels of MDR1. The existence of a blood-brain barrier is well established and is thought to arise from the formation of tight junctions between brain endothelial cells as well as the action of drug efflux pumps (38, 39).

The importance of MDR1 in the blood-brain barrier was dramatically revealed by an incident involving ivermectin toxicity in knockout mice. In mice, there are two MDR1 isoforms, encoded by *mdr1a/mdr1b*. These differ in their tissue distribution and specificity, and *mdr1a*, *mdr1b*, and combined knockout mice have been created. Ivermectin is routinely used in rodent facilities as an antihelmenthic to control parasitic worms. The day after one mouse colony was given standard ivermectin treatment, all of the homozygous *mdr1* knockout mice were found dead. The level of ivermectin was found to be 100-fold higher in their brains than in the brains of normal mice (40). Normal homozygotes and

mdr1 heterozygotes appeared to have normal drug responses. Homozygous knockouts were viable, but very sensitive to xenobiotics, with the combined *mdr1a/mdr1b* knockouts being the most sensitive (41). Other MDR1 substrates include digoxin and loperamide. Loperamide is related to the sedative narcotics, but is widely used as an antidiarrheal agent, because it does not normally get into the brain. In the MDR knockout mice, loperamide was found to be an addictive sedative because it could not be excluded from the brain (42). The clinical significance of P-glycoprotein in preventing CNS effects of loperamide was demonstrated in a study of quinidine potentiation of the opiate-induced depression of the respiratory response to carbon dioxide rebreathing (43). Quinidine is a known P-glycoprotein inhibitor and interacts with other P-gp substrates. Independent effects on both CNS activity and increased plasma loperamide concentrations were observed during quinidine co-therapy.

Other tissues with high MDR1 concentrations include the apical surface of pancreatic duct cells, the adrenal cortex, and the choroid plexus. In the case of secretory glands, MDR1 may be necessary to protect the gland from its own products and perhaps to assist with their export (e.g., hydrophobic steroids synthesized by the adrenal glands). The choroid plexus is responsible for the secretion of cerebrospinal fluid. It consists of epithelial cells with a basal surface in contact with the blood and an apical surface facing the ventricular space. MDR1 is located on the apical surface of choroid plexus cells, analogous to its location in other tissues. This location does not put MDR1 in a position to protect the brain, since transport across the arachnoid membrane separating the CSF and brain cells is thought to be unimpeded. However, choroid plexus cells have been shown to express MRP on their basolateral surface, consistent with a brain-protective role for this transport protein (44).

Transporters are also critical to target tissue uptake of drugs from the extravascular space. As previously mentioned, transport of drugs between the vascular and extravascular spaces, except in capillaries with tight junctions, is probably by nonmediated diffusion and bulk flow. However, specific transporters are necessary for many drugs to enter target cells and also for transport to their subcellular sites of action. Specific examples include the nucleotide transporter family responsible for antiviral and anticancer drug uptake and the reduced folate carrier that is essential for methotrexate uptake. Many tissues also express the same drug export pumps that occur in the barrier epithelial tissues (e.g., MDR, MRP, MXR), and these may be important in normal tissues, as well as in drug-resistant cancers.

For example, P-gp may contribute to resistance to peptidomimetic HIV protease inhibitors (e.g., indinavir, saquinavir, and nelfinavir) in AIDS patients. These drugs are substrates for P-gp, and this transporter prevents their passage across the blood brain barrier. This has the effect of limiting the access of these drugs to HIV within the central nervous system. Furthermore, lymphocytes and macrophages are among the cell types that normally express P-gp at low levels, including the CD4+ expressing T-lymphocytes, targets of HIV infection. In some cases, protease inhibitor resistance of HIV-infected cells may be due to increased expression of MDR1, rather than mutation of the HIV protease (45).

Much less attention appears to have been paid to the role of transporters in intracellular drug transport than to other processes. Yet some drugs must not only cross external cell membrances, but also penetrate intracellular organelles to reach their site of action. Drugs acting in the nucleus presumably diffuse through the nuclear pore protein complex, if they cannot diffuse across the nuclear double membranes themselves. However, the nuclear pore may selectively control transport of at least some molecules, and can be targeted. For example, a 38-amino-acid-long peptide, which targets the nuclear pore protein transportin, has been used to facilitate DNA delivery into the nucleus of cells *in vitro* (46). Mitochondrial nucleotide transporters are responsible for uptake of antiviral nucleotide drugs into that organelle with resulting side effects due to inhibition of mitochondrial DNA polymerase. This can give rise to the drug-induced mitochondrial myopathy that has been observed for AZT (47) and that caused the clinical trial of the antihepatitis drug fialuridine to be halted (48). Vacuolar ATPases maintain proton gradients across various subcellular compartments. These compartments may able to trap weak bases. A small transporter protein (MTP), isolated from mouse cells, is implicated in the transport of nucleosides, antimetabolites, antibiotics, anthracyclines, and other compounds across endosomal and lysosomal membranes (49).

Role of Transporters in Drug Elimination

Each epithelial barrier tissue displays a similar cellular topology with basal surfaces in communication with the extravascular space and apical surfaces, featuring high surface area brush border membranes that face into extravascular compartments. The topology of transporter expression is similar for at least certain transporters in these cells. Thus, MDR1 is expressed on the apical surface of each of these cells, consistent with a role in drug excretion from mucosal cells back

into the intestinal lumen, from hepatocytes into the bile canaliculus, and from the kidney into the renal tubule duct (24). Other important apical cation transporters in these tissues include the TEA/H$^+$ and guanidinium/H$^+$ proton-coupled antiporters. Protection from hydrophobic cations is a particularly important problem for cell survival. Most cells are negatively polarized inside (ca. –70 mV). Hydrophobic cations will accumulate spontaneously within these cells by simple diffusion. Active transport pumps are necessary to expel undesirable materials back out of the cell and out of the body. The overall pH gradient across the renal tubule cell (blood = pH 7.4, internally = pH 7.2, and tubule fluid = pH 6.7) also facilitates the net export of weak bases. In some tissues, such as liver, uptake through the basolateral (sinusoidal) membrane may be facilitated. Two organic cation transporters (Type I and Type II) and a noncharge selective multispecific carrier have been identified in this organ.

Organic anion transport is also important. MRP is located on both the apical (canalicular) and basal (sinusoidal) surfaces of hepatocytes. Anionic drugs and conjugated drugs are excreted both to blood, where they are cleared by the kidney, and to the bile. Renal clearance of anions presents the converse problem to organic cation accumulation. That is, an active transport system is necessary to accumulate anions into the renal tubule cell from the blood (50). This is facilitated by a two-stage secondary pump. In the first stage, the primary sodium gradient is used to drive coupled uptake of sodium and alpha-ketoglutarate. The alpha-ketoglutarate gradient is then used to drive organic anion uptake by a coupled antiport mechanism. Export of organic anions on the brush border membrane into the tubule fluid is facilitated and potential-dependent.

Role of Transporters in Drug Interactions

Interactions involving digoxin and other drugs that have a low therapeutic index are the most clinically significant. Digoxin is a substrate for P-gp, and clinically significant digoxin toxicity has been reported in patients who have been treated simultaneously with quinidine, verapamil, or amiodarone. In one study, co-administration of quinidine reduced both the renal and nonrenal clearance of digoxin to the extent that total clearance was reduced by 35% (9). Digoxin is not metabolized extensively, and studies in cell culture and in knockout mice demonstrate that both these clearance mechanisms appear to be mediated primarily by P-gp (51). CNS levels of digoxin in wild type but not *mdr1a* knockout mice also were increased by this interaction with quinidine, suggesting effects on

P-gp transport in the blood-brain barrier as well. In a controlled study, wherein maintenance dose digoxin therapy was initially established, addition of verapamil was shown to increase plasma digoxin levels 60 to 90% (52). In addition to increasing bioavailability, verapamil was shown to decrease renal clearance of digoxin, apparently through inhibition of renal tubular P-gp. The conclusion from this study is that the dose of digoxin should be reduced and retitrated when verapamil co-therapy is instituted. Studies of hospital records suggest the need for adjustment of digoxin dose in over half of patients who are treated simultaneously with quinidine or amiodarone (53).

The growing use of herbal and other dietary supplements by the population suggests that an increase in dietary supplement–drug interactions may occur. For example, St. John's wort (*Hypericum perforatum*) was shown to decrease the digoxin AUC by 25% after 10 days of treatment (54). The effect appears to reflect induction of P-gp expression. Whether the active component leading to induction is the same or different from hypericin (one of the putative active antidepressant components of St. John's wort) is not known. A significant number of other herbal supplement–drug interactions are known, including life-threatening interactions with anticoagulants (55). It is not clear whether the effect is on metabolism or transport.

P-gp Inhibition as an Adjunct to Treating Chemotherapy-resistant Cancers

Recognition of the importance of drug resistance efflux pumps has motivated a number of attempts to improve drug therapy by specific co-administration of P-gp inhibitors. Since the therapeutic index of verapamil, cyclosporine, and other marketed P-gp inhibitors is too narrow, dexverapamil and valspodar are among a number of new compounds that are being synthesized and evaluated for this specific purpose. So far, the co-administration of P-gp inhibitors and anticancer drugs has yielded mixed results. This reflects in part the natural history of the cancers being treated and the existence of multiple resistance mechanisms.

An extensive survey of MDR1 mRNA expression levels in cancer patient tissue samples and normal controls suggested that three types of MDR1 behavior may be distinguished in different cancer cells (56, 57): 1) MDR1 is normally expressed in transporting epithelium, liver, colon, kidney, pancreas, and adrenal gland. Expression of MDR1 remains high in cancers derived from these tissues. 2) Cancer cells derived from other tissues that normally do not express MDR1 may be induced to express it when selected by drug treatment. This appears to result from clonal selection for resist-

ant cells during the initial phase of drug treatment and leads to patient relapse during the course of an initially successful therapy. Such responses are commonly seen in leukemias, lymphomas, breast, and ovarian cancers. Promoter analysis has shown that *P-gp* expression is induced by xenobiotics. 3) Cancer cells that normally do not express MDR1 may acquire expression in the absence of drug selection by undergoing significant DNA changes that completely alter the normal regulatory mechanisms of the cell. Examples include chronic myeologenous leukemia (CML), sarcomas, and neuroblastomas. Expression of MDR1 may coincide with transformation of the cancer to a more malignant form such as occurs during the blast crisis phase in CML. In the chronic phase of CML the cancer is susceptible to chemotherapy, but in the blast phase becomes resistant.

The responses of these three cancer types were found to differ during clinical trials of MDR1 inhibitors (58). For the first class, MDR1 inhibition has had little effect on the efficacy of the cancer therapy. It appears that too many other transporters and drug resistance mechanisms are present in such front-line defense organs such as kidney, liver, and intestine. For the second class, at least transiently improved responses to anticancer drugs have been seen with MDR1 inhibitor co-therapy. However, a second relapse is seen as other transport and resistance mechanisms become active. In the SWOG trial for acute nonlymphocytic leukemia, results were most promising when MDR1 inhibitor co-therapy was begun with the initial course of chemotherapy (59).

In a novel twist on the idea of altering P-gp function in cancer patients, experiments have examined the potential of using *mdr1* gene therapy to selectively protect hematopoietic cells from the side effects of cancer therapy (60, 61). Using a retroviral vector, a mutant *mdr1* gene (F983A), which is resistant to the P-gp inhibitor trans-(E)-flupentixol, was transfected into bone marrow cells. This allowed the cells to survive increased doses of daunomycin and vinblastine. Treatment of target cells under the same conditions with the P-gp inhibitor increased their sensitivity to the drugs without compromising the protection of the mutant *mdr1* transfected cells.

Role of Transporters in Microbial Drug Resistance

Bacterial cells are similar to mammalian cells in that they bear an internal negative charge and naturally accumulate organic cations. Transport systems apparently evolved long ago to eliminate natural cationic toxins. Mechanisms of drug uptake in bacteria utilize outer membrane (OM) porins, periplasmic binding proteins, and inner membrane (IM) pumps (62). Relatively selective channels may be used by some antibiotics (e.g., imipenem), and nutrient transporters may be used by others (e.g., aminoglycosides). The discovery of resistance due to reduced uptake has been a key to understanding the role of specific transporters in antibiotic transport. Antibiotics that mimic siderophores (e.g., by including catechol groups) utilize uptake mechanisms used by bacteria for uptake of iron. Such agents and modes of drug delivery have been "naturally selected" by antibiotic drug screening programs. Only recently has structure-based drug design been explored in an attempt to take explicit advantage of these systems. Notably, the FepA and Fhu siderophore transporters were until recently the only active transport systems for which high resolution structures had been determined (1).

In addition to mutations that alter drug uptake, several systems are known to confer bacterial drug resistance by enhancing drug efflux (e.g., resistance to tetracyclines, quinolones, and macrolides). These include transporters in the MF family (e.g., TetA), the RND family (AcrAB, EmrAB, TolC), the small multidrug resistance pumps (SMR), and the ABC family (63). These systems have highly varied membrane topologies, subunit structures, and bioenergetics. Of particular interest is the LmrA gene product, which appears to be an ABC type half-transporter similar to MXR and a potentially ideal candidate for biophysical and mechanistic studies.

PHARMACOGENETICS AND PHARMACOGENOMICS OF TRANSPORTERS[1]

Pharmacogenetics

There appear to be few well-documented examples of genetic polymorphisms responsible for conferring altered pharmacokinetic or pharmacodynamic properties due to altered transporter function. In a report from the Gottesman laboratory (64), sequences were

[1] The terms pharmacogenetics and pharmacogenomics mean different things to different people. Unfortunately in the field of transporters, the term has been co-opted by the indexers to cover papers dealing with the evolution of microbial drug resistance. The National Institute of General Medical Sciences has launched a research program in pharmacogenetics to define the genetic component underlying individual variations in drug response. See: http://www.nigms.nih.gov/funding/pharmacogenetics.html for RFA-GM-00-003 and PA-99-016, indicating NIH interest in this research area.

compared of MDR1 cDNAs cloned from normal human adrenal gland and from a colchicine-selected multidrug resistant cell-line derived from an epidermoid carcinoma. Nine nucleotide sequence differences were noted, but only two altered the coding sequence. A variation, TT=>GA at NT544-545 (Gly185Val) was shown to be associated with an enhanced resistance to colchicine, relative to other MDR substrates, and was thought to arise during selection of the cells. A second variation, G=>T at NT2677 (Ser893Ala), was thought to reflect a naturally occurring, nonselected genetic polymorphism. However, cancer cells are known to undergo numerous, and often severe, genetic alterations, which may be amplified by selection. It is difficult to know whether the Ser893Ala variation occurs in identical tissues of normal healthy individuals, and whether it has any effect on drug transport.

The NT2677 polymorphism was used by Mickley et al. (65) to examine the allelic expression of MDR1 in normal tissues, unselected and drug-selected cell lines, and in malignant lymphomas. In normal tissue samples 43% were heterozygous, 42% were homozygous for G, and 15% were homozygous for T ($n = 83$), and expression from each allele was similar. In drug-selected cells and relapsed lymphomas, expression of only one allele at an elevated level was frequently found.

Hoffmeyer et al. (66) used overlapping PCR primers to examine much of the MDR1 sequence in genomic DNA isolated from healthy normal volunteers. MDR1 expression was assayed in duodenal biopsy samples by immunohistochemistry and Western blotting, and *in vivo* intestinal P-gp activity was estimated using digoxin as a marker. Fifteen polymorphisms were identified among 24 individuals. Seven were located within introns, three were at wobble positions that did not alter the coded amino acid, one was in the 5'-noncoding region, and one occurred just prior to the initiator methionine site. Three resulted in amino acid substitutions (Asn21Asp, Phe103Leu, Ser450Asn). Oddly, the NT2677 polymorphism was not detected in this sample. Only the polymorphism C/T at wobble position NT3435 was correlated with altered MDR1 function. Levels of expression were two-fold lower and plasma digoxin levels were significantly higher in homozygous T-allele subjects. Heterozygotes were intermediate. It is most likely that this effect reflects changes in mRNA processing, rather than other effects on expression. In a sample of 188 individuals, 48.9% were heterozygous and 22.4% were homozygous for the T-allele. Because this variation is widely occurring, it may contribute to the need to individualize digoxin dosage in patients treated with this drug.

Of the five human P-gp polymorphisms affecting the protein sequence, none are in the substrate binding regions. However, small variations in substrate specificity have been observed. The most common *coding* polymorphism occurs at a rate of 4% homozygous and 20% heterozygous. In work with experimental animals, comparisons between *mdr1a* genes of mouse strains that are inherently resistant or sensitive to ivermectin neurotoxicity revealed a specific restriction fragment length polymorphism (RFLP) that is predictive of the observed phenotype (67).

In the nucleotide transporter family, human CNT1 (SPNT) from kidney was shown to differ from human CNT2 from small intestine in only a single R75S substitution (68). However, it is difficult to determine whether this difference is due to a polymorphic variation in the individuals from whom the cell lines were derived or to tissue specific differences in the mRNAs from which the sequenced cDNA clones were derived.

As discussed in Chapter 4, the intestinal hPEPT-1 transporter plays a role in absorption of peptide-like cephalosporin antibiotics and other drugs. Interindividual variations in hPEPT-1 may account for the large interindividual variations in bioavailability that have been observed (69).

In the past decade, a large number of polymorphisms in various CYP450 isoenzymes have been discovered. There is no reason to think that this gene is unique in its genetic diversity. With increased scrutiny of the normal human population, undoubtedly a significant number of variations in transporter gene sequences will be discovered. Individual variation in a transporter function is already clearly established as important in cancer therapy and may be expected to play a role in other therapies, both as a target of drug action and a mediator of drug delivery to other targets.

Pharmacogenomics of Drug Transport

Pharmacogenomic approaches are being applied to reveal the rich diversity of transporters present in the rapidly growing database of sequences (69–71). Classifications of transporter genes may be constructed based on translocation mechanism (transporter or channel), origin, topology, domain structures, energetics (passive or active), energy source (ATPase, H^+- or Na^+-coupled secondary pump), substrate specificity, sequences, and three-dimensional structure. Widely applied sequence analysis tools include BLAST (Basic Local Alignment Search Tool) and INCA (Integrative Neighborhood Cluster Analysis). Sadée et al. (69) have applied these methods to examine relationships in the H^+/dipeptide, facilitative glucose, sodium/glucose, sodium/nucleoside, amino acid transporter, sodium neurotransmitter symporter, and ABC transporter families in species ranging from bacteria to mammals.

The two human family members, hPEPT-1 and hPEPT-2, have already been described. Saier et al. (72–75) have developed a system of transporter classification (T.C. number) analogous to the Enzyme Commission (E.C. number) system for uniquely identifying enzymes. Transporters are organized by:

W = type and energy source
X = transporter family or superfamily
Y = transporter subfamily
Z = substrate(s) transported

Each transporter is assigned a unique identifier: T.C. #W.X.Y.Z. The authors have constructed a database that organizes data derived from the 18+ organisms for which completely sequenced genomes are available and conducted extensive cross-species analyses. A total of 81 distinct families were identified. Two superfamilies, the ABC and the MF superfamilies, account for 50% of all microbial transporters. Probable functions could be ascribed to 80 to 90% of the putative transport proteins. The number of transporters is roughly proportional to genome size, and the patterns of transporter usage are correlated with microbial physiology and ecological niche. These data also yield insight into the evolutionary origins of membrane transporters and into the origins of bacterial multidrug resistance. Certainly, evolution of the four major drug transporter types occurred in four major stages well before human development of antibiotic therapy. However, proliferation of substrate-specific pumps has occurred frequently and is ongoing.

The Institute for Genome Research (Rockville, MD) has also completed analyses of several recently completed genomes (76, 77). They have allowed an estimate of the number of transporters in the genomes and defined the minimal set of transporter functions necessary for different metabolic lifestyles. The TIGR website (78) provides access to annotated sequences of human transporter genes and transcripts as well as cDNAs, through the Expressed Gene Anatomy Database (EGAD). Sadée (79) has begun the Human Membrane Transporter Database. This database includes information on transporter families, sequences, tissue distributions, and substrates/drugs transported. For example, all transporters expressed in human kidney can be easily retrieved. Thus far, approximately 250 human membrane transporters are known, including 100 putative ABC family transporters. Estimates of the total number of transporters in the human genome range from 500 to 2500 (e.g., perhaps 4 to 5% of the proteome). It is expected that many of these transporters can recognize drugs and therefore might affect the drug response in the body.

An extension of the genomic approach is the concept of structural genomics. The premise here is that proteins are even more clearly conserved in three-dimensional structure than in linear sequence. By determining the structures of proteins, whose functions may be unknown, they can be placed in appropriate families that maximize the ability to recognize sequence and probable functional homology. Substrate binding sites and ligand specificities might be recognizable through computerized docking calculations. A feedback loop is anticipated in that the selection of targets for structure determination will be guided by the best possible *a priori* clustering of sequences. The objective is to put every sequence within good homology modeling distance of a known experimentally determined high resolution (X-ray, NMR, or EM) structural model. Regrettably, most proponents of this effort put membrane proteins aside at the outset as being too difficult for high-throughput structure solution. However, at least three groups are known to be working on crystallizing P-gp. It may be hoped that with initial breakthroughs in the membrane transporter class, additional workers will join the fray.[2]

EXPERIMENTAL METHODS FOR STUDYING DRUG TRANSPORT

In vivo Methods for Measuring Drug Transport

If a drug concentrates in a particular tissue compartment, the drug must exhibit either specific or nonspecific preferential partitioning or binding to that tissue and/or there must be mechanisms that specifically increase transport of drug into the compartment. Methods for measuring distribution and transport *in vivo* include: 1) tissue sampling/biopsy; 2) autoradiography; 3) cannulation and perfusion; 4) radiological and magnetic resonance imaging; and 5) microdialysis. Because the spatial resolution of these methods is not sufficient to resolve intracellular spaces, the transport of drug across most sampling points will reflect transport across more than one cell type (e.g., epithelial and endothelial) and permeation through additional layers of tissue (e.g., muscle, basement membrane, interstitial space). However, the rate-determining transport membrane sometimes can be inferred by examining transport from both directions across a macroscopic tissue barrier.

[2] Structural Genomics Initiatives; see: http://www.nigms.nih.gov/funding/psi.html for information on government support for this effort.

The most basic experiment consists of dosing a drug, collecting tissue samples some time later, and analyzing them for drug content using a suitable assay. This may be one of the chemical or immunological assays described in Chapter 12 or it may entail some form of direct visualization. For example, the first observations on the blood-brain barrier were made by Paul Ehrlich who visualized exclusion of trypan blue. Currently, autoradiography is used to visualize the distribution of radiolabeled drug (80). For example, it was possible to use autoradiography to obtain a direct image of camptothecin distribution (81).

In animal models, *in vivo* or *in situ* methods have been devised to perfuse and sample virtually every anatomical compartment and its adjacent blood and lymphatic vessels (82). Limited perfusion studies are possible even in human subjects. For example, in Chapter 4 results were described from studies in which a multichannel intubation device was used to isolate a segment of the intestine by using inflatable balloons to block the lumen at the either end of the segment. Separate tubes allowed for delivery of drug and sampling of material from this intestinal segment. The permeability of the intestinal mucosa was estimated by measuring the disappearance of drug from the isolated segment. In some studies, biopsies of the intestinal mucosa have been performed that allow explicit demonstration of uptake into brush border cells. Such methods for assessing drug permeability can be compared with *in vitro* methods or with direct measurement drug bioavailability in human subjects (see Figure 4.5) (83, 84).

Radiological methods that utilize contrast enhancing agents permit drug distribution and selective permeability to be visualized *in vivo*. For example, radio-opaque, iodine-containing contrast dyes used to image the kidney and computer-assisted tomography (CAT scans) used to detect brain injury depend on the selective concentration of dye by the kidney tubule and exclusion of dye from undamaged brain tissue by the intact blood-brain barrier. Radiolabeled drugs also are used to study drug distribution by single photon emission computed tomography (SPECT) or positron emission tomography (PET). The selective intracellular concentration of ^{99m}Tc-sestamibi into mitochondria, and the high concentration of these organelles within cardiac muscle, make it possible to use this agent to image cardiac perfusion (85). ^{99m}Tc-Sestamibi is excluded from tissues bearing drug efflux pumps and has been validated for use in assessing the drug-resistance of breast tumors and the likelihood of patient response to chemotherapy (86). In addition, PET imaging of ^{11}C-labeled verapamil uptake from implanted tumors has demonstrated in rats the potential clinical utility of this technique for localizing and distinguishing drug-sensitive from drug-resistant cancers (87). The same labeled materials and imaging techniques can be applied in imaging P-gp-mediated blood-brain barrier exclusion of ^{11}C-verapamil. The ability to image the *in vivo* distribution of radiolabeled verapamil provides a bridge to imaging the *in vivo* transport of other drugs that are P-gp substrates. Because the transport of verapamil by P-gp is well characterized, it is now commonly used as a P-gp marker, and competition with other drugs may be detected by altered verapamil distribution.

Microdialysis has been described in Chapter 9 as a method for sampling from selected organs or tissues using an in-dwelling cannula, the tip of which houses a semipermeable dialysis membrane. This allows small molecules to diffuse from interstitial fluid into the cannula, while excluding macromolecules and bulk material flow. A dialysis fluid is fed to the tip and returned to microanalytical equipment via concentric tubes. The method is useful for measuring concentrations of *free* (as opposed to total) amounts of compounds *in vivo*. It has been used extensively to study concentrations of endogenous neurotransmitters and drugs in the brain and cerebrospinal fluid compartments. An advantage of the method is that long-term monitoring in normally active animal models is possible; a disadvantage is that calibration of the absolute amounts is difficult and sampling can be limited by diffusion within the tissue being sampled (88). Application of this method to analysis of codeine transport across the blood-brain barrier in rats revealed that the drug rapidly reached distribution equilibrium with equal unbound concentrations in blood and brain (89).

In vitro Methods for Measuring Drug Transport

Because *in vivo* permeability data are difficult and expensive to obtain, these methods do not lend themselves to screening large numbers of compounds. Furthermore, it is often difficult to isolate and control variables to gain mechanistic information from *in vivo* studies. Therefore, a battery of perfused organ, isolated tissue, and cell-culture methods have been developed. In addition to the Caco-2 cell model that was developed to mimic the transport relevant to gastrointestinal drug absorption (see Chapter 4), there is a whole range of other less frequently employed *in vitro* methods for studying nasal, pulmonary, sublingual, buccal, rectal, vaginal, and transdermal drug delivery. *In vitro* methods also have been developed to estimate renal and hepatic clearance and permeability across the blood brain barrier. Such methods have become an essential part of pharmaceutical industry drug discovery and development programs (82).

An important tool for measuring transport *in vitro* is the Ussing chamber, first developed for measuring ion fluxes across frog skin preparations (90). In this device, a piece of excised tissue separates two fluid chambers. In the most advanced versions, the compositions of the two chambers can be carefully controlled and replenished or sampled by perfusion, and the temperature, transmembrane pressure differential, electrical potential, conductivity, and pH can be measured and controlled (91). Studies are typically conducted on opened segments of intestine from which muscle layers may or may not be removed. Another method commonly used to assess gastrointestinal uptake is the everted gut-sac model. In this method, a segment of intestine is turned inside out and the ends are tied shut so that the absorptive mucosal layer may be placed in contact with a solution of drug. Drug uptake from the bath and/or uptake into the gut-sac can be measured. Good correlations have been obtained between Ussing chamber and everted gut-sac data on rodent intestine samples and human *in vivo* permeability data (92).

Mechanistic studies usually rely on measurements of uptake by vesicles or by cells in culture. Vesicles may be isolated from tissues or cells (e.g., secretory vesicles, mitochondria, outer membrane fragments), or may be prepared by reconstitution of purified proteins with phospholipids. Uptake/efflux measurements with nonattached cells or vesicles can be accomplished using filtration or centrifugation methods. The "oil-stop" method can be used to facilitate rapid, clean separation of cells or vesicles from the extracellular fluid. This method has been used to analyze the kinetics of doxorubicin transport in sensitive and resistant acute myelocytic leukemia cell lines (93). For surface adherent cells, uptake may be assessed by sampling the culture fluid as a function of time or by analyzing the cells after washing away the culture fluid. Analysis is facilitated by the use of radiotracer. For strongly colored (e.g., trypan blue), or fluorescent compounds (e.g., mitoxantrone, rhodamine) uptake is readily quantitated microscopically in either attached or unattached cells. With confocal microscopic methods, it is possible to image selective subcellular compartmentation (94).

Monolayer cell cultures that are adherent to freely permeable (0.45–3.0 micron pore size) supporting membranes have become a most important system for measuring transport. Epithelial cells, such as the Caco-2 colon carcinoma-derived cell line or the MDCKII canine kidney cell line, will grow on such membranes to form a confluent monolayer with tight junctions between neighboring cells. This is demonstrated by the measurement of a high electrical impedance across the monolayer. Furthermore, the cells are oriented with their apical, brush border surfaces exposed to the culture medium and their basal surfaces in contact with the supporting membrane. Sample wells have been devised to grow these membranes between two fluid compartments that can be independently controlled and monitored. Transport of drugs can be measured in either the apical to basal or the basal to apical direction. This system is highly amenable to high-throughput screening and allows bioavailability issues to be considered early in the drug discovery and development process (82).

Wielinga et al. (95) have devised a sample holder for monolayer cell cultures to fit a standard fluorometer and provide effective stirring of both compartments in contact with the membrane. This has allowed them to obtain reliable kinetic data on transport of the fluorescent compounds daunorubicin and idarubicin. Fluorescein isothiocyanate (FITC)-labeled dextran was included as a marker for bulk solvent flow across the membrane and the transmembrane conductivity was also measured. By flipping the membrane upside down, they could measure transport in either direction. They also tested the effect of P-gp inhibitors such as valspodar. The results allowed them to dissect in detail the various components of transport across an MDCKII cell monolayer. They were able to discern two transport pathways: 1) a paracellular route representing leakage through tight junctions; and 2) a transcellular route with distinguishable rates for uptake from the basolateral and apical sides. They further concluded that transcellular transport in the apical to basal direction represented passive diffusion, but that transport in the basal to apical direction involved P-gp-mediated active transport.

Molecular Biology Methods for Studying Drug Transport

Much of what has been learned about drug transporters has been derived from the application of molecular biology to study cells in culture. A few recent examples illustrate the general approach. The Fojo and Bates laboratories (94) have isolated the *mxr* (mitoxantrone resistance gene) from cells of patients with resistant tumors. Cells were grown under progressively selective conditions providing clonal resistance to mitoxantrone in the presence of verapamil to exclude cells with elevated MDR levels. Isolation of differentially expressed mRNA as cDNA and cDNA sequencing identified a new drug resistance gene. Northern analysis was used to examine mRNA expression levels, and Southern analysis was used to exam-

ine gene copy number, which was elevated in some cases. Quantitative PCR was used to analyze expression levels in nonselected sensitive and resistant cell lines. Ross et al. (96, 97) followed a somewhat different approach to isolate a breast-cancer-resistant protein (BCRP) gene from the same initial cell lines. In this case, selection was for doxorubicin resistance in the presence of verapamil. Transfection of nonselected cells with the isolated gene conferred resistance not only to doxorubicin, but also to mitoxantrone and daunorubicin. *In vitro* fluorescence measurements demonstrated decreased drug uptake (e.g., duanorubicin) and increased efflux (e.g., rhodamine test). Northern and Southern analysis demonstrated elevated mRNA and/or gene copy numbers in various resistant patient tumor cell lines. Comparison of the sequences led to the conclusion that the *bcrp* and *mxr* genes are the same.

Work by Kruh and colleagues (98) illustrates the power of the emerging human genome in identifying drug transport genes. The canalicular multispecific organic anion transporter (cMOAT), which is a member of the MRP family, had previously been isolated. PCR with nonstringent primers identified an additional form (MOAT-B). A homology search against the expressed sequence tag (EST) database of the Institute for Genome Research yielded two more family members and partial clones that could be used to isolate more complete cDNAs. Tissue specific expression was examined by RNA blot analysis against a Clontech human tissue expression library. The chromosomal location of the genes was determined by fluorescence *in situ* hybridization (FISH) in normal human lymphocytes. These results demonstrate the extreme rapidity with which drug transport genes can now be identified. Other cell culture and molecular biology methods that have been applied include expression cloning in *Xenopus* oocytes, homologous hybridization, cloning by RT-PCR with degenerate primers, and cloning by functional complementation.

Once new drug resistance cDNAs and genes have been isolated and sequenced, several techniques can be used to analyze the sequence: homology searches against existing databases (BLAST), hydropathy analysis (Kyte–Dolittle plots) to identify probable transmembrane spanning helices, sequence-based structure motif recognition, and homology modeling to known protein structures. These methods may suggest whether the new gene is a transporter and if it is related to previously known transporters.

Functional, biochemical, and biophysical characterization of isolated genes may be considerably harder. Ideally, this will include expression of transport activity *in vitro*, examination of substrate structure/activity profiles and co-substrates (e.g., GSH, ATP, H^+, Na^+), the actions of inhibitors and uncouplers, determination of tissue distribution through EST database searches, RNA expression level measurements, antibody-based quantitation and *in situ* detection, phenotypic characterization in knockout rodents, subcellular localization by microscopy; isolation, purification, and reconstitution; structural characterization by electron microscopy, X-ray crystallography, NMR spectroscopy; and elucidation of the mechanism of substrate transport and energy coupling. The goal of such enzymological studies is to eventually be able to develop selective inhibitors or utilize transporters in drug delivery through rational drug design. Relatively few membrane transport proteins have been structurally characterized (1). Some of the best understood examples to date are the lactose permease (a paradigm for the multifacilitator transporter family) and the Ca^{++} P-type ATPase (which is a primary ion pump). Other structurally well-characterized transport proteins include the bacterial porins and siderophore receptor proteins that were previously discussed.

References

1. Pang DC, Amidon GL, Preusch PC, Sadée W. Meeting report: Second AAPS-NIH frontier symposium—Membrane transporters and drug therapy, April 8–10,1999. PharmSci (AAPS Serial on the Internet) 1999;1:48K. (Internet at: http://www.pharmsci.org/journal.)
2. Hediger MA, Meier PJ, Murer H. Membrane transporters: New perspectives in drug delivery and drug targeting—International conference, August 9–12, 1999. (Program Internet at: http://pharmaconference.bwh.harvard.edu.)
3. Amidon GL, Sadée W, editors. Membrane transporters as drug targets. New York: Kluwer Academic/Plenum Publishers; 1999.
4. Friedman MH. Principles and models of biological transport. New York: Springer-Verlag; 1986.
5. Stein WD. Channels, carriers, and pumps: An introduction to membrane transport, New York: Academic Press; 1990.
6. Hancock REW. Bacterial transport as an import mechanism and target for antimicrobials. In: Georgopapadakou NH, editor. Drug transport in antimicrobial and anticancer chemotherapy. New York: Marcel Dekker, Inc.; 1995. p. 289–306.
7. Fournier RL. Basic transport phenomena in biomedical engineering. Philadelphia: Taylor & Frances Publishers; 1999.
8. Lakshminarayanaiah N. Equations of membrane biophysics. New York: Academic Press; 1984.
9. Hager WD, Fenster P, Mayersohn M, Perrier D, Graves P, Marcus FI, et al. Digoxin-quinidine interaction. N Engl J Med 1979;300:1238–41.
10. Bassolino-Klimas D, Alper HE, Stouch TR. Solute diffusion in lipid bilayer membranes: An atomic level study by molecular dynamics simulation. Biochemistry 1993;32:12624–37.
11. Bassolino D, Alper H, Stouch TR. Drug-membrane interactions studied by molecular dynamics simulation: Size dependence of diffusion. Drug Des Discov 1996;13:135–41.
12. Hansch C, Leo A. Exploring QSAR fundamentals and applications in chemistry and biology. Washington, DC: American Chemical Society; 1995.
13. Austel B, Kutter R. Absorption, distribution, and metabolism of drugs. In: Toplis JG, editor. Quantitative structure activity relationships. Medicinal Chemistry Monographs, vol 19. New York: Academic Press; 1983. p. 437–96.
14. Chopra I. Tetracycline uptake and efflux in bacteria. In: Georgopapadakou NH, editor. Drug transport in antimicrobial and anticancer chemotherapy. New York: Marcel Dekker, Inc.; 1995. p. 221–44.
15. Vasey PA, Kaye SB, Morrison R, Twelves C, Wilson P, Duncan R, et al. Phase I clinical and pharmacokinetic study of PK1 [N-(2-hydroxypropyl)-methacylamide copolymer doxorubicin]: First member of a new class of chemotherapeutic agents-drug polymer conjugates. Clin Cancer Res 1999;5:83–94.
16. Abdellaoui K, Boustta M, Morjani H, Vert M. Uptake and intracellular distribution of 4-amino-fluorescein-labelled poly(L-lysine citramide imide) in K562 cells. J Drug Target 1998;5:193–206.
17. Swaan PW. Recent advances in intestinal macromolecular drug delivery via receptor-mediated transport pathways. Pharm Res 1998;15:826–34.
18. Whelton A, Solez K. Aminoglycoside nephrotoxicity—A tale of two transports. J Lab Clin Med 1982;99:148–55.
19. Bickel U, Pardridge WM. Vector-mediated delivery of opiod peptides to the brain. In: Rapaka RS, editor. Membranes and barriers: Targeted drug delivery. NIDA Res Monograph 154, NIH Pub. #95-3889. p. 28–46.
20. Pardridge WM, Wu D, Sakane T. Combined use of carboxyl-directed protein pegylation and vector-mediated blood-brain barrier drug delivery system optimizes brain uptake of brain-derived neurotrophic factor following intravenous administration. Pharm Res 1998;15:576–82.
21. Fei Y-J, Ganapathy V, Leibach F. Molecular and structural features of the proton-coupled oligopeptide transporter superfamily. Prog Nucleic Acid Res Mol Biol 1998:58:239–61.
22. Wang J, Schaner ME, Thomassen S, Su S-F, Piquette-Miller M, Giacomini KM. Functional and molecular characteristics of Na^+-dependent nucleoside transporters. Pharm Res 1997;14:1524–31.
23. Cass CE. Nucleoside transport. In: Georgopapadakou NH, editor. Drug transport in antimicrobial and anticancer chemotherapy. New York: Marcel Dekker, Inc.; 1995. p. 408–51.
24. Zhang L, Brett CM, Giacomini KM. Role of organic cation transporters in drug absorption and elimination. Annu Rev Pharmacol Toxicol 1998;38:431–60.
25. Silverman JA, Schrenk D. Hepatic canalicular membrane 4: Expression of the multidrug resistance genes in the liver. FASEB J 1997;11:308–13.
26. Muller M, de Vries EGE, Jansen PLM. Role of multidrug resistance protein (MRP) in glutathione S-conjugate transport in mammalian cells. J Hepatol 1996;24(suppl 1):100–8.
27. Madon J, Eckhardt U, Gerloff T, Stieger B, Meier PJ. Functional expression of the rat liver canalicular isoform of the multidrug resistance-associated protein. FEBS Lett 1997;406:75–8.
28. Meier PJ, Eckhardt U, Schroeder A, Hagenbuch B, Stieger B. Substrate specificity of sinusoidal bile acid and organic anion uptake systems in rat and human liver. Hepatology 1997;26:1667–77.
29. Surendran N, Covitz KM, Han H, Sadée W, Oh GM, Amidon GL, et al. Evidence for overlapping substrate specificity between large neutral amino acid (LNAA) and dipeptide (hPEPT1) transporters for PD 158473, an NMDA antagonist. Pharm Res 1999;16:391–5.
30. Ambudkar SV, Pastan I, Gottesman MM. Cellular and biochemical aspects of multidrug resistance. In: Georgopapadakou NH, editor. Drug transport in antimicrobial and anticancer chemotherapy. New York: Marcel Dekker, Inc.; 1995. p. 525–47.
31. Ambudkar SV, Dey S, Hrycyna CA, Ramachandra M, Pastan I, Gottesman MM. Biochemical, cellular, and pharmacological

aspects of the multidrug transporter. Annu Rev Pharmacol Toxicol 1999;39:361–98.

32. Armstrong SR, Zhang H, Tabernero L, Hermodson M, Stauffacher CV. Crystal structure of the N-terminal ATP binding cassette of the ribose ABC transporter. American Crystallographic Association Meeting, July 18–23, 1998. Abstract #W0252. (Internet at: http://www.hwi.buffalo.edu/ACA/ACA98/abstracts/text/W0252.htm1.)

33. Han H, de Vrueh RL, Rhie JK, Covitz KM, Smith PL, Lee CP, et al. 5′-Amino acid esters of antiviral nucleosides, acyclovir, and AZT are absorbed by the intestinal PEPT1 peptide transporter. Pharm Res 1998;15:1154–9.

34. Yu DK. The contribution P-glycoprotein to pharmacokinetic drug-drug interactions. J Clin Pharmacol 1999;39:1203–11.

35. Gramatte T, Oertel R. Intestinal secretion of intravenous talinolol is inhibited by luminal R-verapamil. Clin Pharmacol Ther 1999;66:239–45.

36. Eagling VA, Profit L, Black DJ. Inhibition of the CYP3A4-mediated metabolism and P-glycoprotein-mediated transport of the HIV-1 protease inhibitor saquinavir by grapefruit juice components. Br J Clin Pharmacol 1999;48:543–52.

37 Soldner A, Christians U, Susanto M, Wacher VJ, Silverman JA, Benet LZ. Grapefruit juice activates P-glycoprotein-mediated drug transport. Pharm Res 1999;16:478–85.

38. Bradbury MWB, editor. Physiology and pharmacology of the blood-brain barrier. Handbook of experimental pharmacology, vol 103. New York: Springer-Verlag, 1992.

39. Davson H, Segal M. Physiology of the cerebrospinal fluid and blood-brain barrier. Boca Raton: CRC Press, 1996. p. 8.

40. Schinkel AH, Smit JJ, van Tellingen O, Beijnen JH, Wagenaar E, van Deemter L, et al. Disruption of the mouse *mdr1a* P-glycoprotein gene leads to deficiency in the blood brain barrier and to increased sensitivity to drugs. Cell 1994;77:491–502.

41. Schinkel AH, Mayer U, Wagenaar E, Mol CA, van Deemter L, Smit JJ, et al. Normal viability and altered pharmacokinetics in mice lacking mdr1-type (drug-transporting) P-glycoproteins. Proc Natl Acad Sci USA 1997;94:4028–33.

42. Schinkel AH, Wagenaar E, Mol CA, van Deemter L. P-glycoprotein in the blood-brain barrier of mice influences the brain penetration and pharmacological activity of many drugs. J Clin Invest 1996;97:2517–24.

43. Sadeque AJM, Wandel C, He H, Shah S, Wood AJJ. Increased drug delivery to the brain by P-glycoprotein inhibition. Clin Pharmacol Ther 2000;68:231–7.

44. Rao VV, Dahlheimer JL, Bardgett ME, Snyder AZ, Finch RA, Sartorelli AC, et al. Choroid plexus epithelial expression of MDR1 P-glycoprotein and multidrug resistance-associated protein contribute to the blood-cerebrospinal fluid drug-permeability barrier. Proc Natl Acad Sci USA 1999;96:3900–5.

45. Lee CGL, Gottesman MM. HIV-1 protease inhibitors and the MDR1 multidrug transporter. J Clin Invest 1998;101:287–8.

46. Subramanian A, Ranganathan P, Diamond SL. Nuclear targeting peptide scaffolds for lipofection of nondividing mammalian cells. Nat Biotechnol 1999;17:873–7.

47. Gerschenson M, Erhart SW, Paik CY, St Claire MC, Nagashima K, Skopets B, et al. Fetal mitochondrial heart and skeletal muscle damage in *Erythrocebus patas* monkeys exposed in utero to 3′-azido-3′-deoxythymidine. AIDS Res Hum Retroviruses 2000;16:635–44.

48. McKenzie R, Fried MW, Sallie R, Conjeevaram H, Di Bisceglie AM, Park Y, et al. Hepatic failure and lactic acidosis due to fialuridine (FIAU), an investigational nucleoside analogue for chronic hepatitis B. N Engl J Med 1995;333:1099–105.

49. Cabrita MA, Hobman TC, Hogue DL, King KM, Cass CE. Mouse transporter protein, a membrane protein that regulates cellular

multidrug resistance, is localized to lysosomes. Cancer Res 1999;59:4890–7.

50. Pritchard JB, Miller DS. Renal secretion of organic anions and cations. Kidney Int 1996;49:1649–54.

51. Fromm MF, Kim RB, Stein CM, Wilkinson GR, Roden DM. Inhibition of P-glycoprotein-mediated drug transport: A unifying mechanism to explain the interaction between digoxin and quinidine. Circulation 1999;99:552–7.

52. Verschraagen M, Koks CH, Schellens JH, Beijnen JH. P-glycoprotein system as a determinant of drug interactions: The case of digoxin-verapamil. Pharmacol Res 1999;40:301–6.

53. Freitag D, Bebee R, Sunderland B. Digoxin-quinidine and digoxin-amiodarone interactions: Frequency of occurrence and monitoring in Australian repatriation hospitals. J Clin Pharm Ther 1995;20:179–83.

54. Johne A, Brockmoller J, Bauer S, Maurer A, Langheinrich M, Roots I. Pharmacokinetic interaction of digoxin with an herbal extract from St. John's wort (*Hypericum perforatum*). Clin Pharmacol Ther 1999;66:338–45.

55. Fugh-Berman A. Herb-drug interactions. Lancet 2000;355:134–8. See also erratum and comment: Lancet 2000;355:1019–20.

56. Goldstein LJ, Gottesman MM, Pastan I. Expression of MDR1 gene in human cancer. Cancer Treat Res 1991;57:101–19.

57. Goldstein LJ, Pastan I, Gottesman MM. Multidrug resistance in human cancers. Crit Rev Oncol Hematol 1992;12:243–53.

58. Wilson WH, Bates SE, Fojo A, Bryant G, Zhan Z, Regis J, et al. Controlled trial of dexverapamil, a modulator of multidrug resistance, in lymphomas refractory to EPOCH chemotherapy. J Clin Oncol 1995;12:1995–2004.

59. Leith CP, Kopecky KJ, Chen IM, Eijdems L, Slovak ML, McConnell TS, et al. Frequency and clinical significance of the expression of multidrug resistance proteins MDR1/P-glycoprotein, MRP1, and LRP in acute myeloid leukemia: A Southwest Oncology Group study. Blood 1999;94:1086–99.

60. Licht T, Pastan I, Gottesman MM, Herrmann F. The multidrug-resistance gene in gene therapy of cancer and hematopoietic disorders. Ann Hematol 1996;72:184–93.

61. Hafkemeyer P, Licht T, Pastan I, Gottesman MM. Chemoprotection of hematopoietic cells by a mutant P-glycoprotein resistant to a potent chemosensitizer of multidrug-resistant cancers. Hum Gene Ther 2000;11:555–65.

62. Georgopapadakou NH, editor. Drug transport in antimicrobial and anticancer chemotherapy, New York: Marcel Dekker, Inc.; 1995.

63. Lewis K. Multidrug resistance efflux. In: Broome-Smith JK, Baumberg S, Stirling CJ, Ward FB, editors. Transport of molecules across microbial membranes. 58th Symp. of the Society for General Microbiology, University of Leeds, September 1999. London: Cambridge University Press, 1999. p. 15–40.

64. Kioka N, Tsubota J, Kakehi Y, Komano T, Gottesman MM, Pastan I, et al. P-glycoprotein gene (MDR1) cDNA from human adrenal: Normal P-glycoprotein carries Gly185 with an altered pattern of multidrug resistance. Biochem Biophys Res Commun 1989;162:224–31.

65. Mickley LA, Lee JS, Weng Z, Zhan Z, Alvarez M, Wilson W et al. Genetic polymorphism in MDR-1: A tool for examining allelic expression in normal cells, unselected and drug-selected cells, and human tumors. Blood 1998;91:1749–56.

66. Hoffmeyer S, Burk O, von Richter O, Arnold HP, Brockmoller J, Johne A, et al. Functional polymorphisms of the human multidrug-resistance gene: Multiple sequence variations and correlation of one allele with P-glycoprotein expression and activity in vivo. Proc Natl Acad Sci USA 2000;97:3473–78.

67. Umbenhauer DR, Lankas GR, Pippert TR, Wise LD, Cartwright ME, Hall SJ, et al. Identification of a P-glycoprotein-deficient sub-

population in the CF-1 mouse strain using a restriction fragment length polymorphism. Toxicol Appl Pharmacol 1997;146:88–94.

68. Ritzel MW, Yao SY, Ng AM, Mackey RJ, Cass CE, Young JD. Molecular cloning, functional expression and chromosomal localization of a cDNA encoding a human Na⁺/nucleoside cotransporter (hCNT2) selective for purine nucleosides and uridine. Mol Membr Biol 1998;15:203–11.

69. Sadée W, Graul RC, Lee AY. Classification of membrane transporters. In: Amidon GL, Sadée W, editors. Membrane transporters as drug targets. New York: Kluwer Academic/Plenum Publishers; 1999. p. 29–58.

70. Sadée W. Genomics and drugs: finding the optimal drug for the right patient. Pharm Res 1998;15:959–63.

71. Evans WE, Relling MV. Pharmacogenomics: translating functional genomics into rational therapeutics. Science 1999;286:487–91.

72. Saier MH Jr, Paulsen IT, Sliwinski MK, Pao SS, Skurray RA, Nikaido H. Evolutionary origins of multidrug and drug-specific efflux pumps in bacteria. FASEB J 1998;12:265–74.

73. Saier MH Jr, Tseng T-T. Evolutionary origins of transmembrane transport systems. In: Transport of molecules across microbial membranes. 58th Symposium of the Society for General Microbiology, University of Leeds, September 1999. London: Cambridge University Press; 1999. p, 252–74. (See also Internet at: http://www.biology.ucsd.edu/~msaier/transport/titlepage.html.)

74. Paulsen IT, Sliwinski MK, Saier MH Jr. Microbial genome analyses: Global comparisons of transport capabilities based on phylogenies, bioenergetics and substrate specificities. J Mol Biol 1998;277:573–92. (See also Internet at: http://www.biology.ucsd.edu/~ipaulsen/transport/index2.html.)

75. Paulsen IT, Sliwinski MK, Nelissen B, Goffeau A, Saier MH Jr. Unified inventory of established and putative transporters encoded within the complete genome of Saccharomyces cerevisiae. FEBS Lett 1998;430:116–25.

76. Clayton RA, White O, Ketchum KA, Venter JC. The first genome from the third domain of life. Nature 1997;387:459–62.

77. Fraser CM, Norris SJ, Weinstock GM, White O, Sutton GG, Dodson R, et al. Complete genome sequence of Treponema pallidum, the syphilis spirochete. Science 1998;281:375–88.

78. Internet at: www.tigr.org. A list of known human transporters is given under the heading EGAD Cellular Roles/Metabolism/egad_scripts/role_seq_id_list.spl?Transport: http://www.tigr.org/docs/tigr-scripts/egadscripts/roleseqidlist.spl?role=transport&cat=2.

79. Internet at: http://128.218.190.183:81/transporter.

80. Coe RA. Quantitative whole-body autoradiography. Regul Toxicol Pharmacol 2000;31:S1–3.

81. Liehr JG, Ahmed AE, Giovanella BC. Pharmacokinetics of camptothecins administered orally. Ann NY Acad Sci 1996;803:157–63.

82. Borchardt RT, Smith PL, Wilson G, editors. Models for assessing drug absorption and metabolism. New York: Plenum Press;1996.

83. Lennernäs H. Human jejunal effective permeability and its correlation with preclinical drug absorption models. J Pharm Pharmacol 1997;49:627–38.

84. Barthe L, Woodley J, Houin G. Gastrointestinal absorption of drugs: Methods and studies. Fundam Clin Pharmacol 1999;13:154–68.

85. Crane P, Laliberte R, Heminway S, Thoolen M, Orlandi C. Effect of mitochondrial viability and metabolism on technetium-99m-sestamibi myocardial retention. Eur J Nucl Med 1993;20:20–5.

86. Luker GD, Fracasso PM, Dobkin J, Piwnica-Worms D. Modulation of the multidrug resistance P-glycoprotein: detection with technetium-99m-sestamibi in vivo. J Nucl Med 1997;38:369–72.

87. Hendrikse NH, de Vries EG, Eriks-Fluks L, van der Graaf WT, Hospers GA, Willemsen AT, et al. A new in vivo method to study P-glycoprotein transport in tumors and the blood brain barrier. Cancer Res 1999;59:2411–16.

88. de Lange EC, Danhof M, de Boer AG, Breimer DD. Methodological considerations of intracerebral microdialysis in pharmacokinetic studies on drug transport across the blood-brain barrier. Brain Res Brain Res Rev 1997;25:27–49.

89. Xie R, Hammarlund-Udenaes M. Blood-brain barrier equilibration of codeine in rats studied with microdialysis. Pharm Res 1998;15:570–5.

90. Ussing HH. Transport of ions across cellular membranes. Physiol Rev 1949;29:127–55.

91. For example, see: Harvard Apparatus, Inc., catalog, online, p. M78. Vertical Ussing and Horizontal Diffusion Chamber System. Internet at: http://www.harvardapparatus.com/pdf-files/B2K_M078.pdf.

92. Lennernäs H. Human intestinal permeability. J Pharm Sci 1998;87:403–10.

93. Dordal MS, Winter JN, Atkinson AJ Jr. Kinetic analysis of P-glycoprotein-mediated doxorubicin efflux. J Pharmacol Exp Ther 1992;263:762–6.

94. Miyake K, Mickley L, Litman T, Zhan Z, Robey R, Cristensen B, et al. Molecular cloning of cDNAs which are highly overexpressed in mitoxantrone-resistant cells: demonstration of homology to ABC transport genes. Cancer Res 1999;59:8–13.

95. Wielinga PR, de Waal E, Westerhoff HV, Lankelma J. In vitro transepithelial drug transport by on-line measurement: cellular control of paracellular and transcellular transport. J Pharm Sci 1999;88:1340–7.

96. Doyle LA, Yang W, Abruzzo LV, Krogmann T, Gao Y, Rishi AK, et al. A multidrug resistance transporter from human MCF-7 breast cancer cells. Proc Natl Acad Sci USA 1998;95:15665–70.

97. Ross DD, Yang W, Abruzzo LV, Dalton WS, Schneider E, Lage H, et al. Atypical multidrug resistance: breast cancer resistance protein messenger RNA expression in mitoxantrone-selected cell lines. J Natl Cancer Inst 1999;91:429–33.

98. Belinsky MG, Bain LJ, Balsara BB, Testa JR, Kruh GD. Characterization of MOAT-C and MOAT-D, new members of the MRP/cMOAT subfamily of transporter proteins. J Natl Cancer Inst 1998;90:1735–41.

PART III

ASSESSMENT OF DRUG EFFECTS

CHAPTER

17

Physiological and Laboratory Markers of Drug Effect

ARTHUR J. ATKINSON, JR.

Clinical Center, National Institutes of Health, Bethesda, Maryland

BIOLOGICAL MARKERS OF DRUG EFFECT

The selection and measurement of relevant drug effects are increasingly important parts of clinical pharmacology. Traditionally, the efficacy and safety of drug therapy have been assessed using *clinical endpoints,* such as survival, onset of serious morbidity or symptomatic response. Nonetheless, these endpoints have obvious disadvantages as useful measures in monitoring the response of individual patients to existing drug therapy, and increase the duration and cost of the clinical trials that are needed to evaluate potential new drugs. These constraints have provided the impetus for identifying more accessible response markers or *biomarkers* that could be assessed more easily and rapidly than more definitive clinical endpoints. In some cases, these biomarkers have served as *surrogate endpoints* and have provided the basis for regulatory approval of new drugs under the conditions stipulated in the following excerpt from the Code of Federal Regulations:

> FDA may grant marketing approval for a new drug product on the basis of adequate and well-controlled trials establishing that the drug product has an effect on a surrogate endpoint that is reasonably likely, based on epidemiologic, therapeutic, pathophysiologic, or other evidence, to predict clinical benefit or on the basis of an effect on a clinical endpoint other than survival or irreversible morbidity. *Title 21, Section 314.50, Subpart H of the Code of Federal Regulations (1)*

Examples of some commonly used biomarkers and surrogate endpoints are listed along with clinical endpoints for several therapeutic classes in Table 17.1.

In a number of clinical trials, initial conclusions based on the response of candidate surrogate endpoints were not borne out by the subsequent clinical response. These unexpected results have fueled concerns that many proposed surrogate endpoints may

TABLE 17.1   Examples of Biomarkers and Surrogate Endpoints

Therapeutic class	Biomarker/ surrogate	Clinical endpoint
Physiologic markers		
Antihypertensive drugs	↓ Blood pressure	↓ Stroke
Drugs for glaucoma	↓ Intraocular pressure	Preservation of vision
Drugs for osteoporosis	↑ Bone density	↓ Fracture rate
Antiarrhythmic drugs	↓ Arrhythmias	↑ Survival
Laboratory markers		
Antibiotics	Negative culture	Clinical cure
Antiretroviral drugs	↑ CD4 count, ↓ Viral RNA	↑ Survival
Antidiabetic drugs	↓ Blood glucose	↓ Morbidity
Lipid-lowering drugs	↓ Cholesterol	↓ Coronary artery disease
Drugs for prostate cancer	↓ Prostate-specific antigen	Tumor response

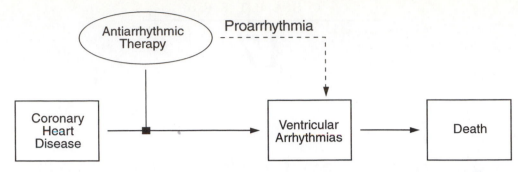

FIGURE 17.1 Path diagram illustrating the potential of adverse proarrhythmic effects of antiarrhythmic drug therapy *(broken line and arrow)* to outweigh the potential benefit of suppressing ventricular arrhythmias in patients with coronary heart disease.

not accurately predict meaningful clinical outcomes (2, 3, 4). One of the most notable examples is provided by the Cardiac Arrhythmia Suppression Trial (CAST) in which a dichotomy was found between suppression of ventricular ectopy and increased mortality in patients who received long-term therapy with antiarrhythmic drugs (5). The impetus for the trial was provided by the fact that patients who have sustained a myocardial infarction, and subsequently have ventricular ectopy with more than 10 premature ventricular depolarizations per hour, have a four-fold increase in mortality rate. A total of 1498 patients were entered in the trial and were randomized to receive encainide, flecainide, or placebo. However, after a mean treatment period of 10 months, the safety monitoring board stopped the trial because 63 patients died while receiving these antiarrhythmic drugs, whereas only 26 placebo-treated patients died ($P = 0.0001$). Although complete understanding of the mechanisms underlying the excess mortality is lacking, it is presumed that the adverse proarrhythmic effects of drug therapy outweighed the benefit provided by suppression of arrhythmias resulting from underlying cardiac disease (Figure 17.1). Supporting this interpretation is the finding that patients receiving antiarrhythmic drugs had an increased incidence of fatal arrhythmias and shock after recurrent myocardial infarction.

Further controversy surrounding biomarkers and surrogate endpoints stems from ambiguity in the terminology that has been used by members of the different disciplines that are engaged in the design, conduct, analysis, and regulatory evaluation of clinical trials. For this reason, a number of proposals have been made to clarify this terminology (4, 6). A synthesis of these proposals is presented in Table 17.2. A hierarchy is implicit in this sequence of definitions in that relatively few biomarkers are robust enough to serve as surrogate endpoints. For example, blood pressure and serum

cholesterol concentrations are the only surrogate endpoints that are currently used in the United States as the basis for approval of cardiovascular drugs (4).

Although an intermediate endpoint is associated with clinical benefit, this benefit may be more than offset by the adverse effects of drug therapy when the ultimate outcome is considered. For example, ventricular ectopy traditionally has been regarded as a harbinger of life-threatening ventricular fibrillation in the setting of acute myocardial infarction. This provided a rationale for administering lidocaine to patients whose myocardial infarction was accompanied by ventricular ectopy (7). More recent studies have confirmed that this intervention does reduce the incidence of ventricular fibrillation in these patients (8). However, two meta-analyses of several studies have indicated that this use of lidocaine therapy actually worsens patient

TABLE 17.2   Definition of Biomarker and Endpoint Terms

Biological marker (Biomarker)	A physical sign or laboratory measurement that occurs in association with a pathological process and has putative diagnostic and/or prognostic utility.
Surrogate endpoint	A biomarker that is intended to serve as a substitute for a clinically meaningful endpoint and is expected to predict the effect of a therapeutic intervention.
Clinical endpoint	A clinically meaningful measure of how a patient feels, functions, or survives.
Intermediate endpoint	A clinical endpoint that is not the ultimate outcome, but is nonetheless of real clinical benefit.
Ultimate outcome	A clinical endpoint such as survival, onset of serious morbidity, or symptomatic response that captures the benefits and risks of an intervention.

survival (9, 10). As a result of these analyses, some authors now recommend that prophylactic lidocaine therapy no longer be routine for patients with acute myocardial infarction who demonstrate even high-grade ventricular ectopy (11).

IDENTIFICATION AND EVALUATION OF BIOMARKERS

Most of the biomarkers listed in Table 17.1 were identified in studies of pathophysiology and epidemiology that demonstrated an association between the marker and the presence or prognosis of the underlying clinical condition. For example, clinical and epidemiological observations led to the conclusion that elevated blood pressure was associated with an increased risk of atherosclerotic cardiovascular disease, heart failure, stroke, and kidney failure (12). Pathophysiologic studies in humans and animal models were particularly helpful in establishing a firm linkage between hypertension and cerebral hemorrhage and infarction (13). A more recent epidemiologic study has demonstrated that the risk of stroke and coronary heart disease is correlated with the extent of diastolic blood pressure elevation (14). In the aggregate, this considerable evidence supports the *biological plausibility* of using blood pressure as a surrogate endpoint. In clinical practice, the measurement of blood pressure is used to diagnose hypertension, estimate its severity, and monitor response to antihypertensive therapy.

Further support for using blood pressure as a surrogate endpoint is provided by the concordance of evidence from a number of clinical trials in which blood pressure lowering with low-dose diuretics and β-blockers was shown to reduce the incidence of stroke, coronary artery disease, and congestive heart failure in hypertensive patients (15). Of particular interest is a meta-analysis that was conducted to compare the extent of blood pressure reduction achieved in different clinical trials with the maximum benefit that was anticipated on epidemiolgic grounds (Table 17.3) (16). The fall in stroke incidence anticipated for a 5- to 6-mm/Hg average reduction in diastolic blood pressure was fully realized with only 2 to 3 years of antihypertensive therapy. However, the reduction in coronary heart disease risk was substantially less than the maximum anticipated benefit, perhaps reflecting the fact that atherosclerosis is a chronic and largely irreversible process.

More recently, it has been shown that hypokalemia and other dose-related adverse metabolic effects of thiazide diuretics increase the risk of sudden death and negate the cardiovascular benefit of blood pressure

TABLE 17.3   Incidence Change Resulting from a 5–6-mm Hg Change in Diastolic Blood Pressure[a]

| | Clinical trial results | | Epidemiologic expectations |
	Observed result	95% CI	95% CI
Stroke	42%	33–50%	35–40%
Coronary heart disease	14%	4–22%	20–25%

[a] Data from Collins R, Peto R, Mac Mahon S, et al. Lancet 1990;335:827–38.

lowering when high doses of these drugs are prescribed (17). Hence, another explanation for the apparent inability of antihypertensive therapy to lower mortality in patients with coronary heart disease is that high thiazide doses were used in many of the trials that were analyzed. As pointed out by Temple (2), this explanation is supported by the results of a trial of antihypertensive therapy in elderly patients with isolated systolic hypertension (18). In this study, only low doses of a thiazide diuretic were prescribed and a 4-mm Hg average fall in diastolic blood pressure was associated with a 36% reduction in the 5-year incidence of stroke and a 25% reduction in the incidence of coronary heart disease. Similar concerns have been raised about the clinical efficacy of antihypertensive therapy with short-acting calcium channel blocking drugs, which lower blood pressure but have been found to increase the risk of myocardial infarction in hypertensive patients (19). These observations emphasize the point, diagrammed in Figure 17.2, that sole reliance on even a well-established surrogate endpoint can lead to erroneous conclusions when beneficial effects on the surrogate are outweighed by unexpected adverse effects.

Figure 17.2 also emphasizes that it is inherently more difficult to demonstrate the benefit of antihypertensive therapy in preventing coronary heart disease than stroke because, in the former case, therapy is directed against only one of many predisposing risk factors. To deal with the complexity of this problem, Shatzkin and colleagues (20) have proposed a means for calculating the extent to which response measured by the clinical endpoint can be attributed to a biomarker. The formula for calculating this *attributable proportion (AP)* is:

$$AP = S\left(1 - \frac{1}{R}\right)$$

where S is the sensitivity, the proportion of patients with the clinical endpoint who are biomarker positive,

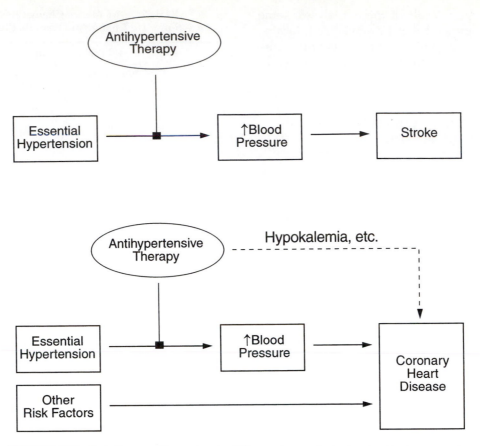

FIGURE 17.2 Path diagrams illustrating the difference in complexity involved in demonstrating the efficacy of antihypertensive therapy in reducing the incidence of stroke and coronary heart disease. The anticipated benefit in reducing the incidence of coronary heart disease is offset by the deleterious effects of some antihypertensive drug regimens. In addition, hypertension is just one of many factors that contribute to the risk of developing coronary heart disease.

and R is the relative risk, the incidence of the clinical endpoint in patients who are biomarker positive divided by the incidence in those who are biomarker negative. More elaborate analyses also have been proposed for estimating the proportion of treatment effect explained by a biomarker (21, 22).

Ideally a biomarker would capture the full relationship between a given therapy and a clinical endpoint before being relied on to serve as a surrogate endpoint (23). However, this expectation seems unrealistic, as illustrated by the complexity of the relationship between hypertension, antihypertensive therapy, and the incidence of coronary heart disease (Figure 17.2). In view of this uncertainty, regulatory acceptance of a biomarker as a surrogate for a clinical endpoint is to some extent dependent on a risk/benefit assessment that includes the availability of alternative effective therapy, the difficulty of obtaining clinical endpoint data, and the safety data base of the drug in question (4).

USES OF BIOMARKERS AND SURROGATE ENDPOINTS

A high level of stringency is required when the response of a biomarker to drug therapy is proposed as a surrogate for a clinical endpoint and is intended to be used as the basis for regulatory approval of an application to market a new drug. On the other hand, biomarkers need not be validated thoroughly in order to play an important role in facilitating our understanding of disease mechanisms and natural history, expediting the development of new drugs, and improving the quality of patient care. In addition, the emphasis placed on using biomarkers to evaluate therapeutic efficacy has obscured the equally important role that they can play in evaluating the toxic potential of drug therapy. For example, drugs that prolong the electrocardiographic QT interval frequently cause potentially fatal *torsades de pointes* arrhythmia (24). Blood level measurements can serve as a biomarker

TABLE 17.4 Some Applications of Biomarkers and Surrogate Endpoints

Predevelopment studies of target illness

Used to correlate with diagnosis and prognosis

Used to help elucidate pathophysiology of disease

Preclinical drug development

Used to confirm proposed pharmacologic activity *in vivo*

Used to explore plasma level-response relationships in animal studies

Phase I–II clinical studies

Used to demonstrate pharmacologic activity in humans

Used to define dose or plasma level-response relationships

Phase III clinical studies

Used as a basis for stratifying patient groups

Used for compliance and safety monitoring

Used as basis for interim analysis of patient response

Used as basis for conditional regulatory approval

Phase IV clinical studies

Used in studies designed to establish new indications for marketed drugs

Used as a basis for regulatory approval of formulation changes and of generic drugs

Application in clinical practice

Used to establish diagnosis and prognosis

Used as an aid in selecting therapy

Used to monitor response to treatment

---

for toxicity as well as efficacy, both in the initial stages of drug development and in subsequent clinical use.

Some applications of biomarkers are outlined in Table 17.4. Many, but not all biomarker applications are part of the drug development process that was diagrammed in Figure 5.1. Studies to provide an epidemiologic and pathophysiologic basis for biomarkers have been alluded to already, and these generally precede their use is drug development. In preclinical and early clinical development, biomarkers can provide evidence of *in vivo* pharmacologic activity and can define the dose or range of plasma concentrations that is likely to be effective in subsequent studies

In large-scale clinical trials, biomarkers such as CD4 count may be useful for patient stratification (25). Blood levels and toxicity biomarkers also could be used for safety monitoring. Biomarkers used as efficacy measures in exploratory Phase II clinical trials may be helpful in reaching a go/no-go decision regarding further development of a particular drug. Here, as in earlier phases of drug development, the extent of validation of a biomarker is of concern primarily to the sponsor. However, a more stringent stan-

dard of validity is required in a pivotal Phase III trial of a new drug if a biomarker is proposed as a surrogate endpoint to be used as the basis for regulatory approval. In fact, even when regulatory approval is based on results obtained with a surrogate endpoint, that approval is contingent on subsequent verification of clinical benefit (1). Similar considerations apply to Phase IV studies that are designed to establish additional clinical indications for a marketed drug. As described in Chapter 4, blood level measurements of new product formulations and generic drug products are relied on as a surrogate for formal efficacy studies in establishing bioequivalence. In addition, as discussed in Chapter 2, drug levels are used to guide dose adjustment and monitor therapy with drugs that have a narrow therapeutic index and no readily observable clinical endpoint. Measurements of blood pressure, intraocular pressure, serum total cholesterol, and prostate-specific antigen are among the many biomarkers that are used in routine clinical practice for establishing diagnosis and prognosis, selecting therapy, and subsequent patient monitoring.

Use of Serum Cholesterol as a Biomarker and Surrogate Endpoint

Although serum cholesterol measurements are an accepted surrogate endpoint for lipid-lowering therapy, there is a long history of controversy regarding the value of this therapy in preventing coronary heart disease (26). Epidemiologic studies provided initial evidence that elevated serum cholesterol concentrations were associated with an increased risk of death from coronary heart disease (Figure 17.3) (27). This relationship was confirmed by studies conducted in a number of animal models (28). Taken together, this evidence provided strong support for the hypothesis that reducing cholesterol levels would lower morbidity and mortality from coronary heart disease. Accordingly, serum cholesterol has played an important role as a biomarker in the clinical development of inhibitors of 3-hydroxy-3-methylglutaryl coenzyme A (HMG-CoA) reductase and other lipid lowering agents. This experience illustrates both some important uses of biomarkers and some of the continuing pitfalls surrounding their role as surrogate endpoints.

Role of Serum Cholesterol in the Simvastatin Development Program

Measurements of serum cholesterol were used in a Phase II dose-ranging study in which simvastatin doses, ranging from 2.5 to 40 mg once daily to 1.25 to 40 mg twice daily, were administered to 43 patients

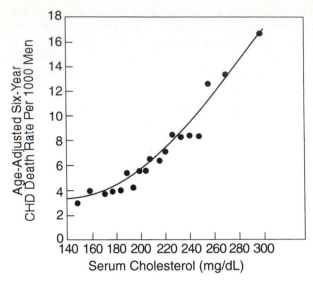

FIGURE 17.3 Relation of serum cholesterol to coronary heart disease death in a population of 361,662 men aged 35–57. The average duration of follow-up was 6 years. (Reproduced with permission from Gotto AM Jr, LaRosa JC, Hunninghake D, Grundy SM, Wilson PW, Clarkson TB, Hay JW, Goodman DS. Circulation 1990;81:1721–33.)

with heterozygous familial hypercholesterolemia (29). The study duration was only 6 weeks and only four study centers were needed for patient recruitment. Based on the results shown in Figure 17.4, it was concluded that simvastatin had suitable efficacy whether given once or twice daily, and that 20 mg/day represented an appropriate starting point for dosing in subsequent studies. These results were then incorporated

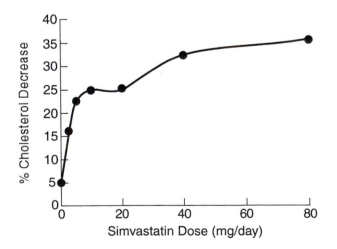

FIGURE 17.4 Results of a study that established the dose-response relationship between simvastatin dose and the percentage of reduction in serum cholesterol levels in patients with heterozygous familial hypercholesterolemia.

in a definitive randomized, placebo-controlled Phase III trial in which 4444 patients with coronary heart disease were followed in 94 centers for a median of 5.4 years (30). Patients receiving simvastatin were initially treated with a daily dose of 20 mg that subsequently was adjusted as needed to lower serum cholesterol concentrations to the range of 117 to 200 mg/dL. The study demonstrated that simvastatin therapy reduced total cholesterol by a mean of 25% during the study (average LDL cholesterol reduction was 34%), and was associated with a 34% reduction in the incidence of major coronary events. Total mortality was 30% less for patients who were treated with simvastatin than for those who received placebo.

The inclusion of clinical endpoints in this larger Phase III study provided the first definite evidence that lipid-lowering therapy could reduce total mortality in patients with coronary heart disease. Subgroup analysis subsequently indicated that the relationship between lowering LDL cholesterol and reducing major clinical events was curvilinear in that decreases in cholesterol level resulted in continuing but progressively smaller reductions in major coronary events (31). This is consistent with the epidemiologic findings shown in Figure 17.3, and supports clinical practice guidelines that recommend lowering LDL cholesterol levels to or below 100 mg/dL for patients who have established coronary heart disease and to less than 130 mg/dL for high-risk patents whose cholesterol levels are elevated (32).

Unanticipated Consequences of Cholesterol-lowering Therapy

Of particular interest are the results of the West of Scotland Coronary Prevention Study in which the relationship between the observed incidence of coronary heart disease events was compared with that predicted from an equation that incorporates cholesterol levels, smoking history, diabetes, blood pressure, and other risk factors that were known at the time (33). These results, shown in Figure 17.5, indicate that the predicted and observed event rates in patients who received placebo were similar. On the other hand, coronary event rates in pravastatin-treated patients were consistently lower than those that were predicted. This finding suggests that pravastatin provides therapeutic benefits that extend beyond lipid lowering. Indeed, most studies with HMG-CoA reductase inhibitors have demonstrated a more rapid onset of therapeutic benefit than would be expected from their lipid-lowering properties (34). In this regard, pravastatin therapy recently has been shown to reduce plasma concentrations of C-reactive protein, a biomarker for systemic inflammation (35). The magni-

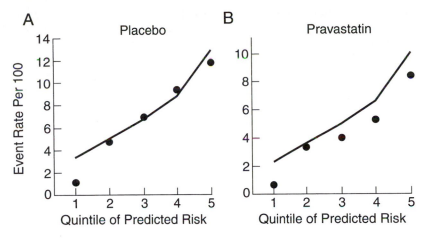

FIGURE 17.5 Comparison of observed risk of a coronary heart disease event *(circles)* and predicted risk *(lines)* for patients receiving either placebo or pravastatin over the 4.4-year duration of the West of Scotland Coronary Prevention Study. (Reproduced with permission from West of Scotland Coronary Prevention Group. Circulation 1998;97:1440–5.

tude of this effect also appears to be unrelated to the extent of lipid lowering. The potential significance of this finding is underscored by the fact that the combination of C-reactive protein and lipid measurements predicts relative risk of myocardial infarction better than when either biomarker is used alone (36).

It is relatively uncommon for the clinical benefit of therapeutic interventions to exceed predictions based on biomarker response. Far more often, unanticipated adverse effects diminish or nullify the clinical benefits expected from drug effects on a biomarker. For example, probucol, a drug structurally unrelated to HMG CoA inhibitors, exerted pronounced lipid-lowering effects and received marketing approval in the 1970s, even though long-term survival studies were not conducted. Probucol also was known to prolong the electrocardiographic QT interval. In a scenario reminiscent of that encountered with antiarrhythmic drugs (Figure 17.1), subsequent investigations indicated that this drug was proarrhythmic in that it caused *torsades de pointes* ventricular tachycardia (37). Therefore, it is hazardous to assume *a priori* that any drug that lowers cholesterol will also improve patient survival.

Other Biomarker Applications and Future Developments

Laboratory biomarkers are playing an increasingly important role in managing patients with cancer or with human immunodeficiency virus type 1 (HIV-1) infection. Most of these biomarkers are used to establish prognosis and monitor response to therapy or disease progression. Relatively few of them, such as prostate-specific antigen, have had diagnostic utility.

Because tumor biomarkers play a critical role in patient management, their marketing in the United States is regulated by the Food and Drug Administration under the Medical Device Law (38). Currently, candidate tumor markers are evaluated with respect to their analytical sensitivity and specificity and the robustness of the cutoff value that is chosen to distinguish positive from negative test results. Different antibody assays for the same tumor biomarkers can give different results, in part because tumor antigen proteins have several distinct epitopes protruding from their surface (39). Therefore, studies are required to compare new and old versions of a given tumor biomarker assay (38). The AIDS Clinical Trials Group has implemented similarly rigorous programs for standardization and quality control of biomarker measurements in patients with HIV-1 infection (40).

In some cases, it has been useful to monitor the rate of change of serial laboratory biomarker measurements. More than 30 years ago, weekly measurements of the steady-state ratio of cerebrospinal fluid (CSF) to blood glucose concentrations (R_{CSF}) were used to monitor the response to therapy of patients with cryptococcal meningitis (41). Meningeal infection with *C. neoformans* disrupts carrier-mediated facilitated diffusion of glucose between blood and CSF and results in initially low R_{CSF} values in these patients (41, 42). With effective therapy, R_{CSF} was found to rise at a rate of 0.013 ± 0.002 (± SD) per day until it reached the normal range of 0.45 to 0.65. In one patient, a decline in R_{CSF} during therapy preceded clinical evidence of deterioration. More recently, measurements of tumor biomarker half-life have been shown to be useful in assessing the efficacy of therapeutic interventions, and tumor biomarker doubling time has been used to evaluate the probability of metastasis or tumor recurrence (39).

Measurement of both CD4 lymphocytes and viral load are currently regarded as somewhat independent biomarkers of disease progression rate in patients infected with HIV-1 (43, 44). It has been found that serial measurements are more informative than a single measurement of viral load in that failure to account for the evolution of viral load can lead to underestimates of progression risk (45). In addition, analysis of the kinetics of HIV-1 viral load and turnover of peripheral blood mononuclear cells has provided fundamental insight into viral replication rates and the need for long-term therapy with even highly active antiretroviral drug regimens (46, 47). Finally, both increases in CD4 lymphocyte count and reductions in viral load have attained surrogate endpoint status and have been used as the basis for accelerated approval of several antiretroviral drugs. However, no single marker has been shown to explain fully the spectrum of clinical response to therapeutic intervention (40).

So far we have considered biomarkers whose validity has either been somewhat established or discredited by their use in clinical practice or clinical trials. However, Rolan (48) has emphasized the important fact that the degree of innovation represented by a biomarker generally varies inversely with the extent of its validation. This is a consequence of the fact that prior use in clinical trials is an important component of biomarker evaluation. Innovative but incompletely evaluated biomarkers are particularly likely to play an important role in exploratory studies of a new drug candidate. For example, positron emission tomography was used in an innovative dose-ranging study to demonstrate that a 0.48 mg/kg dose of a reversible monamine oxidase type B (MAO-B) inhibitor was needed to achieve more than 90% blockade of irreversible L-[^{11}C]deprenyl binding to central nervous system MAO-B (49). Here blockade of irreversible L-[^{11}C]deprenyl binding was used as the biomarker, and it was estimated that a 1-year Phase II study in patients with Parkinson's disease would have been required had conventional clinical endpoints been used for dose-ranging studies.

In the near future, it is likely that proteomics and genomics will expand the current repertoire of biomarkers. For example, it was found in the area of cholesterol-lowering therapy that the Taq1B polymorphism in the *CETP* gene that codes for cholesterol ester transfer protein (CETP) affects not only the rate of progression of coronary atherosclerois but also the extent to which patients benefit from pravastatin therapy (50). Coronary narrowing appears to progress more rapidly in B1 homozygotes than in B2 homozygotes, with heterozygotes having an intermediate rate

of progression. On the other hand, pravastatin reduced the rate of progression most markedly in B1 heterozygotes, somewhat less in heterozygotes, and not at all in B2 heterozygotes, even though the extent of cholesterol lowering was similar in all three groups. Hence, this genetic marker appears to have great potential in the selection of patients for future clinical trials of lipid-lowering therapy or as a co-variate in the analysis of these trials, and as a basis for selecting patients for therapy with pravastatin, and presumably other HMG-CoA reductase inhibitors.

Although it is expected that most disease states will be characterized by a typical gene expression pattern in one or more tissues of relevance, the pathophysiology of most common diseases is multifactorial. For this reason, the expression pattern of multiple genes frequently will be needed to develop a "signature" that could be used to confirm diagnosis, establish prognosis, choose the most appropriate therapy for an individual patient, and monitor patient response (51). Accordingly, future developments in pharmacogenomics are likely to incorporate the use of microarrays that can analyze the differential expression of as many as 10,000 genes in a single experiment (52, 53). The use of microarray technology poses a substantial bioinformatic challenge, but progress already is being made in developing relational database management systems that can store, process, and analyze the data that will be generated by high-throughput pharmacogenomic methods (54–55). Despite the technical challenges that remain, advances in pharmacogenomics and bioinformatics have the potential to provide panels of relevant biomarkers that can transform the drug development process and eventually establish an allele-specific basis for medical diagnosis and patient therapy (54).

References

1. Code of Federal Regulations, Title 21, Vol. 5, Parts 300 to 499. Washington, DC: U.S. Government Printing Office; April 1, 1997.
2. Temple RJ. A regulatory authority's opinion about surrogate endpoints. In: Nimmo WS, Tucker GT, editors. Clinical measurement in drug evaluation. New York: J Wiley; 1995.
3. Fleming TR, DeMets DL. Surrogate end points in clinical trials: Are we being misled? Ann Intern Med 1996;125:605–13.
4. Temple R. Are surrogate markers adequate to assess cardiovascular disease drugs? JAMA 1999;282:790–5.
5. Echt DS, Liebson PR, Mitchell B, Peters RW, Obias-Manno D, Barker AH, Arensberg D, Baker A, Friedman L, Greene L, Huther ML, Richardson DW, CAST Investigators. Mortality and morbidity of patients receiving encainide, flecainide or placebo: The cardiac arrhythmia suppression trial. N Engl J Med 1991;324:781–8.
6. NIH Definitions Working Group. Biomarkers and surrogate endpoints in clinical research: definitions and conceptual model. In: Downing GL, editor. Biomarkers and surrogate endpoints: Clinical research and applications. Amsterdam: Elsevier; 2000. p. 1–9.

7. Lown B, Fakharo AM, Hood WB, Thorn GW. The coronary care unit: New perspectives and directions. JAMA 1967;199:188–98.

8. Lie KI, Wellens HJ, van Capelle FJ, Durrer D. Lidocaine in the prevention of primary ventricular fibrillation: A double-blind, randomized study of 212 consecutive patients. N Engl J Med 1974;291:1324–6.

9. MacMahon S, Collins R, Peto R, Koster RW, Yusuf S. Effects of prophylactic lidocaine in suspected acute myocardial infarction: An overview of results from the randomized controlled trials. JAMA 1988;260:1910–16.

10. Hine LK, Laird N, Hewitt P, Chalmers TC. Meta-analytic evidence against prophylactic use of lidocaine in acute myocardial infarction. Arch Intern Med 1989;149:2694–8.

11. Campbell RWF. Arrhythmia prevention in the hospital phase of acute myocardial infarction. In: Califf RM, Mark DB, Wagner GS, editors. Acute coronary care. 2nd ed. St. Louis: Mosby-Year Book; 1995. p. 371–6.

12. Chobanian AV. The influence of hypertension and other hemodynamic factors in atherogenesis. Prog Cardiovasc Dis 1983;26:177–96.

13. Russell RWR. How does blood-pressure cause storke? Lancet 1975;ii:1283–5.

14. MacMahon S, Peto R, Cutler J, Collins R, Sorlie P, Neaton J, Abbott R, Godwin J, Dyer A, Stamler J. Blood pressure, stroke, and coronary heart disease: Part I, prolonged differences in blood pressure: prospective observational studies corrected for the regression dilution bias. Lancet 1990;335:765–74.

15. Psaty BM, Smith NL, Siscovick DS, Koepsell TD, Weiss NS, Heckbert SR, Lemaitre RN, Wagner EH, Furberg CD. Health outcomes associated with antihypertensive therapies used as first-line agents: A systematic review and meta-analysis. JAMA 1997;277:739–45.

16. Collins R, Peto R, MacMahon S, Hebert P, Fiebach NH, Eberlein KA, Godwin J, Qizilbash N, Taylor JO, Hennekens CH. Blood pressure, stroke, and coronary heart disease: Part 2, short-term reductions in blood pressure: Overview of randomized drug trials in their epidemiological context. Lancet 1990;335:827–38.

17. Siscovick DS, Raghunathan TE, Psaty BM, Koepsell TD, Wicklund KG, Lin X, Cobb L, Rautaharju PM, Copass MK, Wagner EH. Diuretic therapy for hypertension and the risk of primary cardiac arrest. N Engl J Med 1994;330:1852–7.

18. SHEP Cooperative Research Group. Prevention of stroke by antihypertensive drug treatment in older persons with isolated systolic hypertension: Final results of the systolic hypertension in the elderly program (SHEP). JAMA 1991;265:3255–64.

19. Furberg CD, Psaty BM, Meyer JV. Dose-related increase in mortality in patients with coronary heart disease. Circulation 1995;92:1326–31.

20. Shatzkin A, Freedman LS, Schiffman MH, Dawsey SM. Validation of intermediate end points in cancer research. J Natl Cancer Inst 1990;82:1746–52.

21. Freedman LS, Graubard BI. Statistical validation of intermediate endpoints for chronic diseases. Stat Med 1992;11:167–78.

22. Lin DY, Fleming TR, De Gruttola V. Estimating the proportion of treatment effect explained by a surrogate marker. Stat Med 1997;16:1515–27.

23. Prentice RL. Surrogate endpoints in clinical trials: Definition and operational criteria. Stat Med 1989;8:431–40.

24. Woosley RL, Chen Y, Freiman JP, Gillis RA. Mechanism of the cardiotoxic actions of terfenadine. JAMA 1993;269:1532–6.

25. Miller V, Mocroft A, Reiss P, Katlama C, Papadopoulos AI, Katzenstein T, van Lunzen J, Antunes F, Phillips AN, Lundgren JD, for the EuroSIDA Study Group. Relations among CD4 lymphocyte nadir, antiretroviral therapy, and HIV-1 disease progression: Results from the EuroSIDA study. Ann Intern Med 1999;130:570–7.

26. Davey Smith G, Pekkanen J. Should there be a moratorium on the use of cholesterol lowering drugs? BMJ 1992;304:431–4.

27. Gotto AM Jr, LaRosa JC, Hunninghake D, Grundy SM, Wilson PW, Clarkson TB, Hay JW, Goodman DS. The cholesterol facts: A summary of the evidence relating dietary fats, serum cholesterol, and coronary heart disease: a joint statement by the American Heart Association and the National Heart, Lung, and Blood Institute. Circulation 1990;81:1721–33.

28. Wissler RW, Vesselinovitch D. Can atherosclerotic plaques regress? Anatomic and biochemical evidence from nonhuman animal models. Am J Cardiol 1990;65:33F–40F.

29. Mol MJTM, Erkelens DW, Gevers Leuven JA, Schouten JA, Stalenhoef AFH. Effects of synvinolin (MK-733) on plasma lipids in familial hypercholesterolaemia. Lancet 1986;ii:936–9.

30. Scandinavian Simvastatin Survival Study Group. Randomised trial of cholesterol lowering in 4444 patients with coronary heart disease: The Scandinavian Simvastatin Survival Study (4S). Lancet 1994;344:1383–9.

31. Pedersen TR, Olsson AG, Færgeman O, Kjekshus J, Wedel H, Berg K, Wilhelmsen L, Haghfelt T, Thorgeirson G, Pyörälä K, Miettinen T, Christophersen B, Tobert JA, Musliner TA, Cook TJ, for the Scandinavian Simvastatin Survival Study Group. Lipoprotein changes and reduction in the incidence of major coronary heart disease events in the Scandinavian Simvastatin Survival Study. Circulation 97:1998;1453–60.

32. Grundy SM. Statin trials and goals of cholesterol-lowering therapy. Circulation 1998;97:1436–9.

33. West of Scotland Coronary Prevention Study Group. Influence of pravastatin and plasma lipids on clinical events in the West of Scotland Coronary Prevention Study (WOSCOPS). Circulation 1998;97:1440–5.

34. Vaughan CJ, Murphy MB, Buckley BM. Statins do more than just lower cholesterol. Lancet 1996;348:1079–82.

35. Ridker PM, Rifai N, Pfeffer MA, Sacks F, Braunwald E, for the Cholesterol and Recurrent Events (CARE) Investigators. Long-term effects of pravastatin on plasma concentration of C-reactive protein. Circulation 1999;100:230–5.

36. Ridker PM. Evaluating novel cardiovascular risk factors: Can we better predict heart attacks? Ann Intern Med 1999;130:933–7.

37. Reinoehl J, Frankovich D, Machado C, Kawasaki R, Baga JJ, Pires LA, Steinman RT, Fromm BS, Lehmann MH. Probucol-associated tachyarrhythmic events and QT prolongation: Importance of gender. Am Heart J 1996;131:1184–91.

38. Aziz KJ. Tumor markers: Reclassification and new approaches to evaluation. Adv Clin Chem 1999;33:169–99.

39. Bidart J-M, Thuillier F, Augereau C, Chalas J, Daver A, Jacob N, Labrousse F, Voitot H. Kinetics of serum tumor marker concentrations and usefulness in clinical monitoring. Clin Chem 1999;45:1695–707.

40. Mildvan D, Landay A, De Gruttola V, Machado SG, Kagan J. An approach to the validation of markers for use in AIDS clinical trials. Clin Infect Dis 1997;24:764–74.

41. Atkinson AJ Jr. The cerebrospinal fluid glucose concentration. Steady state and kinetic studies in patients with cryptococcal meningitis. Am Rev Resp Dis 1969;99:59–66.

42. Atkinson AJ Jr, Weiss MF. Kinetics of blood-cerebrospinal fluid glucose transfer in the normal dog. Am J Physiol 1969;216:1120–6.

43. O'Brien WA, Hartigan PM, Martin D, Esinhart J, Hill A, Benoit S, Rubin M, Simberkoff MS, Hamilton JD, the Veterans Affairs Cooperative Study Group on AIDS. Changes in plasma HIV-1 RNA and CD4+ lymphocyte counts and the risk of progression to AIDS. N Engl J Med 1996;334:426–31.

44. Engels EA, Rosenberg PS, O'Brien TR, Goedert JJ, for the Multicenter Hemophilia Cohort Study. Plasma HIV viral load in patients with hemophilia and late-stage HIV disease: A measure of current immune suppression. Ann Intern Med 1999;131:256–64.

45. O'Brien TR, Rosenberg PS, Yellin F, Goedert JJ. Longitudinal HIV-1 RNA levels in a cohort of homosexual men. J Acquir Immune Defic Syndr Hum Retrovirol 1998;18:155–61.

46. Ho DD, Neumann AU, Perelson AS, Chen W, Leonard JM, Markowitz M. Rapid turnover of plasma virions and CD4 lymphocytes in HIV-1 infection. Nature 1995;373:123–6.

47. Perelson AS, Essunger P, Cao Y, Vesanen M, Hurley A, Saksela K, Markowitz M, Ho DD. Decay characteristics of HIV-1 infected compartments during combination therapy. Nature 1997;387:188–91.

48. Rolan P. The contribution of clinical pharmacology surrogates and models to drug development—A critical appraisal. Br J Clin Pharmacol 1997;44:219–25.

49. Bench CJ, Price GW, Lammertsma AA, Cremer JC, Luthra SK, Turton D, Dolan RJ, Kettler R, Dingemanse J, Da Prada M, Biziere K, McClelland GR, Jamieson VL, Wood ND, Frackowiak RSJ. Measurement of human cerebral monamine oxidase type B (MAO-B) activity with positron emission tomography (PET): A dose ranging study with the reversible inhibitor Ro 19–6327. Br J Clin Pharmacol 1991;40:169–73.

50. Kuivenhoven JA, Jukema JW, Zwinderman AH, de Knijff, P, McPherson R, Bruschke AVG, Lie KI, Kastelein JJP, for the Regression Growth Evaluation Statin Study Group. The role of a common variant of the cholesterol ester transfer protein gene in the progression of coronary atherosclerosis. N Engl J Med 1998;338:86–93.

51. Van Ommen GJB, Bakker E, den Dunnen JT. The human genome project and the future of diagnostics, treatment, and prevention. Lancet 1999;354(suppl 1):5–10.

52. Debouck C, Goodfellow PN. DNA microarrays in drug discovery and development. Nat Genet 1999;21:48–50.

53. Hiltunen MO, Niemi M, Ylä-Herttuala S. Functional genomics and DNA array techniques in atherosclerosis research. Curr Opin Lipidol 1999;10:515–9.

54. Braxton S, Bedilion T. The integration of microarray information in the drug development process. Curr Opin Biotechnol 1998;9:643–9.

55. Carlisle AJ, Prabhu VV, Elkahloun A, Hudson J, Trent JM, Linehan WM, et al. Development of a prostate cDNA microarray and statistical gene expression analysis package. Mol Carcinogen 2000;28:12–22.

56. Scherf U, Ross DT, Waltham M, Smith LH, Lee JK, Tanabe L, et al. A gene expression database for the molecular pharmacology of cancer. Nat Genet 2000;24:236–44.

Dose-Effect and Concentration-Effect Analysis

ELIZABETH S. LOWE AND FRANK M. BALIS

*Pharmacology and Experimental Therapeutics Section, Pediatric Oncology Branch, National Cancer Institute,
National Institutes of Health, Bethesda, Maryland*

BACKGROUND

The intensity and duration of a drug's pharmacological effect are proportional to the dose of the drug administered and the concentration of the drug at its site of action. This simple fundamental principle of pharmacology has a pervasive influence on our approach to the study and use of drugs from the basic research laboratory to the management of patients receiving drug therapy in the clinic. *Pharmacodynamics* is the discipline that quantifies the relationship between drug concentration at the site of drug action and the drug's pharmacological effect. A drug's pharmacological effect can be monitored and quantified at several levels, including at a molecular or cellular level *in vitro,* in a tissue or organ *in vitro* or *in vivo*, or in the whole organism. The endpoint that is used to measure effect may differ at each level even for the same drug, and at the organism level the overall pharmacological effect may be the sum of multiple drug effects and the physiologic response of the organism to these drug effects.

A drug effect endpoint, such as change in blood pressure, that is measured on a continuous scale is termed a *graded* dose-effect relationship, whereas an all-or-none endpoint, such as alive or dead, is termed a *quantal* dose-effect relationship. Graded dose-effect relationships can be measured in a single biological unit that is exposed to a range of doses and dose or drug concentration is related to the *intensity* of the effect. Quantal dose-effect relationships are measured in a population of subjects that are treated with a range of doses and the dose is related to the *frequency* of the all-or-none effect at each dose level.

Figure 18.1 illustrates a graded dose-effect relationship for recombinant human erythropoietin (rhEPO) in patients with end-stage renal disease (1). Erythropoietin, which is produced by the kidney in response to hypoxia, is a naturally occurring hematopoietic growth factor that stimulates bone marrow production of red blood cells. Patients with end-stage renal disease are deficient in erythropoietin and, as a result, they are usually severely anemic and transfusion dependent. In this dose-finding study, 18 patients with end-stage renal disease and baseline hematocrit < 20% were treated with rhEPO at doses ranging from 1.5 to 500 units/kg in cohorts of three to five patients per dose level. The effect of the rhEPO is measured as the peak absolute increment in the hematocrit. At the lowest dose levels (1.5 and 5 units/kg), there was no effect on hematocrit, but starting at a dose of 15 units/kg, the hematocrit increased by 4% to 22% as the rhEPO dose increased. The shape of the dose-effect curve is a rectangular hyperbola, which asymptotically approaches a maximum effect. This means that, at higher doses, there is a "diminishing return" because the incremental increase in hematocrit is smaller with each incremental increase in rhEPO dose.

DRUG-RECEPTOR INTERACTIONS

The pharmacological effects of rhEPO and most drugs result from their noncovalent interaction with

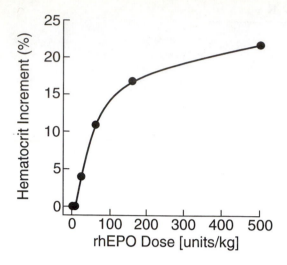

FIGURE 18.1 Dose-effect curve for recombinant human erythropoietin in patients with end-stage renal disease. Each point represents the mean absolute increase in hematocrit in a cohort of three to five patients. (Adapted from data published by Eschbach JW, Egrie JC, Downing MR, et al. N Engl J Med 1987;316:73–8.)

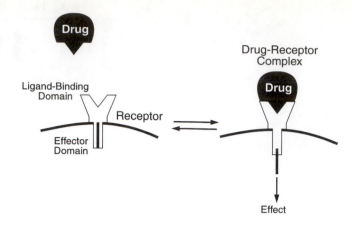

FIGURE 18.2 Drug-receptor interaction. A drug molecule binds reversibly to the ligand-binding domain of a receptor on the cell surface and the receptor propagates the signal into the cell via its effector domain resulting in a pharmacological effect.

receptors (Figure 18.2). A receptor can be any cellular macromolecule to which a drug selectively binds to initiate its pharmacological effect. Cellular proteins are the most important class of drug receptors, especially cellular proteins that are receptors for endogenous regulatory ligands, such as hormones, growth factors, and neurotransmitters. The drug's chemical structure is the primary determinant of the class of receptors with which the drug will interact. Receptors on the cell surface have two functional domains—a *ligand-binding domain* that is the drug binding site and an *effector domain* that propagates a signal and results in an effect (Figure 18.2). The interaction of a drug and its receptor is reversible and conforms to the *law of mass action*:

$$C + R \underset{k_2}{\overset{k_1}{\rightleftharpoons}} C - R$$

where C is the free drug concentration at the site of action, R is the concentration of unoccupied receptor in tissue, $C - R$ is the concentration of receptors occupied by drug, and k_1 and k_2 are the proportionality constants for the formation and dissociation of the drug-receptor complex.

Receptor Occupation Theory

The receptor *occupation theory* of drug action equates drug effect to receptor occupancy. The intensity of drug effect is proportional to the number of receptors that are occupied by drug and the maximum effect occurs when all receptors are occupied by drug.

The relationship between drug effect and the concentration of free drug at the site of action *(C)* can be described at equilibrium by the following equation:

$$\text{Effect} = \frac{\text{Maximum Effect} \cdot C}{K_D + C}$$

where Maximum Effect is the intensity of the pharmacological effect that occurs when all the receptors are occupied, and K_D, which equals k_2/k_1, is the equilibrium dissociation constant of the drug-receptor complex. The dissociation constant (K_D) is also a measure of the affinity of a drug for its receptor, analogous to the Michaelis–Menten constant (K_m), which is a measure of the affinity of a substrate for its enzyme. The expression $C/(K_D + C)$ in this equation represents the fraction of receptors that are occupied with drug. When $C >> K_D$, the expression equals 1 (i.e., all the receptors are occupied with drug), and the Effect = Maximum Effect.

The equation relating a drug's pharmacological effect to its concentration describes a hyperbolic function that is shown graphically in Figure 18.3A. As free drug concentration increases, the drug effect asymptotically approaches the maximum effect. When the free drug concentration on the x-axis is transformed to a logarithmic scale, the dose-effect curve becomes sigmoidal, with a central segment that is nearly log-linear (Figure 18.3B). Semilog dose-effect curves allow for a better assessment of the dose-effect relationship at low doses and of a wide range of doses on the same plot. The EC_{50} is the dose at which 50% of the maximum effect is produced or the concentration of drug at which the drug is half-maximally effective. On a semilogarithmic plot, the EC_{50} is located at the midpoint or

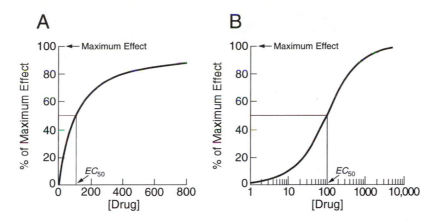

FIGURE 18.3   Dose-effect curves plotted using a linear *(Panel A)* or logarithmic *(Panel B)* scale for drug dose/concentration on the x-axis. The function relating effect to dose/concentration is based on the receptor occupation theory described in the text. The relationship is nonlinear and with each increment in dose/concentration there is diminishing increment in effect. EC_{50} is the dose/concentration producing half of the maximum effect.

inflection point of the curve. When the relationship between receptor occupancy and effect is linear, the K_D = EC_{50}. If there is amplification between receptor occupancy and effect, such as if the receptor has catalytic activity when the receptor ligand is bound, then the EC_{50} lies to the left of the K_D.

Receptor-mediated Effects

Figure 18.4A shows dose-effect curves for the types of pharmacological effects that can be elicited when a drug interacts with its receptor. Drugs that interact with a receptor and elicit the same stimulatory effect as the receptor's endogenous ligand are called *agonists*. An agonist that produces less than the maximum effect at doses or concentrations that saturate the receptor is a *partial agonist*. An *antagonist* binds to a receptor, but produces no effect. Antagonists produce their pharmacological effects by inhibiting the action of an agonist that binds to the same receptor.

Dose-effect curves are also useful for studying pharmacodynamic drug interactions (Figure 18.4B). A

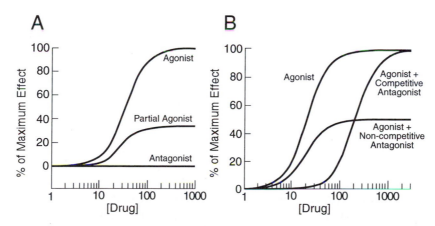

FIGURE 18.4   *Panel A:* Dose-effect curves describing the types of pharmacological effects produced when a drug interacts with its receptor. An *agonist* produces the maximum stimulatory effect, a *partial agonist* produces less than the maximum stimulatory effect, and an *antagonist* elicits no effect, but inhibits the effect of an agonist. *Panel B:* Dose-effect curves for the combination of an agonist and antagonist. A competitive antagonist reduces the potency of the agonist, but not the maximum effect. A noncompetitive antagonist reduces the efficacy (maximum effect), but does not alter the potency of the agonist.

competitive antagonist binds to the same binding site as the agonist, and the competitive antagonist can be displaced from the binding site by an excess of the agonist. Therefore, the maximum effect of an agonist can still be achieved in the presence of a competitive antagonist, if a sufficient dose or concentration of the agonist is used. The competitive antagonist lowers the potency of the agonist, but does not alter its efficacy. A *noncompetitive antagonist* binds irreversibly to the same binding site as the agonist, or it interacts with other components of the receptor to diminish or eliminate the effect of the drug binding to the receptor. A noncompetitive antagonist prevents the agonist, at any concentration, from producing its maximum effect. Typically, a dose-effect curve with this type of interaction will reveal a reduced apparent efficacy, but the potency of the drug is unchanged.

THE GRADED DOSE-EFFECT RELATIONSHIP

The drug-receptor concept of drug action and the receptor occupation theory describe a graded dose-effect relationship, in which the responding system is capable of showing progressively increasing effect with increasing dose or drug concentration. Graded dose-effect relationships are measured by exposing a single subject or a specific organ or tissue to increasing amounts of drug and quantifying the resulting effect on a continuous scale. Although the dose-effect curve can take on a variety of shapes, the classical graded dose-effect curve is the rectangular hyperbola (Figure 18.3) that was described previously.

Figure 18.5 demonstrates a graded concentration-effect study of an intravenous infusion of lidocaine at a rate of 8.35 mg/min in patients with neuropathic pain (2). The severity of pain was measured using a visual analog pain scale (0 to 10) at 10-minute intervals, and blood levels of lidocaine were also measured at 10-minute intervals. Patients had a median pain score of 7 prior to the initiation of therapy, and the maximal effect, no pain, had a score of 0. The concentration-effect curve for lidocaine is very steep. The pain decreased over a concentration range of 0.62 μg/mL. This steep concentration-effect curve indicates that the response to intravenous lidocaine is characterized by a precipitous break in pain over a narrow range in lidocaine concentrations.

Dose-Effect Parameters

Potency and *efficacy* are parameters that are derived from graded dose-effect curves and can be used to com-

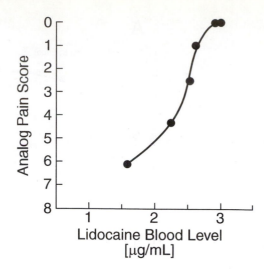

FIGURE 18.5 Graded concentration-effect curve for intravenous lidocaine in patients with neuropathic pain. Pain was scored from 0 to 10 with an analog pain scale. The median pretreatment pain score was 7 and a score of 0 meant no pain. Blood levels of lidocaine were measured every 10 minutes and pain was scored at the same time points. The graph relates the blood level of lidocaine to the severity of pain. (Reproduced with permission from Ferrante FM, Paggioli J, Cherukuri S, Arthur GR. Anesth Analg 1996;82:91–7.)

pare drugs that elicit the same pharmacological effect. Potency, which is a measure of the sensitivity of a target organ or tissue to the drugs, is a relative term that relates the amount of one drug required to produce a desired level of effect to the amount of a different drug required to produce the same effect. On the semilogarithmic graded dose-effect plot, the curve of the more potent agent is to the left, and the EC_{50} is lower. A drug's potency is influenced by its affinity for its receptor. In Figure 18.6, Drug A is more potent than Drug B.

Figure 18.7 shows the *in vitro* dose-effect curves for two thiopurine analogs, thioguanine and mercaptopurine. The thiopurines are antimetabolites that are used in the treatment of acute leukemia. Both drugs have multiple sites of action, but their primary mechanism of action is felt to be the result of their incorporation into DNA strands. Effect is measured as the percentage of leukemic cells killed in the presence of drug compared to untreated controls for three different leukemic cell lines *in vitro* (3). The dose-effect curves show that thioguanine is approximately 10-fold more potent than mercaptopurine, despite the fact that they have very similar chemical structures and are converted to the same active intracellular metabolite (deoxy-thioguanosine triphosphate) prior to their incorporation into DNA. The two drugs appear to have similar efficacy in this *in vitro* study. Considerable weight is placed on these *in vitro* concentration-effect studies for anticancer drugs because it has not

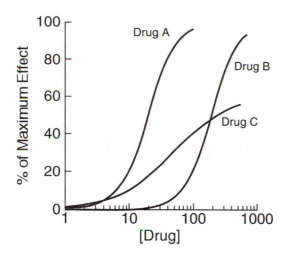

FIGURE 18.6 Evaluation of the relative potency and efficacy of drugs that produce the same pharmacological effect. Drug A is more potent than Drug B, and drugs A and B are more efficacious than drug C.

been possible to define therapeutic concentrations *in vivo* in animal models or patients.

Efficacy is the drug property that allows the receptor-bound drug to produce its pharmacological effect. The relative efficacy of two drugs that elicit the same effect can be measured by comparing the maximum effects of the drugs. In Figure 18.6, Drugs A and B are more efficacious than Drug C. *Intrinsic activity* (α), which is a proportionality factor that relates drug

effect in a specific tissue to receptor occupancy, has become a standard parameter for quantifying the ability of a drug to produce a response:

$$\text{Effect} = \alpha \cdot \left(\frac{\text{Maximum Effect} \cdot \text{Dose}}{K_D + \text{Dose}} \right)$$

The value for intrinsic activity ranges from 1 for a full agonist to 0 for an antagonist, and the fractional values between these extremes represent partial agonists. Intrinsic activity is a property of both the drug and the tissue in which drug effect is measured.

Comparing the dose-effect curves of drugs that produce the same pharmacological effect can also provide information about the site of action of the drugs. Drugs A and B in Figure 18.6 have parallel dose-effect curves with identical shapes and the same level of maximal response. This suggests, but does not prove, that these two drugs act through the same receptor. Conversely, Drugs A and C have nonparallel dose-response curves, suggesting that they have different sites of action.

Dose-Effect and Site of Drug Action

Graded concentration-effect studies may be useful for establishing the mechanism of action of a drug at a molecular or biochemical level by assessing the drug-receptor interaction. The xanthine analog, theophylline, which is a potent relaxant of bronchial smooth muscle, is used for the treatment of asthma. However, theophylline has a narrow therapeutic range, and at concentrations above this therapeutic range patients can experience vomiting, tremor, seizures, and cardiac arrhythmias. Theophylline interacts with multiple receptors that could account for its antiasthmatic effect and its toxicity. Theophylline is an adenosine receptor antagonist and it inhibits phosphodiesterase (PDE). These two mechanisms have been proposed as the basis for the pharmacological effects of theophylline and other xanthines.

In Figure 18.8, the drug concentration that is required to elicit relaxation of tracheal smooth muscle in isolated guinea pig tracheal segments *in vitro* for a series of xanthine analogs, including theophylline, is related to the drug concentration required to antagonize the A1-adenosine receptor (Figure 18.8A) or inhibit brain soluble PDE (Figure 18.8B) (4). The relative potencies of these xanthine analogs as adenosine receptor antagonists do not correlate with their potencies as tracheal relaxants. However, there is an association between PDE inhibition and tracheal relaxant activity, suggesting that PDE inhibition is the primary site of drug action. This type of graded concentration-

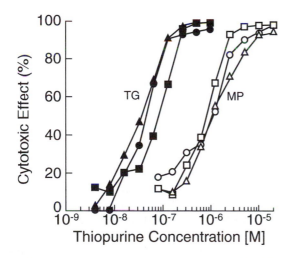

FIGURE 18.7 Concentration-effect curves for the thiopurine analogs, mercaptopurine (MP, *open symbols*) and thioguanine (TG, *closed symbols*). Effect is the percentage of cells killed *in vitro* relative to an untreated control in MOLT 4 *(squares)*, CCRF-CEM *(triangles)* and Wilson *(circles)* leukemia cell lines. TG is 10-fold more potent than MP. (Reproduced with permission from Adamson PC, Poplack DG, Balis FM. Leukemia Res 1994;18:805–10.)

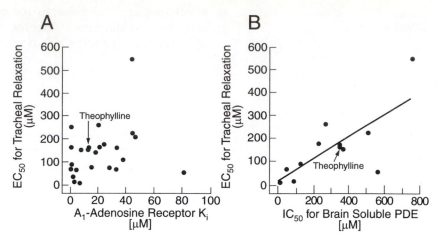

FIGURE 18.8 Correlation between concentration-effect at the tissue level measured by EC_{50} for relaxation of guinea pig trachea and concentration-effect at the receptor level for antagonism of the A1-adenosine receptor *(Panel A)* and inhibition of phosphodiesterase *(Panel B)* for a series of xanthine analogs, including theophylline. The correlation between EC_{50} for tracheal relaxation and IC_{50} for phosphodiesterase inhibition suggests that phosphodiesterase inhibition is the primary site of action for the antiasthmatic effects of these drugs. (Reproduced with permission from Brackett LE, Shamim MT, Daley JW. Biochem Pharmacol 1990;39:1897–904.)

effect analysis can lead to the development of more selective agents. In this case, xanthine analogs that are more potent PDE inhibitors and weaker adenosine receptor antagonists may be more effective and less toxic anti-asthmatics.

THE QUANTAL DOSE-EFFECT RELATIONSHIP

Whereas a graded dose-effect relationship relates drug dose/concentration to the intensity of a drug's effect measured on a continuous scale in a single biological unit, the *quantal* dose-effect relationship relates dose to the frequency of the all-or-none effect in a population of subjects. The minimally effective dose, or *threshold dose,* of the drug that evokes the all-or-none effect is identified by gradually increasing the dose in each subject. When displayed graphically as a frequency distribution histogram with threshold dose levels as the independent variable (x-axis) and the number of subjects who respond at each threshold dose level on the y-axis, the quantal dose-effect curve assumes a normal frequency distribution or bell-shaped curve (Figure 18.9A). The threshold dose level at which the effect occurs with maximum frequency is in the middle portion of the dose range. For most drugs, a wide range of threshold doses are required to produce the all-or-none effect in a population of subjects. This variability results from differences in drug

disposition (pharmacokinetics) and end-organ or tissue sensitivity to the drug (pharmacodynamics) within the population.

A quantal dose-effect relationship can also be graphically displayed as a cumulative dose-effect curve, in which the cumulative percentage of subjects experiencing an effect is plotted as a function of the threshold dose. The normal frequency distribution in Figure 18.9A takes on a sigmoidal shape when the same data are plotted as a cumulative dose-effect curve (Figure 18.9B). The median effective dose (ED_{50}) for the quantal dose-effect relationship is the dose at which 50% of the population on the cumulative dose-effect curve responds to the drug. The cumulative dose-effect curve reflects the manner in which most quantal dose-effect studies are performed in a population of subjects. It is usually not practical to define the threshold dose for each subject by gradually increasing the dose in each subject in human or animal trials. Therefore, in most studies, groups of subjects are treated at each different dose level, and the fraction of subjects who respond at each dose level represents the cumulative proportion of subjects whose threshold dose is at or below the administered dose. This is equivalent to the cumulative distribution.

When administered to an organism, a drug produces a desired therapeutic effect, but it is also likely to produce at least one toxic effect. As a result, a single dose-effect curve does not adequately characterize the full spectrum of effects from the drug. The toxic effects

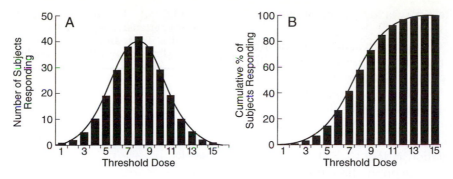

FIGURE 18.9 Population-based, quantal dose-effect curves plotted in *Panel A* as a frequency histogram relating the threshold dose that is required to produce an all-or-none effect to the number of subjects responding at each threshold dose; and in *Panel B* as a cumulative distribution, in which the cumulative fraction of subjects responding at each dose is plotted as a function of the dose.

of a drug can also be described by separate quantal dose-effect curves, and the safety of a drug depends on the degree of separation between the dose that produces the therapeutic effect and the dose that produces unacceptable toxic effects.

Cardiotoxicity, which can lead to congestive heart failure and death, is a toxic effect of the anticancer drug, doxorubicin. A cumulative dose-effect analysis demonstrated that doxorubicin cardiotoxicity is related to the lifetime dose of the drug (Figure 18.10) and provided the basis for the definition of safe lifetime dose levels (5). The lifetime dose of doxorubicin is now limited to less than 400 to 450 mg/m², which is associated with a <5% risk of developing congestive heart failure.

Therapeutic Indices

Therapeutic indices quantify the relative safety of a drug and can be estimated from the cumulative quantal dose-effect curves of a drug's therapeutic and toxic effects. Figure 18.11 shows the doses that are used in the calculation of these indices.

The *therapeutic ratio* $[TD_{50}/ED_{50}]$ is a ratio of the dose at which 50% of subjects experience the toxic effect to the dose at which 50% of patients experience the therapeutic effect. A therapeutic ratio of 2.5 means that approximately 2.5 times as much drug is required to cause toxicity in half of the subjects than is needed to produce a therapeutic effect in the same proportion of subjects. However, this ratio of toxic to therapeutic dose may not be consistent across the entire dose

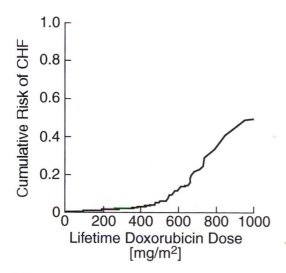

FIGURE 18.10 Cumulative risk of developing congestive heart failure as a function of the lifetime dose of doxorubicin. (Reproduced with permission from Von Hoff DD, Layard MW, Basa P, et al. Ann Intern Med 1979;91:710–7.)

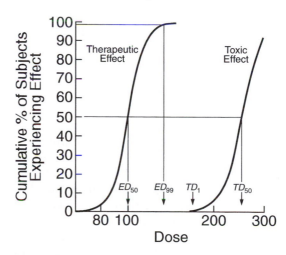

FIGURE 18.11 Cumulative quantal dose-effect curves for a drug's therapeutic and toxic effects. The ED_{50} and ED_{99} are the doses required to produce the drug's therapeutic effect in 50% and 99% of the population, respectively. The TD_1 and TD_{50} are the doses that cause the toxic effect in 1% and 50% of the population, respectively.

range if the dose-effect curves for the therapeutic and toxic effects are not parallel.

The goal of drug therapy is to achieve the desired therapeutic effect in all patients without producing toxic effects in any patients. Therefore, an index that uses the lowest toxic and highest therapeutic doses is more consistent with this goal than the therapeutic ratio. The *certainty safety factor* (CSF) is the ratio of TD_1/ED_{99}. A CSF>1 indicates that the dose effective in 99% of the population is less than the dose that would be toxic in 1% of the population. If the CSF <1, there is overlap between the maximally effective (ED_{99}) and minimally toxic (TD_1) doses. Unlike the therapeutic ratio, this measure is independent of the shapes of the cumulative quantal dose-effect curves for the therapeutic and toxic effects. The *standard safety margin* $\{[(TD_1 - ED_{99})/ED_{99}] \times 100\}$ also uses TD_1 and ED_{99} but is expressed as the percentage by which the ED_{99} must be increased before the TD_1 is reached.

Dose-Effect and Defining Optimal Dose

Characterization of the dose-effect relationship is an important component of clinical trials performed during the initial stages of clinical drug development. These early trials frequently follow a dose-escalation design in which increasing dose levels of drug are administered to cohorts of subjects until the maximal effect is achieved or dose-limiting toxicity is encountered. The optimal dose is identified from these dose-effect relationships for the therapeutic and toxic effects.

Johnston (6) reviewed the dose-finding studies of a variety of antihypertensive agents and compared the initial recommended dosage range from these dose-finding studies with the lowest effective dose identified in subsequent randomized clinical trials and the currently recommended dose (Table 18.1). Based on this dose-effect meta-analysis, he concluded that many antihypertensive agents were introduced into clinical practice at excessively high doses. He attributed this to reliance on a dose-escalation trial design in which the dose was escalated too rapidly, resulting in a failure to define the lower part of the dose-effect relationship. In many of the cases, the initial dose produced the maximum therapeutic effect, but the dose continued to be escalated without any clear evidence of increased efficacy. The initial recommended doses often appeared to be on the plateau of the dose-effect curve rather than in the desired range; at these higher doses, there is very little added benefit but a significantly greater risk for toxicity. A current trend is to avoid this pitfall by identifying the minimum dose required for satisfactory effect (MDSE) (7).

TABLE 18.1 Comparison of Recommended Doses for Antihypertensive Agents Based on Initial Dose-Finding Clinical Trials and Subsequent Experience in Clinical Practice and Randomized Clinical Trials.[a]

Drug	Dose range (mg)		Lowest effective dose (mg)
	Early studies	Present	
Propranolol	160–5000	160–320	80
Atenolol	100–2000	50–100	25
Hydrochlorothiazide	50–400	25–50	12.5
Captropril	75–1000	50–150	37.5
Methyldopa	500–6000	500–3000	750

[a] Data from Johnson GD. Pharmacol Ther 1992;55:53–93).

For anticancer drugs, tumor response is often related to *dose intensity,* and this dose-effect relationship is the basis for the use of the maximum tolerated dose and shortening the dosing interval of anticancer drugs. Dose intensity, or dose rate, is the amount of drug administered within a defined period of time (e.g., mg/week). The strong relationship between doxorubicin dose intensity and the percentage of patients with osteogenic sarcoma who achieved greater than 90% tumor necrosis is shown in Figure 18.12 (8). A dose intensity analysis such as this one is useful in defining the optimal dose of an

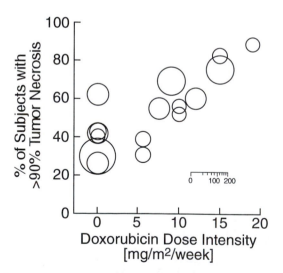

FIGURE 18.12 Dose intensity meta-analysis for doxorubicin in osteosarcoma. Each bubble represents a separate clinical trial and the size of the bubble is proportional to the number of patients treated on the trial. Doxorubicin was administered prior to definitive surgical resection and effect is > 90% necrosis of tumor in the resected specimen. Dose intensity or dose rate is measured in mg/m²/week. (Reproduced with permission from Smith MA, Ungerleider RS, Horowitz ME, et al. J Natl Cancer Inst 1991;83:1460–70.)

anticancer drug if a relationship between dose and therapeutic effect is observed.

PHARMACODYNAMIC MODELS

Pharmacodynamic models mathematically relate a drug's pharmacological effect to its concentration at the effect site. Examples of the types of pharmacodynamic models that have been employed include the fixed effect model, maximum effect models (E_{max} and sigmoid E_{max}), and linear and log-linear models (9). Unlike pharmacokinetic models, pharmacodynamic models are time independent. However, these models can be linked to pharmacokinetic models as discussed in Chapter 19.

Fixed-effect Model

The fixed-effect pharmacodynamic model is a simple model that relates drug concentration to a pharmacological effect that is either present or absent, such as sleep, or a defined cutoff for a continuous effect, such as diastolic blood pressure < 90 mm Hg in a patient with hypertension. The specific pharmacological effect is present when the drug concentration is greater than a threshold level required to produce the effect, and the effect is absent when the drug concentration is below the threshold. This threshold concentration varies among individuals and the fixed effect model quantifies the likelihood or probability that a given concentration will produce an all-or-none effect based on the population distribution of threshold concentrations. This model is used primarily in the clinical setting. For example, based on a study correlating digoxin levels with toxicity, the probability of toxicity is 50% at a digoxin level of 3 ng/mL (10).

Maximum-effect (E_{max} and Sigmoid E_{max}) Models

Although the maximum effect pharmacodynamic models are empirically based, they do incorporate the concept of a maximum effect predicted by the drug-receptor interactions described earlier. The Hill equation, which takes the same form as the equation describing drug effect as a function of receptor occupancy, relates a continuous drug effect to the drug concentration at the effect site as shown:

$$\text{Effect} = \frac{E_{max} \cdot C^n}{EC_{50}^n + C^n}$$

where E_{max} is the maximum effect, EC_{50} is the drug concentration producing 50% of E_{max}, C is the drug

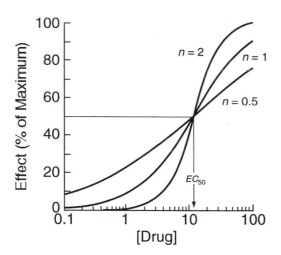

FIGURE 18.13 Sigmoid E_{max} pharmacodynamic model relating drug effect to the drug concentration at the effect site. The three curves show the effect of the exponential Hill constant *(n)* on the slope of the sigmoid curves.

concentration, and the exponential constant, *n* (the Hill constant), controls the slope of the resulting sigmoid-shaped curve, as shown in Figure 18.13 (11). If there is a baseline effect in the absence of drug, the Effect term in the equation can be expressed as the absolute or percentage change from baseline. Maximum effect models describe a hyperbolic relationship between drug concentration and effect such that there is no effect in the absence of drug, there is a maximum effect (E_{max}) when concentrations approach infinity, and there is a diminishing increment in effect as the concentration rises above the EC_{50}.

The E_{max} model is a simpler form of the sigmoid E_{max} model with a slope factor $n = 1$, so that:

$$\text{Effect} = \frac{E_{max} \cdot C}{EC_{50} + C}$$

In Figure 18.14, the E_{max} model is used to quantify the relationship between theophylline serum level and improvement in pulmonary function as measured by the increase in FEV_1 in six patients who were treated with placebo and three incremental doses of theophylline (12).

Linear and Log-linear Model

In the linear model concentration-effect relationships are described by the equation:

$$\text{Effect} = E_0 + \sigma C$$

where E_0 is the baseline effect prior to treatment, σ is the slope of the line, and C is the drug concentration. Although the linear model will predict no effect when

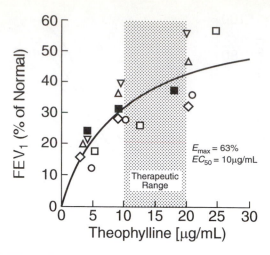

FIGURE 18.14 Theophylline pharmacodynamics in patients with asthma. Effect, which was measured as improvement in FEV_1, is related to the serum drug level in six patients, who were studied after placebo and three incremental doses of theophylline. An E_{max} model is fit to the concentration-effect data. Based on this analysis, a therapeutic range of 10 to 20 μg/mL was proposed *(shaded area)*. (Adapted from data published by Mitenko PA, Ogilvie RI. N Engl J Med 1973;289:600–3.)

drug concentrations are zero, it cannot predict a maximum effect. Therefore, for many effects, this model is only applicable over a narrow concentration range. At low drug concentrations ($<<EC_{50}$), the slope will approach the value of E_{max}/E_{50}.

When the maximum effect models are plotted on a semilog scale, the sigmoidal curves are log-linear within the range of 20% to 80% of the maximum effect, and can be described by the *log-linear model* (Effect = $\sigma \cdot \log C + I$, where I is the intercept). The disadvantages of this approach are that the pharmacologic effect cannot be predicted when the drug concentration is zero because of the logarithmic function, and the maximum effect cannot be predicted at very high concentrations. For example, the data shown in Figure 18.14 were linearized in the original article by plotting them with a logarithmic abscissa (12). This linearized version of the figure unfortunately obscured the fact that theophylline levels above 15 μg/mL result in relatively little gain in therapeutic efficacy. Thus maximum-effect models, which do not have these limitations, may be preferable to the linear models over a broad drug concentration range. Although simpler linear models are necessary when responses are linear over narrow concentration ranges, semilogarithmic plots should not be used to linearize curvilinear dose response relationships.

CONCLUSION

The dose- or concentration-effect relationship is a central tenet of pharmacology. Dose-effect studies contribute to our understanding of the site of action of a drug, the selection of a dose and dosing schedule, the determination of an agent's potency and efficacy, and the elucidation of drug interactions. An essential aspect of the preclinical and clinical evaluation of any new drug is the careful delineation of the dose-effect relationship over the anticipated dosing range for the drug's therapeutic and toxic effects. More rational individualized dosing regimens that incorporate adaptive dosing, therapeutic drug monitoring, and the determination of risk/benefit from therapeutic indices have evolved from the integration of our knowledge of pharmacokinetics and pharmacodynamics.

References

1. Eschbach JW, Egrie JC, Downing MR, Browne JK, Adamson JW. Correction of the anemia of end-stage renal disease with recombinant human erythropoietin: Results of a combined phase I and II clinical trial. N Engl J Med 1987;316:73–8.
2. Ferrante FM, Paggioli J, Cherukuri S, Arthur GR. The analgesic response to intravenous lidocaine in the treatment of neuropathic pain. Anesthes Analges 1996;82:91–7.
3. Adamson PC, Poplack DG, Balis FM. The cytotoxicity of thioguanine vs mercaptopurine in acute lymphoblastic leukemia. Leukemia Res 1994;18:805–10.
4. Brackett LE, Shamim MT, Daley JW. Activities of caffeine, theophylline, and enprofylline analogs as tracheal relaxants. Biochem Pharmacol 1990;39:1897–904.
5. Von Hoff DD, Layard MW, Basa P, Davis HL, Von Hoff AL, Rozencweig M, et al. Risk factors for doxorubicin-induced congestive heart failure. Ann Intern Med 1979;91:710–7.
6. Johnston GD. Dose-response relationships with antihypertensive drugs. Pharmacol Ther 1992;55:53–93.
7. Rolan P. The contribution of clinical pharmacology surrogates and models to drug development—A critical appraisal. Br J Clin Pharmacol 1997;44:219–25.
8. Smith MA, Ungerleider RS, Horowitz ME, Simon R. Influence of doxorubicin dose intensity on response and outcome for patients with osteogenic sarcoma and Ewing's sarcoma. J Natl Cancer Inst 1991;83:1460–70.
9. Holford NHG, Sheiner LB. Pharmacokinetic and pharmacodynamic modeling in vivo. CRC Crit Rev Bioengineer 1981;5:273–322.
10. Piergies AA, Worwag EM, Atkinson AJ Jr. A concurrent audit of high digoxin plasma levels. Clin Pharmacol Ther 1994;55:353–8.
11. Wagner JG. Kinetics of pharmacologic response. J Theor Biol 1968;20:173–201.
12. Mitenko PA, Ogilvie RI. Rational intravenous doses of theophylline. N Engl J Med 1973;289:600–3.

19

Kinetic Analysis
of Pharmacologic Effect

ARTHUR J. ATKINSON, JR.

Clinical Center, National Institutes of Health, Bethesda, Maryland

A reversible pharmacologic response to a drug dose frequently occurs perceptibly later than would be expected from the plasma level profile of the drug. In many instances this temporal dissociation can be characterized by conducting a pharmacokinetic-pharmacodynamic analysis of repeated drug plasma level and effect measurements. Two basic conceptual approaches have been developed for analyzing hysteresis between drug plasma levels and pharmacodynamic response (1). In the first approach, the pharmacologic effect is considered a direct consequence of drug action and the delay in response is thought to reflect the time required for the drug to reach its site of pharmacologic action, or *biophase*. Alternatively, the drug receptor interaction may initiate a series of downstream biochemical events that account for the observed time lag. In the second approach, the drug is thought to act indirectly to alter the synthesis or degradation of some factor, usually an endogenous compound, that mediates the drug effect. With each approach, the basic relationships between drug concentration and intensity of effect that were described in Chapter 18 can be applied to the pharmacodynamic analysis.

ANALYSIS OF DIRECT PHARMACOLOGIC EFFECTS

In some cases it is biologically plausible to identify as the site of drug action one of the compartments used to characterize the kinetics of drug distribution. As described in Chapter 3, Sherwin et al. (2) noted that the time course of insulin-stimulated glucose utilization parallels expected insulin concentrations in the slowly equilibrating compartment of a three-compartment model of insulin distribution (Figure 3.3). Since this compartment is composed largely of skeletal muscle interstitial fluid (3), it is reasonable to conclude that this pharmacokinetic compartment is also the site of this particular insulin effect. In a study of digoxin pharmacokinetics and inotropic effects, Kramer et al. (4) observed that there is a close relationship between the time course of these effects and estimated digoxin concentrations in the slowly equilibrating peripheral compartment of a three-compartment pharmacokinetic model. Although the heart constitutes only a small fraction of total body muscle mass, there is some physiological justification for identifying myocardium as a component of this compartment. On the other hand, the authors were correct in emphasizing that the time course of inotropic response could also reflect a delay due to the time required for the cascade of digoxin-initiated intracellular events to result in increased myocardial contractile force. In this regard, models in which the effects of lysergic acid diethylamide on arithmetic performance appear to emanate from a peripheral compartment of a pharmacokinetic model would appear to result from coincidence and do not have an obvious physiological rationale (5, 6).

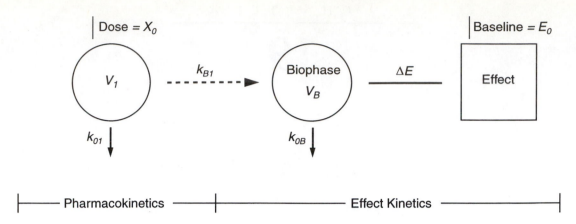

FIGURE 19.1 A direct pharmacokinetic effect model in which the kinetics of drug distribution and elimination are modeled with a single compartment (V_1) that receives a bolus input dose $X_{(0)}$ and has an elimination rate constant k_{01}. Plasma concentrations are linked to a biophase compartment (V_B), and ΔE transduces drug concentrations in the biophase compartment into changes in the observed effect (E). The baseline value for the effect is given by E_0 so that $E = E_0 \pm \Delta E$. The time course of the observed effects is governed by the rate constant k_{0B}. The arrow linking V_1 and V_B is dotted to indicate that no mass transfer occurs between these compartments and that k_{B1} is not an independent parameter of the system (see text).

Analyses Incorporating a Biophase Compartment

Since only a small fraction of an administered drug dose actually binds to receptors or in other ways produces an observed response, it is reasonable to suppose that the biophase may have kinetic properties that are distinct from those of the splanchnic and somatic tissues that, as discussed in Chapter 3, primarily govern the overall drug distribution process. This was first appreciated by Segre (7), who introduced the concept of a separate biophase compartment to explain the fact that the pressor effects of norephinephrine lagged appreciably behind its concentration profile in blood. Hull et al. (8) and Sheiner et al. (9) independently incorporated a biophase compartment in their pharmacokinetic-pharmacodynamic studies of the linkage between plasma concentrations of neuromuscular blocking drugs and their skeletal muscle paralyzing effects.

Figure 19.1 is a schematic diagram of a pharmacokinetic-pharmacodynamic model in which a biophase compartment links drug concentrations in plasma to observed pharmacological effects. The mathematical characteristics of this biophase compartment have been described in detail by Sheiner et al. (9) and by Holford and Sheiner (10). In Figure 19.1, the pharmacokinetics of drug distribution and elimination are characterized by a single compartment (V_1). Since no drug actually passes from V_1 to V_B, and this compartment merely serves as a forcing function with respect to the biophase, the differential equation for drug in V_1 can be written as:

$$dX/dt = -k_{01} X$$

The differential equation for drug in the biophase compartment is:

$$dB/dt = k_{B1} X - k_{0B} B \tag{19.1}$$

Expressing these in Laplace notation (see Appendix I) gives the following two simultaneous equations:

$$sX(s) - X_0 = -k_{01}X(s) \quad \text{or} \quad X(s) = \frac{X_0}{s + k_{01}} \tag{19.2}$$

and:

$$sB(s) = k_{B1}X(s) - k_{0B}B(s) \quad \text{or} \quad B(s) = \frac{k_{B1}X(s)}{s + k_{0B}} \tag{19.3}$$

Substituting $X(s)$ as defined by Equation 19.2 into Equation 19.3 yields:

$$B(s) = \frac{X_0 k_{B1}}{(s + k_{0B})(s + k_{0B})}$$

Taking the inverse Laplace transform of this expression for the general case when $k_{01} \neq k_{0B}$:

$$B(s) = \frac{X_0 k_{B1}}{(k_{0B} - k_{01})} \left(e^{-k_{01}t} - e^{-k_{0B}t} \right) \tag{19.4}$$

From Equation 19.1, we see that at steady state:

$$k_{B1} X_{SS} = k_{0B} B_{SS}$$

where X_{SS} and B_{SS} are the respective steady state values for X and B. To interpret biophase concentration-related effects in terms of their equivalent steady-state plasma concentrations, we equate their steady-state concentrations by letting $B_{SS} = X_{SS}$ and $V_B = V_1$. Therefore, $k_{B1} = k_{0B}$, and Equation 19.4 can be rewritten to describe biophase concentrations as:

$$[B] = \frac{X_0 k_{0B}}{V_1(k_{0B} - k_{01})} \left(e^{-k_{01}t} - e^{-k_{0B}t}\right) \qquad (19.5)$$

Under these conditions k_{0B} is the only parameter that characterizes the biophase compartment that is not obtained from the conventional kinetic analysis of drug distribution and elimination.

Incorporation of Pharmacodynamic Models

The approaches described in Chapter 18 that are used to relate steady-state plasma concentrations of drug to observed pharmacologic effects can also be applied in pharmacokinetic-pharmacodynamic analysis.

Linear Response Models

If the relationship between change in effect (ΔE) and biophase concentration is linear, biophase concentrations can be related to ΔE by a constant (σ) such that:

$$\Delta E = \sigma[B] \qquad (19.6)$$

Biophase concentrations then are related to observations made on the effect variable (*E*) as follows:

$$E = E_0 \pm \sigma[B] \qquad (19.7)$$

where E_0 is the baseline observed effect and $\pm$ denotes that the change in effect can either add to or subtract from the baseline value.

Blood pressure and electrocardiographic QT interval are examples of effects in which pharmacokinetic-pharmacodynamic analysis usually incorporates a linear response model (11, 12). It was shown in one study in which linear response models were used that the blood-pressure-lowering effects and blockade of transmission across sympathetic ganglia caused by *N*-acetylprocainamide followed a similar time course (11). This pharmacokinetic-pharmacodynamic analysis was used to provide supporting evidence for the conclusion that the observed hypotensive effect of the drug was mediated by its ganglionic blocking action. This detailed analysis in dogs was also shown to characterize the intensity and time course of the hypotensive effects of *N*-acetylprocainamide in a human subject.

E_{max} Models

The apparent linear relationship between biophase concentration and pharmacologic response usually reflects the fact that effects have been analyzed over only a very limited concentration range (10). In many cases, an E_{max} model is required to analyze more pronounced effects, such as the blood pressure response of cats to norepinephrine that was the concentration-effect relationship initially analyzed by Segre (7). For the E_{max} model, ΔE in Equation 19.6 is described by:

$$\Delta E = \frac{E_0}{EC_{50} + [B]} \qquad (19.8)$$

The linear response model defines this relationship adequately as long as biophase drug concentrations, $[B]$, are substantially less than the EC_{50}. However, the decision to use an E_{max} rather than a linear model is determined by the available data rather than by theoretical considerations. For example, in one study of QT interval prolongation by an antiarrhythmic drug, a linear effect model was satisfactory for analyzing the response of four patients, but an E_{max} model was required to analyze the exaggerated response of a fifth patient (13).

Although the mathematical form of the E_{max} model is physiologically realistic (7), no physiological significance has been assigned to E_{max} and EC_{50} estimates in most applications of this model. Nonetheless, E_{max} values in some cases may provide an indication of the maximal degree to which a particular intervention can affect enzyme or receptor activity. It also may be possible to find similarities between EC_{50} values and drug-binding affinity. For example, ε-aminocaproic acid is a lysine analog that has clot-stabilizing antifibrinolytic effects because it binds to lysine binding sites on plasminogen, preventing its attachment to fibrin. A study of ε-aminocaproic acid kinetics and antifibrinolytic effects in human subjects provided an IC_{50} estimate, analogous to EC_{50} in Equation 19.8, of 63.0 ± 19.7 μg/mL which was similar to the *in vitro* estimate of 0.55 mM or 72 μg/mL for the ε-aminocaproic acid-plasminogen dissociation constant (14). In fact, these results represent an oversimplification of physiological reality since plasminogen has one high-affinity and four low-affinity sites that bind ε-aminocaproic acid (15).

Sigmoid E_{max} Models

In some cases, Equation 19.8 will need to be modified to account for the fact that the biophase concentration-response relationship is sigmoid rather than hyperbolic. This modification was necessary in analyzing the pharmacokinetics and effects of *d*-tubocurarine

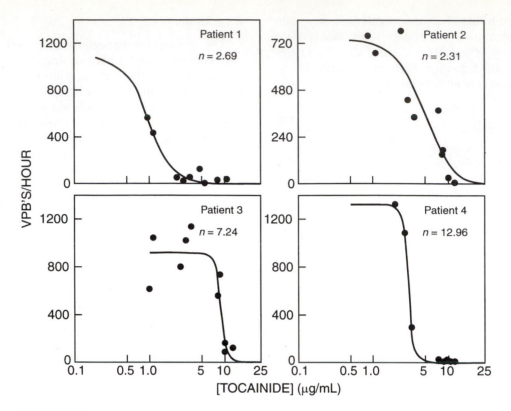

FIGURE 19.2   Relationship between plasma concentrations of tocainide and suppression of ventricular premature beats (VPBs) for four representative patients. The relationship between VPB frequency and tocainide concentrations shown by the solid curves was obtained from a nonlinear least-squares regression analysis of the data using Equation 19.8. The estimate of n for each patient can be compared with the shape of the tocainide concentration-antiarrhythmic response curve. (Reproduced with permission from Meffin PJ, Winkle RA, Blaschke TF, Fitzgerald J, Harrison DC. Clin Pharmacol Ther 1977;22:42–57.)

(9). In this case, the following equation was used to relate estimated biophase concentrations of d-tubocurarine to the degree of skeletal muscle paralysis (ΔE), ranging from normal function to complete paralysis $(E_{max} = 1)$ caused by this drug:

$$\Delta E = \frac{E_{max}}{EC_{50}^{n} + [B]^{n}} [B]^{n} \qquad (19.9)$$

Equation 19.9 was developed initially by Hill (16) to analyze the oxygen-binding affinity of hemoglobin. For normal human hemoglobins and those of most other mammalian species, n has values ranging from 2.8 to 3.0 (17). This reflects cooperative subunit interactions between the four heme elements of the hemoglobin tetramer. Proteins such as myoglobin that have a single heme subunit and tetrameric hemoglobins such as hemoglobin H that lack subunit cooperativity have n values of 1.0. On the other hand, if oxygenation of one hemoglobin subunit caused an infinite increase in the oxygen-binding affinity of the other subunits, n would

equal 4. Therefore, the n values for normal hemoglobins indicate that there is strong but not infinite cooperativity in oxygen binding by the four heme subunits.

Wagner (18) first proposed using the Hill equation to analyze the relationship between drug concentration and pharmacologic response. However, the physiologic significance of n values estimated in pharmacokinetic-pharmacodynamic studies is far less well understood than it is in the case of oxygen binding to hemoglobin. Accordingly, n is currently regarded in these studies as simply an empirical parameter that confers sigmoidicity and steepness to the relationship between biophase concentrations and pharmacologic effect. This is illustrated by Figure 19.2 in which Equation 19.8 was used to analyze the relationship between tocainide plasma concentration and antiarrhythmic response (19). It can be seen from this figure that the shape of the concentration-response curves approximates that of a step function as n values increase. In fact, pharmacokinetic-pharmacodynamic models can be developed for *quantal responses* simply by fixing n at an arbitrary large value, such as 20 (10). In that case, the EC_{50} parameter estimate will indicate the threshold concentration of drug needed to provide the quantal response.

Sigmoid E_{max} models have been particularly useful in the pharmacokinetic-pharmacodynamic analysis of anesthetic drugs (20). Waveform analyses of electroencephalographic (EEG) morphology have served as biomarkers for anesthetic effects, and show characteristic changes that are different for barbiturates, benzodiazepines, and opiates. Since it often is impossible to conduct clinical studies of these agents at steady state, pharmacokinetic-pharmacodynamic investigations have been performed under conditions in which drug plasma concentrations and effects are constantly changing. The time lag between changes in drug concentration and effect has been analyzed using a biophase compartment, such as that shown in Figure 19.1.

Of practical clinical importance is the role that pharmacokinetic-pharmacodynamic analysis played in optimizing dosing guidelines for using midazolam as an intravenous anesthetic agent (20). Drug approval was based on results of traditional studies from which it was estimated that midazolam was no more than twice as potent as diazepam, the benzodiazepine with which clinicians had the greatest familiarity (21). However, after considerable patient morbidity and mortality was encountered in routine clinical practice, pharmacokinetic-pharmacodynamic studies provided a significantly greater estimate of midazolam relative potency (22). The EEG effect chosen in comparing midazolam with diazepam was total voltage from 0 to 30 Hz, as obtained from aperiodic waveform analysis. The results summarized in Table 19.1 show that the two agents have similar E_{max} values, indicating similar efficacy, but that the EC_{50} of midazolam is 5.5 times that of diazepam, demonstrating that midazolam is that much more potent than diazepam. In addition, the equilibration half life between plasma and the biophase compartment, calculated as:

$$t_{1/2(k_{0B})} = \frac{0.693}{k_{0B}}$$

is three times longer for midazolam than for diazepam. This suggests that repeat doses of midazolam should be spaced at a longer interval than for diazepam (20). No physiological significance has been attached to the values of n that were obtained in these studies. However, investigations in rats have demonstrated a correlation between the EC_{50} of EEG effects and estimates of K_i obtained from in vitro studies of the ability of a series of benzodiazepines to displace $[^3H]$flumazenil from benzodiazepine receptors (Figure 19.3) (23).

Changes in the Relationship between Biophase Concentration and Drug Effect

So far we have considered examples in which the relationship between drug concentration in the biophase compartment and pharmacologic response is time invariant and independent of route of drug administration. The potential impact of active drug metabolites on this relationship is illustrated by a study of the ability of quinidine to prolong the QT interval (24). Pharmacokinetic-pharmacodynamic analyses using a biophase compartment and linear response model indicated that, at any given biophase concentration of quinidine, the QT interval was more prolonged after oral than after intravenous administration. This discrepancy was attributed to formation of pharmacologically active metabolites of quinidine during first-pass metabolism of orally administered drug.

Tolerance can also affect drug response during a pharmacokinetic-pharmacodynamic study. Pharmacologic tolerance is suggested by a diminution of response despite maintenance of constant biophase concentrations of drug. There is now general agreement that tolerance develops rapidly to the cardiovascular and euphoric effects of cocaine (25, 26). This phenomenon was best characterized by studies in which a bolus injection of cocaine was followed by an exponentially tapering infusion, so that relatively constant plasma concentrations were maintained while pharmacologic effects were observed (27). A biophase compartment and linear response model were used for pharmacokinetic-pharmacodynamic analysis of both the cardiovascular and euphoric effects of cocaine. Function generators were used to characterize the acute development of tolerance by reducing effect intensity, σ in Equation 19.6. Subjective evaluation of cocaine-induced euphoria declined to baseline with an average half-life of 66 minutes. However, the increase in heart rate that followed cocaine administration decreased with a 31-minute average half-life from its

TABLE 19.1 Comparison of Parameters Describing Midazolam and Diazepam Effect Kinetics[a]

	$t_{1/2(k_{0B})}$(min)	$E_{max}(\mu V)$	EC_{50}(ng/mL)	n
Midazolam	5.6	141	171	1.8
Diazepam	1.9	137	946	1.7

[a] Parametric analysis results from Bührer et al. Clin Pharmacol Ther 1990;48:555–67.

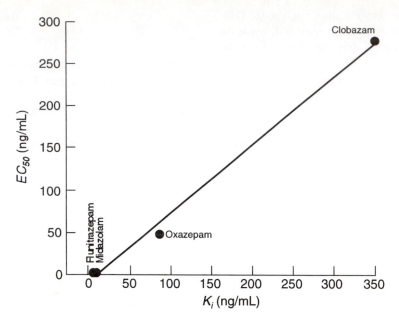

FIGURE 19.3 Relationship in rats between the EC_{50} of EEG effects (averaged amplitude in the 11.5–30 Hz frequency band) and estimates of K_i obtained from *in vitro* studies of the ability of four benzodiazepines to displace [³H]flumazenil from benzodiazepine receptors on brain tissue homogenates. Estimates of EC_{50} were based on free benzodiazepine concentrations not bound to plasma proteins. (Data from Mandema JW, et al. J Pharmacol Exp Ther 1991;257:472–8.)

peak to a plateau that averaged 33% of peak values. Changes in blood pressure paralleled the increase and subsequent decline in heart rate (25).

Sensitization refers to an increase in pharmacologic response despite maintenance of constant biophase concentrations of drug. Adverse clinical consequences of sensitization are observed perhaps most commonly following abrupt withdrawal of β-adrenergic blocking drug therapy in patients with coronary heart disease and include ventricular arrhythmias, worsening of angina, and myocardial infarction (28). Although several mechanisms have been proposed, these adverse events primarily reflect the fact that chronic therapy with β-adrenergic receptor blocking drugs causes an increase in the number of available β-adrenergic receptors, a phenomenon termed *up-regulation* (28, 29). When therapy with β-adrenergic receptor blocking drugs is stopped abruptly, the decline in up-regulated receptors lags behind the elimination of the receptor blocking drug, resulting in a period of exaggerated response to normal circulating catecholamine levels. Using data describing the time course of receptor up-regulation in lymphocytes, Lima et al. (30) have developed a kinetic model of the fractional increase in β-adrenergic receptors that occurs with the institution of β-adrenergic receptor blocking drug therapy, and of its subsequent decline when this therapy is stopped. A

modification of Equation 19.8 was used to characterize the initial intensity of β-adrenergic receptor agonist-induced chronotropic response in the presence of a β-adrenergic receptor antagonist. Supersensitivity was then modeled by simply multiplying this estimate of initial response by the expected increase in β-adrenergic receptor density.

ANALYSIS OF INDIRECT PHARMACOLOGIC EFFECTS

In some cases, effects are mediated by an endogenous substance, and drugs modulate these effects indirectly by either affecting the production or elimination of this response mediator (Figure 19.4). If the formation rate (P) of the mediator (M) is regarded as a zero-order process and the elimination rate of the mediator is regarded as first order, the following equation describes the mass balance of the mediator:

$$dM/dt = P - k_e M \qquad (19.10)$$

where k_e is the first-order elimination rate constant. Indirectly acting drugs can then be modeled as exerting their effects by altering initial values of either P or k_e. Implicit in Equation 19.10 is the fact that the rate of onset of effect is governed by the elimination rate of the mediator.

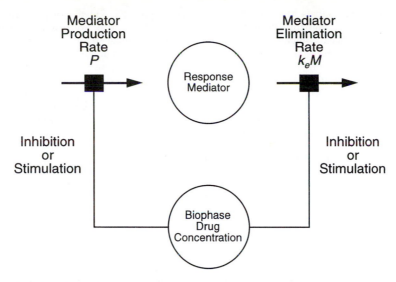

FIGURE 19.4　Basic concept of indirect pharmacodynamic response models. Observed effects are mediated by an endogenous substance *(response mediator)*. Indirectly acting drugs modulate these effects by either inhibiting or stimulating the production or elimination of this response mediator. This accounts for the fact that the development of these drug effects is delayed beyond the time required for the drug to reach its pharmacologic site of action *(biophase)*.

Warfarin is a classic example of a drug that exerts its anticoagulant effects indirectly by blocking synthesis of vitamin K-dependent clotting factors (factors II, VII, IX, and X). This effect can be analyzed by adding to Equation 19.10 a forcing function (f_c) to relate the degree of inhibition of clotting factor synthesis to the plasma level of warfarin that is obtained (10):

$$dM/dt = P \cdot f_c - k_e M \qquad (19.11)$$

Nagashima et al. (31) developed a model in which the forcing function was modeled as proportional to the logarithm of the warfarin concentration in plasma. However, Pitsiu et al. (32) subsequently found that the Hill equation is more suitable for modeling the relationship between plasma concentrations of *S*-warfarin, the active isomer of warfarin, and anticoagulant effect.

Any of the pharmacodynamic models that we have described for direct pharmacologic effects can serve as forcing functions in Equation 19.11, and model choice is guided best by an understanding of the mechanism of drug action and by the information content of the available data (1, 10). For example, Sharma and Jusko (1) have selected the following modification of the E_{max} model to illustrate the general use of a forcing function to model inhibition of either mediator synthesis or elimination:

$$f_c = 1 - \frac{I_{max}\,[B]}{IC_{50} + [B]}$$

where I_{max} is the maximal fractional degree of inhibition provided by any drug concentration [B] and IC_{50} is the concentration required for half-maximal inhibitory effect. The corresponding forcing function for stimulatory drug effects would be given by:

$$f_c = 1 + \frac{I_{max}\,[B]}{IC_{50} + [B]}$$

In addition to warfarin, Sharma and Jusko (1) have listed a large number of other drugs that have indirect pharmacologic effects. These range from H_2–receptor antagonists, diuretics, and bronchodilators to corticosteroids, nonsteroidal anti-inflammatory drugs, and interferon. Finally, it should be emphasized that most pharmacokinetic-pharmacodynamic studies have dealt with acute drug effects. Study of long-term drug effects requires incorporation of a disease progression model into the analysis, and this will be the subject of the next chapter.

References

1. Sharma A, Jusko WJ. Characteristics of indirect pharmacodynamic models and applications to clinical drug responses. Br J Clin Pharmacol 1998;45:229–39.
2. Sherwin RS, Kramer KJ, Tobin JD, Insel PA, Liljenquist JE, Berman M, Andres R. A model of the kinetics of insulin in man. J Clin Invest 1974;53:1481–92.
3. Steil GM, Meador MA, Bergman RN. Thoracic duct lymph. Relative contribution from splanchnic and muscle tissue. Diabetes 1993;42:720–31.

4. Kramer WG, Kolibash AJ, Lewis RP, Bathala MS, Visconti JA, Reuning RH. Pharmacokinetics of digoxin: Relationship between response intensity and predicted compartmental drug levels in man. J Pharmacokinet Biopharm 1979;7:47–61.

5. Wagner JG, Aghajanian GK, Bing OHL. Correlation of performance test scores with "tissue concentration" of lysergic acid diethylamide in human subjects. Clin Pharmacol Ther 1968;9:635–8.

6. Levy G, Gibaldi M, Jusko WJ. Multicompartmental pharmacokinetic models and pharmacologic effects. J Pharm Sci 1969;58:422–4.

7. Segre G. Kinetics of interaction between drugs and biological systems. Farmaco Ed Sci 1968;23:907–18.

8. Hull CJ, Van Beem HBH, McLeod K, Sibbald A, Watson MJ. A pharmacodynamic model for pancuronium. Br J Anaesth 1978;50:1113–23.

9. Sheiner LB, Stanski DR, Vozeh S, Miller RD, Ham J. Simultaneous modeling of pharmacokinetics and pharmacodynamics: Application to d-tubocurarine. Clin Pharmacol Ther 1979;25:358–71.

10. Holford NHG, Sheiner LB. Pharmacokinetic and pharmacodynamic modeling in vivo. CRC Crit Rev Bioengineer 1981;5:273–322.

11. Eudeikis JR, Henthorn TK, Lertora JJL, Atkinson AJ Jr, Chao GC, Kushner W. Kinetic analysis of the vasodilator and ganglionic blocking actions of N-acetylprocainamide. J Cardiovasc Pharmacol 1982;4:303–9.

12. Thibonnier M, Holford NH, Upton RA, Blume CD, Williams RL. Pharmacokinetic-pharmacodynamic analysis of unbound disopyramide directly measured in serial plasma samples in man. J Pharmacokinet Biopharm 1984;12:559–73.

13. Piergies AA, Ruo TI, Jansyn EM, Belknap SM, Atkinson AJ Jr. Effect kinetics of N-acetylprocainamide-induced QT interval prolongation. Clin Pharmacol Ther 1987;42:107–12.

14. Frederiksen MC, Bowsher DJ, Ruo TI, Henthorn TK, Ts'ao C-H, Green D, Atkinson AJ Jr. Kinetics of epsilon-aminocaproic acid distribution, elimination, and antifibrinolytic effects in normal subjects. Clin Pharmacol Ther 1984;35:387–93.

15. Markus G, DePasquale JL, Wissler FC. Quantitative determination of the binding of ε-aminocaproic acid to native plasminogen. J Biol Chem 1978;253:727–32.

16. Hill AV. The possible effects of the aggregation of the molecules of hemoglobin on its dissociation curves. J Physiol 1910;40:iv–vii.

17. Bunn HF, Forget BG, Ranney HM. Human hemoglobins. Philadelphia: WB Saunders; 1977. p. 35–41.

18. Wagner JG. Kinetics of pharmacologic response: I. Proposed relationships between response and drug concentration in the intact animal and man. J Theor Biol 1968;20:173–201.

19. Meffin PJ, Winkle RA, Blaschke TF, Fitzgerald J, Harrison DC. Response optimization of drug dosage: Antiarrhythmic studies with tocainide. Clin Pharmacol Ther 1977;22:42–57.

20. Stanski DR. Pharmacodynamic modeling of anesthetic EEG drug effects. Annu Rev Pharmacol Toxicol 1992;32:423–47.

21. Magni VC, Frost RA, Leung JWC, Cotton PB. A randomized comparison of midazolam and diazepam for sedation in upper gastrointestinal endoscopy. Br J Anaesth 1983;55:1095–101.

22. Bührer M, Maitre PO, Crevoisier C, Stanski DR. Electroencephalographic effects of benzodiazepines. II. Pharmacodynamic modeling of the electroencephalographic effects of midazolam and diazepam. Clin Pharmacol Ther 1990;48:555–67.

23. Mandema JW, Sansom LN, Dios-Vièitez MC, Hollander-Jansen M, Danhof M. Pharmacokinetic-pharmacodynamic modeling of the electroencephalographic effects of benzodiazepines. Correlation with receptor binding and anticonvulsant activity. J Pharmacol Exp Ther 1991;257:472–8.

24. Holford NG, Coates PE, Guentert TW, Riegelman S, Sheiner LB. The effect of quinidine and its metabolites on the electrocardiogram and systolic time intervals: Concentration-effect relationships. Br J Clin Pharmacol 1981;11:187–95.

25. Ambre JJ. Acute tolerance to pressor effects of cocaine in humans. Ther Drug Monit 1993;15:537–40.

26. Foltin RW, Fischman MW, Levin FR. Cardiovascular effects of cocaine in humans: laboratory studies. Drug Alcohol Depend 1995;37:193–210.

27. Ambre JJ, Belknap SM, Nelson J, Ruo TI, Shin S-G, Atkinson AJ Jr. Acute tolerance to cocaine in humans. Clin Pharmacol Ther 1988;44:1–8.

28. Nattel S, Rangno RE, Van Loon G. Mechanism of propranolol withdrawal phenomenon. Circulation 1979;59:1158–64.

29. Houston MC, Hodge R. Beta-adrenergic blocker withdrawal syndromes in hypertension and other cardiovascular diseases. Am Heart J 1988;116:515–23.

30. Lima JJ, Krukenmyer JJ, Boudoulas H. Drug- or hormone-induced adaptation: Model of adrenergic hypersensitivity. J Pharamacokinet Biopharm 1989;17:347–64.

31. Nagashima R, O'Reilly RA, Levy G. Kinetics of pharmacologic effects in man: The anticoagulant action of warfarin. Clin Pharmacol Ther 1969;10:22–35.

32. Pitsiu M, Parker EM, Aarons L, Rowland M. Population pharmacokinetics and pharmacodynamics of warfarin in healthy young adults. Eur J Pharm Sci 1993;1:151–7.

20

Disease Progress Models

NICHOLAS H. G. HOLFORD*, DIANE R. MOULD†, AND CARL C. PECK†

*Division of Pharmacology and Clinical Pharmacology, University of Auckland, Auckland, New Zealand,
†Center for Drug Development Science, Georgetown University Medical Center, Washington, D.C.

CLINICAL PHARMACOLOGY AND DISEASE PROGRESS

Clinical pharmacology, like many disciplines, can be viewed from several perspectives. In the context of a clinical trial of a therapeutic agent, clinical pharmacology provides a conceptual framework for relating drug treatment to responses observed in a clinical trial. In the context of simulation and modeling, it is useful to think of clinical pharmacology as a model itself—that is, the combination of disease progress and drug action.

$$\text{Clinical Pharmacology} = \text{Disease Progress} + \text{Drug Action} \qquad (20.1)$$

Disease progress refers to the evolution of a disease over time. Specifically, it can be used to describe the time course of a biomarker or clinical outcome reflecting the status of a disease. The status is a reflection of the state of the disease at a point in time. The disease status may improve or worsen over time, or may be a cyclical phenomenon (e.g., malarial quartan fever or seasonal affective disorder). Therefore, a model of disease progress is a mathematical expression that describes the expected changes in status over time.

Drug action refers to all the pharmacokinetic and pharmacodynamic processes involved in producing a drug effect on the disease. The effect of the drug is assumed to influence the disease status. Pharmacokinetic and pharmacodynamic drug properties are the major attributes determining drug action and its effect on the time course of progression of the disease. Disease progress models can be extended to include terms that account for the changes in disease progress that

are affected by drug treatment. We call such a combined model the clinical pharmacology model for the drug (Equation 20.1).

DISEASE PROGRESS MODELS

In this chapter, we examine the basic elements of clinical pharmacology models for use in describing the time course of disease progress and the changes in progress in response to treatment. These models have two components: the first describes the disease progress without therapeutic intervention and the second defines the change in progress as a result of treatment.

"No Progress" Model

The simplest model of disease progress assumes there is no change in disease status during the period of observation. Previously, this has been reflected in simple pharmacodynamic models, such as those described in Chapter 19, by the constant "baseline effect" parameter, often symbolized by E_0 (1). A constant baseline is a common assumption made in the design and analysis of clinical trials. Such an analysis ignores the progression of disease during the course of the trial by comparing the effect of drug treatment groups at similar points in time. This is a reflection of a "minimalist" approach to clinical trial design and analysis that seeks only to falsify the null hypothesis and not to learn by an informative description of the observed phenomena (2, 3). The assumption that there is no change in disease status over time does not allow the analyst to infer anything about the effect of the drug on the rate of disease progress.

Linear Progress Model

The linear disease progress model (Equation 20.2) assumes a constant rate of change of a biomarker or clinical outcome that reflects the disease status (S) at any time, t, from the initial observation of the patient—for example, at the time of entry into a clinical trial. It can be defined in terms of a baseline disease status (S_0) and a slope (α), that reflects the change from baseline status with time.

$$S(t) = S_0 + \alpha \cdot t \qquad (20.2)$$

Using this model as a basis to describe the effect of drug on the time course of disease progress, three drug effect patterns are possible. Treatment can change the patient status without affecting the rate of progress (offset pattern), it can alter the rate of progress of the disease (slope pattern), or it can do both of these things (combined slope and offset pattern):

Offset Pattern

We define a drug-induced shift upwards or downwards without a change in slope of the disease status line as the offset pattern. The effect of the drug, E_{OFF}, can be thought of as modifying the baseline parameter S_0 as shown in Equation 20.3.

$$S(t) = S_0 + E_{OFF}(C_{e,A}) + \alpha \cdot t \qquad (20.3)$$

This model can be used to describe a nonpersistent drug effect (sometimes termed symptomatic)—for example, lowering of blood pressure by an antihypertensive agent that persists during periods of exposure to the drug, but with a return to pre-treatment status on cessation of therapy. The onset of drug effect may be delayed by adding an effect compartment to the drug action part of the model, which incorporates more realism by making active drug concentrations at the effect site $(C_{e,A})$ delayed in relation to plasma drug concentrations (4).

Slope Pattern

We define a drug-induced increase or decrease in the rate of progression of disease status as the slope pattern. The effect of the drug, E_{SLOPE}, can be thought of as modifying the slope parameter α as shown in Equation 20.4.

$$S(t) = S_0 + [E_{SLOPE}(C_{e,A}) + \alpha] \cdot t \qquad (20.4)$$

Compared to the offset pattern, this model can be used to describe a more permanent (disease-modifying),

protective drug effect—for example, slowing the progression of a disease such as rheumatoid arthritis. In this case, the cessation of therapy would not be expected to result in a return to pre-treatment status. In general, we might expect some delay in the onset of effect (predicted by $C_{e,A}$), but an instantaneous effect model to describe the drug effect on the slope parameter may be sufficient because changes in status tend to develop slowly when the slope changes.

Combined Offset and Slope Pattern

Both an offset effect and a slope effect may be combined to describe the changes in disease status (Equation 20.5).

$$S(t) = S_0 + E_{OFF}(C_{e,A}) + [E_{SLOPE}(C_{e,A}) + \alpha] \cdot t \qquad (20.5)$$

Figure 20.1 illustrates the offset and slope models and the combination of both types of effect. The offset pattern of drug effect provides an explicit definition of a temporary or symptomatic effect of a drug. In contrast, the slope pattern of drug effect defines a drug with a disease-modifying, protective effect. The pattern of disease progress in the absence of drug is usually referred to as the natural history of the disease (Figure 20.1). A study by Griggs et al. (5) reporting temporary increases in muscle strength of muscular dystrophy patients treated with prednisone illustrates an application of the offset drug effect pattern (Figure 20.2).

Figure 20.3 shows a similar offset pattern of the effect of zidovudine in CD4 cell measurements in HIV

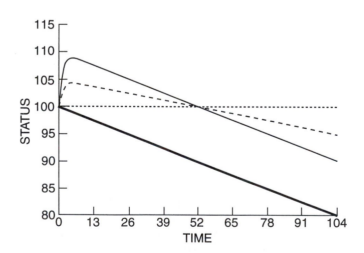

FIGURE 20.1 The *thick line* depicts the natural course of disease progress without therapeutic intervention (Equation 20.2). The *thin line* describes an offset pattern ("symptomatic") as a consequence of treatment (Equation 20.3). The *dotted line* reflects a slope pattern with a change in the rate of progress of the disease ("protective") (Equation 20.4). The *dashed line* shows the combination of both offset and slope patterns (Equation 20.5).

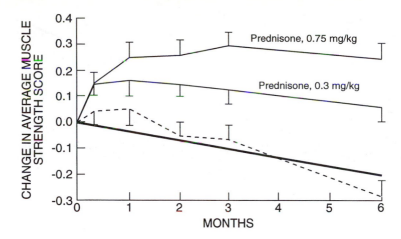

FIGURE 20.2 Example of linear disease progress and offset drug effect pattern when prednisone is used to treat muscular dystrophy. The *thick line* is the expected natural history of progressive loss of muscle strength. The *dashed line* shows the transient improvement due to the placebo response. The thin lines demonstrate the delayed offset pattern of drug effect at two doses of prednisone. (Reproduced with permission from Griggs RC, Moxley RT 3rd, Mendell JR, Fenichel GM, Brooke MH, Pestronik A, et al. Arch Neurol 1991;48:383–8.)

patients (6). However, in this case, the model of disease progress uses functions that are not simply straight lines under placebo (polynomial, Equation 20.6) and zidovudine treatment (combined polynomial and exponential, Equation 20.7).

$$Placebo\ (t) = CD4_0 - k_1 \cdot t - k_2 \cdot t^2 \qquad (20.6)$$

$$Treatment\ (t) = [B + (k_5 \cdot CD4_0) + (k_6 \cdot CD4_0{}^2)]$$
$$\cdot\ (e^{-k_3 \cdot t} - e^{-k_4 \cdot t}) \qquad (20.7)$$

Models for multiple periods of treatment with placebo and active drug (with different doses) have been used with a disease progress model to describe

the response to tacrine in Alzheimer's disease. Figure 20.4 shows the placebo and active treatment components as well as the disease progress model (7). The predicted time course of response in patients with Alzheimer's disease in a complex clinical trial design combining disease progress, placebo, and tacrine effects is shown in Figure 20.5 (8). In this figure, the upper curve reflects the expected patient status, which would reflect a combination of disease progress and the effect of placebo on the time course of disease progress. In the lower curve, the sequential effects of varying treatments including doses of

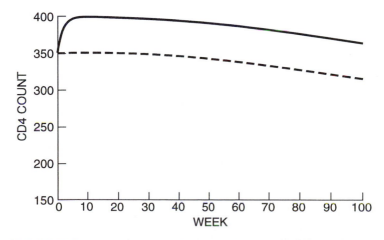

FIGURE 20.3 Time course of CD4 count in placebo *(dashed line)* and zidovudine *(solid line)* treated patients. (Reproduced with permission from Sale M, Sheiner LB, Volberding P, Blaschke TF. Clin Pharmacol Ther 1993;54:556–66.)

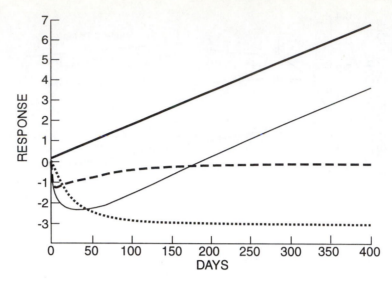

FIGURE 20.4   Models of Alzheimer's disease progress *(thick line)*, placebo effect *(dashed line)* and drug effect *(dotted line)*, in absence of disease progress, and combined (drug plus placebo) response to active drug in the presence of disease progress *(thin line)*. Drug effect is assessed by subtracting placebo response and disease progress from the combined response that is observed with drug therapy. (Reproduced with permission from Holford NHG. Population models for Alzheimer's and Parkinson's disease. In: Aarons L, Balant LP, editors. The population approach: measuring and managing variability in response, concentration and dose. Brussels: COST B1 European Commission; 1997. p. 97–104.)

placebo (P), 40 and 80 mg/day of tacrine were simulated. The difference between the control and active groups increases notably over the duration of the trial. This underscores the point that it is essential to incorporate appropriate models of disease progress as well as to account for placebo effect during any clinical trial simulation.

Finally, a disease progress model can reflect more complex drug action phenomena such as a drug concentration-effect delay, tolerance, and rebound to both

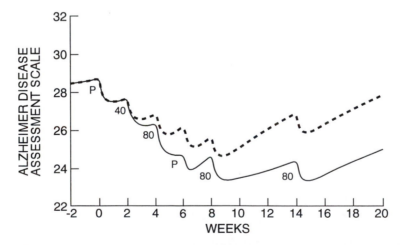

FIGURE 20.5   The *upper curve* shows the time course of predicted responses in a patient receiving placebo treatments as part of the three-part trial design used to evaluate tacrine in Alzheimer's disease. The *lower curve* shows the simulated response in a patient receiving a particular sequence of placebo (P) followed by tacrine (40 or 80 mg/day). (Reproduced with permission from Holford NH, Peace KE. Proc Natl Acad Sci USA 1992;89:11466–70.)

placebo and active treatments can be made using a linear offset model. These effects can be accounted for by including the appropriate terms. For instance, a delay to onset can be accounted for by the addition of an effect compartment, and tolerance and rebound effects can be described by the addition of a precursor pool compartment, which would limit the effect of drug activity.

Asymptotic Progress Model

Zero Asymptote

A common pattern of disease progress provides for the patient's return to health or recovery. For example, the time course of postoperative pain can be expected to start at a baseline state, which would be expected to involve intense levels of pain. However, over a few days the level of pain experienced by the patient would be expected to decrease until eventually pain is no longer perceived. This recovery can be approximated by an exponential model with an asymptote of zero, indicating the absence of pain. As shown in Equation 20.8, the parameters of this model are the baseline pain status S_0 and the half-life of progression, T_{prog}:

$$S(t) = S_0 \cdot e^{-\ln 2/T_{prog} \cdot t} \qquad (20.8)$$

The asymptote model is particularly useful for illustrating one of the primary potential drawbacks of not accounting for disease progress. Because patients are expected to improve over time, a simple minimalist approach to the comparison of different drug effects would be expected to be dependent on the time of comparative assessment. If the comparison were made at a point in time when recovery has largely occurred, the difference between treatments would probably be undetectable.

As with the linear model of disease progress, the consequences of therapeutic intervention on the asymptotic model of disease progress can be described by including terms to account for the expected action of a drug. Drugs may exert an immediate and transient symptomatic effect, they may act to alter the progress of the disease, such as shortening the time to recovery, or they may do both.

Zero Asymptote Offset Model Pattern

As shown in Equation 20.9, drug action models based on the zero asymptote model can be extended to include an offset term $[E_{OFF}(C_{e,A})]$ in the model of progress describing symptomatic benefit such as the relief of pain from a simple analgesic.

$$S(t) = E_{OFF}(C_{e,A}) + S_0 \cdot e^{-\ln 2/T_{prog} \cdot t} \qquad (20.9)$$

As with the offset model for the linear disease progress model, the effect of drug would be expected to disappear on cessation of therapy in this offset model. Again, a delay to the onset of drug effect can be incorporated with the use of an effect compartment component.

Zero Asymptote Slope Pattern

In addition, an exponentially progressing pattern of disease progress (parameterised by a half-life) can reflect a protective benefit of drug treatment if the therapeutic intervention enhances the return to the normal state or shortens the half-life of the recovery process. Equation 20.10 describes the protective benefit.

$$S(t) = S_0 \cdot e^{-\ln 2/[E_{TP}(C_{e,A}) + T_{prog}] \cdot t} \qquad (20.10)$$

Combined Offset and Slope Pattern

The effects of a therapeutic agent (E_{TP}) on the progress of a disease may include both an immediate palliative effect and a reduction in the overall recovery time. Equation 20.11 describes the combination of these actions on the zero-asymptote disease progress model:

$$S(t) = E_{OFF}(C_{e,A}) + S_0 \cdot e^{-\ln 2/[E_{TP}(C_{e,A}) + T_{prog}] \cdot t} \qquad (20.11)$$

Figure 20.6 illustrates the expected changes in the progress of a disease, which can be described using the zero-asymptote model.

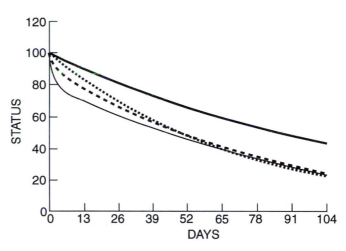

FIGURE 20.6 Patterns of drug effect with the zero-asymptote progress model. The *thick line* describes the normal expected time course of recovery without therapeutic intervention. The *thin line* shows the change when a drug that affects symptoms is administered. The *dotted line* illustrates the expected time course of disease when an agent is given that hastens recovery (protective) and the *dashed line* describes the expected results from administering an agent that exhibits both an immediate symptomatic effect and a protective effect on the time course of disease progress.

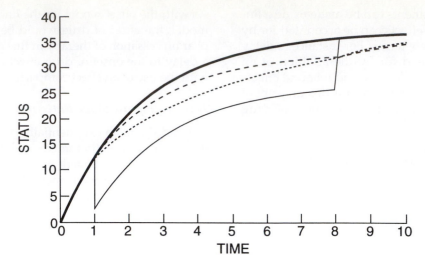

FIGURE 20.7 Non-zero asymptote model with natural history *(thick line)*, off-set pattern *(thin line)*, and two types of protective pattern drug effects: S_{ss}—effect on steady state burned out state *(dashed line)*, and T_{prog}—effect on half-life of disease progress *(dotted line)*.

Nonzero Asymptote

Another pattern of disease progress encompasses reaching a "burned out" state (S_{SS}). This state is thought to happen when diseases such as rheumatoid arthritis reach a point when disease processes damage tissue beyond repair by any therapeutic means. This irreversibly damaged state can be described by another exponential model. Since the onset of the disease process is usually not known, the model can be expressed as follows where t is time after the start of observing the disease from a baseline state (S_0) and the half-life of progression is T_{prog}.

$$S(t) = S_0 \cdot e^{-\ln 2 / T_{prog} \cdot t} + S_{SS} \cdot (1 - e^{-\ln 2 / T_{prog} \cdot t}) \quad (20.12)$$

Offset Pattern

Therapeutic treatment can affect disease status without altering the time to reach a "burned out" steady-state status, S_{SS}. This improvement in patient status would be expected to be transient and dependent on continual drug exposure. Equation 20.13 describes the effect of adding a drug that has a symptomatic effect ($E_{OFF}(C_{e,A})$) on patient status.

$$S(t) = E_{OFF}(C_{e,A}) + S_0 \cdot e^{-\ln 2 / T_{prog} \cdot t} \\ + S_{SS} \cdot (1 - e^{-\ln 2 / T_{prog} \cdot t}) \quad (20.13)$$

Slope Pattern

Additional models for drug effects on the nonzero asymptote model include two patterns of protective drug effects. These assume a drug effect changing either the burned out state, S_{SS}:

$$S(t) = S_0 \cdot e^{-\ln 2 / T_{prog} \cdot t} + [E_{OFF}(C_{e,A}) + S_{SS}] \\ \cdot (1 - e^{-\ln 2 / T_{prog} \cdot t}) \quad (20.14)$$

or affecting the half-life of progression, T_{prog}.

$$S(t) = S_0 \cdot e^{-\ln 2 / [E(C_{e,A}) + T_{prog}] \cdot t} \\ + S_{SS} \cdot (1 - e^{-\ln 2 / [E(C_{e,A}) + T_{prog}] \cdot t}) \quad (20.15)$$

Offset and Slope Patterns

Figure 20.7 illustrates the nonzero asymptote model with all three patterns of disease progress influenced by drug effect. Drug exposure starts at 1.0 time units and is stopped at 8.0 time units. In Equation 20.16 the effects of symptomatic improvement and the two functions describing the action of drug on both the burned out state and on the time to reach this state have been included.

$$S(t) = E_{OFF}(C_{e,A}) + S_0 \cdot e^{-\ln 2 / [E_{TP}(C_{e,A}) + T_{prog}] \cdot t} \\ + [E_{SS}(C_{e,A}) + S_{SS}] \cdot (1 - e^{-\ln 2 / [E_{TP}(C_{e,A}) + T_{prog}] \cdot t}) \quad (20.16)$$

Physiological Effect Models

The time course of drug effect can often be understood in terms of drug-induced changes in the processes controlling synthesis rate (R_{syn}) or elimination of a physiological mediator (9, 10). These models can be readily extended to describe disease progress by incorporating a time-varying change *(PDI)* in either

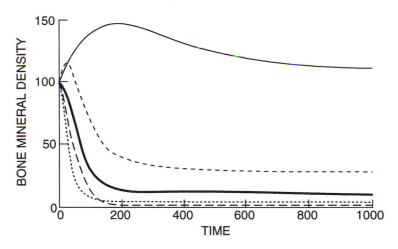

FIGURE 20.8   Disease progress due to a time varying increase in the rate of loss of a physiological mediator of the response. The *thick line* shows the time course of response in the untreated state with an increase in the loss of physiological mediator. If the response was change in bone mass from a baseline of 100 at time zero then the rate of bone loss would be increased by a factor of 10 reaching a new steady state after 200 time units. The time to steady state is determined both by the time course of change in rate of bone loss and the turnover time of bone. The other four lines show the patterns expected from four different kinds of drug effect. Potentially therapeutic effects are inhibition of bone loss *(thin line)* and stimulation of bone synthesis *(upper broken line)*. Deleterious drug effects are inhibition of synthesis *(lower broken line)* and stimulation of bone loss *(dotted line)*.

synthesis or elimination. For example, if the rate constant (k_{loss}) describing loss of a physiological mediator starts from a baseline state, $k_{loss\,0}$, and decreases with a half-life of $T50_{loss}$, then the time course of the disease state can be described by solving the differential equation given in Equation 20.17:

$$\frac{dS}{dt} = R_{syn} - k_{loss} \cdot PDI \cdot S \qquad (20.17)$$

where,

$$k_{loss} = k_{loss\,0} \cdot [1 + (MaxProg - 1) \cdot (1 - e^{\ln 2/T\,50_{loss} \cdot t})] \quad (20.18)$$

$MaxProg$ is a parameter that determines the fractional change in $k_{loss\,0}$ at infinite time. The effect of a drug might be to inhibit loss, in which case PDI would be modeled by Equation 20.19, where $C_{e,A}$ is the effect site concentration and $C50$ is the value of $C_{e,A}$ causing a 50% inhibition of loss.

$$PDI = 1 - \frac{C_{e,A}}{C50 + C_{e,A}} \qquad (20.19)$$

Figure 20.8 illustrates the four basic drug effect patterns when the input or output parameter changes with an exponential time course. As an example of this type of disease progress model, consider postmenopausal osteoporosis reflected by the net loss of bone mass after

the menopause. Bone loss may be due to decreased formation or increased resorption of bone. Figure 20.9 illustrates the time course of bone mass change due to increased bone loss and the effect of administering a drug to reduce that loss. For example, raloxifene has been shown to be beneficial in women with postmenopausal osteoporosis (11). The pattern of increase in bone mineral density observed after treatment with raloxifene or placebo resembles the curves shown in Figure 20.10. However, the treatment duration in this data set was too short to identify the actual mechanism of raloxifene effect on disease progress.

Growth Models

Another approach to modeling the course of disease progress is to use a growth function. The growth function might be used to describe something such as tumor growth or bacterial cell increase, where growth is dependent on the number of cells dividing actively. A simple function that can be used to describe the growth of a response R is given in Equation 20.20 (12, 13)

$$\frac{dR}{dt} = k_{growth} \cdot R - k_{death} \cdot R \qquad (20.20)$$

The solution to this equation describes an exponential increase in cell count with time.

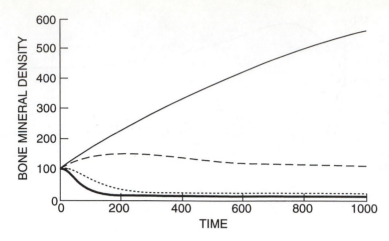

FIGURE 20.9 The pattern and time course of response to treatment is crucially dependent on the dose. This shows the same model as that illustrated in Figure 8 without treatment *(thick line)* and with three different dose rates of a drug which reduces the rate of loss of physiological substance *(dotted line = dose rate of 10, broken line = dose rate of 100, thin line = dose rate of 1000).*

As with the other physiological models, the effect of drug treatment may be realized by slowing the growth rate (k_{growth}) or increasing the cell death rate k_{death}). In the latter case, this effect can be incorporated by including a term for the effect of drug concentration ($C_{e,A}$) on the rate constant for cell decrease, as shown in Equation 20.21.

$$\frac{dR}{dt} = k_{growth} \cdot R - k_{death} \cdot R \cdot C_{e,A} \qquad (20.21)$$

A more realistic refinement of the simple cell growth model would describe cells that, through mutation or other processes, may become resistant to drug treatment. The change of cell characteristic from a responsive to an unresponsive state can be either reversible or irreversible. Equations 20.22 and 20.23 describe the reversible case, which may be reflective of cells moving between sensitive phases (R_S) and phases that are not sensitive to therapeutic intervention (R_R) (14):

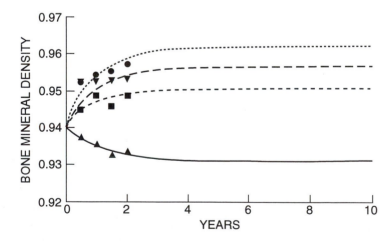

FIGURE 20.10 Bone mineral density change with placebo and three doses of raloxifene. Symbols indicate observed responses to placebo (▲) and daily doses of 30 mg (■), 60 mg (▼) and 150 mg (●). Curves show predictions assuming disease progress is due to increased loss and raloxifene reduces loss. The model is the same as that shown in Figures 20.8 and 20.9. (Curves fit to lumbar spine data from Delmas PD, Bjarnason NH, Mitlak BH, Ravoux A-C, Shah AS, Huster WJ, et al. N Engl J Med 1997;337:1641–7.)

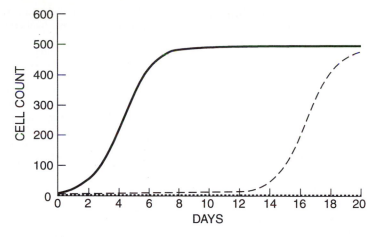

FIGURE 20.11 Growth curves for responsive cells exposed to three different treatment regimens: untreated *(thick line)*, inadequately treated with a low drug dose *(broken line)*, and adequately treated with a higher drug dose *(dotted line)*. The curves show that cell regrowth following inadequate treatment is rapid.

$$\frac{dR_S}{dt} = k_{growth} \cdot R_S - k_{SR} \cdot R_S + k_{RS} \cdot R_R - k_{death} \cdot R_S \quad (20.22)$$

and

$$\frac{dR_R}{dt} = k_{SR} \cdot R_S - k_{RS} \cdot R_R \quad (20.23)$$

where the rates of transformation to and from the resistant state are indicated by k_{SR} and k_{RS}, respectively.

Another series of functions frequently used to describe growth kinetics are the Gompertz functions (15). These functions are unique in that they describe a rapid initial rapid rate of growth (β), followed by a slower phase of growth until a finite limit (β_{max}) is reached. This behavior makes the Gompertz functions particularly useful for describing disease progress in which there is a maximum level of impairment associated with the disease (e.g., a burned-out state). Consequently, Gompertz functions have been used to describe the pharmacodynamics of antibacterial agents (16), as well as other systems in which growth kinetics are important. The following pair of equations (Equations 20.24 and 20.25) describe a Gompertz function of cell growth in which the cells oscillate between a therapeutically sensitive state (R_S) and a resistant state (R_R). The effect of drug concentration $(C_{e,A})$ is described using an E_{max} equation that acts to reduce the number of responsive cells in the system by increasing loss (k_{SO}) independently of transformation to or from the resistant state:

$$\frac{dR_S}{dt} = k_{RS} \cdot R_R + \beta \cdot R_S (\beta_{max} - R_S)$$
$$- \left[k_{SR} + \left(1 + \frac{E_{max} \cdot C_{e,A}}{EC50 + C_{e,A}}\right) \cdot k_{SO} \right] \cdot R_S \quad (20.24)$$

$$\frac{dR_{SR}}{dt} = k_{SR} \cdot R_S - k_{RS} \cdot R_R \quad (20.25)$$

Figure 20.11 shows the expected pattern of growth of cells in three different treatment groups. In the low-dose treatment group, cell regrowth is expected to be rapid.

CONCLUSION

The use of models to describe disease progress is an important tool that allows the analyst to appropriately evaluate the effects of drug treatment on the time course of disease. In the "learning versus confirming" paradigm (3), inclusion of models for disease progress can focus attention more clearly on the objectives of a clinical trial. In early, "learning phase" studies, the model of disease progress can be developed and the mechanism of drug action is elucidated. Subsequently, clinical trials can be designed to account for variability in the natural history of disease, which increases the statistical power to distinguish between the effects of different treatments and thus "confirm" the effectiveness of the drug. Once the disease progress model has been defined and an effect of the drug on progress has been accepted, study designs can be defined that optimize clinical activity. In some cases, the mechanism of action of the drug may suggest innovative combination therapies or novel treatment approaches that would not have been considered without knowledge of the disease and the effect of drug on disease progress.

In this chapter, we have described some examples of models that can be used to depict the natural history of disease. We have also suggested modifications to these models that can be used to account for the effect of drug treatment. The development of an appropriate model for disease progress is ideally a team-based approach. It requires the input of clinical experts as to the validity of the status measure used to describe the progress of the disease, statisticians to advise on the inferences that can be drawn from clinical trial observations, and pharmacometricians to determine the appropriateness and utility of the clinical pharmacology model for predicting the response to treatment and to provide guidance to the patient and prescriber on how to use the drug safely and effectively.

References

1. Holford NHG, Sheiner LB. Understanding the dose effect relationship: clinical application of pharmacokinetic-pharmacodynamic models. Clin Pharmacokinet 1981;6:429–53.
2. Sheiner LB. Clinical pharmacology and the choice between theory and empiricism. Clin Pharmacol Ther 1989;46:605–15.
3. Sheiner LB. Learning versus confirming in clinical drug development. Clin Pharmacol Ther 1997;61:275–91.
4. Holford NHG, Sheiner LB. Kinetics of pharmacologic response. Pharmacol Ther 1982;16:143–66.
5. Griggs RC, Moxley RT 3rd, Mendell JR, Fenichel GM, Brooke MH, Pestronik A, et al. Prednisone in Duchenne dystrophy. A randomized, controlled trial defining the time course and dose response. Clinical Investigation of Duchenne Dystrophy Group. Arch Neurol 1991;48:383–8.
6. Sale M, Sheiner LB, Volberding P, Blaschke TF. Zidovudine response relationships in early human immunodeficiency virus infection. Clin Pharmacol Ther 1993;54:556–66.
7. Holford NHG. Population models for Alzheimer's and Parkinson's disease. In: Aarons L, Balant LP, editors. The population approach: measuring and managing variability in response, concentration and dose. Brussels: COST B1 European Commission; 1997. p. 97–104.
8. Holford NH, Peace KE. Methodologic aspects of a population pharmacodynamic model for cognitive effects in Alzheimer patients treated with tacrine. Proc Natl Acad Sci USA 1992;89:11466–70.
9. Holford NHG. Physiological alternatives to the effect compartment model. In: D'Argenio DZ, editor. Advanced methods of pharmacokinetic and pharmacodynamic systems analysis. New York: Plenum Press; 1991. p. 55–68.
10. Dayneka NL, Garg V, Jusko WJ. Comparison of four basic models of indirect pharmacodynamic response. J Pharmacokinet Biopharm 1993;21:457–78.
11. Delmas PD, Bjarnason NH, Mitlak BH, Ravoux A-C, Shah AS, Huster WJ, et al. Effects of raloxifene on bone mineral density, serum cholesterol concentrations, and uterine endometrium in postmenopausal women. N Engl J Med 1997;337:1641–7.
12. Jusko W. Pharmacodynamics of chemotherapeutic effects: dose-time-response relationships for phase-nonspecific agents. J Pharm Sci 1971;60:892–5.
13. Zhi J, Nightingale CH, Quintilliani R. A pharmacodynamic model for the activity of antibiotics against microorganisms under nonsaturable conditions. J Pharm Sci 1986;75:1063–7.
14. Jusko W. A pharmacodynamic model for cell-cycle-specific chemotherapeutic agents. J Pharmacokinet Biopharm 1973;1:175–200.
15. Royston P. A useful monotonic non-linear model with applications in medicine and epidemiology. Stat Med 2000;19:2053–66.
16. Yano Y, Oguma T, Nagata H, Sasaki S. Application of a logistic growth model to pharmacodynamic analysis of in vitro bacteriocidal kinetics. J Pharm Sci 1998;87:1177–83.

OPTIMIZING AND EVALUATING PATIENT THERAPY

21

Pharmacological Differences between Men and Women

MARY J. BERG

Division of Clinical and Administrative Pharmacy, University of Iowa College of Pharmacy, Iowa City, Iowa

If most drugs had been developed in mixed gender populations, then the extent to which these issues contribute to gender-related variability in drug response would be clearer. However, women were systematically excluded from many clinical trials until relatively recently, and gender-related differences in drug response have only been sporadically reported (1).

The introduction of women's health as an issue in the 1980s not only began to examine disease and conditions specific to women, but also started to ask the question whether women and men responded the same or differently to medication. This also raised questions regarding proper dosing of medicines for members of different ethnic groups. Therefore, the whole issue of women's health extends beyond its origins just 20 years ago. Accordingly, this chapter will focus on pharmacological differences and similarities between men and women in the context of their ethnic grouping. In accordance with currently accepted usage, those differences that reflect biological differences between men and women that are hormonal or reproductive in nature will be referred to as *sex differences*, whereas cultural differences, such as differences in smoking behavior, will be referred to as *gender differences* (2).

The study of a pharmacological agent, such as a prescription medicine, an over-the-counter drug, or even an alternative medicine, such as St. John's wort, requires an interdisciplinary approach involving many disciplines. The following basic areas of pharmacokinetics, pharmacodynamics, pharmacogenetics, chronopharmacology, modulators, and biologic/molecular markers must be incorporated to ensure that safe and efficacious medications are developed (1). It is known that adverse drug events are more prevalent in women than in men (3). Reasons for this include not only sex differences in hormonal levels and in pharmacokinetics and pharmacodynamics but gender differences in that there is a higher rate of medication use in women, and different reporting rates between men and women. Drug–drug, drug–nutrient, drug–herbal, and drug–smoking interactions may also alter pharmacokinetics and lead to possible adverse drug events.

PHARMACOKINETICS

The first medication to be sex analyzed for pharmacokinetic differences was antipyrine in 1971 (4). This drug is eliminated entirely by hepatic metabolism, and this study showed that the half-life of antipyrine was shorter in women than in men. A subsequent study concluded that the clearance of this drug is the same for women and men only on day 5 of the menstrual cycle (5). The next drug to be sex analyzed was acetaminophen, which was studied from the late 1970s through the early 1980s. The clearance of this drug was

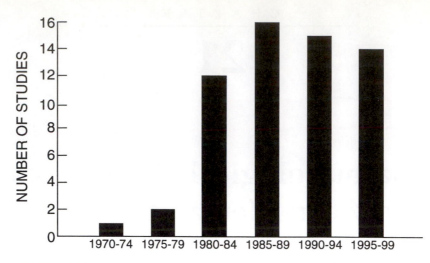

FIGURE 21.1   Reporting of sex-analyzed pharmacokinetic studies of drugs in various therapeutic classes from 1970 through 1999. (Data from Berg MJ. J Gender-Spec Med 1999;2:18–20.)

faster in men than in women. In the 1980s, the first group of drugs, benzodiazepines, was examined for sex-specific differences in pharmacokinetics and it is at this time that the reporting of sex-analyzed pharmacokinetic studies began to approach its current level (Figure 21.1). Conduct of these studies has been facilitated by the passage of the NIH Revitalization Act of 1993 and the issuance of FDA guidelines in the same year (4). However, in 2000, the General Accounting Office (GAO) report stated that the NIH had increased the number of women in clinical trials, but that further analysis for sex differences was needed (6).

ABSORPTION

Absorption encompasses not only the absorption of medications from the gastrointestinal tract, but also absorption from muscle, subcutaneous fat, and lung. Unfortunately, only a few examples in the literature document differences between men and women in drug absorption. Life stages are particularly important in considering absorption of a chemical entity. For example, gastrointestinal absorption of calcium is decreased in menopause. However, it can be reversed with estrogen hormone replacement therapy (7, 8).

It has been shown that gastric emptying of solids is slower in women than in men, and this could slow drug absorption from distal gastrointestinal sites (9). The mechanism is unknown, but it may be related to differences in steroid hormone levels. Gastric acidity can play an important role in drug dissolution, and it

is known that women have a higher gastric pH than men. In one study of aspirin bioavailability in men and women, it was found that aspirin was absorbed more rapidly in women, but that there was no sex difference in the extent of aspirin absorption (10). Women may also have different levels of gastrointestinal enzyme activity. For example, women have less aspirin esterase activity in the gut. As a result there is less first-pass metabolism of aspirin in women, which in another study accounted for having increased aspirin bioavailability (11). Therefore, there is conflicting data regarding sex differences in the bioavailability of even this commonly used drug.

Sex differences in other gastrointestinal enzymes may account for important differences between men and women in first-pass metabolism and bioavailability. For example, women have less alcohol dehydrogenase in the gut and this partly explains why women have higher blood alcohol levels than men after consuming the same amount of ethyl alcohol (12). Both men and women express CYP3A4 enzyme in the gut as well as in the liver. Sex differences in the activity of this enzyme in the liver have been documented (13). Since the extent of CYP3A4 expression in the gut and liver can also differ, it is possible that sex differences noted after intravenous administration of CYP3A4 substrates will not be the same as after oral administration. For example, sex differences in intestinal CYP3A4 activity appear to account for the fact that verapamil bioavailability is higher in women than in men, although both sexes clear this drug at a similar rate after intravenous administration (14).

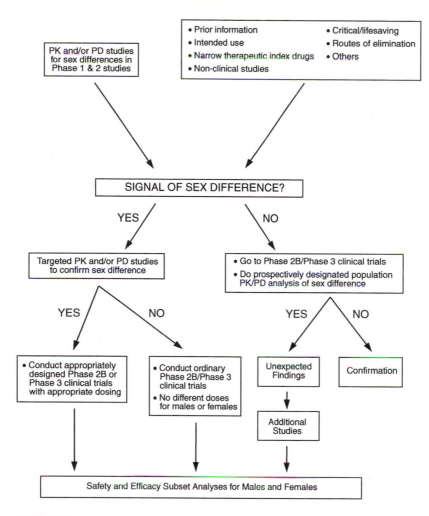

FIGURE 21.2 Decision tree for thinking about ways to assess sex differences during the development of medical products. [Modified from Gender studies in product development: Scientific issues and approaches. Executive summary. U.S. FDA, 1999. (Internet at http://www.fda.gov/womens/Executive.html).]

It is known that grapefruit juice affects CYP3A4 in the gut by irreversibly inhibiting this enzyme for at least three days and this can increase the bioavailability of drugs from 30 to 300%. The specific chemical entity responsible for this enzyme inhibition in the gut is still debated. Possible chemical entities include naringin (the most prevalent flavanoid in grapefruit juice), bergamottin, quercetin, and kaemferol (15–17). As yet there have been no sex-specific analyses of this food–drug interaction.

Sex differences in intramuscular absorption may be due to differences in regional blood flow. A study with the lysine salt of aspirin showed that women absorbed the drug at a slower rate than men (10). However, the possibility of drug injection into subcutaneous fat rather than muscle should be considered when studies of this type are being evaluated.

DISTRIBUTION

Distribution includes both drug binding to plasma proteins and transfer between the intravascular space and peripheral tissues. Body weight, muscle mass, and fat are major determinants of drug distribution volume and women generally differ from men in both body weight and composition.

Sex differences in drug binding to plasma proteins in the blood have not been studied extensively. It appears that drug binding to albumin is not greatly influenced by sex (18). However, there may be age-related changes (19). In certain disease states the amount of this protein decreases markedly (20). Many basic drugs, and to a lesser extent acidic and neutral drugs, are bound to α_1-acid-glycoprotein. Estrogen decreases α_1-acid-glycoprotein levels, presumably accounting for the fact that drugs bind less extensively to this protein in women than in men. Alpha$_1$-acid-glycoprotein is an acute-phase reactant and plasma concentrations of this protein usually increase in disease states or inflammatory conditions (20). Other plasma proteins that drugs may bind to include corticosteroid-binding globulin, sex-hormone binding globulin, and various lipoproteins, and sex influences the plasma concentrations of all of these (19).

Fat constitutes a greater proportion of body weight in women than in men. Hence, the distribution volume of lipophilic drugs will be greater in women than in men when normalized on a liter per kilogram body weight (L/kg) basis. Lipophilic medications such as diazepam, nitrazepam, and chlordiazepoxide have larger L/kg volumes of distribution in women than men (21–25). Since muscle constitutes a lower proportion of body mass in women than in men, total body water and the distribution volume of hydrophilic drugs will be lower in women than in men on a L/kg basis. Since the distribution volume of ethanol, a hydrophilic drug, is smaller in women than in men, this explains why they have higher peak alcohol blood levels after a drink. Muscle mass also declines with age with the result that older men and women have smaller distribution volumes of bromazepam than either sex of younger individuals (26).

HEPATIC METABOLISM

Sex Differences in Metabolic Pathways

Although it is tempting to assume that structurally related compounds that exhibit the same mechanism of action are also pharmacokinetically the same, this certainly is not true in all cases. Perhaps the best example of this complexity is provided by the benzodiazepines. Among the members of this group, oxidation is greater in women than in men for alprazolam, diazepam, and desmethyldiazepam; reduction is the same for men and women for bromazepam, lorazepam, nitrazepam, and triazolam; and conjugation is greater for men than women for chlordiazepoxide, oxazepam, and temazepam. Some clarification can be provided by focusing on sex differences that occur in the specific Phase I and Phase II metabolic pathways that were described in Chapter 11.

Phase I Metabolic Pathways

Pharmacogenetic studies now play an integral role in our understanding of drug metabolism, and to date primary emphasis has been placed on Phase I reactions. Accumulated data has shown that the activity of some drug-metabolizing enzymes is affected not only by ethnicity but by sex (27). As discussed in Chapter 11, the six members of the cytochrome P450 enzyme superfamily that have been implicated in Phase I drug metabolism are CYP1A2, CYP2C9, CYP2C19, CYP2D6, CYP2E1, and CYP3A4.

The CYP3A4 isoenzyme metabolizes greater than 50% of drugs and its activity in the liver is greater in young women than in young men by a ratio of 1.4:1 (28, 29). It was thought that CYP3A4 exhibited no genetic polymorphism (30–32), since a study done in comparing the elimination kinetics of triazolam, a CYP3A4 substrate, showed no difference between Southern Asian and Caucasian males (33). However, when 6β-hydroxycortisol, a specific marker for CYP3A4 activity, was measured in women, it was found that Asian women had two to three times less activity than Caucasian women throughout the menstrual cycle (34). Because CYP3A4 activity is regulated by sex hormones, it is not surprising that differences have also been reported between premenopausal and postmenopausal women (35). Therefore, hormonal state as well as ethnicity must be considered in evaluating the activity of this isoenzyme. Of the drugs metabolized by CYP3A4, erythromycin, prednisolone, methylprednisolone, diazepam, verapamil, and tirilazad all have clearances that are higher in women than in men. On the other hand, no sex differences in clearance or conflicting data have been reported for dapsone, nifedipine (one-third of the women were taking oral contraceptives), alfentanil, and cyclosporine (13, 30–32). The reason for this discrepancy is unclear.

The CYP2D6 isoenzyme metabolizes more than 40 drugs in current use, including antidepressasnts, antiarrhythmics, analgesics, and beta-blockers. As discussed in Chapter 13, the CYP2D6 isoenzyme is polymorphic with poor metabolizers composing 5 to 10% of Caucasian populations but only about 2% of African or Asian populations. There is no evidence of a sex-related difference in the incidence of the poor metabolizer phenotype. Of the drugs metabolized by this isoenzyme, there was no sex difference in desipramine clearance when normalized for weight (36). Although both clomipramine and desipramine have been reported to have clearances that are greater in males than females, the reported clomipramine clearance unfortunately was not normalized for weight whereas desipramine clearance was (37).

The CYP2C19 isoenzyme, like CYP2D6, shows polymorphism. There is large interethnic variation with poor metabolizers constituting 12 to 25% of Asians, and 2 to 5% of African Americans and Caucasians (1, 38). The effect of sex on CYP2C19 activity is population specific. Thus, there is no evidence of a sex-related difference in CYP2C19 activity in poor metabolizers or in Caucasian or North Indian extensive metabolizers (38). However, Chinese women who are extensive metabolizers have greater CYP2C19 activity than men (39), whereas Jewish Israeli and African-American men have greater CYP2C19 activity than women (40).

The CYP2C9 isoenzyme shows phenotypic variation, but little information is available. There is interethnic variation in the incidence of poor metabolizers between Caucasians and Chinese. However, the incidence of the poor metabolizer phenotype is too low to identify sex differences, and reports on sex differences in the activity of CYP2C9 are conflicting (13).

The CYP1A2 isoenzyme is less active in women than men. It is responsible for oxidation of both caffeine and theophylline (1, 13). There is little information available about sex differences in the activity of CYP2E1, and even less about the other Phase I enzymes, called non-P450 monoxygenases (27, 28).

Phase II Metabolic Pathways

Sex differences also have been identified in drug conjugation reactions that are classified as Phase II (Chapter 11). Glucuronide conjugates of diflunisal, oxazepam, and temazepam are formed by UDP-glucuronosyltransferase (41–44). For oxazepam and temazepam, the ratio of clearance in men versus women is 1.5:1 (13). The clearance of acetaminophen, which undergoes both glucuronidation and sulfate conjugation, is also 22% greater in men than in women. However, the glucuronidation of clofibric acid and ibuprofen shows no sex differences (45, 46). Salicylic acid undergoes glycine conjugation and its clearance is greater in women than in men (11). Less is known about sex differences for other drug-metabolizing enzymes that are involved in Phase II reactions (1).

Multiple Metabolic Pathways

Although we have associated a number of drugs with a specific metabolic pathway, the metabolism of many drugs actually involves multiple pathways operating either in series or in parallel. Thus, many drugs are first oxidized in a Phase I reaction that is followed by Phase II conjugation (13). It also is common for several isoenzymes to be involved in the Phase I metabolism of a drug. For example, ring oxidation of propranolol is mediated by CYP2D6. Both CYP1A and CYP2C participate in side-chain cleavage, and propranolol is also glucuronidated (13, 47, 48). Therefore, sex differences in both Phase I and II metabolic pathways

provide a number of reasons why propranolol concentration is higher in women than in men.

Drug Metabolism Interactions of Particular Importance to Women

As shown in Table 21.1, concomitant administration of oral contraceptives can increase the clearance of some drugs, decrease the clearance of some drugs, and have no effect on the clearance of others (13). Clearance increases primarily reflect the ability of oral contraceptives to increase the activity of glucuronyltransferase. The mechanism by which oral contraceptives decrease

TABLE 21.1 Effects of Oral Contraceptives on Drug Metabolism[a]

Drug	Change in clearance
Increase in drug clearance	**Percent increase**
Acetaminophen	41–61
Clofibric Acid	48
Lorazepam	0–273
Morphine	90
Oxazepam	157
Salicylic Acid	41–46
Temazepam	62
Decrease in drug clearance	**Percent decrease**
Alprazolam	0–22
Antipyrine	21–38
Amitryptiline	88
Caffeine	43
Cholordiazepoxide	34–60
Cyclosporine	126
Diazepam	40
Imipramine	50
Metoprolol	41
Nitrazepam	26
Phenytoin	67
Prednisolone	30–84
Theophylline	29
Triazolam	32
No effect on clearance	
Acebutolol	
Bromazepam	
Ethanol	
Meperidine	
Oxprenolol	
Phenylbutazone	
Propranolol	

[a] Data from Harris RZ, Benet LZ, Schwartz JB. Drugs 1995;50:222–39.

drug metabolism is unknown and it is not known to what extent the estrogen or the progesterone components of oral contraceptives participate in these interactions (49). Drug metabolism interactions resulting from hormone replacement therapy also warrant consideration, but little data are available (50–55).

Women use herbal products and dietary supplements more frequently than men. As more and more patients are combining these alternative therapies with conventional pharmaceuticals, drug–herb and drug–nutrient interactions are becoming increasingly important (56–62). The complexity of the situation is illustrated by the fact that St. John's wort, or its hypericum extract, contains at least seven groups of chemical compounds. These include, napthodianthrons (hypericin and pseudohypericin), flavenoids (quercetin, hyperoside, and rutin), biflavones, tannic acid, phenylpropanes, and hyperforin. It is known that hypericin induces CYP1A2, which would affect theophylline metabolism, and that quercetin induces P-glycoprotein. St. John's wort interacts with indinavir, a protease inhibitor that is metabolized by CYP3A4, with the result that therapeutic response to this drug is compromised because its plasma concentrations are decreased. St. John's wort has also been reported to decrease the concentration of cyclosporine, a CYP3A4 and P-glycoprotein substrate, in heart-transplant patients (59). Because sex steroids are metabolized by CYP3A4, one would expect plasma concentrations of oral contraceptives also to decrease in patients taking St. John's wort. Therefore, women who wish to take this herbal remedy should be advised to use an alternative birth control method. This herb also decreases the concentration of digoxin, presumably because it induces P-glycoprotein that decreases absorption and increases excretion of this drug. It has been observed that, although it involves a different mechanism, the interaction potential of hypericum extract may be quantitatively comparable to that of grapefruit juice. (59).

In the United States, a higher percentage of women now smoke than men. Smoking increases CYP1A2 activity and therefore increases the clearance of caffeine and theophylline. The effect on caffeine clearance is greater in men than in women, but the opposite is true for theophylline (63–64).

RENAL EXCRETION

Three processes are considered in evaluating the renal excretion of drugs: glomerular filtration rate, tubular secretion, and tubular reabsorption. Glomerular filtration rate is not influenced by sex. Although the Cockcroft and Gault equation that is used to estimate glomerular filtration rate includes a multiplier of 0.85 for women (65), this only reflects the fact that women have a lower rate of creatinine synthesis per Kg body weight than men because their muscle mass is proportionately smaller (see Chapter 1). There is little data regarding sex differences in tubular secretion. In one study, it was found that the tubular secretion of amantadine normally was similar in men and women, but was inhibited by quinine and quinidine in men but not in women (66). Tubular secretion of amantadine is mediated by P-glycoprotein and both quinine and quinidine are known inhibitors of this efflux pump. As yet, no sex-specific analysis of the activity of P-glycoprotein has been reported. Finally, there has been no evaluation of sex differences in the renal tubular reabsorption of drugs.

CHRONOPHARMACOLOGY, MENSTRUAL CYCLE, AND MENOPAUSE

Chronopharmacology concerns itself with the effects of biological rhythms on drugs. Although little work has been done in this area, it is known that disease states and therapeutic responses are not time invariant (67, 68). Chronopharmacokinetics also includes the impact of circadian rhythms on hepatic drug metabolism (69). The highest activity for the P450 system, oxidative reactions, and glucuronide conjugation is during the waking hours while the highest activity for sulfate and glutathione conjugation is during the resting period. It has been assumed that the need for medications is the same over 24 hours. In the future, drug dosing schedules may be optimized based on an understanding of chronopharmacology. To data, cefodizime (70) and lorazepam (71) are the only two drugs for which there has been a sex-based analysis of chronopharmacology. For example, when cefodizime was administered intravenously four times per day, the plasma concentrations of the drug were less in women at 1200 and 1800 hours while the renal excretion was greater at those times for women as compared to men. For the morning oral dose (0700), women taking lorazepam had a faster absorption rate (k_a) and half-life than men. For the evening oral dose (1900 hours), there was no sex difference in these parameters and AUCs were not significantly different.

Chronopharmacology also includes the impact of the menstrual cycle on drug pharmacokinetics and pharmacodynamics (70). The menstrual cycle includes the follicular, ovulatory, and luteal phases that are accompanied by substantial hormonal changes. Therefore, it cannot be assume that a premenopausal woman has the same kinetic profile as a man in the same age range. There have been few studies that have encompassed all different phases of the menstrual cycle. During ovulation, absorption of ethanol and salicylates is decreased, while clearance of acetaminophen, antipyrine, and methaqualone is increased. In the luteal phase, the clearance of caffeine and theophylline is decreased. However, it is known that the clearance of phenytoin is increased in the luteal phase prior to menses and this may cause women to become preictal. The metabolic ratio of debrisoquine, a probe for CYP2D6 metabolic phenotyping, is significantly lower in the luteal phase as compared to the follicular and ovulatory phases. Drugs not affected by the menstural cycle include alprazolam, carbamazepine, dextromethorphan, ethylmorphine, lithium, midazolam, nitrazepam, phenazone, phenobarbital, propranolol, tobramycin, and zidovudine. However, no generalizations can be made at this point about whether the menstrual cycle affects particular isoenzymes more than others, or affects certain aspects of the oral absorption or renal excretion of drugs.

American women spend one-third of their life in menopause, a time when plasma levels of estrogen and progesterone are greatly reduced (1, 13). The metabolic clearance of a number of drugs has been shown to decline in postmenopausal women, whereas decreases were not found in men of corresponding age. For example, the elimination clearance of alfentanil, a CYP3A4 substrate, is decreased in older women, but does not change with age in men (73, 74). The same is seen for S-verapamil (54), and tirilazad (34), which are also metabolized by CYP3A4. Piroxicam, which is metabolized by CYP2C19 and other pathways, shows the same pattern as the other three medications (13). Prednisolone shows a decreased clearance in menopausal women (49). As previously mentioned, calcium absorption is decreased in menopause and this may explain changes in the absorption of drugs that have similar absorptive profiles as this mineral. As described in Chapter 5, the renal clearance of many drugs also decreases with age in parallel with a gradual decline in renal function.

PHARMACODYNAMICS

There are few sex-analyzed studies of pharmacodynamics and even fewer that combine pharmacokinetics and pharmacodynamics. The most information to date has been provided on the cardiovascular effects of drugs, followed by pharmacodynamic studies of analgesics, immunosuppressants, and antidepressants.

Cardiovascular Effects

Perhaps the most dramatic example of sex differences in pharmacologic response is given by the greater risk that women have of developing the life-threatening ventricular arrhythmia called *torsades de pointes* after taking certain medications (75). Women have a risk of developing *torsades de pointes* from these medications that is at least twice as great as that of men (75–78). The demonstration that *torsades de pointes* is an important side effect of terfenadine first attracted widespread attention to the severity of this problem and led to the withdrawal of this nonsedating antihistamine from the market in 1998. Other drugs that increase the risk of *torsades de pointes* include those listed in Table 21.2.

Terfenadine and presumably other drugs that cause *torsades de pointes* block the delayed rectifier potassium current, which initially lengthens the electrocardiographic QT interval (79). More than 40 drugs in current use have been shown to lengthen the QT interval and have the presumed potential to cause *torsades de pointes*. However, *torsades de pointes* does not occur in every patient who is treated with these drugs, and other factors that may predispose to this arrhythmia include hypokalemia, hypomagnesmia, and hypothyroidism (75, 80, 81). Women appear to be at an increased risk of *torsades de pointes* because the heart

TABLE 21.2   Drugs Reported to Have Caused Torsades de Pointes[a]

Antiarrhythmics	
Amiodarone	Ibutilide
Disopyramide	Procainamide
Dofetilide	Quinidine
Flecainide	Sotalol
Antibiotics and anti-infectives	
Erythromycin	Pentamidine
Halofantrine	Sparlfloxacin
Antidepressants and antipsychotics	
Haloperidol	Thioridazine
Antihistamines	
Astemizole[b]	Terfenadine[b]
Other	
Cisapride[b]	Felbamate
Bepridil	Probucol[b]
Droperidol	

[a] Data from Woosley, RL. Internet at http://dml.georgetown.edu/depts/pharmacology/torsades.html.

[b] These drugs have been removed from the U.S. market.

rate-corrected QT interval in women is longer than it is in men (82). The length of the QT interval is similar in males and females at birth, but shortens in males at puberty. Females have an increased incidence of *torsades de pointes* only after puberty and the risk of this arrhythmia shows no sex difference before adolescence. These observations are consistent with the fact that sex hormones affect potassium channel activity. Thus, estrogens have a down-regulating effect on potassium-channel activity and androgens may be responsible for the QT interval shortening that is seen in postpubertal males (75, 78, 83).

Quinidine also causes *torsades de pointes* and, in a retrospective review of cases dating back to 1962, the observed prevalence of this arrhythmia in females was 60% as compared with an expected 43% (75). It has been shown that the pharmacokinetics of qunidine are similar in men and women, but that there is a pharmacodynamic difference in that the QT interval is longer in women than in men who are treated with this drug (84). Similarly, women have three times the risk of developing *torsades de pointes* while receiving sotalol (77, 85, 86). It is particularly instructive that *torsades de pointes* was not noted in the initial clinical safety studies of the lipid-lowering drug probucol, even though QT prolongation was described. However, these safety studies were confined to male patients and *torsades de pointes* was first reported to be a serious side effect of this drug only when studies that included both men and women were reviewed (87).

Propranolol provides another important example of a cardiovascular drug that combines sex differences in pharmacokinetics and in pharmacodynamics. In the Beta-Blocker Heart Attack Trial, equal doses of propranolol were given to both sexes, but women were found to have higher plasma concentrations of this drug than men (1, 48, 88). However, when an isoproterenol challenge infusion was used to assess the actual degree of β-adrenoreceptor blockade, it was found that women had a lower sensitivity to propranolol that compensated for their higher plasma concentration (89, 90). These offsetting pharmacokinetic and pharmacodynamic effects negated the need to reduce propranolol doses in women, an action that could reduce the overall effectiveness of the drug in this sex.

Sex differences in patient response were also noted in a trial that was designed to assess the efficacy of aspirin and dipyridamole in preventing recurrence of stroke in men versus women (91). It was found that there were fewer strokes and a marked reduction in mortality in males but much less of an effect in females. There appears to be a biochemical basis for the finding that aspirin was much less effective in treating women than men. *In vitro* studies have shown that when the same amounts of aspirin were added to the blood of males and females, platelet aggregation decreased more in men than in women (92). Further investigation indicated that when aspirin was added to blood from orchiectomized subjects there was only a modest change in platelet aggregation. However, when testosterone was also added to these blood samples, platelet aggregation was similar to that seen with blood from non-orchiectomized males. Therefore, testosterone appears to play in important role in aspirin-mediated inhibition of platelet aggregation.

Pain

Women respond differently to kappa opioids than men (93). For example, higher doses of morphine must be administered to men than to women in order to provide equivalent relief from postoperative pain. Analgesia may be due to interactions between opioid and steroid receptors or differences in the production of metabolites (94). Another study showed seven women (three in the follicular phase and four in the luteal phase) had greater respiratory depression than the nine men in the same age range. Pharmacodynamic differences were a more important cause of these results than differences in pharmacokinetics (95). On the other hand, standard doses of ibuprofen appeared to be more effective in men than in women when they were challenged with different degrees of earlobe pain (96). This difference in response also could not be attributed to sex differences in pharmacokinetics.

Immunology and Immunosuppression

Although women are more susceptible than men to autoimmune diseases, there are few sex-analyzed studies of immunosuppressant therapy in patients with these disorders (97). However, studies of heart transplantation outcome have shown that women experience more episodes of organ rejection than men (98). This may be due to sex differences in the pharmacokinetics and pharmacodynamics of immunosuppressant drugs. For example, cyclosporine, prednisolone, and methylprednisolone are frequently administered to these patients as immunosuppressants and these drugs are metabolized by the CYP3A4 isoenzyme, which is more active in women than in men. In addition, the length of survival after heart transplantation is inversely correlated with the length of time that is required to withdraw patients from maintenance corticosteroid therapy (99). Since it is more difficult to withdraw steroid therapy from women than from men, this also might account for their decreased survival.

In a sex-analyzed study of methylprednisolone pharmacokinetics and pharmacodynamics in healthy volunteers, it was found that women cleared the drug faster than men, but that women were more sensitive to suppression of endogenous cortisol production (100). The *IC50* value for cortisol suppression in women was 17 times lower than in men. However, these pharmacokinetic and pharmacodynamic sex differences were offsetting so that the net response to a given dose of methylprednisolone was similar in both men and women. This scenario is reminiscent of the offsetting pharmacokinetic and pharmacodynamic sex effects that were encountered with propranolol in the Beta-Blocker Heart Attack Trial.

SUMMARY

There is little data on pharmacokinetic differences between men and women, and even less documentation of sex differences in different ethnic groups. In addition, relatively few studies are sex analyzed for both pharmacokinetic and pharmacodynamic differences. Since mandated by law in 1993, the National Institutes of Health has made good progress in sponsoring sex-analyzed studies. As a result of an interdisciplinary meeting held in 1995, the Food and Drug Administration also has developed the algorithm shown in Figure 21.2 for sex-based analysis of pharmaceutical development studies (1, 101). This excellent algorithm incorporates both basic and applied data to detect sex differences and should be used by the pharmaceutical industry, since the science to date shows clearly that for some medications there are important pharmacological differences between men and women.

References

1. Berg MJ, Ketley JN, Merkatz R, Mittelman A. Pharmacologic issues. In: Agenda for research on women's health for the 21st century. A report of the task force on the NIH women's health research agenda for the 21st century, vol 2. Bethesda, MD: NIH Publication No. 99-4386; 1999. p. 147–66.
2. Kim JS, Nafziger AN. Is it sex or is it gender? Clin Pharmacol Ther 2000;68:1–3.
3. Kando JC, Yonkers KA, Cole JO. Gender as a risk factor for adverse events to medication. Drugs 1995;50:1–6.
4. Berg, MJ. Drugs, vitamins and gender. J Gender Specific Med 1999;2:18–20.
5. Nayak VK, Kshirsagar A, Desai NK, Satoskar RS. Influence of menstrual cycle on antipyrine pharmacokinetics in healthy Indian female volunteers. Br J Clin Pharmacol 1988;26:604–6.
6. U.S. General Accounting Office. GAO Report to Congressional Requesters. Women's health. NIH has increased its efforts to include women in research. Washington, DC. Publication No GAO/HEHS-00-96, May 2000.
7. Arjmandi BH, Salih MA, Herbert DC, Sims SH, Kalu DN. Evidence for estrogen receptor-linked calcium transport in the intestine. Bone Miner 1993;21:63–74.
8. Gennari C, Agnussdei D, Nardi P, Civitelli R. Estrogen preserves a normal intestinal responsiveness to 1,25-dihydroxyvitamin D_3 in oophorectomized women. J Clin Endocrinol Metab 1990;71:1288–93.
9. Datz FL, Christian PE, Moore J. Gender-related differences in gastric emptying. Nucl Med 1987;28:1204–7.
10. Aarons L, Hopkins K, Rowland M, Brossel S, Thiercelin JF. Route of administration and sex differences in the pharmacokinetics of aspirin, administered as its lysine salt. Pharm Res 1989;6:660–6.
11. Ho PC, Triggs EJ, Bourne DW, Heazlewood VJ. The effects of age and sex on the disposition of acetylsalicylic acid and its metabolites. Br J Clin Pharmacol 1985;19:675–84.
12. Seitz HK, Egerer G, Srianowsk UA, Waldherr R, Eckey R, Agarwal DP, et al. Human gastric alcohol dehydragenase activity: effect of age, sex and alcoholism. Gut 1993;34:1433–7.
13. Harris RZ, Benet LZ, Schwartz JB. Gender effects in pharmacokinetics and pharmacodynamics. Drugs 1995;50:222–39.
14. Krecic-Shepard ME, Barnas CR, Slimko J, Jones MP, Schwartz JB. Gender-specific effects on verapamil pharmacokinetics and pharmacodynamics in humans. J Clin Pharmacol 2000;40:219–30.
15. Krishna KH, Hayes KN, Sinz MW, Woolf TF, Hollenberg PF. Inactivation of cytochrome P450-3A4 by bergamottin, a component of grapefruit juice. Clin Res Toxicol 1998;11:252–7.
16. Bailey DG, Malcolm J, Arnold O, Spence JD. Grapefruit juice-drug interactions. Br J Clin Pharmacol 1998;46:101–10.
17. Takanaga H, Ohnishi A, Murankani H, Matsuo H, Higuchi S, Urae A, et al. Relationship between time after intake of grapefruit juice and the effect on pharmacokinetics and pharmacodynamics of nisoldipine in healthy subjects. Clin Pharmacol Ther 2000;67:201–14.
18. Verbeeck RK, Cardinal J-A, Wallace SM. Effect of age and sex on the plasma binding of acidic and basic drugs. Eur J Clin Pharmacol 1984;27:91–7.
19. Wilson K. Sex-related differences in drug disposition in man. Clin Pharmacokinet 1984;9:189–202.
20. MacKichan JJ. Influence of protein binding and use of unbound (free) drug concentrations. In: Evans WE, Schentag JJ, Jusko WJ, editors. Applied pharmacokinetics: Principles of therapeutic drug monitoring. 3rd ed. Vancouver, WA: Applied Therapeutics; 1992. p. 5-1–5-48.
21. Routledge PA, Stargel WW, Kitchell BB, Barchowsky A, Shand DG. Sex-related differences in the plasma protein binding of lignocaine and diazepam. Br J Clin Pharmacol 1981;11:245–50.
22. Abel JG, Sellers, EM, Naranjo CA, Shaw J, Kadar, D, Romach MK. Inter- and intra-subject variation in diazepam free-fraction. Clin Pharmacol Ther 1979;26:247–55.
23. Roberts RK, Desmond PV, Wilkinson GR, Schenker S. Disposition of chlordiazepoxide: sex differences and effects of oral contraceptives. Clin Pharmacol Ther 1979;25:826–31.
24. Ochs HR, Greenblatt DJ, Divoll M. Abernethy DR, Feyerabend H. Dengler HJ. Diazepam kinetics in relation to age and sex. Pharmacology 1981;23:24–30.
25. Greenblatt DJ, Abernethy DR, Locniskar A, Ochs HR, Harmatz JS, Shader RI. Age, sex and nitrazepam kinetics: relation to antipyrine disposition. Clin Pharmacol Ther 1985;38:697–703.
26. Ochs HR, Greenblatt DJ, Friedman H, Burstein ES, Locniskar A, Harmatz JS, Shader RI. Bromazepam pharmacokinetics: influence of age, gender, oral contraceptives, cimetidene, and propranolol. Clin Pharmacol Ther 1987;41:562–70.

27. Bonate PL. Gender-related differences in xenobiotic metabolism. J Clin Pharmacol 1991;31:684–90.
28. Wrighton SA, Stevens JC. The human hepatic cytochrome P450 involved in drug metabolism. Crit Rev Toxicol 1992;22:1–21.
29. Watkins PB, Wrighton SA, Maurel P, Schuetz EG, Mendez-Picon G, Parker GA, et al. Identification of an inducible form of cytochrome P450 in human liver. Proc Natl Acad Sci USA 1985;82:6310–14.
30. May DG, Porter J, Wilkinson GR, Branch RA. Frequency distribution of dapsone N-hydrolase, a putative probe for P4503A4 activity in a white population. Clin Pharmacol Ther 1994;55:492–500.
31. Ahsan CH, Renwick AG, Macklin B. Challenor VF, Waller DG, George CF. Ethnic differences in the pharmacokinetics of oral nifedipine. Br J Clin Pharmacol 1991;31:399–403.
32. Ahsan CH, Renwick AG, Waller DG, Challenor VF, George CF, Amanullah M. The influence of dose and ethnic origins on the pharmacokinetics of nifedipine. Clin Pharmacol Ther 1993;54:329–38.
33. Kinirons MT, Lang CC, Ho HB, Ghebreselasie K, Shay S, Robin DW, Wood AJ. Triazolam pharmacokinetics and pharmacodynamics in Caucasians and Southern Asians: ethnicity and CYP3A4 activity. Br J Clin Pharmacol 1996;41:69–72.
34. Lin Y, Anderson GD, Kantor E, Ojemann LM, Wilensky AJ. Differences in the urinary excretion of 6-beta-hydroxycortisol/cortisol between Asian and Caucasian women. J Clin Pharmacol 1999;39:578–82.
35. Hulst LK, Fleishaker JC, Peters GR, Harry JD, Wright DM, Ward P. Effect of age and gender on tirilazad pharmacokinetics in humans. Clin Pharmacol Ther 1994;55:378–84.
36. Abernethy DR, Greenblatt DJ, Shader RI. Imipramine and desipramine disposition in the elderly. J Pharmacol Exp Ther 1985;232:183–8.
37. Gex-Fabry M, Balant-Gorgia AE, Balant LP, Garrone G. Clomipramine metabolism: Model-based analysis of variability factors from drug monitoring data. Clin Pharmacokinet 1990;19:241–55.
38. Lamba JK, Dhiman RK, Kohli KK. *CYP2C19* genetic mutations in North Indians. Clin Pharmacol Ther 2000;68:328–35.
39. Xie HG, Huang SL, Xu ZH, Xiao ZS, He N, Zhou HH. Evidence for the effect of gender on activity of (S)-mephenytoin 4′-hydroxylase (CYP2C19) in a Chinese population. Pharmacogenetics 1997;7:115–9.
40. Sviri S, Shpizen S, Leitersdorf E, Levy M, Caraco Y. Phenotypic-genotypic analysis of CYP2C19 in the Jewish Israeli population. Clin Pharmacol Ther 1999;65:275–82.
41. Greenblatt DJ, Divoll M, Harmatz JS, Shader R. Oxazepam kinetics: effects of age and sex. J Pharmacol Exp Ther 1980;215:86–91.
42. Divoll M, Greenblatt DJ, Harmatz JS, Shader R. Effects of age and gender on disposition of temazepam. J Pharm Sci 1981;10:1104–7.
43. Miners JO, Attwood J, Birkett DJ. Influence of sex and oral contraceptive steroids on paracetamol metabolism. Br J Clin Pharmacol 1983;16:503–9.
44. Macdonald JI, Herman RJ, Verbeeck RK. Sex-difference and the effects of smoking and oral contraceptive steroids on the kinetics of diflunisal. Eur J Clin Pharmacol 1990;38:175–9.
45. Miners JO, Robson RA, Birkett DJ. Gender and oral contraceptive steroids as determinants of drug glucuronidation: effects on clofibric acid elimination. Br J Clin Pharmacol 1984;18:240–3.
46. Greenblatt DJ, Abernethy DR, Matlis R, Harmatz JS, Shader RI. Absorption and distribution of ibuprofen in the elderly. Arthritis Rheum 1984;27:1066–9.
47. Berg MJ. Status of research on gender differences. Gender-related health issues: An international perspective. In: Berg MJ, Francke G, Rollings M, editors. Washington: American Pharmaceutical Association; 1996. p. 37–68.
48. Walle T, Walle K, Cowart D, Conradi EC. Pathway-selective sex differences in the metabolic clearances of propranolol in human subjects. Clin Pharmacol Ther 1989;46:257–63.
49. Laine K, Tybring G, Bertilsson L. No sex-related differences but significant inhibition by oral contraceptives of CYP2C19 activity as measured by the probe drugs mephenytoin and omeprazole in healthy Swedish white subjects. Clin Pharmacol Ther 2000;68:151–9.
50. Gustavson LE, Benet LZ. Menopause pharmacodynamics and pharmacokinetics. Exp Gerontol 1994;29:437–44.
51. Harris RZ, Tsunoda SM, Mroczkowski P, Wong H, Benet LZ. The effects of menopause and hormone replacement therapies on prednisolone and erythromycin pharmacokinetics. Clin Pharmacol Ther 1996;59:429–35.
52. Gustavson LE, Legler UF, Benet LZ. Impairment of prednisolone disposition in women taking oral contraceptives or conjugated estrogens. J Clin Endocrinol Metab 1986;62:234–7.
53. Holazo AA, Winkler MB, Patel IH. Effects of age, gender and oral contraceptives on intramuscular midazolam pharmacokinetics. J Clin Pharmacol 1988;28:1040–5.
54. Greenblatt DJ, Abernethy DR, Locniskar A, Harmatz JS, Limjuco RA, Shader RI. Effect of age, gender and obesity on midazolam kinetics. Anesthesiology 1984;61:27–36.
55. Schwartz JB, Capili H, Daughtery J. Aging of women alters S-verapamil pharmacokinetics and pharmacodynamics. Clin Pharmacol Ther 1994;55:509–17.
56. Ernest E. Second thoughts about safety of St. John's wort. Lancet 1993;354:2014–6.
57. Piscitelli SC, Burstein AH, Chaitt D, Alfaro RM, Falloon J. Indinavir concentrations and St. John's wort [letter]. Lancet 355;2000:547–8.
58. Fugh-Berman A. Herb-drug interactions. Lancet 2000;355:134–8.
59. Johne A, Brockmöller J, Bauer S, Maurer A, Langheinrich M, Roots I. Pharmacokinetic interaction of digoxin with an herbal extract from St. John's wort (*Hypericum perforatum*). Clin Pharmacol Ther 1999;66:338–45.
60. Risk of drug interactions with St. John's wort and indinavir and other drugs. FDA Public Health Advisory, Rockville, MD, 2000. (Internet at http://www.fda.gov/cder/drug/advisory/stjwort.htm.)
61. Ruschitzka F, Meier PJ, Turina M, Luscher TF, Noll G. Acute heart transplant rejection due to St. John's wort. Lancet 2000;355:548–9.
62. Roby CA, Anderson GB, Kantor E, Dryer DA, Burstein AH. St. John's wort: Effect on CYP3A4 activity. Clin Pharmacol Ther 2000;67:451–7.
63. Carrillo JA, Benitez J. CYP1A2 activity, gender and smoking as variables influencing the toxicity of caffeine. Br J Clin Pharmacol 1996;41:605–8.
64. Jennings TS, Nafziger AN, Davidson ML, Bertino JS Jr. Gender differences in hepatic induction and inhibition of theophylline pharmacokinetics and metabolism. J Lab Clin Med 1993;122:208–16.
65. Cockroft DW, Gault MH. Prediction of creatinine clearance from serum creatinine. Nephron 1976;16:31–41.
66. Gaudry SE, Sitar DS, Smyth DD, McKenzie JK, Aoki FY. Gender and age as factors in the inhibition of renal clearance of amantadine by quinine and quinidine. Clin Pharmacol Ther 1993;54:23–7.
67. Lemmer B. Circadian rhythm in blood pressure: signal transduction, regulatory mechanisms and cardiovascular medication. In: Lemmer B, editor. From the biological clock to chronopharmacology. Stuttgart: Medpharm Scientific Publishers; 1996. p.91–117.

68. Reinberg AE, Ashkenazi IE. Chronopharmacology: Should we individualize drug treatments. In: Lemmer B, editor. From the biological clock to chronopharmacology. Stuttgart: Medpharm Scientific Publishers; 1996. p. 71–89.

69. Labrecque G, Belanger PM. Biological rhythms in the absorption, distribution, metabolism and excretion of drugs. Pharmacol Ther 1991;52:95–107.

70. Jonkman JH, Reinberg A. Oosterhuis B, de Noord OE, Kerkhof FA, Motohashi Y, et al. Dosing time and sex-related differences in the pharmacokinetics of cefodizime and in the circadian cortisol rhythm. Chronobiologia 1988;15:89–102.

71. Bruguerolle B, Bouvenot G, Bartolin R, Descottes C. Temporal and sex-related variations of lorazepam pharmacokinetics. Int J Clin Pharmacol Ther Toxicol 1985;23:352–4.

72. Berg MJ. Drugs in the menstrual cycle. J Gender-Spec Med 1998;3:17–9.

73. Lemmens HJM, Burm AGL, Hennis PJ, Gladines MP, Bovill JG. Influence of age on the pharmacokinetics of alfentanil. Gender dependence. Clin Pharmacokinet 1990;19:416–22.

74. Rubio A, Cox C. Sex, age and alfentanil pharmacokinetics. Clin Pharmacokinet 1991;21:81–2.

75. Ebert SN, Liu X-K, Woosley RL. Female gender as a risk factor for drug-induced cardiac arrhythmias: evaluation of clinical and experimental evidence. J Women's Health 1998;7:547–57.

76. Woosley RL. Drugs that prolong the Q-T interval and/or induce *torsades de pointes*. Washington, DC, Georgetown, 2000. (Internet at http://dml.georgetown.edu/depts/pharmacology/torsades.html.)

77. Makkar RR, Fromm BS, Steinman RT, Meissner MD, Lehmann MH. Female gender as a risk factor for torsades de pointes associated with cardiovascular drugs. JAMA 1993;270:2590–7.

78. Drici MD, Knollmann BC, Wang WX, Woosley RL, Cardiac actions of erythromycin: influence of female sex. JAMA 1998;280:1774–6.

79. Woosley RL, Chen Y, Freiman JP, Gillis RA. Mechanism of the cardiotoxic actions of terfenadine. JAMA 1993;269:1532–6.

80. Kumar A, Bhandari AK, Rahimtoola SH. Torsades de pointes and marked QT prolongation in association with hypothyroidism. Ann Intern Med 1987;106:712–3.

81. Bagchi N, Brown R, Parish RF. Thyroid dysfunction in adults over age 55 years. A study in an urban US community. Arch Intern Med 1990;150:785–7.

82. Bazett HC. An analysis of the time-relations of electrocardiograms. Heart 1919;7:353–70.

83. Drici MD, Burklow TR, Haridasse V, Glazer RI, Woosley RL. Sex hormones prolong the QT interval and down-regulate potassium channel expression in the rabbit heart. Circulation 1996;94:1471–4.

84. Roden DM, Woosley RL, Primm RK. Incidence and clinical features of the quinidine-associated long QT syndrome: implications for patient care. Am Heart J 1986;111:1088–93.

85. Lehmann MH, Hardy S, Archibald D, Quart B, MacNeil DJ. Sex difference in risk of torsades de pointes with d,l-sotalol. Circulation 1996;94:2535–41.

86. Pratt CM, Camm AJ, Cooper W, Friedman PL, MacNeil DJ, Moulton KM, et al. Mortality in the survival with oral D-sotalol (SWORD) trial: why did patients die? Am J Cardiol 1998;81:869–76.

87. Reinoehl J, Frankovich D, Machado C, Kawasaki R, Baga JJ, Pires LA, et al. Probucol-associated tachyarrhythmic events and QT prolongation: importance of gender. Am Heart J 1996;131:1184–91.

88. Walle T, Byington RP, Furberg CD, McIntyre KM, Vokanas PS. Biologic determinants of propranolol disposition: results from 1308 patients in the Beta-Blocker Heart Attack Trial. Clin Pharmacol Ther 1985;38:509–18.

89. Flockhart DA, Drici MD, Samuel C, Abernethy DR, Woosley RL. Effects of gender on propranolol pharmacokinetics and pharmacodynamics [abstract]. FASEB J 1996;10:A429.

90. Berg MJ. Pharmacokinetics and pharmacodynamics of cardiovascular drugs. J Gender-Spec Med 1999;2:22–4.

91. Sivenius J, Laakso M, Penttila IM, Smets P, Lowenthal A, Riekkinen PJ. The European stroke prevention study: Results according to sex. Neurology 1991;41:1189–92.

92. Spranger M, Aspey BS, Harrison MJ. Sex differences in antithrombotic effect of aspirin. Stroke 1989;20:34–7.

93. Gear RW, Miaskowski C, Gordon NC, Paul SM, Heller PH, Levine JD. Kappa-opioids produce significantly greater analgesia in women than in men. Nat Med 1996;2:1248–50.

94. Mercadante S, Casucio A, Pumo S, Fulfaro F. Factors influencing the opioid response in advanced cancer patients with pain followed at home: the effects of age and gender. Support Care Center 2000;8:123–30.

95. Sarton E, Teppema L, Dahan A. Sex differences in morphine-induced ventilatory depression reside within the peripheral chemoreflex loop. Anesthesiology 1999;90:1329–38.

96. Walker J, Carmody JJ. Experimental pain in healthy human subjects: Gender differences in nociception and a response to ibuprofen. Anesth Analg 1998;86:1257–62.

97. Legato MJ. Gender-specific physiology: how real is it? How important is it? Int J Fertil Womens Med 1997;42:19–29.

98. Esmore D, Keogh A, Spratt P, Jones B, Chang V. Heart transplantation in females. J Heart Lung Transplant 1991;10:335–41.

99. Taylor DO, Briston MR, O'Connell JB, Price GD, Hammond EH, Doty DB, et al. Improved long-term survival after heart transplantation predicted by successful early withdrawal from maintenance corticosteroid therapy. J Heart Lung Transplant 1996;15:1039–46.

100. Lew KH, Ludwig EA, Milad MA, Donovan K, Middleton E Jr, Ferry JJ, et al. Gender-based effects on methylprednisolone pharmacokinetics and pharmacodynamics. Clin Pharmacol Ther 1993;54:402–14.

101. Gender studies in product development: scientific issues and approaches. Executive Summary. Rockville, MD: U.S. Food and Drug Administration; 1999. (Internet at http://www.fda.gov/womens/Executive.html.)

Drug Therapy in Pregnant and Nursing Women

CATHERINE S. STIKA AND MARILYNN C. FREDERIKSEN

Department of Obstetrics and Gynecology, Northwestern University Medical School, Chicago, Illinois

The pregnant woman is perhaps the last true therapeutic orphan. Because of the ethical, medico-legal, and fetal safety concerns regarding pregnant women, few pharmacokinetic, pharmacodynamic, or clinical trials are conducted during pregnancy. The majority of drugs that are marketed in the United States, therefore, carry the statement in their labeling that:

> There are, however, no adequate and well-controlled studies in pregnant women. Because animal reproductive studies are not always predictive of human response, this drug should be used during pregnancy only if clearly needed. (1)

This places the burden squarely on the practitioner to assess the risks and benefits of a particular agent in a given clinical situation. The risk most often considered is the fetal risk of teratogenesis, or drug-induced malformation, irrespective of the gestational age during the pregnancy when therapy is initiated. Pregnant women are more often than not left untreated in an attempt to avoid any perceived fetal risk related to use of a pharmacologic agent, and the effect of untreated maternal disease on either the pregnancy outcome or the offspring is not always considered. Issues of appropriate dosage and frequency of administration are often not evaluated, so that the usual adult dose is prescribed without thought to any changes dictated by physiologic differences between nonpregnant and pregnant women.

There are two compelling reasons for studying drugs and drug therapy during pregnancy. The first relates to the changing age of reproduction. Pregnancy was once mainly undertaken by healthy, younger women, yet the age of reproduction now includes women ranging in age from 10 to approximately 50, and with *in vitro* fertilization and egg donation even older women undertake pregnancy. Moreover, the age of a woman's first pregnancy has been steadily rising in the United States, with an increasing number of first pregnancies occurring after age 30 (2). The expansion of the reproductive age range, coupled with the occurrence of pregnancy later in life, increase the number of women who may require drug therapy for diseases present prior to pregnancy and who may need to continue therapy during pregnancy. Knowledge of drug therapy during pregnancy is needed if these women with underlying diseases are to be optimally treated.

The second reason supporting the need to study drugs during pregnancy relates to the physiologic changes that occur with gestation. To accommodate fetal growth and development, and perhaps provide a measure of safety for the woman, pregnancy alters a woman's underlying physiology. This altered physiology can affect the pharmacokinetics of drugs. The changes may increase drug distribution volume, decrease drug binding to plasma proteins, alter peak drug concentration and time to peak drug concentration, and cause variations in either hepatic and/or renal drug clearance. Extrapolation of pharmacokinetic data from drug studies largely conducted in nonpregnant subjects to pregnant women fails to account for the impact of physiologic changes that occur during pregnancy. This disregard for the changes in

277

maternal physiology may affect drug efficacy and ultimately impact the overall pregnancy outcome.

PREGNANCY PHYSIOLOGY POTENTIALLY ALTERING PHARMACOKINETICS

Rather than present a list of the many changes in maternal physiology that occur during pregnancy, the focus here is to select those changes that have the greatest potential to alter the absorption, distribution, and elimination of drugs in pregnant women.

Pregnancy may affect the bioavailability of drugs because gastric emptying is delayed (3) and gastrointestinal transit time is prolonged (4), largely due to the action of progesterone on smooth muscle activity. There is also a decrease in gastric acid secretion that results in a correspondingly higher gastric pH (5).

There are multiple physiological changes in pregnant women that may affect the distribution volume of drugs. In some cases, it is possible to correlate pregnancy-associated changes in distribution volume with changes in extracellular fluid space (ECF), total body water (TBW), and drug binding to plasma proteins using the following equation that was developed in Chapter 3:

$$V_d = \text{ECF} + f_U (\text{TBW} - \text{ECF}) \qquad (22.1)$$

where f_U is the fraction of unbound drug.

By the sixth to eighth week of pregnancy, plasma volume has expanded and continues to increase until approximately 32 to 34 weeks of pregnancy (6). For a singleton gestation, this increase in plasma volume is 1200–1300 mL or approximately 40% higher than the plasma volume of nonpregnant women. Plasma volume expansion is even greater for multiple gestations (7). There are also significant increases in ECF and TBW that vary somewhat with patient weight. These changes in body fluid spaces are summarized in Table 22.1 (8, 9).

Because the concentration of plasma albumin decreases during pregnancy (10, 11), protein binding of drugs often is reduced. The fall in albumin concentration from 4.2 gm/dL in the nonpregnant woman to 3.6 gm/dL in the midtrimester of pregnancy (Figure 22.1) has long been attributed to a dilutional effect of plasma volume expansion. However, a more likely explanation is that this decrease represents either a reduction in the rate of albumin synthesis or an increase in its rate of clearance (see Equation 1.1). Additional support for this explanation is provided by the fact that the plasma concentrations of total protein (10) and α_1-acid glycoprotein (12), which binds many basic drugs, are relatively unchanged during pregnancy.

TABLE 22.1 Body Fluid Spaces in Pregnant and Nonpregnant Women[a]

	Weight (kg)	Plasma volume (mL/kg)	ECF space (L/kg)	TBW (L/kg)	Ref.
Nonpregnant		49			6
	<70		0.189	0.516	8
	70–80		0.156	0.415	8
	>80		0.151	0.389	8
Pregnant		67			6
	<70		0.257	0.572	9
	70–80		0.255	0.514	9
	>80		0.240	0.454	9

[a] Modified from Frederiksen MC, et al. Clin Pharmacol Ther 1986;40:321–8.

Pregnancy is also associated with a partially compensated respiratory alkalosis that may affect the protein binding of some drugs. Respiratory changes in pregnancy include a fall in arterial partial pressure of carbon dioxide to 30.9 mm Hg, most likely due to the effect of progesterone (13, 14). In compensation, serum bicarbonate falls and maternal serum pH increases slightly to 7.44 (13).

Pregnancy-associated increases in plasma volume are accompanied by an increase in cardiac output, which in the third trimester is at least 30 to 50% above normal (15). Cardiac output begins to increase early in pregnancy, and by 8 weeks' gestation can be as much as 50% greater than in the nonpregnant state. Cardiac output then continues to increase until term. Early in pregnancy, increased stroke volume accounts for this increase in cardiac output. However, later in pregnancy, the changes in cardiac output are the result of both elevated maternal heart rate and a continued increase in stroke volume (16).

Regional blood flow changes in pregnant women can also affect drug distribution and elimination. These include an increase in blood flow to the uterus, kidneys, skin, and mammary glands, and a compensatory decrease in skeletal muscle blood flow. At term, blood flow to the uterus represents about 20 to 25% of cardiac output and renal blood flow is 20% of cardiac output (17). Blood flow to the skin is increased to dissipate heat production by the fetus (18). Mammary blood flow is increased during pregnancy in preparation for lactation postpartum (19). Hepatic blood flow measured in L/min does not appear to change during pregnancy (Figure 22.2). However, expressed as a percentage of cardiac output, hepatic blood flow is lower during pregnancy than in the nonpregnant condition

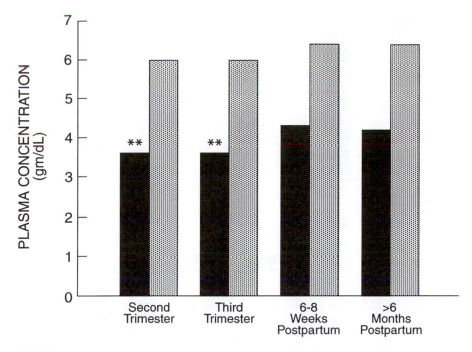

FIGURE 22.1 Albumin *(solid bars)* and total protein *(stippled bars)* concentrations during the second and third trimesters of pregnancy and in the postpartum period. Albumin concentrations are reduced significantly during pregnancy when compared to > 6 months postpartum values (** = *P* < .01). (Data from Frederiksen MC, et al. Clin Pharmacol Ther 1986;40:321–8.)

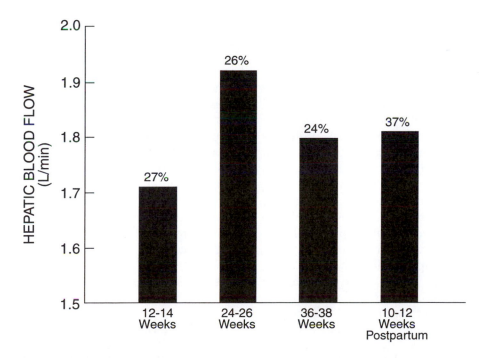

FIGURE 22.2 Hepatic blood flow expressed in L/min *(bars)* and as percent of cardiac output *(numbers above bars)* during pregnancy and in the postpartum period. Although the absolute value of hepatic blood flow is unchanged, it comprises a significantly lower percentage of cardiac output during pregnancy than postpartum. (Data from Robson SC, et al. Br J Obstet Gynaecol 1990;97:720–4.)

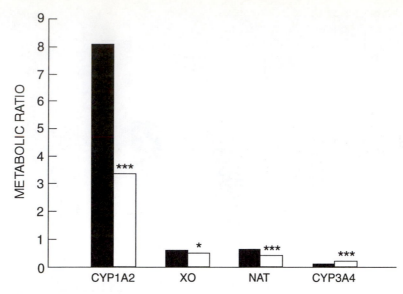

FIGURE 22.3   Paired comparisons of measured ratios of caffeine metabolites to parent drug in non-pregnant *(solid bars)* and pregnant *(open bars)* women. Comparisons were made of the metabolic activities of CYP 1A2, xanthine oxidase (XO), N-acetyltransferase (NAT) and CYP3A4 (* = $P < .05$,*** = $P < .005$). (Data from Bologa M, et al. J Pharmacol Exp Ther 1991;257:735–40.)

because of the increased blood flow to the uterus and kidneys (20). Similarly, a decreased proportion of cardiac output is available to skeletal muscle and perhaps other vascular beds.

Glomerular filtration rate is increased as early as the sixth week of gestation, and continues to rise gradually well into the third trimester (21). This is reflected in an increase in inulin and creatinine clearance during pregnancy and in an increased renal clearance of drugs. Little is known about any effects of normal pregnancy on the renal tubular secretion or resorption of drugs. However, the tubular resorption of glucose appears to be unchanged by pregnancy (22).

The activity of hepatic drug metabolizing enzymes also changes during pregnancy and can affect drug elimination clearance. Pregnancy is an estrogenic state; however, progesterone, the hormone responsible for sustaining gestation, as well as other placental hormones, can also be responsible for hepatic enzymatic activity changes. For example, *N*-demethylation activity has been shown to be inhibited by progesterone (23). Bologa et al. (24) administered caffeine as a metabolic probe to pregnant and nonpregnant women and found that CYP1A2, xanthine oxidase, and *N*-acetyltransferase activities were decreased, but that CYP3A4-mediated 8-hydroxylation was increased during pregnancy (Figure 22.3). Although Wadelius et al. (25) found that CYP2D6 activity was increased during pregnancy in individuals who are homozygous and heterozygous extensive metabolizers of dex-

tromethorphan, the activity of this enzyme appeared to be decreased in homozygous poor metabolizers.

Most of these physiologic changes begin early in gestation but are most pronounced in the third trimester of pregnancy. During labor and delivery, further physiologic changes occur. Maternal cardiac output increases (26), regional blood flows change, and there is a virtual cessation of gastrointestinal activity. The onset of uterine contractions also affects the placental blood flow and drug distribution to the fetus. In the postpartum period, maternal pregnancy changes are sustained with elevated cardiac output, decreased plasma albumin concentration, and increased glomerular filtration rate (27, 28). Some changes in hepatic enzyme activity may rapidly reverse within 24 hours of delivery, while others may return to normal only gradually over the first months after delivery (29). Cardiovascular physiologic changes are sustained as long as 12 weeks postpartum (30). During the puerperium there appears to be great variability between individuals that is largely unstudied.

PHARMACOKINETIC STUDIES ILLUSTRATING MATERNAL PHYSIOLOGIC CHANGES DURING PREGNANCY

Although an exhaustive survey of pharmacokinetic studies is not possible, the purpose here is to present illustrative studies that best demonstrate the effects of maternal physiologic changes on the pharmacokinetics of drugs and potentially dosing and drug efficacy.

Results of Selected Pharmacokinetic Studies in Pregnant Women

Ampicillin

The pharmacokinetics of both intravenously and orally administered ampicillin were studied serially in 26 women who served as their own controls (31). This study combined data from women whose pregnancies ranged from 13 to 33 weeks' gestation, which blurred assessment of the effects of the progression of changes in maternal physiology that occurs during the second and third trimester of pregnancy. Perhaps because both intravenous and oral doses need to be administered, ampicillin is the only medication for which bioavailability has been examined during pregnancy. Although ampicillin is poorly absorbed, no difference in the extent of ampicillin absorption or in time to peak drug concentrations was seen between pregnant and nonpregnant women. However, peak levels were lower than in nonpregnant women. Although this study demonstrated an absolute increase in the volume of distribution with ampicillin, it did not include an analysis of the effect of the change in maternal weight on the volume of distribution. Both renal and total elimination clearance of ampicillin increased by approximately 50% during pregnancy and resulted in correspondingly lower plasma concentrations. Another study of ampicillin pharmacokinetics in the third trimester of pregnancy showed an increase in the steady-state volume of distribution on a L/kg basis (32). Unfortunately, these authors used male controls as an historic reference population.

Caffeine

The pharmacokinetics of caffeine also were studied serially during and after pregnancy (33). In oral pharmacokinetic studies, V_d/F showed no change when calculated on a L/kg basis to take into account the change in weight during and after pregnancy. Caffeine is a CYP1A2 substrate and elimination clearance, estimated as CL/F, was decreased by a factor of two by midgestation and by a factor of three in the third trimester compared to the postpartum period (33).

Theophylline

The pharmacokinetics of intravenously administered theophylline pharmacokinetics have been studied serially in women during and after pregnancy (11). During the second and third trimesters of pregnancy, theophylline binding to plasma proteins was reduced

TABLE 22.2 Comparison of Expected with Measured Values of Theophylline Distribution Volume[a]

	$V_{d(ss)}$[b]	
	Expected (L)	Measured (L)
Pregnant		
24–26 Weeks	32.0 ± 2.0	30.3 ± 6.6
36–38 Weeks	37.9 ± 1.9	36.8 ± 4.2
Postpartum		
6–8 Weeks	28.0 ± 1.1	28.4 ± 3.0
>6 Months	26.9 ± 2.3	30.7 ± 4.4

[a] Data from Frederiksen MC, et al. Clin Pharmacol Ther 1986;40:321–8.
[b] Mean values for five women $\pm$ S.D.

to 11 and 13% of total plasma concentrations, respectively, compared with 28% 6 months postpartum. A subsequent study demonstrated that albumin binding sites for theophylline are actually increased during pregnancy, but the binding affinity constant is significantly lower during pregnancy than in the nonpregnant state (34). Steady-state distribution volume was increased during the second and third trimesters of pregnancy. As shown in Table 22.2, the increases were similar to what was predicted from Equation 22.1 using measured values for protein binding and the estimates of extracellular fluid volume and total body water shown in Table 22.1. On the other hand, these pregnancy-associated changes failed to reach statistical significance when distribution volume was normalized simply for patient weight.

Renal clearance of theophylline paralleled the pregnancy associated increase in creatinine clearance and accounted for 30 and 28% of total theophylline elimination in the second and third trimesters, respectively, compared to only 16% 6 months postpartum. As shown in Figure 22.4, the intrinsic clearance of theophylline, also a CYP1A2 substrate, was reduced substantially during pregnancy. Hepatic clearance showed substantially less change because of the pregnancy-associated decrease in theophylline binding to plasma proteins. As a result of the offsetting changes in renal and hepatic clearance, total elimination clearance of theophylline in the third trimester of pregnancy averaged 86% of its value 6 months postpartum. Although this reduction in elimination clearance was not statistically significant, it combined with the increase in theophylline distribution volume to significantly increase theophylline elimination half-life from an average of 4.4 hours in the nonpregnant state (6 months postpartum) to 6.5 hours in the third trimester of pregnancy.

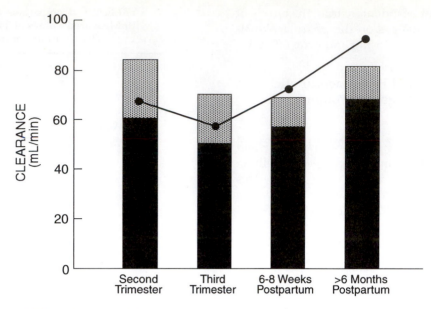

FIGURE 22.4 Theophylline clearance measured during the second and third trimesters of pregnancy and in the postpartum period. During pregnancy, the substantial drop in the intrinsic hepatic clearance (●) of this CYP1A2 substrate is attenuated by decreased theophylline binding to plasma proteins and increased glomerular filtration rate so that overall elimination clearance, consisting of the sum of hepatic clearance *(solid bars)* and renal clearance *(stippled bars)*, is relatively unaffected. (Data from Frederiksen MC, et al. Clin Pharmacol Ther 1986;40:321–8.)

Cefuroxime

The pharmacokinetics of intravenously administered cefuroxime were studied serially in seven women during pregnancy, at delivery, and in the remote postpartum period (35). Distribution volume ($V_{d(extrap)}$) during pregnancy and at delivery approximated the expected ECF shown in Table 22.1. However, the difference in these volumes and the postpartum value was not statistically significant and no change is observed when the distribution volumes are normalized for patient weight. On the other hand, cefuroxime is largely eliminated by renal excretion, and renal clearance was significantly greater during pregnancy than that measured either at delivery or in nonpregnant women. As a result, plasma cefuroxime concentrations resulting from a 750-mg dose were significantly lower during pregnancy.

Methadone

The pharmacokinetics of orally administered methadone were studied serially in nine women at 20–24 weeks and 35–40 weeks of pregnancy and at 1–4 weeks and 8–9 weeks postpartum (36). There was no significant change in methadone binding to plasma proteins during pregnancy. During pregnancy, renal clearance was approximately twice its value in the post-

partum periods. However, renal clearance contributed only minimally to total methadone clearance and this change did not reach statistical significance. On the other hand, estimates of *CL/F* during pregnancy were also doubled and this change was both statistically and clinically significant, resulting in a corresponding lowering of methadone plasma levels and symptoms of methadone withdrawal in some women near the end of gestation. Methadone is a CYP3A4 substrate and the authors concluded that increased metabolic clearance rather than decreased bioavailability was responsible for the decrease in *CL/F*.

Anticonvulsants

The plasma concentrations of most anticonvulsant drugs have been shown to decrease during pregnancy. This is in large part a reflection of the decrease in protein binding that is well documented for phenytoin (37, 38), carbamazepine (38), and phenobarbital (39). However, these drugs are restrictively eliminated and unbound concentrations of carbamazepine (38, 40) and phenobarbital (39) remain unchanged during pregnancy, reflecting the fact that their intrinsic clearance is unchanged. On the other hand, Tomson et al. (38) monitored phenytoin plasma levels serially in 36 women during the first and second trimesters of pregnancy and in the nonpregnant state. Intrinsic clearance

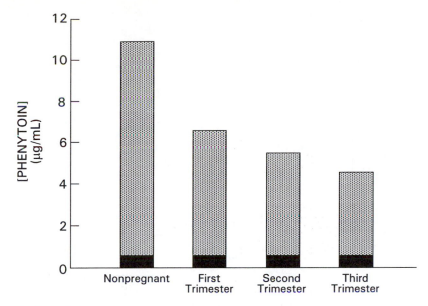

FIGURE 22.5   Total *(solid plus stippled bars)* and free *(solid bars)* plasma concentrations of phenytoin in nonpregnant and pregnant women (Data from Tomson T, et al. Epilepsia 1994;35:122–30.)

was increased in the third trimester of pregnancy and unbound plasma concentrations were significantly lower than in the nonpregnant state (Figure 22.5).

Other Drugs

The clearance of a number of other drugs that are eliminated primarily by renal excretion has also been shown to increase during pregnancy. For example, the pharmacokinetics of subcutaneously administered enoxaprin, a low molecular weight heparin, were studied serially in 13 women at 12–15 weeks and 30–33 weeks gestation and 6–8 weeks postpartum (41). Compared to postpartum values, elimination clearance was increased by approximately 50% in the first gestational study period but was not significantly increased in the later period. In another study, the clearance of tobramycin was shown to peak in the mid-trimester and fall during the third trimester (42).

Plasma concentrations of orally administered nifedipine, another CYP3A4 substrate, have been reported to be decreased in 15 women with pregnancy-induced hypertension who were studied during the third trimester of pregnancy but not subsequently postpartum (43). Estimates of *CL/F* averaged 2.0 L/hr/kg, compared to a value of 0.49 L/hr/kg that was reported in a study of nonpregnant subjects. Another study of nifedipine pharmacokinetics in eight patients with preeclampsia indicated that *CL/F* remains elevated in

the immediate postpartum period, averaging 3.3 L/hr/kg in this clinical setting (44).

First-pass conversion of a prodrug to an active drug has been studied in pregnancy with the drug valacyclovir (45). Orally administered valacyclovir produced three times higher plasma levels of acyclovir than when acyclovir was administered orally. However, the levels achieved with valacyclovir are somewhat lower than that reported in normal volunteers. On the other hand, acyclovir pharmacokinetics were overall similar to what has been reported in nonpregnant women.

Results of Studies During Labor and the Pospartum Period

With the onset of labor, maternal physiology has been shown to differ from the physiology of the antenatal period. Intrapartum cefuroxime clearance is lower than clearance during pregnancy but higher than in the remote postpartum period (35). Morphine clearance is markedly increased during labor, with a corresponding shortening of its elimination half-life (46).

Studies in the postpartum period show greater variability in pharmacokinetic parameters than studies in nonpregnant women or normal volunteers. A study of clindamycin pharmacokinetics demonstrated that there was a 15-fold variation in peak drug concentrations and that t_{max} varied from 1 to 6 hours after oral administration (Figure 22.6) (47). Distribution volume estimates for gentamicin during the postpartum period varied

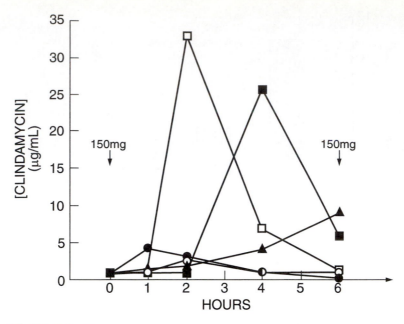

FIGURE 22.6 Plasma concentrations of clindamycin measured in five postpartum women over a 6-hour period after oral administration of a 150-mg dose. (Reproduced with permission from Steen B, Rane A. Br J Clin Pharmacol 1982;13:661–4.)

from 0.1 to 0.5 L/kg, as compared with distribution volume estimates from studies in nonpregnant subjects that ranged from 0.2 to 0.3 L/kg (48).

THE CONDUCT OF DRUG STUDIES IN PREGNANT WOMEN

Studying drugs in pregnancy requires special considerations. Although abstinence from the use of pharmacologic agents is held forth as the ideal during pregnancy, studies have shown that most pregnant women use either prescribed or over-the-counter drugs during pregnancy (49, 50). Ethically, drug studies in pregnancy cannot be done in normal pregnant "volunteers," but only in women who require a drug for a clinical reason. For this reason, study design for these trials must include the ethical argument that the woman would be using the particular agent during pregnancy to treat a medical condition. For FDA approval of drugs specific to pregnancy, such as a tocolytic agents, oxytocic agents, and a drug to treat preeclampsia, studies must be done during pregnancy. However, drugs commonly used by women of childbearing potential, such as antidepressants, asthma medications, antihypertensive agents, and antihistamines also can be justifiably studied during pregnancy. Drugs can be studied not only when given for maternal indications (e.g., hypertension or asthma) but when prescribed for fetal indications (e.g., fetal supraventricular tachycardia).

Some subpopulations of pregnant women, however, often have altered physiology that may affect pharmacokinetics. Therefore, to separate the effects of the specific pathophysiology of the subpopulation on the pharmacokinetics of the drug from those resulting from pregnancy-related changes in general, studies in these women should be designed so that maximal information is obtained. As a first step, population pharmacokinetic techniques can serve as a screening tool to establish the need for further intensive pharmacokinetic studies. For drugs that are chronically administered, these intensive studies should be conducted serially during the second and third trimester of pregnancy and in the postpartum period, so that each woman serves as her own control. Ideally, both an early and a remote postpartum evaluation should be included. However, drugs used only during the peripartum period need only be studied at that time. Studies should incorporate *in vitro* measurements of drug binding to plasma proteins, and use established tracer substances or concurrent non-invasive measures of physiology as reference markers. For bioavailability analysis, the stable isotope method described in Chapter 4 would decrease the number of studies necessary and decrease the biologic variation between studies.

PLACENTAL TRANSFER OF DRUGS

The placenta was long thought to be a barrier to drugs and chemicals administered to the mother. However, the thalidomide tragedy, reported independently by McBride (51) and Lenz (52), showed that the placenta was capable of transferring drugs ingested by the mother to the fetus with the potential for great harm. On the other hand, placental transfer of drugs administered to the mother has been used to treat fetal arrhythmias, congestive heart failure, and other conditions (53).

The placenta develops from a portion of the zygote and thus has the same genetic endowment as the developing fetus (54). The embryonic/fetal component consists of trophoblastic derived chorionic villi that invade the maternal endometrium and are exposed directly to maternal blood in lake-like structures called lacunae. These villi create the large surface area necessary for maternal–fetal transfer in what becomes the intervillous space of the placenta. Here the maternal blood pressure supplies pulsatile blood flow in jet-like streams from the spiral arteries of the endometrium to bathe the chorionic villi and allow for transfer of gases, nutrients, and metabolic products. Biologically, the human placenta is classified as a hemochorial placenta because maternal blood is in direct contact with the fetal chorionic membrane. This membrane determines what is transferred to the fetus.

For the most part, drugs and other substances given to the mother will be transferred to the fetus. Drugs cross the placenta largely by simple diffusion. Factors affecting drug transfer are similar to those affecting transfer across other biological membranes and include the molecular weight, lipid solubility, and degree of ionization of the compound. Generally, drugs and chemicals with a molecular weight of less than 600 traverse the placenta readily, while drugs with a molecular weight larger than 1000 transfer less readily, if at all. Compounds that are uncharged and more lipid soluble are also more readily transferred.

There are factors that affect transfer of drugs and chemicals that are unique to the placenta. The placenta has a pore system that allows for bulk water flow across the placenta and can be responsible for "dragging" small drugs and chemicals across the membrane. Within the placenta there is also a pinocytotic process that is capable of transferring large immunoglobulins to the fetus. Placental tissue has a full complement of cytochrome enzymes capable of metabolizing drugs and chemicals some of which may then transfer more readily to the fetus. The permeability and diffusion properties of the placenta may change as the placenta matures due to a decrease in thickness of the trophoblastic epithelium forming the chorionic membrane.

One of the factors affecting drug transfer to the fetus is the amount of drug delivered to the intervillous space by utero-placental blood flow. Blood flow to the uterus and placenta increases during pregnancy from 50 mL/min at 10 weeks' gestation to 500 to 600 mL/min at term (54). Maternal blood flow to the uterus is also influenced by posture, diseases affecting maternal vasculature, such as hypertension and diabetes, placental size, and uterine contractions. For example, maternal cardiac output and utero-placental blood flow are reduced in the supine position and placental perfusion virtually ceases during a contraction. "Small for gestational age" placentas or those with diffuse calcifications are less efficient at transferring any maternal compounds to the fetus. Diseases, such as diabetes, which can thicken the chorionic membrane, may also potentially affect diffusion of drugs into the fetal circulation.

TERATOGENESIS

During the 38 weeks that constitute human gestation the human conceptus develops from a one-cell zygote to the fully developed newborn infant. This complicated process has a high degree of wastage, with approximately 70% of conceptions lost prior to implantation, 20% lost from spontaneous abortion, and 15% born prematurely. Major congenital abnormalities that are recognized at birth occur in approximately 2 to 3 infants per hundred. Minor anomalies occur in another 7 to 14 infants per hundred. Major birth defects cause 20% of infant mortality and are responsible for the majority of childhood hospitalizations.

From the patient's perspective, a birth defect may be any abnormality of the infant found at birth. This may include birth injuries, such as a cephalohematoma or a brachial plexus injury. However, birth defects are usually considered structural defects of the newborn. Structural defects have been broken down into four major categories: a *malformation*, which is a structural defect caused by an intrinsic problem in embryologic differentiation and/or development; a *disruption*, which is an alteration in shape or structure of a normally differentiated part, such as a limb amputation from an amniotic band or a vascular event; a *deformation*, which is an alteration in the shape or structure of a normally differentiated part, such as a Potter's facies or metatarsus adductus that result from mechanical constraint; and a *dysplasia*, which is a primary defect in cellular organization into tissues (55). A *teratogen* is a chemical substance that can induce a mal-

TABLE 22.3   Human Reproductive Risk

Causes of anomalies	Percent of total anomalies
Chromosomal	5
Single gene	20
Polygenic/multifactorial	65
Environmental	10
Irradiation	<1
Maternal disease	1–2
Infection	2–3
Drugs and chemicals	4–5

TABLE 22.4   Known Human Teratogens

Agent	Teratogenic effect
Carbamazepine	Facial dysmorphogenesis, neural tube defect
Phenytoin	Facial dysmorphogenesis, mental retardation, growth retardation, distal digital hypoplasia
Valproate	Lumbosacral spina bifida, facial dysmorphogenesis
Trimethadione	Facial dysmorphogenesis, intrauterine growth retardation, intrauterine fetal demise, neonatal demise
Coumadin	Nasal hypoplasia, epiphyseal stippling, optic atrophy
Alcohol	Facial dysmorphogenesis, growth retardation, mental retardation
Diethylstilbesterol	Vaginal adenosis, uterine anomalies, vaginal carcinogenesis
Androgens	Masculinization of the female genitalia
Methyl mercury	Growth retardation, severe mental retardation
ACE inhibitors	Oligohydramnios, potential lung hypoplasia, postnatal renal failure
Folic acid antagonists (aminopterin, methotrexate)	Abortion, intrauterine growth retardation, microcephaly, hypoplasia of frontal bones
Thalidomide	Phocomelia
Isotretinoin	CNS anomalies, including optic nerve abnormalities; craniofacial anomalies; cardiovascular malformations, thymic abnormalies
Inorganic iodides	Fetal goiter
Tetracycline	Bone deposits, teeth discoloration
Lithium	Ebstein's anomaly

formation during development. An expansion of the definition includes an adverse effect on the developing fetus either in causing a structural abnormality or altering organ function. This should be distinguished from a *mutagen*, which causes a genetic mutation whose effects cannot be seen for at least a generation.

Underlying causes of birth defects are shown in Table 22.3. It should be appreciated that approximately 90% of birth defects have a genetic component. Birth defects caused by drugs represent the one group of anomalies that can potentially be prevented. However, it is a small list of drugs that have been proven to cause human anomalies (Table 22.4). Potential effects of drugs on the developing fetus include altered structural development during the first trimester producing a dysmorphic infant, altered fetal growth during the second and third trimester of pregnancy, and altered function of organ systems.

Principles of Teratology

The principles of teratology have been articulated by Wilson (56). The first principle is that teratogens act with specificity. A teratogen produces a specific abnormality or constellation of abnormalities. For example, thalidomide produces phocomelia, and valproic acid produces neural tube defects. This specificity also applies to species, because drug effects may be seen in one species and not another. The best example is cortisol, which produces cleft palate in mice, but not in humans.

The next principle is that teratogens demonstrate a dose-effect relationship. Given to the mother at a specific time during gestation, low doses can produce no effect, intermediate doses can produce the characteristic pattern of malformation, and higher doses will be lethal to the embryo. Dose effect-curves for most teratogens are steep, changing from minimal to maximal effect by dose doubling. Increasing the dose beyond that found to be lethal to the embryo will eventually

lead to maternal death. This is used as an endpoint in animal teratogenicity studies.

The third principle is that teratogens must reach the developing conceptus in sufficient amounts to cause their effects. The extent of fetal exposure to drugs and other xenobiotics is determined not only by maternal dose, route of elimination, and placental transfer but by fetal elimination mechanisms. Because the fetal liver is interposed between the umbilical vein and systemic circulation, drugs transferred across the placenta are subject to fetal first-pass metabolism (53). This protective mechanism is compromised by ductus venosus shunting that enables 30 to 70% of umbilical venous blood flow to bypass the liver. After drugs reach the fetal systemic circulation, hepatic metabolism constitutes the primary elimination mechanism and renal excretion is relatively ineffective because the fetal kidney is immature and fetal urine passing into the amniotic fluid is swallowed by the fetus. CYP3A7 is a fetal-specific enzyme that accounts for about one-third of fetal hepatic cytochrome P450. CYP1A1, 2C8, 2D6, and 3A3/4 have also been identified in fetal liver. These enzymes are not only protective, but their presence in fetal tissues other than liver is capable of converting drugs into chemically reactive teratogenic intermediates such as phenytoin epoxide (see Scheme 11.11) (57).

The fourth principle is that the effect that a teratogenic agent has on a developing fetus depends on the stage during development when the fetus is exposed. From conception to implantation there is an all-or-nothing effect, in that the embryo, if exposed to a teratogen, either survives unharmed or dies. This concept developed from Brent's studies of the effects of radiation on the developing embryo and may or may not apply to fetal exposure to chemicals (58). After implantation, during the process of differentiation and embryogenesis, the embryo is very susceptible to teratogens. However, since teratogens are capable of affecting many organ systems, the pattern of anomalies produced depends on which organ systems are differentiating at the time of teratogenic exposure. A difference of one or two days can result in a slightly different pattern of anomalies. After organogenesis, a teratogen can affect the growth of the embryo by producing growth retardation, or changing the size or function of a specific organ. Of particular interest is the effect of psychoactive agents, such as cocaine, crack, or antidepressants, on the developing central nervous system during the second and third trimesters of pregnancy, which can potentially affect the function and behavior of the infant after delivery. Giving a teratogen after the fetus has developed normally has no effect on the development of organs already formed. For example, beginning lithium after cardiac development, or valproic acid after the closure of the neural tube will not produce either drug's characteristic anomalies.

The fifth principle is that susceptibility to teratogens is influenced by the genotype of the mother and fetus. Animal studies have shown that certain animal strains are more susceptible to the production of malformations when exposed to a teratogen than other animal strains. In humans, the fetus homozygous for the recessive allele decreasing epoxide hydrolase activity has an increased risk of developing the full fetal hydantoin syndrome (57). Maternal smoking coupled with a fetus carrying the atypical allele for transforming growth factor increase the risk for the development of cleft lip and palate (59). Single mutant genes or polygenic inheritance may explain why certain fetuses are unusually susceptible to teratogens.

Mechanisms of teratogenesis include genetic interference, gene mutation, chromosomal breakage, interference with cellular function, enzyme inhibition, and altered membrane characteristics. The response of the developing embryo to these insults is failure of cell-cell interaction crucial for development, interference with cell migration, or mechanical cellular disruption. The common endpoint is cell death: teratogenesis causing fewer cells. Most mechanisms of teratogenesis are theoretical, not well understood, and imply a genetic component. One exception is the mechanism of thalidomide teratogenesis. In susceptible species, thalidomide causes oxidative DNA damage. Pretreatment with PBN, a free-radical trapping agent, reduces the occurrence of thalidomide embryopathy, suggesting that the mechanism is free radical-mediated oxidative DNA damage (60).

Measures to Minimize Teratogenic Risk

All new drug applications filed with the Federal Drug Administration include data from developmental and reproductive toxicology (DART) studies. These studies examine the effects of the particular agent on all aspects of reproduction, including oogenesis, spermatogenesis, fertility, and fecundity, as well as effects on litter size, spontaneous resorption, fetal malformation, fetal size, and newborn pup function. Most studies are conducted in mice, rats, and rabbits. All studies are designed with dose escalations and with maternal death as the endpoint. Information from these teratologic experiments with the drug is included in the drug labeling. Most human teratogenic reactions of new drugs have been predicted from animal studies. However, animal data is not always applicable to humans, since most animals have a shorter gestational clock than humans. Species vary in their susceptibility to teratogens, with some animal models being either more or less susceptible to teratogenesis than humans. If an agent does not produce an anomaly in animal studies, it does not prove that the agent is innocuous in humans.

Safety of a drug for use in human pregnancy is demonstrated by observational studies after the drug is marketed. Proof of teratogenicity in humans is supported by the following: a recognizable pattern of anomalies; a higher prevalence of the particular anomaly or anomalies in patients exposed to an agent than in a control population; presence of the agent during the stage of organogenesis of the organ system affected; increased incidence of the anomaly after introduction of the agent; and production of the anomaly in experimental animals by administration of the agent during the appropriate stage of organogenesis. Epidemiologic clues to teratogenesis are often found in case reports of abnormal infants, but these are biased in that an abnormal infant is more likely reported than a normal infant, and the background rate of malformations is high. Better studies are conducted prospectively with an exposed and unexposed control population found before pregnancy outcome is known. Although population-based large cohort studies begun prior to pregnancy are considered the best type, they are expensive to conduct and limited to those agents used at the time of the study.

A general approach to reduce the risk of human teratogenesis includes planning for pregnancy. Prior to conception, women with medical problems should be counseled about medications they chronically use, which ones can safely be continued throughout pregnancy, and which ones should be discontinued. Medications should be evaluated and changed if necessary to decrease teratogenic risk. Plasma level monitoring of unbound concentrations of antiepileptic drugs may be helpful in optimizing seizure control, decreasing the need for multiple drug therapy, and minimizing dosage and fetal risk. Since more than 50% of pregnancies in the United States are unplanned, all women should be treated as potential antenatal patients and counseled regarding use of any new drug in a potential pregnancy. Therefore, when a woman of childbearing potential develops a new medical problem, counseling for pregnancy should be included in management. In general, the use of agents widely used during pregnancy is preferred to newer agents. Just stopping pharmacologic therapy or leaving the issue up to the woman does not help her and may place both the mother and fetus at risk for adverse pregnancy outcome.

When using a known human teratogen, particular attention should be given to prevention of pregnancy. This includes counseling the patient on the fetal effects of the drug being used and on the use of one or more effective forms of contraception. Therapy should be begun with a normal menstrual period or no more than 2 weeks from a negative pregnancy test. When renewing prescriptions for these drugs, it is necessary to verify again that the patient is not pregnant.

DRUG THERAPY OF NURSING MOTHERS

Transfer of drugs into breast milk is bidirectional, reflecting passive diffusion of unbound drug between plasma and blood rather than active secretion. Factors that affect the milk concentration include binding to maternal plasma proteins, protein binding in milk, lipid content of milk, and physiochemical factors of

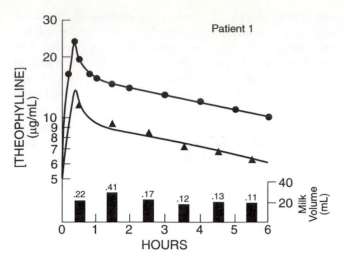

FIGURE 22.7 Kinetic analysis of theophylline plasma (●) and milk (▲) concentrations after intravenous administration of a 3.2 to 5.3 mg/kg aminophylline dose. The solid lines represent the least-squares fit of the measured concentrations. The interval and volume of each milk collection are shown by the solid bars. The milligram recovery of theophylline in each breast-milk collection is shown by the numbers above the bars. (Reproduced with permission from Stec GP, et al. Clin Pharmacol Ther 1980;28:404–8.)

the drug (61). As shown in Figure 22.7, drug concentrations in breast milk are usually less than plasma concentrations and there usually is a fixed ratio between milk and plasma concentrations (62). Concentration-dependent saturation of plasma protein binding precludes calculation of a fixed milk:plasma ratio for a few drugs (Figure 22.8) (63). However, in the usual case, drug concentrations measured in plasma and breast milk are used to calculate a milk:plasma ratio *(M/P)*, from which the daily drug dose to the infant is estimated as follows:

$$\text{Infant Dose/Day} = C_{maternal} \times M/P \times V_{milk} \qquad (22.2)$$

where $C_{maternal}$ is the average maternal plasma concentration of drug during nursing and V_{milk} is the volume of maternal milk ingested each day, usually estimated as 150 mL/kg (61). This estimate of infant dose is often reported as a percentage of administered maternal dose.

Infant blood levels also can be monitored and are usually less than those required for pharmacologic effects. Table 22.5 summarizes representative data for some of the antidepressant drugs that have been used to treat postpartum depression. Based on information similar to that in this table, amitryptyline, nortryptyline and sertraline have been among the antidepressant drugs of choice during breast-feeding (64). Regardless of drug choice, an important clinical point that is a consequence of the bidirectional transfer of

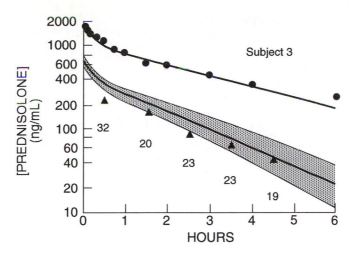

FIGURE 22.8 Kinetic analysis of prednisolone plasma (●) concentrations after intravenous administration of a 50-mg prednisolone dose. The solid lines represent the least-squares fit of the measured plasma concentrations. Measured milk concentrations (▲) are plotted along with the range *(shaded area)* of unbound prednisolone plasma concentrations expected if serum transcortin binding capacity is allowed to vary ± 1 SD from its reported mean. The volume (in milliliters) of each breast milk sample is shown by the numbers below the milk concentrations. (Reproduced with permission from Greenberger PA, et al. Clin Pharmacol Ther 1993;53:324–8.)

TABLE 22.5   Antidepressant Drugs and Breast-Feeding

Drug and (metabolite)	Protein binding (%)	M/P[a]	Infant dose[b] (%)	Detectable in infant plasma	Reported infant toxicity	Ref.
NE reuptake inhibitors[a]						
Amitryptyline	95	0.5–1.6	1.0	No	No	65, 66
(Nortriptyline)	92	0.7–1.1		No[c]		
(E-10-OH-nortriptyline)		0.7		Yes[c]		
Doxepin	15–32	1.1–1.7	2.2	Yes	Respiratory depression	67, 68
(N-desmethyldoxepin)		1.0–1.5		Yes		
Serotonin reuptake inhibitors						
Fluoxetine	>95	0.5–1.5	11	Yes	Colic	69, 70
(Norfluoxetine)	>95	0.6–1.2		Yes		
Sertraline	99	1.9	0.5	Yes	No	71
(N-desmethylsertraline)		1.6		Yes		
Combined reuptake inhibitors						
Venlafaxine	27	4.1	8	No	No	72
(O-desmethylvenlafaxine)	3	3.1		Yes		
Atypical antidepressants						
Bupropion	84	5.8	<1	No	No	73
(Hydroxybupropion)		0.1		No		
(Theohydrobupropion)		1.5		No		
Trazodone	93	0.1	<1	Not measured	No	74

[a] Abbreviations: *M/P* = ratio of concentrations in maternal milk and plasma, NE = norepinephrine.
[b] Expressed as percent of maternal dose for combined parent drug and measured metabolites.
[c] Both nortriptyline and 10-hydroxynortriptyline concentrations have been measured in the serum of nursing infants whose mothers were treated with nortriptyline (75).

drug between plasma and breast milk is that infant dosage can be minimized by breast-feeding just prior to drug administration when maternal serum concentration is lowest (62).

Drugs considered safe for pregnancy are usually safe during the lactation period. Drugs contraindicated during lactation include antineoplastics, immune suppressants, ergot alkaloids, gold, iodine, lithium carbonate, radiopharmaceuticals, social drugs of abuse, and certain antibiotics.

References

1. Zinacef (cefuroxime) labeling, in Physicians' Desk Reference, 54th ed. Montvale, NJ: Medical Economics; 2000. p. 1316.
2. Births: Preliminary data for 1999. National Vital Statistics Reports. vol 48, number 14. Atlanta, GA: Centers for Disease Control; 2000.
3. Hunt JN, Murray FA. Gastric function in pregnancy. J Obstet Gynaecol Br Emp 1958;65:78–83.
4. Parry E, Shields R, Turnbull AC. Transit time in the small intestine in pregnancy. J Obstet Gynaecol Br Commonw 1970;77:900–1.
5. Gryboski WA, Spiro HM. The effect of pregnancy on gastric secretion. N Engl J Med 1976;255:1131–7.
6. Lund CV, Donovan JC. Blood volume during pregnancy: Significance of plasma and red cell volumes. Am J Obstet Gynecol 1967;98:394–403.
7. Hytten F. Blood volume changes in normal pregnancy. Clin Haematol 1985;14:601–12.
8. Petersen VP. Body composition and fluid compartments in normal, obese and underweight human subjects. Acta Med Scand 1957;108:103–11.
9. Plentl AA, Gray MJ. Total body water, sodium space and total exchangeable sodium in normal and toxemic pregnant women. Am J Obstet Gynecol 1959;78:472–8.
10. Mendenhall HW. Serum protein concentrations in pregnancy: I. Concentrations in maternal serum. Am J Obstet Gynecol 1970;106:388–99.
11. Frederiksen MC, Ruo TI, Chow MJ, Atkinson AJ Jr. Theophylline pharmacokinetics in pregnancy. Clin Pharmacol Ther 1986;40:321–8.
12. Wood M, Wood AJJ. Changes in plasma drug binding and α_1-acid glycoprotein in mother and newborn infant. Clin Pharmacol Ther 1981;29:522–6.
13. Lucius H, Gahlenbeck H, Kleine HO, Fabel H, Bartels H. Respiratory functions, buffer system and electrolyte concentrations of blood during human pregnancy. Respir Physiol 1970;9:311–7.
14. Lyons HA, Antonio R. The sensitivity of the respiratory center in pregnancy and after the administration of progesterone. Trans Assoc Am Physicians 1959;72:173–80.
15. Lees MM, Taylor SH, Scott DM, Kerr MR. A study of cardiac output at rest throughout pregnancy. J Obstet Gynaecol Br Commonw 1967;74:319–28.
16. Robson SC, Hunter S, Boys RJ, Dunlop W. Serial study of factors influencing changes in cardiac output during human pregnancy. Am J Physiol 1989; 256:H1060–5.
17. Metcalfe J, Romney SL, Ramsey LH, Burwell CS. Estimation of uterine blood flow in women at term. J Clin Invest 1955;34:1632–8.
18. Ginsburg J, Duncan SL. Peripheral blood flow in normal pregnancy. Cardiovasc Res 1967;1:132–7.
19. Thoresen M, Wesch J. Doppler measurements of changes in human mammary and uterine blood flow during pregnancy and lactation. Acta Obstet Gynecol Scand 1988;67:741–5.
20. Robson SC, Mutch E, Boy RJ, Woodhouse KH. Apparent liver blood flow during pregnancy: A serial study using indocyanine green clearance. Brit J Obstet Gynaecol 1990;97:720–4.
21. Davison JM, Hytten FE. Glomerular filtration during and after pregnancy. J Obstet Gynaecol Br Commonw 1974; 81: 588–95.
22. Davison JM, Hytten FE. The effect of pregnancy on the renal handling of glucose. J Obstet Gynaecol Br Commonw 1975;82:374–81.
23. Gerdin E, Rane A. N-demethylation of ethylmorphine in pregnant and non-pregnant women and in men: an evaluation of the effects of sex steroids. Br J Clin Pharmacol 1992;34:250–5.
24. Bologa M, Tang B, Klein J, Tesoro A, Koren G. Pregnancy-induced changes in drug metabolism in epileptic women. J Pharmacol Exp Ther 1991;257:735–40.
25. Wadelius M, Darj E, Freene G, Rane A. Induction of CYP2D6 in pregnancy. Clin Pharmacol Ther 1997;62:400–7.
26. Lees MM, Scott DH, Kerr MG. Haemodynamic changes associated with labour. J Obstet Gynaecol Br Commonw 1970;77:29–36.
27. Ueland K, Metcalfe J. Circulatory changes in pregnancy. Clin Obstet Gynecol 1975;18:41–50.
28. Sims EAH, Krantz KE. Serial studies of renal function during pregnancy and the puerperium in normal women. J Clin Invest 1958;37:1764–74.
29. Dam M, Christiansen J, Munck O, Mygind KI. Antiepileptic drugs: Metabolism in pregnancy. Clin Pharmacokinet 1979;4:53–62.
30. Capeless EL, Clapp JF. When do cardiovascular parameters return to their preconception values? Am J Obstet Gynecol 1991;165:883–6.
31. Philipson A. Pharmacokinetics of ampicillin during pregnancy. J Infect Dis 1977;136:370–6.
32. Kubacka RT, Johnstone HE, Tan HSI, Reeme PD, Myre SA. Intravenous ampicillin pharmacokinetics in the third trimester of pregnancy. Ther Drug Monit 1983;5:55–60.
33. Aldridge A, Bailey J, Neims AH. The disposition of caffeine during and after pregnancy. Semin Perinatol 1981;5:310–4.
34. Connelly RJ, Ruo TI, Frederiksen MC, Atkinson AJ Jr. Characterization of theophylline binding to serum proteins in nonpregnant and pregnant women. Clin Pharmacol Ther 1990;47:68–72.
35. Philipson A, Stiernstedt G. Pharmacokinetics of cefuroxime in pregnancy. Am J Obstet Gynecol 1982;142:823–8.
36. Pond SM, Kreek MJ, Tong TG, Raghunath J, Benowitz NL. Altered methadone pharmacokinetics in methadone-maintained pregnant women. J Pharmacol Exp Ther 1985;233:1–6.
37. Tomson T, Lindbom U, Ekqvist B, Sundqvist A. Epilepsy in pregnancy: A prospective study of seizure control in relation to free and total plasma concentrations of cabamazepine and phenytoin. Epilepsia 1994:35:122–30.
38. Tomson T, Lindbom U, Ekqvist B, Sundqvist A. Disposition of cabamazepine and phenytoin in pregnancy. Epilepsia 1994:35:131–5.
39. Chen SS, Perucca E. Lee JN, Richens A. Serum protein binding and free concentration of phenytoin and phenobarbitone in pregnancy. Br J Clin Pharmacol 1982;13:547–52.
40. Yerby MS, Friel PN, Miller DQ. Carbamazepine protein binding and disposition in pregnancy. Ther Drug Monit 1985;7:269–73.
41. Casele HL, Laifer SA, Woelders DA, Venkataramanan R. Changes in the pharmacokinetics of the low-molecular-weight heparin enoxaparin sodium during pregnancy. Am J Obstet Gynecol 1999;181:1113–7.
42. Bourget P, Fernandez H, Delouis C, Taburet AM. Pharmacokinetics of tobramycin in pregnant women, safety and efficacy of a once-daily dose regimen. J Clin Pharm Ther 1991;16:167–76.

43. Prevost RR, Aki SA, Whybrew WD, Sibai BM. Oral nifedipine pharmacokinetics in pregnancy-induced hypertension. Pharmacotherapy 1992;12:174–7.

44. Barton JR, Prevost RR, Wilson DA, Whybrew WD, Sibai BM. Nifedipine pharmacokinetics and pharmacodynamics during the immediate postpartum period in patients with preeclampsia. Am J Obstet Gynecol 1991;165:951–4.

45. Kimberlin DF, Weller S, Whitley RJ, Andrews WW, Hauth JC, Lakeman F, et al. Pharmacokinetics of oral valacyclovir and acyclovir in late pregnancy. Am J Obstet Gynecol 1998;179:846–51.

46. Gerdin E, Salmonson T, Lindberg B, Rane A. Maternal kinetics of morphine during labour. J Perinat Med 1990;18:479–87.

47. Steen B, Rane A. Clindamycin passage into human milk. Br J Clin Pharmacol 1982;13:661–4.

48. Del Priore G, Jackson-Stone M, Shim EK, Garfinkel J, Eichmann MA, Frederiksen MC. A comparison of once-daily and eight hour gentamicin dosing in the treatment of postpartum endometritis. Obstet Gynecol 1996;87:994–1000.

49. Nelson MM, Forfar JO. Association between drugs administered during pregnancy and congenital abnormalities of the fetus. Br Med J 1971;1:523–7.

50. Bonati M, Bortolus R, Marchetti F, Romero M, Tognoni G. Drug use in pregnancy: An overview of epidemiological (drug utilization) studies. Eur J Clin Pharmacol 1990;38:325–8.

51. McBride WG. Thalidomide and congenital abnormalities [letter]. Lancet 1961;ii:1358.

52. Lenz W. Kindliche missbildungen nach medikament während der gravidität. Deutsch Med Wschr1961;86:2555–6.

53. Morgan DJ. Drug disposition in mother and foetus. Clin Exp Pharmacol Physiol 1997;24:869–73.

54. Martin CB. The anatomy and circulation of the placenta. In: Barnes AC, editor. Intra-uterine development. Philadelphia: Lea & Febiger; 1968. p. 35–67.

55. Jones KL. Smith's recognizable patterns of human malformation. 5th ed. Philadelphia: WB Saunders; 1997. p. 1–3.

56. Wilson JG. Current status of teratology—General principles and mechanisms derived from animal studies. In: Wilson JG, Fraser FC, editors. Handbook of teratology. Vol. I. General principles and etiology. New York: Plenum Press; 1977. p. 47–74.

57. Buehler BA, Delimont D, van Waes M, Finnell RH. Prenatal prediction of risk of the fetal hydantoin syndrome. N Engl J Med 1990;31:322:1567–72.

58. Brent RL. Radiation teratogenesis. Teratology 1980; 21:281–98.

59. Shaw GM, Wasserman CR, Lammer EJ, O'Malley CD. Murray JC, Basart AM, et al. Orofacial clefts, parental cigarette smoking, and transforming growth factor-alpha gene variants. Am J Hum Genet 1996;58:551–61.

60. Parman T, Wiley MJ, Wells PG. Free radical-mediated oxidative DNA damage in the mechanism of thalidomide teratogenicity. Nat Med 1999;5:582–5.

61. Begg EJ, Atkinson HC, Duffull SB. Prospective evaluation of a model for the prediction of milk:plasma drug concentrations from physicochemical characteristics. Br J Clin Pharmacol 1992;33:501–5.

62. Stec GP, Greenberger P, Ruo TI, Henthorn T, Morita Y, Atkinson AJ Jr, Patterson R. Kinetics of theophylline transfer to breast milk. Clin Pharmacol Ther 1980; 28:404–8.

63. Greenberger PA, Odeh YK, Frederiksen MC, Atkinson AJ Jr. Pharmacokinetics of prednisolone transfer to breast milk. Clin Pharmacol Ther 1993;53:324–8.

64. Wisner KL, Perel JM, Finding RL. Antidepressant treatment during breast-feeding. Am J Psychiatry 1996;153:1132–7.

65. Brixen-Rasmussen L, Halgrener J, Jørgensen A. Amitriptyline and nortriptyline excretion in human breast milk. Psychopharmacology 1982;76:94–5.

66. Breyer-Pfaff U, Entenmann A, Gaertner HJ. Secretion of amitriptyline and metabolites into breast milk [letter]. Am J Psychiatry 1995;152:812–3.

67. Kemp J, Ilett KF, Booth J, Hackett LP. Excretion of doxepin and N-desmethyldoxepin in human milk. Br J Clin Pharmacol 1985;20:497–9.

68. Matheson I, Pande H, Alertsen AR. Respiratory depression caused by N-desmethyldoxipin in breast milk [letter]. Lancet 1985;2:1124.

69. Taddio A, Ito S, Koren G. Excretion of fluoxetine and its metabolite, norfluoxetine, in human breast milk. J Clin Pharmacol 1996;36:42–7.

70. Lester BM, Cucca J, Andreaozzi L, Flanagan P, Oh W. Possible association between fluoxetine hydrochloride and colic in an infant. J Am Acad Child Adolesc Psychiatry 1993,32:1253–5.

71. Kristensen JH, Ilett KF, Dusci LJ, Hackett LP, Yapp P, Wojnar-Horton RE, et al. Distribution and excretion of sertraline and N-desmethylsertraline in human milk. Br J Clin Pharmacol 1998;45:453–7.

72. Ilett KF, Hackett LP, Dusci LJ, Roberts MJ, Kristensen JH, Paech M, et al. Distribution and excretion of venlafaxine and O-desmethylvenlafaxine in human milk. Br J Clin Pharmacol 1998;45:459–62.

73. Briggs GG, Samson JH, Ambrose PJ, Schroeder DH. Excretion of bupropion in breast milk. Ann Pharmacother 1993,27:431–3.

74. Verbeeck RK, Ross SG, McKenna EA. Excretion of trazodone in breast milk. Br J Clin Pharmacol 1986;22:367–70.

75. Wisner KL, Perel JM. Serum nortriptyline levels in nursing mothers and their infants. Am J Psychiatry 1991;148:1234–6.

23

Drug Therapy in Neonates and Pediatric Patients

ELIZABETH FOX AND FRANK M. BALIS

Pharmacology and Experimental Therapeutics Section, Pediatric Oncology Branch, National Cancer Institute,
National Institutes of Health, Bethesda, Maryland

BACKGROUND

The use of drugs in newborns, infants, and children is often based on safety, efficacy, and pharmacological data generated in adults, but the practice of scaling adult drug doses to infants and children based on body weight or body surface area (BSA) does not account for the developmental changes that affect drug pharmacokinetics or target tissue and organ sensitivity to the drug. In fact, this dosing practice has resulted in therapeutic tragedies that illustrate the importance of understanding the effects of ontogeny on drug pharmacokinetics and drug effect and the need for separate clinical trials and pharmacological studies of drugs in pediatric patient populations.

Chloramphenicol Therapy of Newborns

The chloramphenicol-induced gray baby syndrome is an example of the potential dangers inherent in treating newborns based on dosing recommendations for adults. Chloramphenicol is detoxified in the liver primarily through conjugation with glucuronide. Because of its broad spectrum of activity, it was widely used to treat a variety of infections in the 1950s, including nursery infections in neonates. Hospital-acquired bacterial infections in the newborn nursery were often due to less sensitive bacterial strains, consequently premature and full-term infants were treated with adult doses scaled to body weight or doses exceeding those recommended in adults (1). In the late 1950s,

case reports of unexplained deaths in newborns who were receiving chloramphenicol appeared and led to a controlled clinical trial of chloramphenicol therapy in premature newborns who were at high risk of infection because they were born more than 24 hours after spontaneous rupture of membranes. The standard of care for these newborns was empirical treatment with antibiotics but newborns studied in this trial were assigned to one of four groups: 1) no antibiotics, 2) procaine penicillin and streptomycin, 3) chloramphenicol, and 4) all three antibiotics (Table 23.1). Mortality was substantially higher in the newborns receiving chloramphenicol and nearly two-thirds of the newborns receiving chloramphenicol died, compared to the < 20% mortality rate in newborns who did not receive chloramphenicol. In infants weighing more than 2000 gm at birth, 45% receiving chloramphenicol died compared with 2.5% in the nonchloramphenicol-treated groups. This high mortality rate was ascribed to chloramphenicol toxicity (2).

The *gray baby syndrome* refers to a characteristic constellation of physical signs, consisting of vomiting, refusal to feed, respiratory distress (irregular rapid respiration), abdominal distention, periods of cyanosis, passage of loose, green stools, flaccidity, ashen color, hypothermia, vascular collapse, and death (usually by the fifth day of life) that was recognized in the chloramphenicol-treated patients. Fifty-eight percent of the infants who received chloramphenicol and survived had similar signs which completely resolved 24 to 36 hours after discontinuing the drug.

TABLE 23.1 Mortality in Premature Neonates at Increased Risk of Bacterial Infection Who Were Randomized to One of Four Empiric Antibiotic Treatment Groups[a]

	All premature newborns		Good prognosis premature newborns (2001–2500 gm)	
	Number	Deaths	Number	Deaths
No empiric antibiotics	32	6	17	1
Penicillin + streptomycin[b]	33	6	24	0
Chloramphenicol[b]	30	19	16	8
Penicillin + streptomycin + chloramphenicol[b]	31	21	15	6

[a] Reproduced with permission from Burns LE, et al. N Engl J Med 1959;261:1318–21.

[b] Intramuscular doses of antibiotics: procaine penicillin—150,000–600,000 units/day, streptomycin—50 mg/kg/day, chloramphenicol—100–165 mg/kg/day.

Studies of chloramphenicol pharmacokinetics were subsequently performed in newborns and children. High concentrations of chloramphenicol and its metabolites accumulated in newborns who developed toxicity (Figure 23.1A), and presumably accounted for the severe toxicity. This accumulation of drug on a dosing regimen that is tolerable in adults resulted from the reduced capacity of newborns to metabolize chloramphenicol by glucuronide conjugation. When studied at lower doses in a group of children over a wider age range, the rate of chloramphenicol metabo-

lism was found to be highly age dependent. The half-life was 26 hours in the newborns, 10 hours in the infants, and 4 hours in the children (Figure 23.1B) (3).

As demonstrated by chloramphenicol, the pharmacological impact of developmental changes that affect drug disposition are often discovered only after unexpected or severe toxicity in infants and children leads to detailed pharmacological studies. Such therapeutic tragedies could be avoided by performing pediatric pharmacological studies during the drug development process, as exemplified by the clinical development of zidovudine for use in newborns, infants, and children.

Zidovudine Therapy of Newborns, Infants, and Children

Zidovudine is a synthetic nucleoside analog that blocks replication of the human immunodeficiency virus (HIV) by inhibiting reverse transcriptase. The primary indication for zidovudine administration in newborns is the prevention of vertical transmission of HIV. Like chloramphenicol, zidovudine is eliminated in adults primarily by glucuronide conjugation, suggesting that newborns may have a reduced capacity to eliminate zidovudine. However, unlike chloramphenicol, prior to widespread administration of zidovudine to newborns and infants born to HIV-infected mothers, the pharmacology and safety of the drug were carefully studied in this population and age-specific dosing guidelines were developed.

The pharmacokinetic parameters for zidovudine in various age groups are presented in Table 23.2 (4–7).

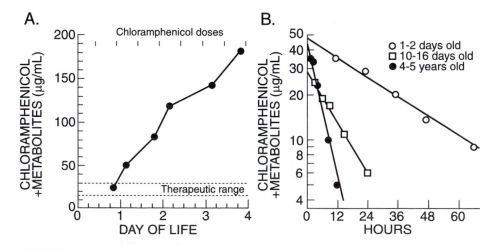

FIGURE 23.1 **(A)** Plasma concentration of chloramphenicol and its metabolites in a newborn who received intravenous chloramphenicol every 12 hours at doses equivalent to those recommended for adults. (Reproduced with permission from Burns LE, et al. N Engl J Med 1959;261:1318–21.) **(B)** The concentration vs. time profile for chloramphenicol in newborns and children demonstrating the age-dependent elimination of chloramphenicol and its metabolites. (Reproduced with permission from Weiss CF, et al. N Engl J Med 1960;262:787–94.)

TABLE 23.2 Zidovudine Pharmacokinetic Parameters for Various Age Groups[a]

Population	Age	CL_E (mL/min/kg)	$T_{1/2}$ (hr)	F (%)
Preterm infants	5.5 days	2.5	7.2	
	17.7 days	4.4	4.4	
Term infants	≤ 14 days	10.9	3.1	89
	≥ 14 days	19.0	1.9	61
Children	1–13 years	24	1.5	68
Adults		21	1.1	63

[a] Data from Klecker RW Jr, et al. Clin Pharmacol Ther 1987;41:407–12; Balis F et al. J Pediatr 1989;114:880–4; Mirochnick M, et al. Antimicrob Agents Chemother 1998;42:808–12; and Boucher FD, et al. J Pediatr 1993;122:137–44.

Newborns cleared zidovudine more slowly than children and adults, and the clearance in preterm newborns is slower than in the full-term infants. Zidovudine clearance rapidly increases over the first few weeks of life, consistent with the up-regulation of glucuronidation pathways in newborns after birth, and by 2 weeks of age approaches values in older children and adults. In addition, the extent of zidovudine absorption *(F)* in newborns ≤ 14 days of age is higher than in older children, presumably because of reduced first-pass metabolism. Based on these studies, a safe and potentially effective dose of zidovudine was defined for term and preterm newborns (6–8).

The pharmacology and safety of zidovudine were also studied in the prenatal and perinatal setting in pregnant women. Based on these studies, a placebo-controlled, double-blind, randomized trial of zidovudine was conducted in HIV-infected pregnant women to determine if zidovudine could block maternal–fetal transmission of HIV. Mothers received 100 mg of zidovudine orally, five times daily; then at the onset of labor and through delivery a continuous intravenous infusion of zidovudine (1 mg/kg/hr). Beginning 8 to 12 hours after birth, full-term newborns were treated with 2 mg/kg of zidovudine orally every 6 hours for 6 weeks. The HIV transmission rate from mother to child was significantly reduced by administering zidovudine before, during, and after delivery. Equally important, newborn infants experienced no substantial adverse events from this regimen (9).

Development of Federal Regulations

Many Food and Drug Administration (FDA) regulations that impact on pediatric drug development and dosing are the result of therapeutic tragedies that occurred in children. The 1938 Food Drug and Cosmetic Act (FDCA), which is described in Chapter 34, was legislated in part due to the deaths of 107 children from sulfanilamide elixir, which contained diethylene glycol as the vehicle. In 1962, the Harris-Kefauver Amendment to the FDCA mandated that drugs had to be safe and effective in the population for which they were marketed. This amendment states that safety and efficacy in one population cannot be assumed for another—specifically, results from studies done in adults cannot be applied to infants or children. The impetus for this amendment was the recognition of fetal malformations from maternal ingestion of thalidomide.

FDA regulations enacted in 1979 were intended to increase the number of drugs available to infants and children through voluntary measures. However, over the next two decades, only 25% of newly marketed drugs had sufficient clinical safety and efficacy data in infants and children (10). In 1994, the FDA requested drug companies to survey existing data that could support labeling for pediatric use of marketed drugs. Only 430 supplements were submitted in response to the 1994 rule, and a majority of the supplements simply added the disclaimer "Safety and effectiveness in pediatric patients have not been established." Only 65 supplements provided enough data to justify new pediatric labeling for all pediatric age groups.

With these voluntary measures, the proportion of new drugs with adequate pediatric labeling has not increased since 1991. Overall, 40% of new drugs were not felt to be of potential use in childhood diseases, but less than half of the remaining 60% had pediatric studies performed or pediatric labeling at the time of approval (10). Failed efforts to gain voluntary compliance have lead to new legislative measures that empower the FDA to require pediatric studies for selected marketed drugs and new drugs that are likely to be used in a substantial number of pediatric patients, or could be an improvement over current treatment of childhood diseases. These new regulations also provide incentives (extension of marketing exclusivity) to drug companies for performing clinical trials in the pediatric population.

The consequences of inadequate pediatric dosing information include a greater risk of toxicity, as occurred with chloramphenicol; ineffective treatment due to underdosing; and an unwillingness of physicians to prescribe newer, potentially more efficacious drugs for children because pediatric dosing recommendations are not available. Appropriate pediatric labeling would help insure the availability of a pediatric formulation that is palatable and acceptable for the intended ages of children and would prevent denial of third-party reimbursement on the basis of a lack of labeling (11).

ONTOGENY AND PHARMACOLOGY

Because clinical investigation of new agents is not uniformly performed in newborns, infants, and children, we have a poor understanding of the effect of ontogeny on the pharmacokinetics and pharmacodynamics of most drugs. However, we can often anticipate age-related differences in pharmacokinetics and the intensity of drug effects based on our knowledge of the maturation process. During childhood, changes in body mass and composition and the maturation of excretory organs have a substantial effect on pharmacokinetics. As with chloramphenicol and zidovudine, the most dramatic changes occur during the first days to months of life. Predicting the effect of growth and development on pharmacodynamics is more difficult because there is less information regarding age-related changes in drug-receptor expression.

The FDA subdivides the pediatric population into five age groups: 1) Preterm newborn infants, 2) term newborn infants (0 to 27 days of age), 3) infants and toddlers (28 days to 23 months), 4) children (2 to 11 years of age), and 5) adolescents (12 to 16 or 18 years of age depending on region). The category of preterm infant is heterogeneous due to the impact of gestational age, unique neonatal diseases, and organ susceptibility to toxicity. Term infants undergo rapid physiologic changes in total body water and renal and hepatic function during the first few days of life. CNS maturation with completion of myelination occurs in the infant and toddler age group. Children experience accelerated skeletal growth, weight gain, psychomotor development, and the onset of puberty, and sexual maturation is achieved during the adolescent period (12). These five pediatric stages are arbitrary groupings and do not necessarily coincide with the periods of greatest physiologic change that affect the clinical pharmacology of drugs.

Drug Absorption

As discussed in Chapter 4, the bioavailability of orally administered drugs is influenced by gastric acid secretion, gastrointestinal motility, intestinal absorptive surface area, bacterial colonization of the gut, and the activity of drug metabolizing enzymes in the intestine and liver that are responsible for presystemic metabolism of drugs. Gastric pH is neutral at birth, but drops to pH 1–3 within hours of birth. Gastric acid secretion then declines on days 10–30, and does not approach adult values until approximately 3 months of age. The lower level of gastric acid secretion in newborns contributes to the increased bioavailability of acid labile drugs, like the penicillins, in newborns (13).

TABLE 23.3   Relative Gastrointestinal Absorption of Selected Drugs in Infants and Adults[a]

Increased in newborns	Infants = adults	Decreased in newborns
Penicillin	Theophylline	Phenytoin
Ampicillin	Sulphonamides	Acetaminophen
Erythromycin		Phenobarbital
Digoxin		
Zidovudine		

[a] Data from Loebstein R, Koren G. Pediatr Rev 1998:19:423–8.

Gastric emptying is delayed and irregular in the newborn, but approaches adult values by 6 to 8 months of age. Intestinal motility is also irregular, and highly dependent on feeding patterns in newborn. In newborns, decreased gastrointestinal motility can delay drug absorption and result in lower peak plasma drug concentrations, but does not alter the fraction of drug absorbed for most drugs. In children, gastrointestinal transit time may be increased (14).

The ratio of absorptive surface area to BSA is greater in infants and children than in adults. Although pancreatic enzyme excretion is low in newborns, malabsorption does not occur and no effect on drug absorption has been observed. The newborn intestine is colonized with bacteria within days of birth, but the spectrum of bacterial flora may change over the first few years of life. The patterns and extent of colonization depend on age, type of delivery, type of feeding, and concurrent drug therapy (15). Compared to adults, the capacity of intestinal bacterial flora to inactivate orally administered digoxin is decreased and digoxin bioavailability is thereby increased in infants less than 2 years old (16). The relative gastrointestinal drug absorption of selected drugs in infants and adults is presented in Table 23.3.

Drug Distribution

Factors that affect drug distribution include the physicochemical properties of the drug, cardiac output, regional blood flow, body composition (e.g., extracellular water and adipose tissue), and the degree of protein and tissue binding. Serum albumin, α_1-acid glycoprotein, and total protein concentrations are lower at birth and during early infancy, but approach adult levels by 1 year of age. Lower plasma protein levels result in lower levels of drug binding to plasma proteins (Table 23.4). Although the absolute differences in the fraction of drug bound may be only 10 to 20%, for highly protein bound drugs this could

TABLE 23.4 Plasma Protein Binding
of Selected Drugs in Cord Blood
and Adult Blood[a]

	Plasma protein binding (%)	
	Cord blood	Adult
Acetaminophen	36.8	47.5
Chloramphenicol	31	42
Morphine	46	66
Phenobarbital	32.4	50.7
Phenytoin	74.4	85.8
Promethazine	69.8	82.7

[a] Data from Kurz H, et al. Eur J Clin Pharmacol 1977;11:469–72.

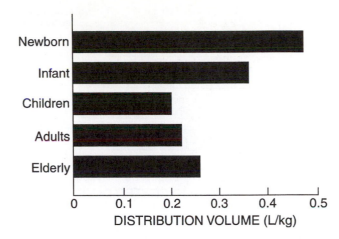

FIGURE 23.3 The distribution volume of sulfisoxazole in newborns, infants, children, and adults. (Data from Routledge P. J Antimicrob Chemother 1994;34(suppl A):19–24.)

make a substantial difference in the free drug concentration in plasma. For example, promethazine is nearly 70% protein bound in cord blood and 83% protein bound in adult blood. This translates into a nearly two-fold higher concentration of free promethazine in cord blood (17). Higher free drug concentrations can enhance drug delivery to tissues. The higher free fraction in newborns also influences the interpretation of plasma drug concentrations relative to the therapeutic range defined in adults, in whom a smaller fraction of the measured total drug concentration is unbound (18).

Body composition, especially water and fat content, are also highly age dependent (Figure 23.2) (19). Total

body water accounts for a larger fraction of body weight in newborns than in older children and adults. There is also a larger fraction of extracellular water at birth. As a result of this change and the decrease in binding to plasma proteins previously described, the apparent distribution volume of the water-soluble drug sulfisoxazole is greater in newborns and infants than in adults when normalized to body weight or surface area (Figure 23.3) (13). Because infants have a higher proportion of body fat than adults, lipid soluble drugs also have a larger distribution volume in them than in older individuals (20).

Drug Metabolism

The capacity of the liver to metabolize drugs is lower at birth, and the rate of development of the various metabolic pathways is highly variable and may be influenced by exposure to drugs *in utero* and postnatally. Generalizations about the rate of maturation of drug metabolizing enzymes systems during infancy and childhood are difficult because of the lack of data, the degree of variability, and the inducibility of some enzyme systems. Oxidative capacity is reduced at birth, but appears to develop over days as evidenced by the decline in the half-life of ibuprofen, which has a half-life greater than 30 hours in premature infants in the first day of life compared with less than 2 hours in children and adults (21). During childhood, oxidative capacity for drugs exceeds that in adults, especially when expressed per kilogram of body weight (13). In contrast, the activity of alcohol dehydrogenase does not approach adult levels until 5 years of age (22). The

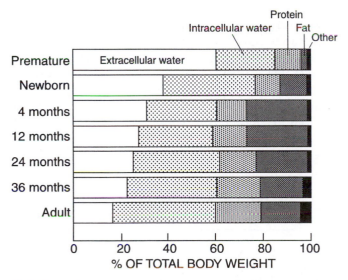

FIGURE 23.2 Age-related changes in body composition. (Reproduced with permission from Kaufman RE, Pediatric pharmacology. In Aranda JV, Yaffe SJ, editors. Pediatric pharmacology, therapeutic principles in practice. Philadelphia: WB Saunders; 1992 p. 212–9.)

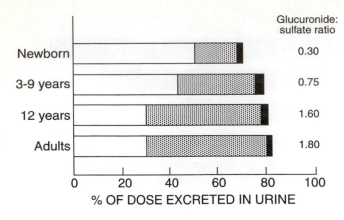

FIGURE 23.4 Percentage of the dose of acetaminophen excreted in the urine as unchanged drug *(solid bars)*, glucuronide conjugate *(stippled bars)*, or sulfate conjugate *(open bars)* in selected age groups. The ratio of glucuronide: sulfate excreted in the urine increases with age. (Reproduced with permission from Miller RP, et al. Clin Pharmacol Ther 1976;19:284–94.)

development of other Phase I reactions (e.g., hydrolysis, demethylation) has not been well characterized (15).

Because of variation in the rate of maturation of drug metabolizing enzymes, the primary metabolic pathway for some drugs may be different in newborns and infants than in adults. For example, the activity of glucuronide conjugation is low at birth and does not approach adult levels until 3 years of age, but sulfate conjugation is active *in utero* and at birth and declines in relative importance with age. Therefore, drugs that are eliminated in adults by glucuronide conjugation may be cleared primarily as sulfate conjugates in newborns and infants (15). This is demonstrated by age-related differences in acetaminophen metabolism. In adults, the glucuronide conjugate is the primary urinary metabolite of acetaminophen, whereas, in newborns, a higher proportion of the dose is excreted as the sulfate conjugate. In young children, both the sulfate conjugate and glucuronide are present in urine (Figure 23.4). Despite these quantitative differences in the metabolic pathways used to inactivate the drug, the overall elimination rate constant for the parent drug was not age dependent. Therefore, in the case of acetaminophen metabolism, sulfate conjugation compensated for the developmental deficiency in glucuronidation (23).

The cytochrome P450 hepatic drug metabolizing enzymes catalyze the biotransformation of a wide variety of compounds. These enzymes are regulated by genetic, environmental, and hormonal factors, and recent evidence suggests that there may also be a developmental component to the regulation of their expression and level of activity (24). For example, CYP3A, which is the primary drug metabolizing cytochrome

P450 subfamily in adults, undergoes functional maturation over the first month of life in full-term newborns (25, 26). CYP3A7 is the major fetal hepatic cytochrome P450 enzyme and can be detected early in fetal development. However, in adults, CYP3A4 and to a lesser extent CYP3A5 are responsible for a majority of the drug metabolism by the cytochrome P450 system (26). CYP1A1 and CYP2E1 are also present early in fetal development and metabolize exogenous toxins and alcohol, respectively. Hepatic CYP2D6, CYP2C8/9, and CYP2C18/19 become active at birth, and CYP1A2 becomes active at 4 to 5 months of age. A detailed description of the cytochrome P450 system and pharmacogenetics can be found in Chapters 11 and 13.

Renal Excretion

Renal function is limited at birth because the kidneys are anatomically and functionally immature. In full-term newborns, glomerular filtration rate (GFR) is 10–15 mL/min/m² and in premature infants the GFR is only 5–10 mL/min/m². GFR doubles by 1 week of age because of a postnatal drop in renal vascular resistance and increase in renal blood flow. GFR reaches adult values by 1 year of age (Figure 23.5) (27, 28). A glomerular/tubular imbalance is present in newborns because glomerular function matures more rapidly than renal tubular secretion. Although renal tubular secretory function is impaired at birth, it also approaches adult values by 1 year of age.

Renal clearance of drugs is delayed in newborns and young infants, necessitating dose reductions (Figure 23.6), but after 8 to 12 months of age, renal excretion of drugs is comparable with that of older children and may even exceed that of adults. In young children, the ratio of renal size relative to BSA is larger than in adults and drug clearance normalized to BSA can exceed that in adults. Because renal clearance is more efficient in children, the dose of aminoglycosides required to achieve effective antibiotic plasma concentrations in children is usually 1.5- to 2-fold higher than in adults. The dosing interval in children also may need to be shorter than in adults (29).

THERAPEUTIC IMPLICATIONS OF GROWTH AND DEVELOPMENT

Drug effect is related to the free drug concentration at the target site and the presence and density of drug receptors at the target site. The free drug concentration at the target site is determined by the dose and pharmacokinetics of the drug. Developmental changes in body composition, level of protein binding, and excre-

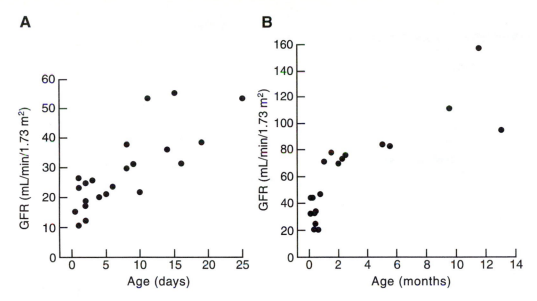

FIGURE 23.5 Glomerular filtration rate (GFR) in newborns **(A)** and through the first year of life **(B)**. When normalized for body surface area, GFR reaches adult values by 1 year of age. (Data from Aperia A, et al. Acta Paediatr Scand 1975;64:393–8; and Guignard J, et al. J Pediatr 1975;87:268–72.)

tory organ function have a significant impact on plasma drug concentration and, therefore, the amount of drug that reaches the target site. These developmental changes must be taken into account when devising a dose and dosing schedule for infants and children of different ages. The rapid changes that occur postnatally may require frequent dose adjustments during the first few days to weeks of life. Antibiotic doses, for example, are frequently increased after the first 7 days of life, to account for the initial rapid increase in renal function. Drug receptor expression over the course of normal growth and development has not been well studied, but could also modulate a drug's effect during infancy and childhood.

Effect on Pharmacokinetics

Developmental changes in liver and kidney excretory function during infancy and childhood may necessitate dose adjustments to achieve a therapeutic drug concentration. For example, theophylline dose recommendations are age specific during childhood to compensate for changes in drug clearance. The overall clearance of theophylline (renal excretion + hepatic metabolism) is markedly slowed in newborns (20 mL/min/kg in preterm newborns), and the recommended dose in this population is 4 mg/kg/day. However, theophylline clearance in children (100 mL/min/kg) is 40% higher than adults (70 mL/min/kg), and children will require higher bodyweight normalized doses than adults (30–33). The effect of age-dependent clearance rate of theophylline on the dose required to maintain a therapeutic drug level is shown in Figure 23.7. In this study, more than 3500 serum theophylline concentrations were measured in 1073 patients who ranged in age from 1 to 73 years (median, 9 years) (33). The dose of sustained release theophylline was adjusted to achieve a serum

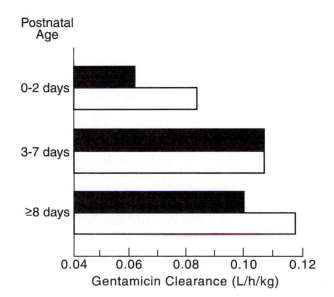

FIGURE 23.6 Plasma clearance of gentamicin in premature (< 37 week gestation, *solid bars*) and full term *(open bars)* newborns at various postnatal ages. (Data from Pons G, et al. Ther Drug Monit 1988;10:42–7.)

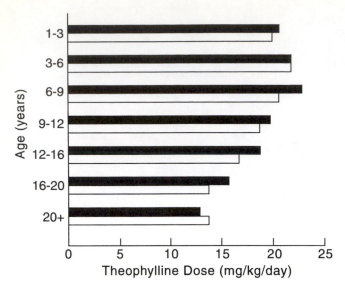

FIGURE 23.7 Effect of age-related clearance of theophylline on the dose of sustained-release theophylline required to maintain a therapeutic drug level (range: 10–20 μg/mL) in males *(solid bars)* and females *(open bars)* across a broad age range. (Reproduced with permission from Milavetz G, et al. J Pediatr 1986109:351–4.)

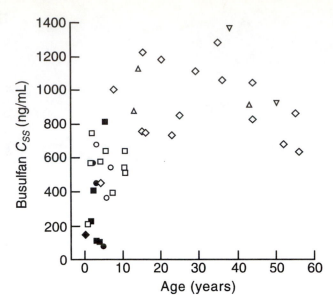

FIGURE 23.8 Plasma busulfan steady state concentrations *(C$_{ss}$)* as a function of age. Patients were treated with 16–30 mg/kg of busulfan in combination with cyclophosphamide prior to bone marrow transplant. *Closed symbols* represent patients who rejected their graft or had a mixed chimera. Patients who experienced grade 0 treatment-related toxicity are designated by *circles*, grade 1 toxicity by *squares*, grade 2 toxicity by *diamonds*, grade 3 toxicity by *upright triangles*, and grade 4 toxicity by *inverted triangles*. Young children had substantially lower C_{ss}, less toxicity, and were at greater risk for graft rejection. (Data from Slattery JT, et al. Bone Marrow Transplant 1995;16:31–42.)

level between 10 and 20 μg/mL. The higher dose required to achieve this therapeutic serum concentration in younger patients is a reflection of lower bioavailablity and more rapid clearance of theophylline than in adults. Females require a lower weight-adjusted dose at an earlier age than males, presumably because they tend to enter puberty at an earlier age than males (34).

There may also be age-dependent changes in the route of elimination of drugs, as illustrated by theophylline. In premature newborns, over 50% of the drug is excreted unchanged in the urine compared with 10% in adults. Although theophylline is *N*-methylated to caffeine in all age groups, the elimination of caffeine is slower in newborns than in adults. Therefore, caffeine is measurable in the serum of the newborn, but by 6 to 12 months of age is metabolized more rapidly and is no longer detectable. Additionally, the metabolism of theophylline by liver cytochrome P450 enzymes increases during infancy. By 2 to 3 years of age the fraction of theophylline excreted unchanged in the urine has dropped to 15%, and theophylline is eliminated primarily by hepatic metabolism throughout adulthood.

Age-dependent clearance of busulfan also has a direct impact on the clinical outcome of patients treated with this anticancer drug. Busulfan is a bifunctional alkylating agent that is an important component of preparative regimens for bone marrow transplantation. In children < 5 years of age, the apparent clearance of busulfan is

two- to three-fold higher than it is in adults, due to enhanced glutathione conjugation (primary route of elimination) in children (35). As a result, steady-state plasma concentrations of busulfan resulting from a standard dose were lower in young children (Figure 23.8). Although the incidence and severity of busulfan-related toxicity were also lower in young children, the graft rejection rate was significantly higher (36).

Differences in the relative size of body organs or tissues between children and adults can also impact the pharmacokinetics of drugs. The liver and kidney are relatively larger in newborns compared to adults. Liver size as a percent of total body weight peaks during early childhood and this coincides with the enhanced clearance of hepatically metabolized drugs, such as theophylline.

The size of the central nervous system (CNS), which is disproportionately larger relative to body size in infants as compared to adults, has a quantifiable effect on drug concentrations achieved in the cerebrospinal fluid (CSF) after intrathecal administration of drugs and influences the dosing of intrathecal therapy in infants and young children. For example, CSF

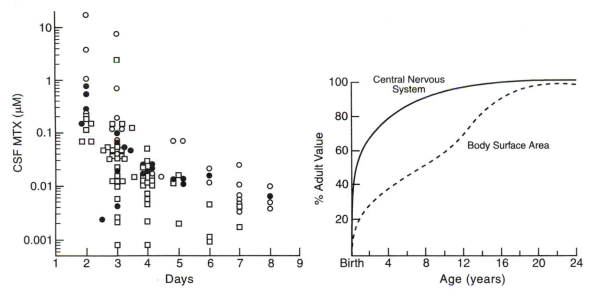

FIGURE 23.9 **(A)** Cerebrospinal fluid (CSF) methotrexate concentrations after an intrathecal dose of 12mg/m². Children (□) and adolescents (●) had lower concentrations than adults (○). Lower concentrations were associated with a higher risk of treatment failure. **(B)** Growth rate of central nervous system volume relative to whole body growth represented by body surface area. (Reproduced with permission from Bleyer WA. Cancer Treat Rep 1977;61:1419–25.)

methotrexate concentrations after an intrathecal dose of 12 mg/m² are age dependent (Figure 23.9A) (37). Higher CSF concentrations were observed in adults, intermediate concentrations in adolescents, and low concentrations in children. The low concentrations in children were also associated with an increased risk of treatment failure. The physiologic reason for this age discrepancy relates to the difference in the rate of growth of the CNS relative to the rest of the body (Figure 23.9B). By 3 years of age, CNS volume is 80% of the adult volume, while BSA, on which the methotrexate dose is based, increases at a slower rate toward the eventual adult value. If the dose of an intrathecally administered drug is calculated based on BSA, young children receive a lower dose relative to their CNS volume than adults. Based on this observation, a pharmacokinetically guided, age-based intrathecal dosing schedule was devised for methotrexate. Patients less than 1 year of age receive 6 mg, patients who are 1 year old receive 8 mg, patients who are 2 years old receive 10 mg, and patients 3 years of age and older receive a 12-mg dose. With this age-adjusted dosing schedule CSF methotrexate concentrations were less variable than with the standard 12 mg/m² dose, even though this adaptive dosing schedule results in a > 50% absolute dose increase in young children and a lower dose in patients older than 10 years (Figure 23.10) (37). The age-adjusted dosing regimen for intrathecal methotrexate has had a significant impact on the efficacy of preventative therapy in children with acute

lymphoblastic leukemia. The overall CNS relapse rate was significantly lower with the new regimen and the greatest improvement occurred in children < 3 years of age (38).

For most systemically administered drugs, specific adaptive dosing methods, such as those developed for intrathecal methotrexate, do not exist, and the dose is

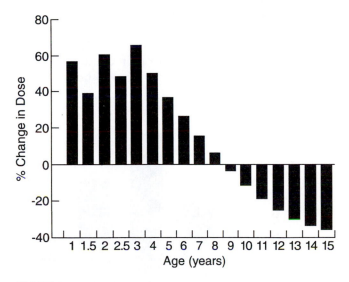

FIGURE 23.10 Percentage change in the dose of intrathecal methotrexate using the age-adjusted dosing schedule (< 1 year, 6 mg; 1 year, 8 mg; 2 years, 10 mg; ≥ 3 years, 12 mg) relative to administering a 12 mg/m² dose adjusted to body surface area (*horizontal line at 0%*).

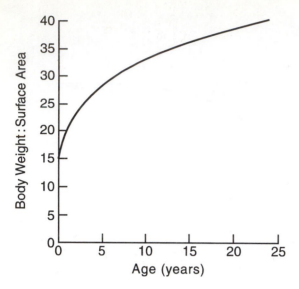

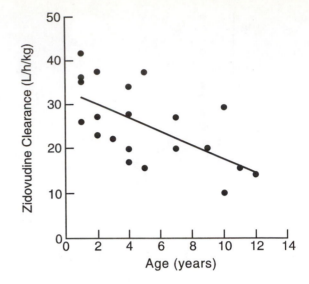

FIGURE 23.11   Relationship between body weight and body surface area (BSA) during childhood and adolescence.

FIGURE 23.12   Relationship between age and zidovudine clearance normalized to body weight. (Data from Balis F, et al. J Pediatr 1989;114:880–4.)

usually scaled to body weight or surface area. Figure 23.11 depicts the relationship between weight and BSA at various ages. BSA is greater relative to weight in newborns, but weight increases more rapidly than BSA during childhood and adolescence. Many physiologic parameters such as cardiac output, blood volume, extracellular fluid volume, GFR, renal blood flow, and metabolic rate are better correlated with BSA than weight. As a general rule, drug doses developed in adults or older children that are normalized to weight will result in a lower dose in infants than when scaling doses normalized to BSA from adults to infants. For example, when normalized to body weight, the clearance of zidovudine is higher in younger than in older children (Figure 23.12), indicating that scaling the dose to body weight

will result in lower serum concentrations at a given dose in the younger age group (5). Clinical experience has shown that dosing according to BSA usually results in more uniform plasma drug concentrations across a broad age range.

Scaling the dose to BSA may not always be the best method for dosing infants. Vincristine is an anticancer drug that causes peripheral neuropathy, and, in clinical trials, younger patients appeared to be more susceptible to this toxicity. Vincristine clearance based on BSA was lower in infants compared to older children and adolescents (Figure 23.13), thus a dose scaled to BSA would result in higher plasma concentrations in younger patients and account for the greater toxicity. For this reason, the vincristine dose for infants is now

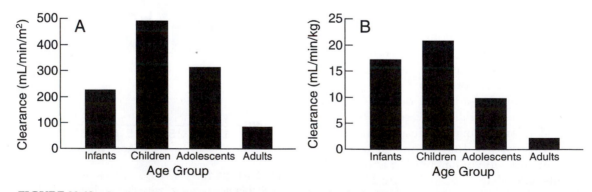

FIGURE 23.13   Comparison of vincristine clearance normalized to body surface area **(A)** with clearance normalized to body weight **(B)** in infants, children, adolescents, and adults. The risk of developing neurotoxicity is greater for infants dosed on the basis of body surface area than when doses are based on body weight. (Reproduced with permission from Crom WR, et al. J Pediatr 1994;125:642–9.)

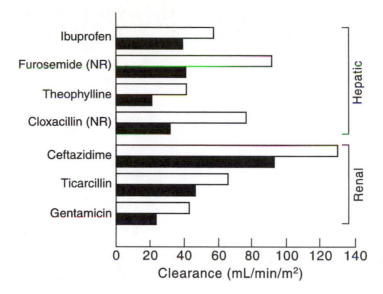

FIGURE 23.14 Comparison of hepatic and renal clearance of selected drugs in children with cystic fibrosis *(open bars)* and controls *(solid bars)*. Clearance is enhanced in patients with cystic fibrosis. NR indicates nonrenal component of total clearance. (Data from Rey E, et al. Clin Pharmacokinet 1998;35:313–29.)

routinely scaled to body weight, resulting in a lower vincristine dose and less toxicity in this age group (39).

Effect on Pharmacodynamics

The effect of normal growth and development on the pharmacodynamics of drugs has been less well studied. Age-dependent variation in receptor number, receptor affinity for drugs, or the responsiveness of the target organ or tissue to receptor occupancy could influence drug effect. Drugs may also alter the growth and development process or express effects that are dependent on the stage of development, such as the enamel dysplasia caused by tetracycline in young children or the depression of linear growth by corticosteroids.

Age-dependent, receptor-mediated drug effects have been observed with dopamine. The effect of dopamine on blood flow (estimated by measuring the pulsatility index by ultrasonography) was assessed in the right renal, superior mesenteric, and middle cerebral arteries in sick premature infants (40). Renal blood flow increased during the dopamine infusion, but mesenteric and cerebral blood flow were not altered. In adults, dopamine does increase blood flow to the intestine, indicating that the lack of response in preterm neonates is related to the immaturity of the mesenteric vascular bed.

Effect of Childhood Diseases

The spectrum of diseases that occur in the pediatric population is also quite different from diseases that afflict adults, and the effect of pediatric diseases on the pharmacokinetics and pharmacodynamics of the drugs used to treat these diseases requires more study. For example, in cystic fibrosis, the major organs associated with drug disposition, including the GI tract, pancreas, heart, liver, and kidney, can be affected. The underlying defect in chloride transport can cause inspissated secretions, leading to tissue damage in these organs and tissues. Surprisingly, the clearance of a wide variety of drugs, including drugs that are metabolized by the liver and those that are excreted by the kidney, is enhanced in patients with cystic fibrosis (Figure 23.14). The exact mechanism of the increased clearance is not clear, but these patients require larger doses of antibiotics to achieve therapeutic plasma drug concentrations than children who do not have cystic fibrosis (41).

CONCLUSIONS

Consideration of the impact of developmental changes occurring throughout the newborn period, infancy, childhood, and adolescence will lead to more rational, safer, and more effective use of drugs in the pediatric population. The examples in this chapter highlight the substantial impact of normal growth and development on the pharmacokinetics and pharmacodynamics of drugs, and emphasize the need for separate detailed clinical studies in newborns and children. To date, pediatric clinical trials have not been systematically performed for either marketed or new drugs because of economic, ethical, and technical factors.

Pediatric diseases are rare relative to adult diseases. Thus, for most drugs, the pediatric market share is small and there has been little financial incentive for pharmaceutical companies to perform studies in children for the purpose of developing specific labeling for childhood disease, either during initial development or after marketing approval has been obtained. New FDA regulations are designed to rectify this situation by requiring testing in pediatric populations and by providing incentives to pharmaceutical companies for completing those studies.[1]

Ethical constraints have also contributed to the hesitancy to perform studies in the pediatric population. Under current federal regulations governing biomedical research, children are afforded special protection. These federal regulations limit research studies that do not provide direct benefit to the pediatric subjects that participate. This means that drug studies can only be performed in children who have the disease that the drug is intended to treat. Thus, unlike initial drug testing in normal adult volunteers, the initial pharmacokinetic and safety testing usually cannot be done in normal pediatric volunteers (42). Compounding this is the fact that it is technically more challenging to perform research in children, especially in newborns in whom the most dramatic developmental changes occur.

The Pediatric Pharmacology Research Unit (PPRU) is a network of experienced clinical investigators committed to facilitating pharmacological research in the pediatric medical community (43). Acting as a consortium, the PPRU has the potential to provide access to a very large population of infants and children with varied diagnoses. The PPRU offers expertise in pediatric pharmacology and in the conduct of biomedical research involving children.[2]

References

1. Lietman P. Chloramphenicol and the neonate-1979 view. Clin Perinatol 1979;6:151–62.
2. Burns LE, Hodgman JE, Cass AB. Fatal circulatory collapse in premature infants receiving chloramphenicol. N Engl J Med 1959;261:1318–21.

---

[1] Additional information on pediatric initiatives by FDA's Center for Drug Evaluation and Research can be found at http://FDA.gov/CDER/pediatric/index.htm.

[2] Information about the Pediatric Pharmacology Research Unit (PPRU) can be found by visiting their link through the National Institute of Child Health and Human Development Center for Research for Mothers and Children; Endocrine, Nutrition and Growth Branch at http://www.nichd.nih.gov/crmc/eng/eng.htm.

3. Weiss CF, Glazko A, Weston JK. Chloramphenicol in the newborn infant. N Engl J Med 1960;262:787–94.
4. Klecker RW Jr, Collins JM, Yarchoan R, Thomas R, Jenkins JF, Broder S, et al. Plasma and cerebrospinal fluid pharmacokinetics of 3′-azido-3′-deoxythymide: A novel pyrimidine analog with potential application for the treatment of patients with AIDS and related diseases. Clin Pharmacol Ther 1987;41:407–12.
5. Balis F, Pizzo P, Eddy J, Wilfert C, McKinney R, Scott G, et al. Pharmacokinetics of zidovudine administered intravenously and orally in children with human immunodeficiency virus infection. J Pediatr 1989;114:880–4.
6. Mirochnick M, Capparelli E, Dankner W, Sperling RS, vanDyke R, Spector SA. Zidovudine pharmacokinetics in premature infants exposed to human immunodeficiency virus. Antimicrob Agents Chemother 1998;42:808–12.
7. Boucher FD, Modlin JF, Weller S, Ruff AA, Mirochnick M, Pelton SP, et al. Phase 1 evaluation of zidovudine administered to infants exposed at birth to the human immunodeficiency virus. J Pediatr 1993;122:137–44.
8. O'Sullivan MJ, Boyer PJ, Scott GB, Parks PW, Weller S, Blum MR, et al. The pharmacokinetics and safety of zidovudine in the third trimester of pregnancy for women infected with human immunodeficiency virus and their infants: Phase I Acquired Immunodeficiency Syndrome Clinical Trial Group Study (protocol 082). Zidovudine Collaborative Working Group. Am J Obstet Gynecol 1993;168:1510–6.
9. Connor EM, Sperling RS, Gelber R, Kiselev P, Scott G, O'Sullivan MJ, et al. Reduction of maternal-infant transmission of human immunodeficiency virus type I with zidovudine treatment. N Engl J Med 1994;331:1173–80.
10. Friedman M, Shalala DE. Regulations requiring manufacturers to assess the safety and effectiveness of new drugs and biological products in pediatric patients (21 CFR Parts 201, 312, 314, and 601). Federal Register 1998;63:66632–72.
11. Wilson T. An update on the therapeutic orphan. Pediatrics 1999;104:585–90.
12. Hubbard W. International Conference on Harmonization; E11: Clinical investigation of medicinal products in the pediatric population. Federal Register 2000;65:19777–81.
13. Routledge P. Pharmacokinetics in children. J Antimicrob Chemother 1994;34(suppl A):19–24.
14. Loebstein R, Koren G. Clinical pharmacology and therapeutic drug monitoring in neonates and children. Pediatr Rev 1998;19:423–8.
15. Reed MD, Besunder JB. Developmental pharmacology: ontogenic basis of drug disposition. Pediatr Clin North Am 1989;36:1053–74.
16. Linday L, Dobkin JF, Wang TC, Butler VP Jr, Saha JR, Lindenbaum R. Digoxin inactivation by the gut flora in infancy and childhood. Pediatrics 1987;79:544–8.
17. Kurz H, Michels H, Stickel HH. Differences in the binding of drugs to plasma proteins from newborn and adult man. II. Eur J Clin Pharmacol 1977;11:469–72.
18. Morselli PL. Clinical pharmacology of the perinatal period and early infancy. Clin Pharmacokinet 1989;17(suppl 1):13–28.
19. Kaufman RE. Pediatric pharmacology. In: Aranda JV, Yaffe SJ, editors. Pediatric pharmacology, therapeutic principles in practice. Philadelphia: WB Saunders; 1992. p. 212–19.
20. Kearns GL, Reed MD. Clinical pharmacokinetics in infancy and children, a reappraisal. Clin Pharmacokinet 1989;17(suppl 1):29–67.
21. Aranda J, Varvarigou A, Beharry K, Bansal R, Bardin C, Modanlou H, et al. Pharmacokinetics and protein binding of intravenous ibuprofen in the premature newborn infant. Acta Paediatr 1997;86:289–93.

22. Pikkarainen PH, Raiha NC. Development of alcohol dehydrogenase activity in human liver. Pediatr Res 1967;1:165–8.

23. Miller RP, Roberts JR, Fischer LJ. Acetaminophen elimination kinetics in neonates, children, and adults. Clin Pharmacol Ther 1976;19:284–94.

24. Kearns G. Pharmacogenetics and development: Are infants and children at increased risk for adverse outcomes? Curr Opin Pediatr 1995;7:220–33.

25. Leeder JS, Adciock K, Gaedigk A, Gotschall R, Wilson JT, Kearns GL. Delayed maturation of cytochrome P450 3A (CYP3A) activity in vivo in the first year of life (abstract). Pediatr Res 2000;47:472A.

26. Oesterheld JR. A review of developmental aspects of cytochrome P450. J Child Adolesc Psychopharmacol 1998;8:161–74.

27. Aperia A, Broberger O, Thodenius K, Zetterstrom R. Development of renal control of salt and fluid homeostasis during the first year of life. Acta Paediatr Scand 1975;64:393–8.

28. Guignard J, Torrado A, Da Cunha O, Gautier E. Glomerular filtration in the first three weeks of life. J Pediatr 1975;87:268–72.

29. Pons G, d'Athis P, Rey E, de Lauture D, Richard MO, Badoual J, et al. Gentamicin monitoring in neonates. Ther Drug Monit 1988;10:42–7.

30. Kraus DM, Fischer JH, Reitz SJ, Kecskes SA, Yeh TF, McCulloch KM, et al. Alterations in theophylline metabolism during the first year of life. Clin Pharmacol Ther 1993;54:351–9.

31. Grygiel JJ, Birkett DJ. Effect of age on patterns of theophylline metabolism. Clin Pharmacol Ther 1980;28:456–62.

32. Ueno K, Tanaka K, Shiokawa M, Horiuchi Y. Age-dependent changes of renal excretion of theophylline in asthmatic children (letter). Ann Pharmacother 1994;28:281–2.

33. Tserng K-Y, Takieddine FN, King KC. Developmental aspects of theophylline metabolism in premature infants. Clin Pharmacol Ther 1983;33:522–8.

34. Milavetz G, Vaughan LM, Weinberger MM, Hendeles L. Evaluation of a scheme for establishing and maintaining dosage of theophylline in ambulatory patients with chronic asthma. J Pediatr 1986;109:351–4.

35. Gibbs J, Murray G, Risler L, Chien JY, Dev R, Slattery JT. Age-dependent tetrahydrothiophenium ion formation in young children and adults receiving high-dose busulfan. Cancer Res 1997;57:5509–16.

36. Slattery J, Sanders JE, Buckner CD, Schaffer RL, Lambert KW, Langer FP, et al. Graft-rejection and toxicity following bone marrow transplantation in relation to busulfan pharmacokinetics. Bone Marrow Transplant 1995;16:31–42.

37. Bleyer WA. Clinical pharmacology of intrathecal methotrexate. II. An improved dosage regimen derived from age-related pharmacokinetics. Cancer Treat Rep 1977;61:1419–25.

38. Bleyer WA, Coccia PF, Sather HN, Level C, Lukens J, Niebrugge DJ, et al. Reduction in central nervous system leukemia with a pharmacokinetically derived intrathecal methotrexate dosage regimen. J Clin Oncol 1983;1:317–25.

39. Crom WR, de Graaf SS, Synold T, Uges DR, Bloemhof H, Rivera G, et al. Pharmacokinetics of vincristine in children and adolescents with acute lymphocytic leukemia. J Pediatr 1994;125:642–9.

40. Seri I, Abbasi S, Wood DC, Gerdes JS. Regional hemodynamic effects of dopamine in the sick preterm neonate. J Pediatr 1998;133:728–34.

41. Rey E, Treluyer T-M, Pons G. Drug disposition in cystic fibrosis. Clin Pharmacokinet 1998;35:313–29.

42. American Academy of Pediatrics Committee on Drugs. Guidelines for the ethical conduct of studies to evaluate drugs in pediatric populations. Pediatrics 1995;95:286–94.

43. Cohen S. The Pediatric Pharmacology Research Unit (PPRU) Network and its role in meeting pediatric labeling needs. Pediatrics 1999;104:644–5.

24

Drug Therapy in the Elderly

DARRELL R. ABERNETHY

Gerontology Research Center, National Institute on Aging, Baltimore, Maryland

INTRODUCTION

A hallmark of aging in humans is the development of multiple coexisting physiological and pathophysiological changes that may benefit from drug therapy. It is not uncommon for an older individual to have 5 to 10 diagnoses, each with proven beneficial therapy (Table 24.1). Examples abound; the presence of hypertension, coronary artery disease, osteoarthritis, osteoporosis, type 2 diabetes mellitus, and treated prostate or breast cancer often coexist in an individual patient. In addition, treatable insomnia, depression, and anxiety may be present, either independently or associated with these medical illnesses. As the number of individuals who are greater than 85 years old dramatically increases, the incidence of Alzheimer's disease and other forms of cognitive impairment for which somewhat effective treatment is available will increase as well (Figure 24.1). This will increase medication exposure and the potential for drug interactions (see Chapter 14) even more. With the availability of medications that are in many instances dramatically effective, it is imperative to understand the impact of multiple concurrent medications (high drug burden) on the older individual.

A number of studies over the past three decades have demonstrated that the likelihood of adverse drug effects increases with the number of drugs prescribed (1, 2). There is a disproportionate increase in both total and severe adverse drug reactions when more than five drugs are co-administered (3). Adverse drug effects also are more likely in older patients when certain drugs such as warfarin, theophylline, or digoxin are among the drugs prescribed. However, the absolute number of drugs the patient concurrently receives is probably the best predictor of an adverse drug event (Figure 24.2) (2).

Further complicating this issue is the fact that the relative therapeutic benefit of treatments such as thrombolytic therapy, hypocholesterolemic therapy, post myocardial infarction β blocker treatment, and angiotensin-converting enzyme inhibitor treatment of congestive heart failure in patients over the age of 75 is similar to that seen in younger patients. Unfortunately, these data create a dilemma in that dramatic therapeutic advances have been made for many illnesses that afflict the elderly, yet administration of multiple medications increases the likelihood of adverse drug events.

PATHOPHYSIOLOGY OF AGING

It is useful to think of the aging process in physiological, not chronological terms. That being said, a chronological definition is often used to stratify the aging population into three groups: *young old*—age 65–75 years; *old*—age 75–85 years; and *old old*—age ≥ 85 years. Nearly all the research that describes pharmacokinetics and pharmacodynamics in older individ-

TABLE 24.1   Age-related Chronic Medical Conditions[a]

| Medical condition | Frequency per 1000 persons in United States | | |
	Age < 45 years	Age 46–64 years	Age > 65 years
Arthritis	30	241	481
Hypertension	129	244	372
Hearing impairment	37	141	321
Heart disease	31	134	295
Diabetes	9	57	99
Visual impairment	19	48	79
Cerebrovascular disease	1	16	63
Constipation	11	19	60

[a] From Zisook S, Downs NS. J Clin Psych 1998;59 (suppl 4):80–91, data from Dorgan CA, editor. Statistical record of health and medicine. New York: International Thompson Publishing Co; 1995.

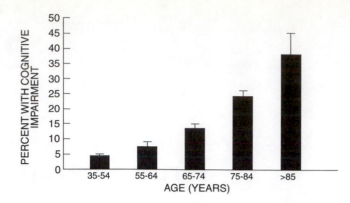

FIGURE 24.1   Age-related impairment in cognitive function as defined by 6 or more errors in the Mini-Mental Status Exam. (Data from Robins LN, Regier, editors. Psychiatric disorders in America: The Epidemiolgic Cachment Area Study. New York: The Free Press; 1991.)

uals has been obtained from study of the young old, that is, age ≤ 75 years. Therefore, the validity of extrapolating these findings to the older age groups may be questioned. In contrast, the data describing adverse drug events in older as compared to younger patients is obtained from patient populations and data bases that include the full age spectrum of the elderly.

The general physiological changes that occur with aging can be characterized as a decrease in maximum performance capacity and loss of homeostatic reserve (4). Although these changes occur in different degrees for each organ system or function, they are present in individuals who are in good health and are accentuated during illness. Placed in the context of response to

drugs, it is most useful to discuss age-related physiological changes that occur in integrated functions. Systemic drug responses are the result of the complex interaction of specific and nonspecific drug effects, and the direct and indirect physiological or pathological responses to these drug effects. The sum of these effects is the pharmacodynamic response that is observed, whether therapeutic or toxic. Therefore, the age-related changes that occur in physiological or psychological function prior to drug exposure are helpful in predicting and describing a particular drug response.

The observed pharmacodynamic response is the result of extent of drug exposure, determined by drug pharmacokinetics (Table 24.2), and sensitivity to a given drug exposure, determined by the state of function of

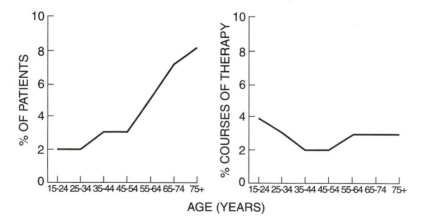

FIGURE 24.2   The relationship of increasing age and likelihood of adverse drug events (*left panel*), and the relationship of increasing age and adverse drug reactions when corrected for number of drugs per patient (*right panel*). (Reproduced with permission from Gurwitz JH, Avorn J. Ann Intern Med 1991;114:956–66.)

TABLE 24.2 Pharmacokinetic Changes in the Elderly

Process	Change with age
Gastrointestinal absorption	—
Drug distribution	
Central compartment volume	— or ↓
Peripheral compartment volume	
Lipophilic drugs	↑↑
Hydrophilic drugs	↓↓
Plasma protein binding	
Binding to albumin	↓
Binding to α_1-acid glycoprotein	— or ↑
Drug elimination	
Renal elimination	↓↓
Hepatic metabolism	
Phase I reactions	
CYP3A	↓
CYP1A2	— or ↓
CYP2D6	— or ↓
CYP2C9	— or ↓
CYP2C19	— or ↓
CYP2E1	— or ↓
Phase II reactions	
Glucuronidation	—
Sulfation	—
Acetylation	—

the effectors of drug response, such as receptor-cellular transduction processes (Figure 24.3). We will discuss the age-related changes that have been described for renal drug elimination and hepatic and extrahepatic drug biotransformations. We will then briefly review the age-related changes that have been described for central nervous system function, autonomic nervous system function, cardiovascular function, and renal function. These functions are selected as each has been rather comprehensively evaluated in the healthy elderly and a great diversity of drugs can have adverse as well as beneficial effects on these functions. We will describe and/or predict the effect of these changes on drug pharmacodynamics at a given drug exposure for drug groups commonly used in older patients. Finally, we discuss drug groups for which increased age confers greater risk for drug toxicity, along with the mechanism when known.

AGE-RELATED CHANGES IN PHARMACOKINETICS

Age-related Changes in Renal Clearance

The most consistent and predictable age-related change in drug pharmacokinetics is that of renal clearance of drugs. Renal function, including renal blood flow, glomerular filtration rate, and active renal tubular secretory processes, all decline with increasing age (5). Although there is considerable variability in this decline, an approximation of the decline in glomerular filtration rate has been usefully characterized by the Cockroft–Gault equation referred to in Chapters 1 and 5 (6). For men, creatinine clearance can be estimated from this equation as follows:

$$CL_{CR} \text{ (mL/min)} = \frac{(140 - \text{age}) (\text{weight in kg})}{72 (\text{serum creatinine in mg/dL})}$$

For women, this estimate should be reduced by 15%. Drugs that are eliminated primarily by glomerular

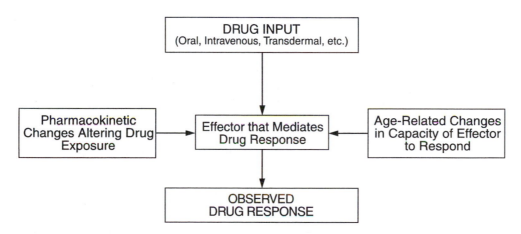

FIGURE 24.3 Observed drug responses in elderly patients represent the combined effects of drug input and age-related pharmacokinetic and pharmacodynamic changes.

TABLE 24.3   Some Drugs with Decreased Clearance in the Elderly

Route of clearance	Representative drugs	
Renal	All aminoglycosides	Sotalol
	Vancomycin	Atenolol
	Digoxin	Dofetilide
	Procainamide	Cimetidine
	Lithium	
Single Phase I metabolic pathway		
CYP3A	Alprazolam	
	Midazolam	
	Triazolam	
	Verapamil	
	Diltiazem	
	Dihydropyridine calcium channel blockers	
	Lidocaine	
CYP2C	Diazepam	
	Phenytoin	
	Celecoxib	
CYP1A2	Theophylline	
Multiple Phase I metabolic pathways	Imipramine	
	Desipramine	
	Trazodone	
	Hexobarbital	
	Flurazepam	

filtration, including aminoglycoside antibiotics, lithium, and digoxin, have an elimination clearance that decreases with age in parallel with the decline in measured or calculated creatinine clearance (7–9).

The renal clearance of drugs undergoing active renal tubular secretion also decreases with aging (Table 24.3). For example, the decrease in renal tubular secretion of cimetidine has been shown to parallel the decrease in creatinine clearance in older patients (10). On the other hand, the renal clearance/creatinine clearance ratio of both procainamide and N-acetylprocainamide decreases in the elderly, indicating that the renal tubular secretion of these drugs declines more rapidly than creatinine clearance (11).

Age-related Changes in Hepatic and Extrahepatic Drug Biotransformations

Drug biotransformations occur in quantitatively important amounts in the liver, gastrointestinal tract,

kidneys, lung, and skin. However, nearly all organs have some metabolic activity. As described in Chapter 11, *in vivo* drug biotransformations are commonly separated into Phase I and Phase II biotransformations. Phase I biotransformations are catalyzed by membrane-bound enzymes found in the endoplasmic reticulum and Phase II biotransformations occur predominantly in the cytosol, with the exception of the UDP-glucuronosyltransferases that are bound to endoplasmic reticulum membranes. Phase I biotransformations are primarily catalyzed by enzymes of the cytochrome P450 monoxygenase system (CYP450), with the important members of this enzyme family for drug biotransformations being CYP3A, CYP2D6, CYP2C, CYP1A2, and CYP2E1.

Phase I biotransformations catalyzed by CYP3A have been shown most consistently to be decreased in aging, with the decrease on the order of 10 to 40%. The drugs studied that are prototype CYP3A substrates and exemplify this are midazolam and triazolam (12, 13). The result of this decrease in drug biotransformation is decreased metabolic clearance and increased exposure to drug of the individual at a given dose. The clinical consequence of this is that older patients treated with a given dose of triazolam experience increased sedation and impaired task performance (14). Quantitatively significant CYP3A activity in the gastrointestinal wall, which catalyzes biotransformation of drugs prior to and during absorption, has been demonstrated. However, it is unknown at present if this activity changes with aging (15). P-glycoprotein in the intestinal wall also has been recognized recently as playing an important role in the absorption of some drugs. However, it is unknown if this is altered in aging as well (16).

There is some suggestion that Phase I biotransformations catalyzed by CYP2C are decreased with age, with modest decreases in clearance of warfarin (CYP2C9) and phenytoin (CYP2C19) reported in older individuals. However, this is much less well established (17, 18). Similarly, Phase I biotransformation by CYP1A2 may be somewhat decreased in older individuals, and decreased theophylline and caffeine clearance have been reported (19). However, this too is not well established.

Phase II biotransformations are little changed with aging, based on studies of glucuronidation, sulfation, and acetylation. Prototype substrates studied for glucuronidation have been lorazepam and oxazepam, for sulfation acetaminophen, and for acetylation isoniazid and procainamide.

As discussed in Chapter 13, genetic polymorphisms for the Phase I enzymes CYP2D6, CYP2C19, and the Phase II enzymes N-acetyltransferase and the methyltransferases, thiopurine methyltransferase, catechol O-methyl transferase, and thiol methyltransferase, may significantly alter exposure to relevant drug substrates. Evaluation of the frequency of polymorphic variants with increasing age has consistently shown that the same frequencies occur in older individuals as in younger individuals.

AGE-RELATED CHANGES IN EFFECTOR SYSTEM FUNCTION

Central Nervous System (CNS)

It is important to separate age-related and disease-related changes in CNS function. The following changes have been noted in the absence of dementing illness, Parkinson's disease, and primary psychiatric disease. Brain aging proceeds in a relatively selective fashion, with the prefrontal cortex and the subcortical monoaminergic nuclei most affected. In the case of the prefrontal cortex, progressive loss of volume with aging is consistently shown. Age-related slowing in mental-processing function is a consistent finding, but the mechanism is uncertain. Aging has been associated with changes in brain activation during encoding and retrieval processes of memory function. Older individuals have more widespread task-related brain activation to conduct the same tasks as compared to younger individuals. One postulate has been that older individuals need to recruit greater brain resources to conduct the same memory function (20). Even in the absence of parkinsonism, the dopaminergic systems are diminished as a function of age. The dopaminergic impairment has been most clearly defined for processes involving dopamine D2 receptors (21).

An important pharmacodynamic principle is that older individuals have increased sensitivity to a given exposure of some CNS depressant drugs. After accounting for age-related pharmacokinetic changes that may cause greater drug exposure at a given dose, the aged individual is more sensitive to the opiate anesthetic induction agents propofol, fentanyl, and alfentanil (22–24). In the case of propofol, the concentration needed to induce anesthesia in a 75-year-old healthy individual was approximately one-half that required for 25-year-old individual (22, 23). The mechanism for this increased pharmacodynamic sensitivity is unknown. A similar increase in pharmacodynamic sensitivity to fentanyl and alfentanil has been described with again a 50% decrease in dose requirement to induce the same degree of drug effect in older individuals (up to 89 years) as compared to younger individuals (24).

These findings for opiates are in contrast to findings with the barbiturate thiopental and the benzodiazepines midazolam and triazolam (14, 25, 26). Although a substantially lower dose of these drugs is needed to induce anesthesia or the same degree of sedation in older than in younger individuals, this is the result of the pharmacokinetic changes of aging. When drug effect is normalized to arterial drug concentration, the concentration effect relationship is similar in the young and the elderly. For ambulatory elderly patients, the clinical consequences of increased exposure to benzodiazepines due to decreased Phase I metabolic clearance can be devastating, with an increased incidence of hip fracture noted in older patients taking long half-life benzodiazepines (27). These drugs (e.g., flurazepam and diazepam) undergo Phase I biotransformation, and the decreased clearance seen in the elderly results in markedly greater drug accumulation, even when taken once daily as a sedative-hypnotic (28, 29).

There are fewer data on adverse effects in older patients caused by neuroleptic and antidepressant drugs. However, as shown in Figure 24.4, it is now clear that older patients have a three- to five-fold higher incidence of tardive dyskinesia than younger patients when "typical" neuroleptics (e.g., phenothiazines and haloperidol) are administered (30–32). Across studies, 10 to 20% of younger patients develop tardive dyskinesia after three years or more of neuroleptic treatment, while 40 to 60% of older patients are affected within the same treatment period (32). It is unknown if this is related to age-dependent pharmacokinetic or pharmacodynamic changes. The newer neuroleptics, such as risperidol and olanzapine, have a much lower incidence of tardive dyskinesia in all patient groups studied and may be of considerable clinical utility for this reason (33). However, it will require some time to definitively establish the spec-

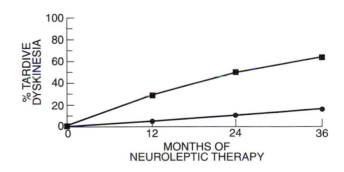

FIGURE 24.4 Cumulative incidence of neuroleptic-induced tardive dyskinesia in old (■) and young (●) adults. (Reproduced with permission from Jeste DV. J Clin Psychiatry 2000;61 (suppl 4):27–32.)

trum of adverse as well as therapeutic effects of these drugs.

There has been less comprehensive analysis of other classes of CNS active drugs, but the general clinical impression is that older patients are more sensitive to side effects and require a lower dose of drug to achieve similar therapeutic benefit. Pharmacokinetic studies of lithium, which undergoes renal elimination, and tricyclic antidepressants, which undergo Phase I biotransformation, show decreased clearance on the basis of the age-related decrease in renal function and the age-related decrease in Phase I drug metabolizing capacity, respectively (8, 34).

Autonomic Nervous System (ANS)

The age-related changes in ANS function are very diverse, and are likely to be associated with many of the age-related changes observed in drug response and toxicity across many therapeutic classes of drugs. Cardiovagal function is diminished, as indicated by age-related decreases in resting heart rate and beat-to-beat heart rate variability. Older individuals have lower vagal tone, as indicated by less increase in heart rate with atropine administration. Other findings consistent with this conclusion are that older individuals have decreased heart rate variation with deep breathing and reduced increases in heart rate in response to standing. Baroreflex function is also impaired in the healthy elderly, and this is accentuated in the presence of illness common in older patients, such as hypertension and diabetes mellitus (35). Cardiac sympathetic function is also altered, as demonstrated by decreased tachycardic response to isoproterenol and increased circulating plasma norepinephrine (36, 37). An integrated response that reflects many of these age-related changes is that of orthostatic hypotension, which is substantially increased in older individuals (38). The degree of orthostatic decrease in blood pressure in older patients may be particularly evident in the postprandial state and may be exacerbated in older patients who are treated with diuretics (39, 40). Thermoregulatory homeostasis is also impaired in the elderly who have a higher thermoreceptor threshold and decreased sweating when perspiration is initiated (35).

Data are sparse that conclusively establish that altered drug effects result from impaired ANS function, perhaps due to the difficulty in ascribing a particular drug effect to a particular ANS function. However, increased orthostatic hypotension seen at baseline is certainly exacerbated by drugs that cause sympathetic blockade, such as typical neuroleptics and tricyclic antidepressants, and is likely to be a con-

tributing factor to the increased incidence of hip fractures noted in patients receiving these drugs (41). Similarly, the anticholinergic effects of many drugs, including antihistamines and neuroleptics, may not only accentuate orthostatic blood pressure changes, but also be associated with greater cognitive impairment in older individuals. Impaired thermoregulation at baseline may also be accentuated by administration of these drugs because they have potent anticholinergic effects that further disable thermoregulatory responses. It is unclear at this time how age-related ANS changes may relate to the cardiac proarrhythmic effects of drugs that prolong the electrocardiographic QT interval. However, there is a clear association of increasing age with the proarrhythmic effects of neuroleptic drugs (42). It is clear that these ANS changes markedly alter systemic cardiovascular responses to drugs such as the alpha-beta adrenergic blocking drug labetalol, which, as shown in Figure 24.5, lowers blood

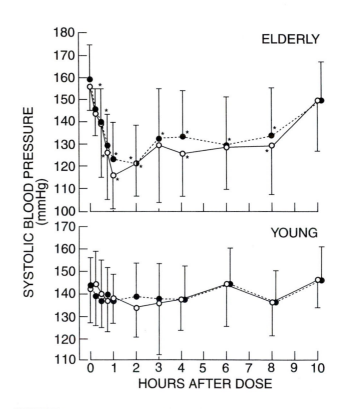

FIGURE 24.5 Comparison of changes in erect (O—O) and sitting (●– –●) systolic blood pressures between elderly (*upper panel*) and young (*lower panel*) hypertensive patients treated with a daily oral labetalol dose of 200 mg. Bars represent the standard deviation from the mean and asterisks indicate values that are significantly different ($P < 0.05$) from the baseline in that posture for the respective group. No differences were noted between sitting and standing blood pressure for either group. (Reproduced with permission from Abernethy DR, Schwartz JB, Plachetka JR, Todd EL, Egan JM. Am J Cardiol 1987;60:697–702.)

pressure to a greater extent in older than in younger hypertensive patients while decreasing heart rate to a much lesser extent (43).

Cardiovascular Function

The age-related changes in cardiovascular function that relate to drug responses are usefully separated into changes in cardiac and changes in peripheral vascular function. But this separation must be made with the understanding that the pharmacodynamic responses seen are generally an integrated function of ANS, cardiac, and peripheral vascular function.

Cardiac output at rest is not substantially changed with age in the absence of superimposed cardiac disease. However, components of the cardiac cycle are indeed changed. Heart rate is decreased, reflecting the decrease in parasympathetic withdrawal noted previously, and perhaps impaired beta-adrenergic and sinoatrial function. Left ventricular mass and left ventricular stroke volume are increased, which allows cardiac output to be maintained in the face of decreased heart rate. However, diastolic relaxation is slowed, making the late left ventricular filling that is associated with atrial contraction a more important determinant of stroke volume in the elderly. Chronotropic response to beta-adrenergic stimulation is impaired, but it is uncertain if this is the cause or the result of increased circulating norepinephrine levels (44). Cellular and molecular mechanisms for these changes have been studied in some detail in animal models and may offer some insight into drug responses. The prolonged left ventricular contraction period and slowed diastolic relaxation may be associated with decreased uptake of calcium by the sarcoplasmic reticulum (45). Many potential mechanisms for the impairment in beta-adrenoceptor function have been suggested but this remains controversial.

The pharmacodynamic consequences of these age-related changes can be substantial. Impaired beta$_1$-adrenergic responsiveness results in a decreased tachycardic response to both direct drug-induced stimulation by drugs, such as isoproterenol (36), and indirect reflex sympathetic stimulation induced by vasodilating drugs, such as the calcium antagonist drug nisoldipine (46). Conversely, the decrease in heart rate caused by beta$_1$-adrenoceptor blockade is reduced in elderly patients (43). Although diastolic relaxation is slowed as a usual consequence of aging, this slowing progresses in many older patients to the extent that symptoms of congestive heart failure occur. As many as 40% of elderly patients with clinical congestive heart failure have normal left ventricular function when it is defined as left ventricular ejection

fraction $\geq 40\%$ (47, 48). These patients are particularly susceptible to loop diuretic-induced intravascular volume depletion that is manifest clinically as increased orthostatic hypotension (49). If the volume depletion is sufficient to decrease vital organ perfusion, other symptoms may occur such as central nervous system depression and decreased renal function (50).

Vascular stiffness increases with age, even in the absence of disease. This may be due to both structural and functional changes, and increased deposition of collagen and other ground substance is evident on microscopic or molecular examination (51). In addition, advanced age alone decreases endothelial-mediated relaxation, even in the absence of concurrent diseases, such as hypertension and hypercholesterolemia, or environmental exposures, such as cigarette smoking, that are associated with impaired vascular endothelial relaxation (52). Not only is beta$_1$-adrenergic function impaired, but beta$_2$-adrenergic mediated peripheral vasodilatation is impaired as well, due to decreased beta-adrenergic vascular relaxation (53). The clinical result of these changes is an increase in pulse pressure, with systolic blood pressure disproportionately increased relative to diastolic blood pressure.

The pharmacodynamic consequences of these age-related cardiovascular changes are quite diverse. With initial administration of a nonselective beta-adrenoceptor blocking drug, the decrease in heart rate is diminished. However, one would predict as well that the beta$_2$-adrenoceptor blockade mediated increase in peripheral vascular resistance would be diminished simultaneously. Clinical data indicate that beta-blocker therapy for hypertension may indeed be somewhat less effective in older hypertensive patients. However the limited data available indicate that beta-blocker therapy is as efficacious in older as in younger patients after myocardial infarction and for the treatment of congestive heart failure. Administration of an alpha-adrenergic blocking drug (e.g., terazosin for the treatment of urinary retention due to prostate hypertrophy) results in greater hypotensive response in older individuals who lack reflex beta adrenergic stimulation (54).

The response of older individuals to calcium channel antagonists is a combination of changes in direct drug effects and age-related alterations in reflex responses to drug effect. Hypotensive responses are maintained because direct arterial vasodilatation remains intact, even though there is the age-related impairment in reflex sympathetic stimulation, as previously noted (55). For verapamil and diltiazem, atrioventricular nodal conduction delay is less in older than in younger individuals, while sinoatrial suppression is greater in the elderly (56, 57). Mechanisms for these changes are unclear, but are thought to entail a complex summation of changes in direct drug effects and age-related ANS and cardiac function changes.

Angiotensin-converting enzyme inhibitors may be less effective in treating hypertension in older than in younger patients (58). The mechanism for this is probably related to the low-renin state and resulting decreased role of the circulating renin-angiotensin-aldosterone axis in maintaining blood pressure in older hypertensive patients (59, 60). Conversely, available data indicate that angiotensin-converting enzyme inhibitors are extremely effective treatment for congestive heart failure in older as well as younger patients (61).

Renal Function

Kidney morphology and renal function have marked changes with aging. These changes have been associated with pharmacokinetic changes (decreased renal drug clearance) and also changes in pharmacodynamics for three drug classes important for the elderly—nonsteroidal antiinflammatory drugs, angiotensin-converting enzyme inhibitors, and diuretics—that each may have responses altered by renal aging.

The anatomic changes associated with aging include a decrease in kidney weight that from the fourth to the ninth decade of life may fall by as much as one-third. This loss of renal mass occurs primarily from the renal cortex, and results in decreased numbers and size of glomeruli. The remaining blood vessels may then produce shunts between afferent and efferent arterioles. The functional result is a decline in glomerular filtration rate that averages 0.75 mL/min/year, but is quite variable. Perhaps as many as one-third of individuals have no decrease in glomerular filtration rate while others have more rapid decreases. Renal plasma flow, measured by para-aminohippurate clearance, decreases more with age than glomerular filtration rate as measured by inulin clearance, and may be decreased as much as 50% in individuals in the ninth decade as compared to the fourth decade of life. The result is that filtration fraction (glomerular filtration rate/renal plasma flow) increases in the elderly (5, 62). These findings also may be related to intrarenal impairment in vascular endothelial vasodilating function as demonstrated by an attenuated vasodilatory response to acetylcholine. Consistent with findings in other vascular beds, intrarenal vasoconstrictive responses to angiotensin II are maintained in the elderly. Circulating atrial natriuretic hormone is increased in older individuals, and

this may be responsible for suppression of renal renin secretion. This suppression leads to decreased basal activation of the renin-angiotensin-aldosterone axis (63). As mentioned previously, the age-associated decrease renal tubular secretion parallels the decrease in glomerular filtration rate for some drugs (10), but occurs more rapidly for others (11). The decrease in renal tubular reabsorption, at least as measured by glucose reabsorption, appears to parallel the decline in glomerular filtration rate. A final impairment in renal tubular function that occurs with aging is manifest as a decreased capacity to concentrate or dilute urine, resulting in an impaired ability to excrete a free-water load and to excrete sodium during states of volume depletion (64).

Altered or accentuated responses to nonsteroidal antiinflammatory drugs in elderly patients include azotemia, decreased glomerular filtration rate, sodium retention, and hyperkalemia (65, 66). A common basis for these adverse effects is likely to rest in part on the increased dependence of the aging kidney on vasodilating prostaglandins that results from the age-related decrease in renal plasma flow. Furthermore, glomerular filtration rate may decrease in older patients to the same extent with selective inhibition of cyclooxygenase-2 as with nonselective cyclooxygenase inhibitors (67, 68). The increased likelihood of sodium retention in older patients may also be associated with the loss of action of vasodilating prostaglandins, decreased glomerular filtration, and decreased renal tubular capacity to concentrate sodium in the decreased urine volume. The increased likelihood of hyperkalemia may reflect a preexisting state of relative hyporeninemic hypoaldosteronism in older individuals, exacerbated either by loss of prostaglandin effect on renin secretion or by increased effective intravascular volume due to drug-induced sodium retention (63–68).

Treatment with angiotensin-converting enzyme inhibitors is also more likely to be associated with hyperkalemia in older individuals (69). Impaired angiotensin II formation limits this potent stimulus for aldosterone secretion, and this is superimposed on the already age-related decrease in activity of the renin-angiotensin-aldosterone axis. The same drug-induced hyporeninemic hypoaldosteronism is predicted for angiotensin receptor blockers. However, to date this has not been documented clincally.

Thiazide diuretic-induced hyponatremia is much more common in older than in younger patients, probably due to thiazide-mediated impairment in renal diluting capacity superimposed on the already present age-related decrease in the capacity to dilute urine. Older studies indicated that this was an extremely common cause of moderate to severe hyponatremia.

However, this may occur less frequently now that lower doses of thiazide diuretics are used to treat hypertension (70–72).

DRUG GROUPS FOR WHICH AGE CONFERS INCREASED RISK FOR TOXICITY

In addition to the adverse pharmacodynamic consequences described, for which there is at least a potential mechanistic understanding, it is more difficult to formulate a mechanistic explanation for a number of drug toxicities that are more frequent in older than younger patients.

Theophylline neurotoxicity and cardiotoxicity are increased in older patients. Although it is unclear whether decreased theophylline clearance and increased exposure in older patients fully explain this apparent sensitivity, clinical reports are uniform in identifying age as a major contributing risk factor for theophylline toxicity (73, 74). This has resulted in much less use of theophylline in older patients.

Isoniazid-induced hepatotoxicity is more likely to occur in individuals who are more than 35 years old (75). Attempts to establish a pharmacokinetic or pharmacogenetic explanation have been unsatisfactory. Nevertheless, this finding led to the subsequent recommendation that isoniazid be withheld from individuals with a positive tuberculin skin test ≥15 mm but no other risk factors (76). Because approximately 5 to 10% of patients with a positive tuberculin test will develop active tuberculosis and elderly individuals are at highest risk, there currently is concern that appropriate chemoprophylaxis is not being made available to individuals who are ≥50 years of age (77). In view of the fact that routine clinical monitoring has reduced the risk of severe hepatotoxicity in recent years, current guidelines do not put an age limit on the use of isoniazid to treat latent tuberculosis but simply discourage tuberculin testing in low-risk individuals (78).

Neuroleptic-induced tardive dyskinesia has been discussed. However, the mechanism for tardive dyskinesia is not well established. It is clear that increased patient age contributes significantly to the risk of developing tardive dyskinesia with the "typical" neuroleptics (32–34).

Nonsteroidal antiinflammatory drugs are probably more likely to induce gastric ulceration in older than in younger patients (79). This may be the result of a decrease in gastric mucosal prostaglandins in the elderly (80) with drug-induced inhibition of gastric prostaglandins being superimposed on this age-related decrease.

CONCLUSIONS

Older patients frequently have multiple coexisting diseases that are often very effectively treated with medications. There is little doubt that the risk of a specific drug therapy, such as angiotensin-converting enzyme inhibitor treatment of patients with congestive heart failure, is in most instances far outweighed by the benefit of therapy. However, the concurrent presence of multiple diseases in older patients results in their being treated with multiple medications, which itself is a risk factor for adverse drug events. Therefore, it is an appropriate generalization to assume that the risk/benefit ratio, or the therapeutic index, of any given therapy is narrowed for older patients. Understanding age-related pathophysiology can in some instances allow for prediction of age-related changes in drug disposition and effect. However, drug therapy continues to be a significant contributor to morbidity and mortality in the elderly (3).

References

1. Smith JW, Seidl LG, Cluff LE. Studies on the epidemiology of adverse drug reactions. V. Clinical factors influencing susceptibility. Ann Intern Med 1966; 65:629–40.
2. Hutchinson TA, Flegel KM, Kramer MS, Leduc DG, Kong HH. Frequency, severity and risk factors for adverse drug reactions in adult outpatients. J Chron Dis 1986;39:533–42.
3. Gurwitz JH, Field TS, Avorn J, McCormick D, Jain S, Eckler M, Benser M, Edmondson AC, Bates DW. Incidence and preventability of adverse drug events in the nursing home setting. Am J Med 2000; 109:87–94.
4. Hall DA. The biomedical basis of gerontology. Littleton, MA: John Wright PSG Inc; 1984.
5. Davies DF, Shock NW. Age changes in glomerular filtration rate, effective renal plasma flow, and tubular excretory capacity in adult males. J Clin Invest 1950; 29:496–507.
6. Cockcroft DW, Gault MH. Prediction of creatinine clearance from serum creatinine. Nephron 1976;16:31–41.
7. Morike K, Schwab M, Klotz U. Use of aminoglycosides in elderly patients: Pharmacokinetic and clinical considerations. Drugs Aging 1997;10:259–77.
8. Sproule BA, Hardy BG, Shulman KI. Differential pharmacokinetics of lithium in elderly patients. Drugs Aging 2000;16:165–77.
9. Cusack B, Kelly J, O'Malley K, Noel J, Lavan J, Horgan J. Digoxin in the elderly: Pharmacokinetic consequences of old age. Clin Pharmacol Ther 1979;25:772–6.
10. Drayer DE, Romankiewicz J, Lorenzo B, Reidenberg MM. Age and renal clearance of cimetidine. Clin Pharmacol Ther 1982;31:45–60.
11. Reidenberg MM, Camacho M, Kluger J, Drayer DE. Aging and renal clearance of procainamide and acetylprocainamide. Clin Pharmacol Ther 1980;28:732–5.
12. Greenblatt DJ, Abernethy DR, Locniskar A, Harmatz JS, Limjuco RA, Shader RI. Effect of age, gender, and obesity on midazolam kinetics. Anesthesiology 1984;61:27–35.
13. Greenblatt DJ, Divoll M, Abernethy DR, Moschitto LJ, Smith RB, Shader RI. Reduced clearance of triazolam in old age: Relation to

antipyrine oxidizing capacity. Br J Clin Pharmacol 1983;15:303–9.

14. Greenblatt DJ, Harmatz JS, Shapiro L, Engelhardt N, Gouthro TA, Shader RI. Sensitivity to triazolam in the elderly. N Engl J Med 1991;324:1691–8.

15. Watkins PB, Wrighton SA, Schuetz EG, Molowa DT, Guzelian PS. Identification of glucocorticoid-inducible cytochromes P-450 in the intestinal mucosa of rats and man. J Clin Invest 1987;80:1029–36.

16. Gatmaitan ZC, Arias IM. Structure and function of P-glycoprotein in normal liver and small intestine. Adv Pharmacol 1993;24:77–97.

17. Shepherd AM, Hewick DS, Moreland TA, Stevenson IH. Age as a determinant of sensitivity to warfarin. Br J Clin Pharmacol 1977;4:315–20.

18. Bauer LA, Blouin RA. Age and phenytoin kinetics in adult epileptics. Clin Pharmacol Ther 1982;31:301–4.

19. Jusko WJ, Gardner MJ, Mangione A, Schentag JJ, Koup JR, Vance JW. Factors affecting theophylline clearances: age, tobacco, marijuana, cirrhosis, congestive heart failure, obesity, oral contraceptives, benzodiazepines, barbiturates, and ethanol. J Pharm Sci 1979;68:1358–66.

20. Raz N. Aging of the brain and its impact on cognitive performance: Integration of structural and functional findings. In: Craik FIM, Salthouse TA, editors. The handbook of aging and cognition. 2nd ed. Mahwah, NJ: Lawrence Erlbaum Associates; 2000. p. 1–90.

21. Volkow ND, Gur RC, Wang G-J, Fowler JS, Moberg PJ, Ding Y-S, Hitzemann R, Smith G, Logan J. Association between decline in brain dopamine activity with age and cognitive and motor impairment in healthy individuals. Am J Psychiatry 1998;155:344–9.

22. Schnider TW, Minto CF, Shafer SL, Gambus PL, Andresen C, Goodale DB, Youngs EJ. The influence of age on propofol pharmacodynamics. Anesthesiology 1999;90:1502–16.

23. Olmos M, Ballester JA, Vidarte A, Elizalde JL, Escobar A. The combined effect of age and premedication on the propofol requirements for induction by target controlled infusion. Anesth Analg 2000;90:1157–61.

24. Scott JC, Stanski DR. Decreased fentanyl and alfentanil dose requirements with age. A simultaneous pharmacokinetic and pharmacodynamic evaluation. J Pharmacol Exp Ther 1987;240:159–66.

25. Stanski DR, Maitre PO. Population pharmacokinetics and pharmacodynamics of thiopental: The effect of age revisited. Anesthesiology 1990;72:412–22.

26. Jacobs JR, Reves JG, Marty J, White WD, Bai SA, Smith LR. Aging increases pharmacodynamic sensitivity to the hypnotic effects of midazolam. Anesth Analg 1995;80:143–8.

27. Ray WA, Griffin MR, Downey W. Benzodiazepines of long and short elimination half-life and the risk of hip fracture. JAMA 1989;262:3303–7.

28. Greenblatt DJ, Shader RI, Abernethy DR. Drug therapy: Current status of benzodiazepines. N Engl J Med 1983;309:354–8,410–6.

29. Greenblatt DJ, Allen MD, Shader RI. Toxicity of high-dose flurazepam in the elderly. Clin Pharmacol Ther 1977;21:355–61.

30. Saltz BL, Woerner MG, Kane JM, Lieberman JA, Alvir JMJ, Bergmann KJ, Blank K, Koblenzer J, Kahaner K. Prospective study of tardive dyskinesia incidence in the elderly. JAMA 1991;266:2402–6.

31. Jeste DV, Caligiuri MP, Paulsen JS, Heaton RK, Lacro JP, Harris J, Bailey A, Fell RL, McAdams LA. Risk of tardive dyskinesia in older patients: A prospective longitudinal study of 266 outpatients. Arch Gen Psychiatry 1995;52:756–65.

32. Woerner MG, Alvir JMJ, Saltz BL, Lieberman JA, Kane JM. Prospective study of tardive dyskinesia in the elderly: Rates and risk factors. Am J Psychiatry 1998;155:1521–8.

33. Jeste DV, Lacro JP, Bailey A, Rockwell E, Harris MJ, Caligiuri MP. Lower incidence of tardive dyskinesia with risperidone compared with haloperidol in older patients. J Am Geriatr Soc 1999;47:716–9.

34. Abernethy DR, Greenblatt DJ, Shader RI. Imipramine and desipramine disposition in the elderly. J Pharmacol Exp Ther 1985;232:183–8.

35. Low PA. The effect of aging on the autonomic nervous system. In: Low PA, editor. Clinical autonomic disorders. 2nd ed. Philadelphia: Lippincott-Raven; 1997. p. 161–75.

36. Vestal RE, Wood AJJ, Shand DG. Reduced beta-adrenoceptor sensitivity in the elderly. Clin Pharmacol Ther 1979;26:181–6.

37. Ziegler MG, Lake CR, Kopin IJ. Plasma noradrenaline increases with age. Nature 1976;261:333–5.

38. Rodstein M, Zeman FD. Postural blood pressure changes in the elderly. J Chronic Dis 1957;6:581–8.

39. Lipsitz LA, Nyquist RP, Wei JY, Rowe JW. Postprandial reduction in blood pressure in the elderly. N Engl J Med 1983;309:81–3.

40. van Kraaij DJW, Jansen RWMM, Gribnau FWJ, Hoefnagels WHL. Diuretic therapy in elderly heart failure patients with and without left ventricular systolic dysfunction. Drugs Aging 2000;16:289–300.

41. Ray WA, Griffin MR, Schaffner W, Baugh DK, Melton LJ. Psychotropic drug use and the risk of hip fracture. N Engl J Med 1987;316:363–9.

42. Reilly JG, Ayis SA, Ferrier IN, Jones SJ, Thomas SHL. QTc-interval abnormalities and psychotropic drug therapy in psychiatric patients. Lancet 2000;355:1048–52.

43. Abernethy DR, Schwartz JB, Plachetka JR, Todd EL, Egan JM. Comparison in young and elderly patients of pharmacodynamics and disposition of labetalol in systemic hypertension. Am J Cardiol 1987;60:697–702.

44. Lakatta EG. Cardiovascular aging research: The next horizons. J Am Geriatr Soc 1999;47:613–25.

45. Maciel LMZ, Polikar R, Rohrer D, Popovich BK, Dillmann WH. Age-induced decreases in the messenger RNA coding for the sarcoplasmic reticulum Ca^{2+}-ATPase of the rat heart. Circ Res 1990;67:230–4.

46. van Harten J, Burggraaf J, Ligthart GJ, van Brummelen P, Breimer DD. Single- and multiple-dose nisoldipine kinetics and effects in the young, the middle-aged, and the elderly. Clin Pharmacol Ther 1989;45:600–7.

47. ACC/AHA Task Force Report. Guidelines for the evaluation and management of heart failure. J Am Coll Cardiol 1995;26:1376–98.

48. Tresch DD. The clinical diagnosis of heart failure in older patients. J Am Geriatr Soc 1997;45:1128–33.

49. Bonow RO, Udelson JE. Left ventricular diastolic dysfunction as a cause of congestive heart failure: Mechanisms and management. Ann Int Med 1992;117:502–10.

50. van Kraaij DJW, Jansen RWMM, Bouwels LHR, Hoefnagels WHL. Furosemide withdrawal improves postprandial hypotension in elderly patients with heart failure and preserved left ventricular systolic function. Arch Intern Med 1999;159:1599–605.

51. Cangiano JL, Martinez-Maldonado M. Isolated systolic hypertension in the elderly. In: Martinez-Maldonado M, editor. Hypertension and renal disease in the elderly. Oxford: Blackwell Scientific Publications; 1992. p. 79–94.

52. Andrawis NS, Jones DS, Abernethy DR. Aging is associated with endothelial dysfunction in the human forearm vasculature. J Am Geriatr Soc 2000;48:193–8.

53. Pan HYM, Hoffman BB, Porshe RA, Blaschke TF. Decline in beta-adrenergic receptor-mediated vascular relaxation with aging in man. J Pharmacol Exp Ther 1986;239:802–7.

54. Hosmane BS, Maurath CJ, Jordan DC, Laddu A. Effect of age and dose on the incidence of adverse events in the treatment of hypertension in patients receiving terazosin. J Clin Pharmacol 1992;32:434–43.

55. Abernethy DR, Gutkowska J, Winterbottom LM. Effects of amlodipine, a long-acting dihydropyridine calcium antagonist in aging hypertension: Pharmacodynamics in relation to disposition. Clin Pharmacol Ther 1990;48:76–86.

56. Abernethy DR, Schwartz JB, Todd EL, Luchi R, Snow E. Verapamil pharmacodynamics and disposition in young versus elderly hypertensive patients. Ann Intern Med 1986;105:329–36.

57. Schwartz JB, Abernethy DR. Responses to intravenous and oral diltiazem in elderly versus younger patients with systemic hypertension. Am J Cardiol 1987;59:1111–7.

58. Verza M, Cacciapuoti F, Spiezia R, D'Avino M, Arpino G, D'Errico S, Sepe J, Varricchio M. Effects of the angiotensin converting enzyme inhibitor enalapril compared with diuretic therapy in elderly hypertensive patients. J Hypertens 1988;6(suppl 1):S97–9.

59. Crane MG, Harris JJ. Effect of aging on renin activity and aldosterone excretion. J Lab Clin Med 1976;87:947–59.

60. Hall JE, Coleman TG, Guyton AC. The renin-angiotensin system: Normal physiology and changes in older hypertensives. J Am Geriatr Soc 1989;37:801–13.

61. Agency for Health Care Policy and Research (AHCPR). Heart failure: Evaluation and treatment of patients with left ventricular systolic dysfunction. J Am Geriatr Soc 1998;46:525–9.

62. Lindeman RD. Overview: Renal physiology and pathophysiology of aging. Am J Kidney Dis 1990;26:275–82.

63. Miller M. Hyponatremia: Age-related risk factors and therapy decisions. Geriatrics 1998;53:32–48.

64. Rowe JW, Minaker KL, Levi M. Pathophysiology and management of electrolyte disturbances in the elderly. In: Martinez-Maldonado M, editor. Hypertension and renal disease in the elderly. Oxford:Blackwell Scientific Publications; 1992. p. 170–84.

65. Gurwitz JH, Avorn J, Ross-Degnan D, Lipsitz LA. Nonsteroidal antiinflammatory drug associated azotemia in the very old. JAMA 1990;264:471–5.

66. Field TS, Gurwitz JH, Glynn RJ, Salive ME, Gaziano JM Taylor JO, Hennekens CH. The renal effects of nonsteroidal anti-inflammatory drugs in older people: Findings from the Established Populations for Epidemiologic Studies of the Elderly. J Am Geriatr Soc 1999;47:507–11.

67. Whelton A, Schulman G, Wallemark C, Drower EJ, Isakson PC, Verburg KM, Geis S. Effects of celecoxib and naproxen on renal function in the elderly. Arch Intern Med 2000;160:1465–70.

68. Swan SK, Rudy DW, Lasseter KC, Ryan CF, Buechel KL, Lambrecht LJ, Pinto MB, Dilzer SC, Obrda O, Sundblad KJ, Gumbs CP, Ebel DL, Quan H, Larson PJ, Schwartz JI, Musliner TA, Gertz BJ, Brater DC, Yao S-L. Effect of cyclooxygenase-2 inhibition on renal function in elderly persons receiving a low salt diet. Ann Intern Med 2000;133:1–9.

69. Reardon LC, Macpherson DS. Hyperkalemia in outpatients using angiotensin-converting enzyme inhibitors. Arch Intern Med 1998;158:26–32.

70. Sunderam SG, Mankikar GD. Hyponatremia in the elderly. Age Ageing 1983;12:77–80.

71. Fichman M, Vorherr H, Kleeman G. Diuretic-induced hyponatremia. Ann Intern Med 1971;75:853–63.

72. Ashraf N, Locksley R, Arieff A. Thiazide-induced hyponatremia associated with death or neurologic damage in outpatients. Am J Med 1981;70:1163–8.

73. Shannon M, Lovejoy FH. The influence of age vs. peak serum concentration on life-threatening events after chronic theophylline intoxication. Arch Intern Med 1990;150:2045–8.

74. Schiff GD, Hedge HK, LaCloche L, Hryhoczuk DO. Inpatient theophylline toxicity: Preventable factors. Ann Intern Med 1991;114:748–53.

75. Kopanoff DE, Snider DE Jr, Caras GJ. Isoniazid-related hepatitis: A U.S. Public Health Service cooperative surveillance study. Am Rev Resp Dis 1979;117:991–1001.

76. American Thoracic Society. Treatment of tuberculosis and tuberculosis infection in adults and children. Am J Respir Crit Care Med 1994;149:1359–74.

77. Sorresso DJ, Mehta JB, Harvill LM, Bentley S. Underutilization of isoniazid chemoprophylaxis in tuberculosis contacts 50 year of age and older. A prospective analysis. Chest 1995;108:706–11.

78. American Thoracic Society. Targeted tuberculin testing and treatment of latent tuberculosis infection. MMWR Morb Mortal Wkly Rep 2000;49(No RR-6):1–51.

79. Gabriel SE, Jaakkimainen L, Bombardier C. Risk for serious gastrointestinal complications related to use of nonsteroidal anti-inflammatory drugs. Ann Intern Med 1991;115:787–96.

80. Cryer B, Lee E, Feldman M. Factors influencing gastroduodenal mucosal prostaglandin concentrations: Roles of smoking and aging. Ann Intern Med 1992;116:636–40.

25

Clinical Analysis of Adverse Drug Reactions

KARIM ANTON CALIS* AND LINDA R. YOUNG†

*Department of Pharmacy, NIH Clinical Center, National Institutes of Health, Bethesda, Maryland,
†Department of Pharmacy Practice and Pharmacoeconomics, University of Tennessee College of Pharmacy, Memphis, Tennessee

INTRODUCTION

Adverse drug reactions (ADRs) represent an important public health problem. Despite efforts to reduce the incidence of medication-related adverse events, morbidity and mortality from drug-induced disease continue to be unacceptably high. Furthermore, methods for ADR detection, evaluation, and monitoring remain inadequate. Although some ADRs are idiosyncratic and unpredictable, others can be anticipated based on knowledge of a medication's clinical pharmacology. In fact, an estimated 30 to 60% of ADRs may be preventable (1–5).

Regrettably, adverse reactions to medications are generally not well studied, and the mechanisms of some remain poorly described. The problem is further exacerbated by the inadequate training that clinicians receive in the basic principles of applied pharmacology and therapeutics. This chapter will focus on the clinical detection of ADRs and on factors that may increase ADR risk.

Epidemiology

Although some adverse drug reactions are minor and resolve without sequelae, others can cause permanent disability or death. ADRs occur commonly, but estimates of incidence vary considerably. This is due to substantial underreporting of ADRs and differences in study methodology, populations studied, and ADR definitions. Adverse drug reactions account for 2.9 to 15.4% of all hospital admissions in the United States (6, 7). The incidence may be highest in the elderly and other compromised populations. Nearly 16% of nursing home residents are hospitalized because of an ADR (8). A significant risk factor for hospitalization is the concomitant use of seven or more medications. ADRs are believed to be the fourth to sixth leading cause of death among hospitalized patients (1). A recent study suggests that an estimated 6.7% of hospitalized patients experience serious adverse drug reactions (defined as those requiring or prolonging hospitalization, are permanently disabling, or result in death) (1). Of 1133 drug-related adverse events reported in a study of more than 30,000 medical records, 19.4% were attributable to an adverse drug reaction (4). The incidence of ADRs in hospitalized HIV-infected patients was reported to be 20% (9). Up to 30% of patients may experience an ADR while hospitalized, of which 3% may be life-threatening, and most receive an average of nine drugs per hospitalization (10). Adverse drug reactions have been reported to increase the length of hospital stay by 2.2 to 4.6 days and to increase hospital costs by more than $2500 per event (11). The economic burden of ADRs has been estimated to be in the billions of dollars annually (12).

Definitions

An adverse drug event is any undesirable experience associated with the use of a medical product in a patient (13). This broad definition includes adverse drug reactions and other events (including medication errors) related to the prescribing, preparation, dispensing, or administration of medications. Karch and Lasagna (14) defined an ADR as any response to a drug that is noxious and unintended and that occurs at doses used in humans for prophylaxis, diagnosis, or therapy, excluding failure to accomplish the intended purpose. The World Health Organization (WHO) adopted a slightly modified version of this definition. According to WHO, an ADR is any response to a drug that is noxious and unintended and that occurs at doses normally used in humans for prophylaxis, diagnosis, or therapy of disease, or for the modification of physiological function (15). Both definitions are limited to reactions caused by medications and purposely exclude therapeutic failures, overdose, drug abuse, noncompliance, and medication errors. The U.S. Food and Drug Administration (FDA) defines an ADR as any undesirable experience associated with the use of a medical product in a patient (16). The FDA defines serious reactions as those that are life-threatening; require intervention to prevent permanent injury; or result in death, initial or prolonged hospitalization, disability, or congenital anomaly.

CLASSIFICATION

Adverse drug reactions can be classified simply according to their onset or severity. ADRs are occasionally classified as acute, sub-acute, or latent. Acute events are those observed within 60 minutes after the administration of a medication and include anaphylactic shock, severe bronchoconstriction, and nausea or vomiting (17). Sub-acute reactions occur within 1 to 24 hours and include maculopapular rash, serum sickness, allergic vasculitis, and antibiotic-associated diarrhea or colitis. Latent reactions require 2 or more days to become apparent and include eczematous eruptions, organ toxicity, and tardive dyskinesia.

ADRs can also be classified as mild, moderate, or severe. Mild reactions, such as dysguesia associated with clarithromycin, are bothersome but may not require a change in therapy. Moderate reactions, such as amphotericin B-induced hypokalemia, often require a change in therapy, additional treatment, or continued hospitalization. Reactions that are disabling or life-threatening, or those that considerably prolong hospitalization, are classified as severe (18).

The classification of Rawlins and Thompson is perhaps the most widely used to describe adverse drug reactions (19). Although this classification system continues to evolve, it serves a useful purpose. Adverse reactions are categorized as Type A or B. Type A reactions are those that extend directly from a drug's pharmacological effects. They are often predictable and dose-dependent and may account for up to two-thirds of all ADRs. Type A reactions also include adverse effects resulting from drug overdose and drug-drug interactions. Sedation caused by an antihistamine or hypotension caused by a beta-adrenergic antagonist are considered Type A reactions. Type B reactions are idiosyncratic or immunologic reactions that are often rare and unpredictable. Examples of Type B reactions include aplastic anemia caused by chloramphenicol or rash induced by beta-lactam antibiotics. Albeit not universally accepted, other authors have extended this classification system to include Types C, D, and E reactions to describe "chemical," delayed, and end-of-treatment reactions, respectively.

Gell and Coombs (20) developed a classification system (Types I through IV) to describe immune-mediated hypersensitivity reactions to medications (Figure 25.1). Immune system components such as intact skin, phagocytes, and complement act as constant barriers to foreign invasion. Lymphocytic and antibody activity are increased after repeated exposure to antigens. Drug molecules or metabolites act as antigens and induce the production of antibodies. Antibodies are produced if lymphocytes are able to recognize the antigenic determinants of foreign particles. Drugs may cause more than one of the four types of hypersensitivity reactions in this classification scheme. For example, as described in Chapter 15, reactions to penicillins can be classified under more than one type based on their clinical presentation and associated laboratory findings.

Type I reactions are IgE-mediated and cause manifestations of allergic symptoms due to the release of immune mediators such as histamine or leukotrienes. They typically occur within minutes of drug exposure and may manifest as generalized pruritus, urticaria, angioedema, anaphylaxis, rhinitis, or conjunctivitis (21). Anaphylaxis can result from exposure to any antigen (e.g., penicillin) and may be fatal in the absence of prompt medical intervention.

Type II reactions involve cytotoxic antibodies (IgG- or IgM-mediated) that react with antigens on the cell surface; the combination then causes cell damage due to the presence of neutrophils and monocytes or com-

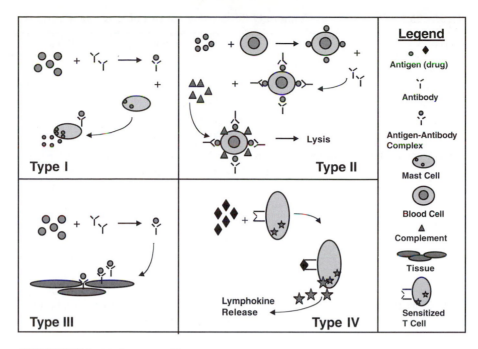

FIGURE 25.1 Mechanisms of hypersensitivity reactions. *Type I:* Antigens bind to antibodies on mast cells causing degranulation and release of histamine and other mediators. *Type II:* Antibodies attach to cell-surface antigens, causing activation of complement or other effector cells (neutrophils, K-lymphocytes, etc.) and resulting in cell damage and cell death. *Type III:* Antigen-antibody complexes are deposited in tissue. *Type IV:* T-cells are sensitized to a specific antigen thereby causing lymphokine release. (Reproduced with permission from Young LR, Wurtzbacher JD, Blankenship CS. Am J Manag Care 1997;3:1884–906.)

plement-induced cell lysis. Examples of Type II reactions are the hemolytic anemias caused by methyldopa or quinine. Acute graft rejection is another Type II hypersensitivity reaction.

Type III reactions are caused by tissue injury due to immune complexes. The antigen-antibody complexes are usually cleared by the immune system; however, repeated contact with antigens can cause the complex to deposit in tissue and result in tissue injury. Serum sickness is the classic example of a Type III reaction. Medications associated with serum sickness include many antibiotics, phenytoin, salicylates, barbiturates, nonsteroidal antiinflammatory drugs, isoniazid, antisera, hydralazine, captopril, and sulfonamides. Procainamide-induced lupus, described in Chapter 15, is also considered a Type III reaction.

Type IV reactions occur when T-cells bind to a specific antigen, thereby causing the release of cytokines. The onset of these reactions may be delayed by more than 12 hours. Topical application of drugs may result in allergic contact dermatitis and photosensitivity. These reactions typically manifest initially as a skin rash and may become systemic on subsequent exposure to the antigen.

CLINICAL DETECTION OF ADRS

Adverse reactions can result from the use of drugs, diagnostic agents, biologicals (including vaccines), nutrients, fluids, electrolytes, and complementary or alternative products. Adverse effects may be attributable to the parent compound, a metabolite, a pharmaceutical excipient, or even a component of the drug delivery system. Occasionally, more than one agent may be involved. Adverse drug reactions, whether expected or not, occur with nearly all medications and have been observed regardless of route or mode of administration. The drug classes most commonly associated with ADRs are listed in Table 25.1.

Some ADRs are caused by most or all medications in a class, while others are agent specific. Nausea, vomiting, and diarrhea have been observed with most antibiotics, yet only chloramphenicol and certain sulfonamide antibiotics have been consistently implicated as causes of aplastic anemia. Some pharmacological effects such as sedation from an antihistamine may be considered adverse effects when they are not intended, but desired effects when they are prescribed

TABLE 25.1   Drug Classes Commonly Reported as Causes of Adverse Reactions

Drug class	Examples of reported adverse reactions
Antimicrobial agents	Diarrhea, rash, pruritus
Antineoplastics	Bone marrow suppression, alopecia, nausea and vomiting
Anticoagulants	Hemorrhage, bruising
Cardiovascular drugs	Heart block, arrhythmias, edema
Antihyperglycemics	Hypoglycemia, diarrhea, gastrointestinal discomfort
Nonsteroidal antiinflammatory drugs	Gastrointestinal ulceration and bleeding, renal insufficiency
Opiate analgesics	Sedation, dizziness, constipation
Diuretics	Hypokalemia, hyperuricemia, hyperglycemia
Diagnostic agents	Hypotension, nephrotoxicity, allergic reactions
Central nervous system agents	Dizziness, drowsiness, headache, hallucination, neuroleptic malignant syndrome, serotonin syndrome

specifically for an indication for which they may be beneficial (e.g., sleeping aid). Several body systems are commonly affected by ADRs and few are spared (Table 25.2). Adverse effects range from nonspecific symptoms to organ-specific toxicity that can be confirmed objectively. Certain medications are widely recognized for selectively targeting specific organs or body systems. For example, the aminoglycoside antibiotics are known to cause nephrotoxicity and ototoxicity; most antineoplastics produce predictable bone marrow suppression, and bleomycin and bulsulfan cause pulmonary fibrosis.

Drug metabolites have been implicated in the pathogenesis of some adverse drug reactions. This is diagrammed in Figure 15.4. The specific chemical mechanisms of adverse reactions involving drug metabolites are described in Chapters 11 and 15.

Herbal products have been identified as a source of serious adverse reactions and interactions (22). Since the passage of the Dietary Supplements Health and Education Act of 1994 (DSHEA), the use of herbal and dietary supplements has increased dramatically in the United States.

Pharmaceutical excipients and drug delivery systems have also been associated with severe allergic and nonallergic adverse reactions (23–25). Excipients are pharmacologically inert substances that include binders, fillers, coloring agents, buffers, lubricants,

TABLE 25.2   Body Systems Commonly Affected by Adverse Drug Reactions

Body system	Examples of reported adverse reactions
Central nervous system	Anxiety, depression, extrapyramidal reactions, ataxia, hyperactivity, insomnia, malaise, pain, vertigo, dystonia, asthenia, seizures
Cardiovascular	Angina, arrhythmias, palpitations, congestive heart failure, syncope, hemorrhage, thrombosis, embolism
Endocrine	Gynecomastia, hypothyroidism, adrenal suppression
Gastrointestinal and hepatic	Gastritis, dyspepsia, dysphagia, colitis, anorexia, hematemesis, pancreatitis, ascites, jaundice, hepatitis
Renal and genitourinary	Vaginitis, hematuria, dysmenorrhea, proteinuria, urinary retention, interstitial nephritis
Hematologic	Blood dyscrasias, anemias, thrombocytopenia
Dermatologic	Pruritus, urticaria, alopecia, bruising, purpura, rash, petechiae
Metabolic	Osteoporosis, fluid, electrolyte, and acid-base disorders
Musculoskeletal	Myalgia, arthralgia, neuropathy, rhabdomyolysis
Respiratory	Bronchospasm, allergic rhinitis, dyspnea, respiratory depression, pulmonary fibrosis, epistaxis, hemoptysis
Sensory	Dysgeusia, impaired vision, ototoxicity, tinnitus, diplopia

detergents, emulsifiers, flavors, solvents, adsorbants, aerosol propellants, stabilizers, and sweeteners. Some of the adverse effects are mild and self-limiting. Lactose in some products may be associated with gastrointestinal complaints and diarrhea in lactose-intolerant patients. Sorbitol-containing liquid preparations can also cause diarrhea. Examples of excipients found to cause morbidity or mortality include the sulfite preservatives, the coloring agent tartrazine, and the polyoxyethylated castor oils (Cremophor®) used as emulsifiers in parenteral products. Para-amino benzoic acid (PABA) and PABA derivatives have been associated with severe allergic reactions. The first major drug-related tragedy in U.S. history was caused by the solvent diethylene glycol found in a formulation of the oral antibiotic sulfanilamide. Exposure to this substance resulted in more than 100 deaths and led to passage of the Food and Drug Act of 1938. Occasionally, even drug formulations themselves have been reported to cause adverse effects. Gastrointestinal irritation, bezoars, and intestinal obstruction have been reported as a result of drug formulations that do not disintegrate or dissolve properly.

Components of drug delivery systems have also been associated with severe reactions. Reports of latex allergy continue to increase as more health care workers are exposed to medical devices that contain this substance, including protective gloves. Incidence of latex sensitization ranges from 1 to 6% of the general population and about 8 to 12% of continuously exposed health care workers (26, 27). Leaching of the plasticizer di-2-ethylhexylphthalate (DEHP) from intravenous drug delivery systems has also been associated with toxicity, particularly in susceptible individuals exposed for long periods.

Risk Factors

Factors believed to contribute to the high incidence of adverse reactions were outlined in Chapter 1. Since many adverse reactions are predictable, recognition and understanding of potential risk factors may be the most critical steps in ADR prevention. Table 25.3 lists the primary ADR risk factors.

Concurrent use of multiple medications is a major ADR risk factor. The potential for clinically significant drug interactions and additive adverse effects increases as the number of medications in a regimen increases (28, 29). In a study of over 9000 hospital admissions, the strongest predictor of ADRs was the large number of concurrent prescription medications (OR = 2.94) (30). Irrational prescribing, inappropriate use, or insufficient monitoring of medications can predispose to adverse outcomes. To minimize the inci-

TABLE 25.3   ADR Risk Factors

Concurrent use of multiple medications

Multiple co-morbid conditions

Drug dose and duration of exposure

Extremes of age (neonates, children, and elderly)

Female sex

Genetic predisposition

Prior history of drug reactions and hypersensitivity

End-organ dysfunction

Altered physiology

Inappropriate medication prescribing, use, or monitoring

Lack of patient education and other system failures

---

dence of adverse reactions, each medication must have a clear indication, and specific therapeutic and toxic endpoints should be established prior to the start of treatment. Factors that contribute to polypharmacy include increasing age, multiple medical conditions, overprescribing, multiple medical providers, absence of a primary care provider, use of multiple pharmacies, frequent drug regimen changes, hoarding of medications, and self-treatment (31). Polypharmacy is of particular concern in the elderly because they are already susceptible to ADRs. Elderly patients often suffer disproportionately from various acute and chronic illnesses and are likely to require more medications (31). They are also more likely than their younger counterparts to have impaired CNS function and to not adhere to the prescribed regimen. Elderly patients in the community use an average of three prescription and nonprescription medications, while those in nursing homes receive an average of five to eight prescription drugs at the same time (32). Patient education and ongoing medication regimen review can minimize the problem of polypharmacy.

The presence of multiple co-morbid conditions (e.g., diabetes, asthma, congestive heart failure, obesity) further increases the risk of ADRs. Such patients may have altered physiology and some degree of end-organ dysfunction (e.g., renal, hepatic, cardiovascular, pulmonary). Conditions such as renal dysfunction may not be readily apparent in the elderly or in those with muscle wasting or malnutrition.

The extent and duration of drug exposure can also predispose to toxicity. This is particularly true for patients with end-organ dysfunction. An estimated 70 to 80% of adverse drug reactions may be dose related (33). Not surprisingly, the medications most commonly associated with adverse reactions are those with narrow therapeutic indices such as digoxin, warfarin, heparin, theophylline, aminoglycosides, and anticonvulsants (34).

Age may be an important risk factor for the development of ADRs, and young children and the elderly may be particularly vulnerable. Despite this risk, documentation of ADRs in these groups is poor, and adverse reactions are often attributed to nondrug causes. Moreover, there is often inadequate experience with medications in these populations because they are often excluded from clinical trials (35).

The incidence of ADRs increases with increasing age (30). In addition to the increased risk posed by polypharmacy and co-morbid conditions, there are important age-related changes in the pharmacokinetic disposition of a number of medications in the elderly (see Chapter 24). Although drug absorption is least likely to be affected, drug distribution, metabolism, and elimination are often altered (36). Age-related decreases in renal function are probably most important. However, changes in body composition, particularly the relative increase in adipose tissue that occurs with aging, may increase the distribution volume of lipid soluble medications, thereby prolonging their half-life and altering peak and trough plasma concentrations. For example, the increased distribution volume of benzodiazepines in elderly patients results in lowered peak and raised trough plasma concentrations after a dose of these drugs. The net effect in the elderly is that these drugs have a reduced efficacy in inducing sleep and an exacerbated posthypnotic hangover effect. Pharmacodynamic changes may also be affected by age, but are not consistently predictable. In general, elderly patients may be more sensitive to the effects of many medications and often require lower initial dosages (32).

Children of all ages also may be particularly susceptible to adverse drug reactions. In a surveillance study of over 10,000 pediatric admissions to several hospitals, 0.2% of admissions to the neonatal intensive care unit were caused by ADRs (37). Twenty-two percent of children with cancer were hospitalized as a result of ADRs. Among all other pediatric admissions studied, 2% were possibly or probably due to ADRs. The drugs most frequently implicated were phenobarbital, aspirin, phenytoin, ampicillin or amoxicillin, theophylline or aminophylline, trimethoprim-sulfamethoxazole, and diphtheria-pertussis-tetanus vaccine. Dosages of some medications begun in childhood (e.g., antiasthmatics, antiepileptics, stimulants, and insulin) may require careful adjustment during adolescence to minimize the risk of ADRs (40). Changes in body weight, drug distribution, and drug clearance can influence drug disposition and affect dosing.

As emphasized in Chapter 23, neonates are especially vulnerable to ADRs because they are sometimes exposed to drugs before birth and have immature renal and hepatic drug clearance capacities. Additionally, there is insufficient information on the clinical pharmacology of many drugs in this age group to guide rational pharmacotherapy (38, 39).

As described in Chapter 21, women appear to be at greater risk for ADRs than men (41–43). Data from the Glaxo Wellcome-Sunnybrook Drug Safety Clinic gathered over a 10-year period suggest that women over 18 years of age experience more ADRs than their age-matched male counterparts (44). More than 77% of all ADRs, including those classified as severe, were reported in women. A recent cohort study evaluating the adverse-event experience with 48 newly marketed drugs in the United Kingdom revealed an incidence per 10,000 patients of 12.9 ADRs in males and 20.6 in females (42). Females over the age of 19 were 43 to 69% more likely than males to experience a suspected ADR. Sex differences in pharmacokinetics and pharmacodynamics, differences in circulating hormone concentrations, and more frequent use of medications that inhibit hepatic metabolism are all cited as possible explanations for the observed differences (43). Women may also use more medications and are more likely to report adverse effects (43). Historically, women have been underrepresented in clinical trials, but this imbalance is reversing as regulations on their participation have changed (41).

Race and ethnicity may also be risk factors for ADRs. Prior personal or family history of ADRs may be predictive of future adverse reactions. Genetic polymorphisms for many metabolic reactions are described in Chapter 13 and have been well documented (45). Prescribing some medications without regard to genetic differences in metabolism can result in therapeutic failures or drug toxicity (45, 46). For example, differences in acetylator phenotype can alter the metabolism of some drugs and influence the risk of certain adverse reactions. Slow acetylators, for example, may be more likely than rapid acetylators to develop hepatotoxicity from isoniazid treatment. The biochemical basis for this difference is described in Chapter 15.

Genetic differences can also influence the likelihood of some drug interactions. For example, co-administration of the antiarrhythmic propafenone to patients being treated with metoprolol substantially reduces metoprolol metabolic clearance in extensive CYP2D6 metabolizers, thereby resulting in exaggerated β-adrenoreceptor blockade and possibly precipitating congestive heart failure, nightmares, and blurred vision. This interaction essentially converts extensive

CYP2D6 metabolizers to poor metabolizers, a phenomenon termed phenocopying, but does not impair metoprolol metabolism in poor metabolizers (45, 47).

Detection Methods

ADRs are sometimes not recognized and often go unreported. In fact, the principal limitation of ADR detection methods is the lack of awareness of what constitutes an ADR. Most ADRs are brought to medical attention by subjective reports and patient complaints. Linkage of a drug with an ADR is most often suspected on the basis of temporal association, but more objective confirmatory evidence is often lacking. Additionally, there are perceived barriers to reporting ADRs, and some clinicians fear that reporting suspected ADRs may expose them to liability. Moreover, many clinicians often fail to attribute new signs or symptoms or changes in laboratory tests or diagnostic studies to drug therapy. Medications should be carefully screened and systematically ruled out as possible causes of any abnormal finding on physical examination or from laboratory tests or diagnostic procedures

Given the perceived failure of spontaneous reporting systems and the paucity of ADR reports, some institutions have instituted more active methods of ADR detection to supplement spontaneous reports. Medication order screening has become a common practice in U.S. hospitals. Manual chart reviews and audits and computer programs are used for retrospective, concurrent, and prospective medication utilization evaluation. Certain events often prompt an evaluation of a suspected adverse reaction. These include abrupt discontinuation of a medication, abrupt dosage reduction, orders for antidotes and emergency medications, orders for special tests or serum drug concentrations, and abnormal results from laboratory tests and medical procedures.

Spontaneous reports to the FDA and drug manufacturers, post-marketing surveillance, and data from ongoing observational studies and clinical trials provide other means for detecting important ADRs that may have not been detected during drug development.

Clinical Evaluation

Clinical evaluation of adverse drug reactions requires careful assessment of the patient and evaluation of pertinent factors. The patient's clinical status and severity of the reaction should be determined promptly in order to fully characterize the event and plan the optimal initial course of action. After obtaining a detailed description of the event, a differential diagnosis can be formulated that considers alternative etiologies. Alternative explanations for the adverse findings (e.g., nondrug causes, exacerbation of preexisting condition, laboratory error) should be carefully evaluated, based on the characteristics of all clinical signs and symptoms. These include severity, extent, temporal factors (onset, duration, frequency), presence of palliative or provoking factors, quality (character or intensity), response to treatment, and other associated findings.

A medical history (including a systematic review of body systems) and a physical examination should be obtained, along with relevant laboratory tests and diagnostic procedures. Relevant patient factors should be noted, including age, race, ethnicity, sex, height, weight, and body composition. Concurrent medical conditions or other factors should be considered that may cause, aggravate, or even mask or confound the manifestations of the reaction. These include such conditions as dehydration, autoimmune disorders, end-organ dysfunction, malnutrition, HIV infection, or pregnancy. Recent invasive medical procedures, treatments (e.g., dialysis), or surgery and any resultant complications (e.g., hypotension, shock, infection) should also be noted. Exposure to contrast material, radiation, or environmental or occupational hazards, and use of tobacco, caffeine, alcohol, and illicit substances should be investigated.

Because of the importance of drug interactions (see Chapter 14), a detailed medication history should be recorded that identifies all prescription, nonprescription, and alternative or complementary medications used by the patient. In addition to medication dosage, other factors that may contribute to the development of adverse reactions include medication administration route, method, site, schedule, rate, and duration. A history of allergies, intolerances, and other medication reactions should be fully investigated. The potential for cross-allergenicity or cross-reactivity should not be overlooked. The possibility of drug-induced laboratory test interference (analytical or physiological) and drug-drug or drug-nutrient interactions should also be explored.

Management of specific adverse reactions is beyond the scope of this chapter. However, it is intuitive that the offending agent should be discontinued if the event is life-threatening or intolerable to the patient, especially when a reasonable alternative exists (48). Palliative and supportive care (e.g., hydration, glucocorticoids, or compresses) may be necessary for management of some adverse reactions. In some cases, specific reversal agents or antidotes are also needed (e.g., flumazenil for benzodiazepines, naloxone for opioids, and protamine for heparin).

Some medications should not be stopped abruptly, and gradual dosage reduction may obviate rebound effects or other complications. In some circumstances, rechallenge with the suspected medication or desensitization may be warranted. Because some adverse reactions are delayed or may have an unpredictable course, careful monitoring and reevaluation are essential.

Causality Assessment

It is often challenging to establish a cause-and-effect relationship between a drug and a specific adverse reaction. This is especially true when appropriate ADR information is incomplete, inconsistent, or altogether lacking. Additional confounding factors include co-administration of other medications, nondrug variables, and concurrent illnesses.

Several methods used to determine causality have been described and compared (49–52). The Naranjo algorithm, perhaps the most commonly accepted causality assessment instrument, is presented in Table

25.4 (53). Most methods of causality evaluation emphasize reproducibility and validity of the data. Reproducibility depends on the precision of the instrument and thereby affects its reliability. Lack of reproducibility results from random error. Reproducibility is achieved when inter- and intraobserver variability are small, or when agreement between observations is high (54, 55). Validity is the extent to which a test accurately measures what it was designed to measure. Lack of validity most often results from experimental error. Validity of a test can be evaluated by measuring its sensitivity and specificity. This is difficult to establish when a gold standard is absent—as is often the case in ADR assessment (54, 55). Causality assessment instruments attempt to quantify information about adverse drug reactions and determine the probability that an ADR was caused by a specific medication. The presence of some or all of the elements listed in Table 25.5 increases the probability of drug culpability in association with an ADR.

A chronological or temporal relationship between the administration of a drug and the development of

---

TABLE 25.4   Naranjo ADR Probability Scale[a]

To assess the adverse drug reaction, please answer the following questionnaire and give the pertinent score

	Yes	No	Do not know	Score
1. Are there previous *conclusive* reports on this reaction?	+1	0	0	____
2. Did the adverse event appear after the suspected drug was administered?	+2	−1	0	____
3. Did the adverse reaction improve when the drug was discontinued or a *specific* antagonist was administered?	+1	0	0	____
4. Did the adverse reactions appear when the drug was readministered?	+2	−1	0	____
5. Are there alternative causes (other than the drug) that could on their own have caused the reaction?	−1	+2	0	____
6. Did the reaction reappear when a placebo was given?	−1	+1	0	____
7. Was the drug detected in the blood (or other fluids) in concentrations known to be toxic?	+1	0	0	____
8. Was the reaction more severe when the dose was increased, or less severe when the dose was decreased?	+1	0	0	____
9. Did the patient have a similar reaction to the same or similar drugs in *any* previous exposure?	+1	0	0	____
10. Was the adverse event confirmed by any objective evidence?	+1	0	0	____
			Total score	____

ADR probability classification based on total score

9	Highly probable
5–8	Probable
1–4	Possible
0	Doubtful

[a] Reproduced with permission from Naranjo CA, Busto U, Sellers EM, Sandor P, Ruiz I, Roberts EA, et al. Clin Pharmacol Ther 1981;30:239–45.

TABLE 25.5   Clinical Evidence Suggestive of Causality

Temporal relationship

Positive dechallenge

Positive rechallenge

Dose-response relationship

Biological plausibility

Absence of alternative etiologies

Objective confirmation

Prior reports of reaction

Past history of reaction to same or related medication

an adverse reaction is essential for establishing causality. The time to onset of reaction must be plausibly related to the administration of the drug. However, because some reactions may not appear for weeks or months after the start of therapy with a medication, they may be erroneously implicated as the cause of the reaction. The presence or absence of alternative etiologies and confounding variables also must be investigated (49, 56). A history of the reaction in a patient receiving the same drug or a similar compound increases the possibility that the association may be causal, and prior reports of similar reactions lend credibility to a cause-and-effect relationship. The absence of prior reports decreases the likelihood but does not eliminate the possibility that the reaction is due to the medication in question. If a precedent cannot be found, the plausibility of the reaction should be based on a consideration of the known clinical pharmacology of the drug (56). Further evidence to support an assertion of drug culpability requires objective data such as abnormally high serum drug concentrations, specific physical examination findings, or other laboratory or diagnostic data characteristic of a drug reaction.

A positive dechallenge (i.e., when a reaction resolves after a drug is discontinued or a specific antagonist is administered) suggests that the medication may be culpable. A positive rechallenge (i.e., when signs or symptoms of the reaction recur after the drug is readministered) provides even more convincing evidence linking the drug to the reaction, but may not be ethically permissible and clinically justifiable. In any case, rechallenge should be done only after dechallenge is complete and signs and symptoms of the reaction have completely abated (57). The probability of a cause-and-effect relationship is further strengthened if the reaction worsens when a higher dose of the medication is administered. To further evaluate the probability of a drug-induced effect,

Naranjo (58) suggests that a placebo challenge be considered.

Reporting Requirements

Documentation and reporting of adverse events are critical steps in the effort to prevent ADRs. Adverse reactions should be clearly described and documented in the medical record. This is mandated by the Joint Commission on Accreditation of Healthcare Organizations (JCAHO) as a method for preventing serious adverse reactions from reexposure to a medication to which a patient may be allergic or intolerant. Most adverse reactions, however, are not properly documented or reported. Despite the importance of spontaneous adverse drug reaction reporting, it is estimated that only one in 10 serious adverse drug reactions is reported to the Food and Drug Administration (FDA). Given the large number of drug prescriptions written each year in the United States, this figure most likely overestimates the number of reports.

The reason most often cited for the lack of adverse event reporting is uncertainty about the causality of an adverse reaction. Although confirmation of an ADR is ideal, it is often not feasible. The FDA readily acknowledges this limitation and continues to encourage the reporting of all *suspected* adverse drug reactions through its MedWatch program. Detailed instructions for reporting adverse events associated with drugs, medical devices, vaccines, and veterinary products can be found at the following URL: http://www.fda.gov/medwatch/report/hcp.htm. The essential components of an ADR report are listed in Table 25.6. The FDA is particularly interested in

TABLE 25.6   Essential Components of an ADR Report

Patient demographics

Suspected product's name and manufacturer

Relevant history and preexisting medical conditions

Other medications or treatments

Detailed description of the adverse event and its management

    Date of onset

      Dates and times that suspected drug was started and stopped

      Dose, frequency, and route/method of drug administration

Outcome of event (e.g., death, disability, prolonged hospitalization)

Relevant laboratory tests or diagnostic findings

Information regarding dechallenge and rechallenge

Presence of confounding variables

Other objective evidence (e.g. reports of similar ADRs)

receiving reports of adverse reactions involving new chemical entities and serious reactions involving any medical product.

Adverse drug reaction data are largely drawn from spontaneous reports to the FDA or pharmaceutical manufacturers, post-marketing surveillance studies, and published case reports or case series. These sources are critical for identifying ADRs that are not detected or clearly characterized during preregistration clinical trials. ADRs are least likely to be detected when they have a low incidence, when drug exposure is minimal or infrequent, when the ADR manifestation or effect has a high background frequency (e.g., common symptom due to causes other than the medication), and when a time or dose relationship are weak or absent (59).

Pharmaceutical manufacturers are required to report serious adverse drug events to the FDA within 15 days of receiving a report. All other reports are submitted on a quarterly basis for the first three years after marketing and annually thereafter. Reports of serious adverse reactions, either during clinical trials or after drug marketing, occasionally result in FDA-mandated inclusion of black box warnings in the product label. These warnings usually are drug specific, but occasionally pertain to an entire pharmacological class of medications. New data relating to drug safety and efficacy also sometimes prompt the FDA to require pharmaceutical manufacturers to disseminate "dear doctor" letters to alert healthcare providers of findings that have the potential for substantial impact on public health. These and other safety notifications can be accessed at the following URL: http://www.fda.gov/medwatch/safety.htm.

ADR DETECTION IN CLINICAL TRIALS

Methodology

Detection of adverse reactions during clinical trials requires careful and systematic evaluation of study participants before, during, and after drug exposure. Objective data must be gathered to determine that study subjects meet all inclusion criteria and do not have any conditions that preclude their participation. Standard laboratory and diagnostic tests are used to establish patients' baseline health and functional status. Such tests should be appropriate for the drug and condition under investigation and should be conducted at predetermined intervals. Typically, serum chemistries and renal, hepatic, hematologic, electrolyte, and mineral panels are included. A complete

medical history (including a review of all body systems) and physical examination and a complete medication history (including allergies and intolerances) should be included. Use of prescription, nonprescription, and alternative and complementary medications by study participants should be specifically documented.

Study protocols should clearly outline how adverse events will be detected, managed, and reported. Study data should be entered on case report forms designed for the study, and a quality-control mechanism for ensuring the accuracy and integrity of the data should be established prior to the start of data collection. Computerized record keeping (i.e., electronic case report forms) can facilitate audits, data management, and data analysis. Adverse drug event questionnaires using extensive checklists of symptoms organized by body system have been developed for use in clinical trials (60). These are typically administered at baseline and at predetermined intervals during and after a study. To increase their utility and allow for comparisons between treatment groups, the questionnaires should be administered by a blinded investigator. Since healthy individuals who are free of illness and not taking medications can occasionally experience symptoms similar to those reported as drug side effects, adequate controls must be used in studies examining adverse drug reactions (61). Comprehensive questionnaires increase the likelihood that patient interviews are conducted in a consistent and nonsuperficial manner. Moreover, they minimize the risk of bias (particularly from focusing on known adverse effects) and can be useful for inter- and intrasubject comparisons. Of course, study participants should be encouraged to report all serious, unexpected, or bothersome symptoms, especially those that persist or require some treatment or intervention.

Toxicity criteria developed by the World Health Organization (WHO) and the National Cancer Institute (NCI) provide guidelines for objectively and systematically categorizing adverse effects according to type and severity grade. NCI's Common Toxicity Criteria (CTC) are particularly useful for studies involving antineoplastic drugs, but are equally applicable to other drug categories. The CTC organizes related adverse events alphabetically according to body system or disease. For example, the "endocrine" category includes specific adverse effects such as gynecomastia and hypothyroidism. Specific criteria are provided for grading the severity of each adverse effect. The CTC can be accessed at the following URL: http://ctep.info.nih.gov/CTC3/default.htm.

Limitations

Despite attempts to screen candidate drugs during the early stages of preclinical development and identify all serious adverse effects during the course of pre-registration clinical trials, some drugs are approved for marketing that later are found to pose unacceptable public health risks. This is not altogether surprising given the limitations of subject enrollment and duration of therapy during the clinical development of new drugs. Given these and other constraints, rare and unusual ADRs often cannot be detected before marketing approval is granted. Uncommon adverse reactions (e.g., those affecting 0.2% of patients or fewer) frequently will not be detected during clinical development (51). For example, it has been estimated that 3000 patients at risk must be studied in order to have 95% certainty in detecting an ADR with an incidence of 1/1000 (62). Given that most drugs are approved despite limited experience in human subjects, a drug such as chloramphenicol, which causes aplastic anemia with an incidence of 1 in 20,000 or less, would likely be approved today without realizing its potential to induce blood dyscrasias.

Even under optimal conditions, some ADRs will not be detected because drug exposure may be limited (i.e., short-term studies). Also, some latent ADRs may go undetected because of superficial monitoring or insufficient follow-up. Occasionally, ADRs may not be detected readily because they manifest slowly and exhibit symptoms that closely resemble those of the underlying condition for which the drug was being used. An example of this is the severe mitochondrial damage and subsequent hepatic injury induced by the synthetic nucleoside analog fialuridine (FIAU) that was being investigated for the treatment of hepatitis B infection (63).

Not only are study participants too few in number to detect uncommon ADRs, but typically they are not representative of the population at large that is likely be exposed to the medication in routine clinical use. Many studies have traditionally excluded children, the elderly, women of childbearing age, and patients with severe forms of the target disease. Moreover, patients with multiple co-morbidities and those taking potentially interacting medications are often not included. It is, therefore, not surprising that even well-designed and impeccably conducted studies yield results that often are not generalizable.

Reporting Requirements

All experimental studies involving human subjects require the approval of an institutional review board (IRB) and ongoing review of study progress. The IRB is specifically charged with the responsibility of safeguarding the rights and welfare of human research subjects. In many cases, the study is monitored by a data and safety monitoring board (DSMB) in cooperation with the IRB. The DSMB reviews all reports of adverse reactions and conducts interim analyses of the data to ensure that study participants are not subjected to excessive risks or denied treatment with an effective medication if one arm of a study is found to be superior to another. Drugs being studied under an investigational new drug application (IND) must conform to criteria set forth by the FDA. Under these criteria, all adverse events must be promptly reported to the FDA, the IRB, and the drug sponsor. Serious adverse events (as defined earlier in this chapter) must be reported within 15 calendar days—7 days if they are life-threatening or result in death. This reporting requirement cannot be waived even if causality (relationship of the event to the research) has not been clearly established. Serious unexpected adverse events (those not described in the approved product label or the investigators' brochure for investigational new drugs) require particular attention.

INFORMATION SOURCES

Information regarding adverse effects of medications is available from many sources and in multiple formats (i.e., print, CD-ROM, online). Table 25.7 lists selected sources of ADR information. To assist in ADR detection, evaluation, and management, critical data regarding adverse reactions are needed (Table 25.8).

This information may be gleaned from specialized ADR resources, texts, and other tertiary sources, including the FDA-approved product label. However, this information must often be augmented using additional data from secondary sources. At minimum, this should include searches of the bibliographic databases from the National Library of Medicine (Medline and Toxline) and Excerpta Medica (Embase).

Primary reports describing adverse reactions and drug-induced diseases include spontaneous reports and other unpublished data available from the manufacturer or the FDA. All reports of adverse reactions reported to the FDA can be retrieved (without identifiers) under the legal authority of the Freedom of Information Act. Anecdotal and descriptive reports of ADRs (including case reports and case series) are occasionally reported in the literature, but are often incomplete and inconclusive. Guidelines for evaluat-

TABLE 25.7   Selected Sources of ADR Information

Tertiary sources	Secondary sources	Primary sources

General drug reference books (e.g., AHFS Drug Information, USP DI Drug Information for the Health Care Professional, Mosby's GenRx, and the Physicians' Desk Reference)	MEDLARS databases (e.g., MEDLINE, TOXLINE, CANCERLIT)
	
	Excerpta Medica (EMBASE)
	
	International Pharmaceutical Abstracts
		Spontaneous reports or unpublished experience
		  Individual clinicians
		  FDA
		  Manufacturer

Medical and pharmacotherapy textbooks	Current Contents	Anecdotal and descriptive reports
		  Case reports
		  Case series

Specialized resources pertaining to ADRs and drug-induced diseases (e.g., Meyler's Side Effects of Drugs, Davies's Textbook of Adverse Drug Reactions)	Biological Abstracts (BIOSIS)
	
	Science Citation Index
		Observational studies
		  Case-control
		  Cross-sectional
		  Cohort

Drug interactions resources (e.g., Drug Interaction Facts, Drug Interactions Analysis and Management, Evaluation of Drug Interacations)	Clin-Alert
	
	Reactions
	
	Cochrane Library
		Experimental and other study designs
		  Clinical trials
		  Meta-analyses

Micromedex databases (e.g., TOMES DRUGDEX, POISINDEX)		
Review articles pertaining to individual ADRs or drug-induced diseases		

ing adverse drug reaction reports have been described (56).

Observational studies, including case-control, cross-sectional, and cohort studies do not establish causality but can reveal associations of risk—the strength of which is measured by relative risk (cohort studies) or odds ratio. Design flaws and bias, however, occasionally render these studies altogether unreliable. Record-linkage studies using large prescription and medical data bases are increasingly being used to gather data regarding ADRs (56, 59). Because they often include information from hundreds of thousands of patient records, well-designed linkage studies have the potential to generate robust epidemiological data. Prospective, randomized, controlled experimental studies (i.e., clinical trials) also can establish causality. These, along with well-designed meta-analyses, are useful for identifying and quantifying certain types of adverse effects. Nonetheless, even these study designs have their limitations.

TABLE 25.8   Essential Elements for Characterizing ADRs

Incidence and prevalence

Mechanism and pathogenesis

Clinical presentation and diagnosis

Time course

Dose relationship

Reversibility

Cross-reactivity/cross-allergenicity

Treatment and prognosis

References

1. Lazarou J, Pomeranz BH, Corey PN. Incidence of adverse drug reactions in hospitalized patients. JAMA 1998;279:1200–5.
2. Dartnell JG, Anderson RP, Chohan V, Galbraith KJ, Lyon ME, Nestor PJ, et al. Hospitalisation for adverse events related to drug therapy: Incidence, avoidability and costs. Med J Aust 1996;164:659–62.
3. Bates DW, Cullen DJ, Laird N, Petersen LA, Small SD, Servi D, et al. Incidence of adverse drug events and potential adverse drug events. Implications for prevention. ADE Prevention Study Group. JAMA 1995;274:29–34.
4. Leape LL, Brennan TA, Laird N, Lawthers AG, Localio AR, Barnes BA, et al. The nature of adverse events in hospitalized patients. Results of the Harvard Medical Practice Study II. N Engl J Med 1991;324:377–84.
5. Shumock GT, Thornton JP, Witte WK. Comparison of pharmacy-based concurrent surveillance and medical record retrospective reporting of adverse drug reactions. Am J Hosp Pharm 1991;48:1974–6.
6. Beard K. Adverse reactions as a cause of hospital admission in the aged. Drugs Aging 1992;2:356–67.
7. Prince BS, Goetz CM, Rihn TL, Olsky M. Drug-related emergency department visits and hospital admissions. Am J Hosp Pharm 1992;49:1696–700.
8. Cooper JW. Adverse drug reaction-related hospitalizations of nursing facility patients: A 4-year study. South Med J 1999;92:485–90.
9. Harb G, Alldredge B, Coleman R, Jacobson M. Pharmacoepidemiology of adverse drug reactions in hospitalized patients

with human immunodeficiency virus disease. J Acquir Immune Defic Syndr 1993;6:919–26.

10. Jick H. Adverse drug reactions: the magnitude of the problem. J Allergy Clin Immunol 1984;74:555–7.

11. Bates DW, Spell N, Cullen DJ, Burdick E, Laird N, Petersen LA, et al. The costs of adverse drug events in hospitalized patients. Adverse Drug Events Prevention Study Group. JAMA 1997;277:307–11.

12. Johnson JA, Bootman JL. Drug-related morbidity and mortality: A cost-of-illness model. Arch Intern Med 1995;155:1949–56.

13. Leape LL. Preventing adverse drug events. Am J Health-Syst Pharm 1995;52:379–82.

14. Karch FE, Lasagna L. Adverse drug reactions. A critical review. JAMA 1975;234:1236–41.

15. Anon. ASHP guidelines on adverse drug reaction monitoring and reporting. Am J Hosp Pharm 1989;46:336–7.

16. Kennedy DL, McGinnis T. Monitoring adverse drug reactions: The FDA's new Medwatch program. P and T 1993;18:833–4, 839–42.

17. Hoigné R, Lawson DH, Weber E. Risk factors for adverse drug reactions—Epidemiological approaches. Eur J Clin Pharmacol 1990;39:321–5.

18. Classen DC, Pestotnik SL, Evans RS, Lloyd JF, Burke JP. Adverse drug events in hospitalized patients. Excess length of stay, extra costs, and attributable mortality. JAMA 1997;277:301–6.

19. Rawlins MD, Thomas SHL. Mechanisms of adverse drug reactions. In: Davies DM, Ferner RE, de Glanville H, editors. Davies's textbook of adverse drug reactions. 5th ed. London: Chapman & Hall Medical; 1998. p. 40–64.

20. Coombs RRA, Gell PGH. Classification of allergic reactions responsible for clinical hypersensitivity and disease. In: Gell PGH, editor. Clinical aspects of immunology. Oxford: Oxford University Press; 1968. p. 575–96.

21. Mathews KP. Clinical spectrum of allergic and pseudoallergic drug reactions. J Allergy Clin Immunol 1984;74:558–66.

22. D'Arcy PF. Adverse reactions and interactions with herbal medicines. Part 2. Drug interactions. Adverse Drug React Toxicol Rev 1993;12:147–62.

23. Uchegbu IF, Florence AT. Adverse drug events related to dosage forms and delivery systems. Drug Saf 1996;14:39–67.

24. Wong YL. Adverse effects of pharmaceutical excipients in drug therapy. Ann Acad Med Singapore 1993;22:99–102.

25. Napke E. Excipients, adverse drug reactions and patients' rights. Can Med Assoc J 1994;151:529–33.

26. Liss GM, Sussman GL, Deal K, Brown S, Cividino M, Siu S, et al. Latex allergy: Epidemiological study of 1351 hospital workers. Occup Environ Med 1997;54:335–42.

27. Liss GM, Sussman GL. Latex sensitization: Occupational versus general population prevalence rates. Am J Ind Med 1999;35:196–200.

28. Clyne KE, German MR. Adverse drug reaction reporting. Focus on cost and prevention. P and T 1992;17:1145–56.

29. French DG. Avoiding adverse drug reactions in the elderly patient: Issues and strategies. Nurse Practitioner 1996;21:90, 96–7, 101–7.

30. Carbonin P, Pahor M, Bernabei R, Sgadari A. Is age an independent risk factor of adverse drug reactions in hospitalized medical patients? J Am Geriatr Soc 1991;39:1093–9.

31. Colley CA, Lucas LM. Polypharmacy: The cure becomes the disease. J Gen Intern Med 1993;8:278–83.

32. Cohen JS. Avoiding adverse reactions. Effective lower-dose drug therapies for older patients. Geriatrics 2000;55:54–6, 59–60, 63–4.

33. Melmon KL. Preventable drug reactions—Causes and cures. N Engl J Med 1971;284:1361–8.

34. Gentry CA, Rodvold KA. How important is therapeutic drug monitoring in the prediction and avoidance of adverse reactions? Drug Saf 1995;12:359–63.

35. Gurwitz JH, Avorn J. The ambiguous relation between aging and adverse drug reactions. Ann Intern Med 1991;114:956–66.

36. Chutka DS, Evans JM, Fleming KC, Mikkelson KG. Drug prescribing for elderly patients. Mayo Clin Proc 1995;70:685–93.

37. Mitchell AA, Lacouture PG, Sheehan JE, Kauffman RE, Shapiro S. Adverse drug reactions in children leading to hospital admission. Pediatrics 1988;82:24–9.

38. Knight M. Adverse drug reactions in neonates. J Clin Pharmacol 1994;34:128–35.

39. Gupta A, Waldhauser LK. Adverse drug reactions from birth to early childhood. Pediatr Clin North Am 1997;44:79–92.

40. Nightingale SL, Hoffman FA. Medwatch and adolescence. J Adolesc Health 1994;15:279–80.

41. Merkatz RB, Temple R, Sobel S, Feiden K, Kessler DA. Women in clinical trials of new drugs. A change in Food and Drug Administration policy. The Working Group on Women in Clinical Trials. N Engl J Med 1993;329:292–6.

42. Martin RM, Biswas PN, Freemantle SN, Pearce GL, Mann RD. Age and sex distribution of suspected adverse drug reactions to newly marketed drugs in general practice in England: analysis of 48 cohort studies. Br J Clin Pharmacol 1998;46:505–11.

43. Kando JC, Yonkers KA, Cole JO. Gender as a risk factor for adverse events to medications. Drugs 1995;50:1–6.

44. Tran C, Knowles SR, Liu BA, Shear NH. Gender differences in adverse drug reactions. J Clin Pharmacol 1998;38:1003–9.

45. Eichelbaum M, Kroemer H, Mikus G. Genetically determined differences in drug metabolism as a risk factor in drug toxicity. Toxicol Lett 1992;64/65:115–22.

46. Lennard MS. Genetically determined adverse drug reactions involving metabolism. Drug Saf 1993;9:60–77.

47. Eichelbaum M. Pharmacokinetic and pharmacodynamic consequences of stereoselective drug metabolism in man. Biochem Pharmacol 1988;37:93–6.

48. Sheffer AL, Pennoyer DS. Management of adverse drug reactions. J Allergy Clin Immunol 1984;74:580–8.

49. Danan G, Benichou C. Causality assessment of adverse reactions to drugs—I. A novel method based on the conclusions of international consensus meetings: Application to drug-induced liver injuries. J Clin Epidemiol 1993;46:1323–30.

50. Miremont G, Haramburu F, Begaud B, Pere JC, Dangoumau J. Adverse drug reactions: Physicians' opinions versus a causality assessment method. Eur J Clin Pharmacol 1994;46:285–9.

51. Michel DJ, Knodel LC. Comparison of three algorithms used to evaluate adverse drug reactions. Am J Hosp Pharm 1986;43:1709–14.

52. Pere JC, Begaud B, Haramburu F, Albin H. Computerized comparison of six adverse drug reaction assessment procedures. Clin Pharmacol Ther 1986;40:451–61.

53. Naranjo CA, Busto U, Sellers EM, Sandor P, Ruiz I, Roberts EA, et al. A method for estimating the probability of adverse drug reactions. Clin Pharmacol Ther 1981;30:239–45.

54. Hutchinson TA, Flegel KM, HoPingKong H, Bloom WS, Kramer MS, Trummer EG. Reasons for disagreement in the standardized assessment of suspected adverse drug reactions. Clin Pharmacol Ther 1983;34:421–6.

55. Hutchinson TA, Lane DA. Assessing methods for causality assessment of suspected adverse drug reactions. J Clin Epidemiol 1989;42:5–16.

56. Lortie FM. Postmarketing surveillance of adverse drug reactions: Problems and solutions. Can Med Assoc J 1986;135:27–32.

57. Girard M. Conclusiveness of rechallenge in the interpretation of adverse drug reactions. Br J Clin Pharmacol 1987;23:73–9.

58. Naranjo CA, Shear NH, Lanctot KL. Advances in the diagnosis of adverse drug reactions. J Clin Pharmacol 1992;32:897–904.

59. Meyboom RHB, Egberts ACG, Edwards IR, Hekster YA, de Koning FHP, Gribnau FWJ. Principles of signal detection in pharmacovigilance. Drug Saf 1997;16:355–65.

60. Corso DM, Pucino F, DeLeo JM, Calis KA, Gallelli JF. Development of a questionnaire for detecting potential adverse drug reactions. Ann Pharmacother 1992;26:890–6.

61. Reidenberg MM, Lowenthal DT. Adverse nondrug reactions. N Engl J Med 1968;279:678–9.

62. Lewis JA. Post-marketing surveillance: how many patients? Trends Pharmacol Sci 1981;2:93–4.

63. McKenzie R, Fried MW, Sallie R, Conjeevaram H, Di Bisceglie AM, Park Y, et al. Hepatic failure and lactic acidosis due to fialuridine (FIAU), an investigational nucleoside analogue for chronic hepatitis B. N Engl J Med 1995;333:1099–105.

26

Quality Assessment of Drug Therapy

CHARLES E. DANIELS

Department of Pharmacy, Clinical Center, National Institutes of Health, Bethesda, Maryland

INTRODUCTION

Each year since 1996, thirty or more new molecular entities have been approved for clinical use by the U.S. Food and Drug Administration (1). Dozens more new combinations and dosage forms have also been approved during that same period. The availability of valuable new agents creates opportunities for improved therapeutic outcomes, but it also involves increased opportunities for inappropriate medication use. The clinical pharmacologist is expected to hold generalized expertise in the use of medications that can be applied across the organization in the clinical practice and in independent and collaborative research activities. Quality assessment and improvement of medication use constitute an important skill set.

The objective of this chapter will be to review medication use quality issues in an institutional context and highlight their impact on patient care and clinical research. It will focus on three themes: understanding the medication use system and organizational interests in medication use; understanding the application of drug use monitoring as a tool to improve medication use; and understanding processes to identify and minimize medication errors.

Adverse Drug Events

Johnson and Bootman (2) projected that costs of $76 billion a year are attributable to medication mis-

use. Adverse drug events (ADEs) are instances in which patient harm results from the use of medication. This includes both adverse drug reactions, which were discussed in Chapter 25, and medication errors, all of which are inherently preventable. A 1999 Institute of Medicine report estimated that 98,000 Americans die each year due to medical error (3). This includes diagnostic mistakes, wrong-site surgery, and other categories of error, including medication errors. Approximately 20% of all medical errors are medication related (4, 5).

A medication error is any preventable event that may cause or lead to inappropriate medication use or patient harm while medication is in the control of a healthcare professional, patient, or consumer (6). Not all medication errors reach the patient. These are often referred to as "near misses." They are not usually considered to be ADEs only because no harm was done. Preventable ADEs are a subset of medication errors, which cause harm to a patient (7). Figure 26.1 depicts the relationship between adverse drug events, medication errors, and adverse drug reactions (8). Because adverse drug reactions are generally unexpected, they are not presently considered a reflection of medication use quality in a classic sense. However, as genetic variances become part of the drug selection consideration, it may be possible to predict and avoid many reactions that have been unexpected in the past. This offers an opportunity to improve the quality of medication use.

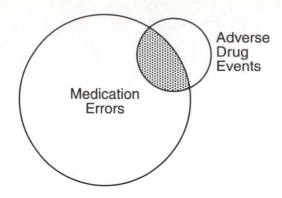

FIGURE 26.1 Diagram showing the relationship between medication errors and adverse drug events. Because some adverse drug events are preventable, they are also considered medication errors (*shaded area*). (Adapted from Bates DW, et al. J Gen Intern Med 1995;10:199–205.)

Medication errors are costly and are a diversion from the intended therapeutic objective. Morbidity or mortality are possible outcomes of medication errors. A 1997 study by Bates et al. (9) found that 6.5 ADEs occur for every 100 nonobstetric hospital admissions, and that 28% of them were preventable. It also was determined that 42% of life-threatening and serious ADEs were preventable. Preventable ADEs were responsible for an increased length of hospital stay of 4.6 days and $5857 per event. The cost for all ADEs was projected to be a cost of $5.6 million per year just for the institution in which the study was conducted. This study demonstrates that safer medication use, with fewer adverse medication events, is a cost-effective target.

The Medication Use Process

Medications are prescribed, distributed, and consumed under the assumption that the therapeutic plan will work as intended to provide the expected outcome. It is clear from previous chapters that there are many biological system issues that will influence the success of the plan. Other organizational and societal system issues also influence the success of the therapeutic plan as profoundly as those biological systems issues. A prescriber writes an order for a medication based on the best available information, the likely diagnosis, and the expected outcome. A pharmacist reviews the requested medication order (prescription), clarifies it based on additional information about the patient or medication (allergies, drug interactions, etc.), prepares the medication for use, counsels the patient about the drug, and gives it to the patient. The patient is respon-

sible for understanding the therapeutic objective, knowing about the drug, creating a daily compliance plan (deciding when to take the drug), watching for good or bad results, and providing feedback to the prescriber or pharmacist regarding planned or unplanned outcomes. This process occurs over a variable period of time, in a system in which the key participants of the process seldom speak with each other. Each action creates an opportunity for success or failure. Is there any wonder that the quality and integrity of the system are compromised on a regular basis?

The medication use system in an institutional setting offers even more complexity, with more chances for error. The five subsystems of the medication system in a hospital are selection and procurement of drugs, drug prescribing, preparation and dispensing, drug administration, and monitoring for medication or related effects (10). Evaluation and improvement of medication use quality require consideration of all these subsystems.

Figure 26.2 is a flowchart of appropriate, safe, effective, and efficient use of medications in the hospital setting (11). It incorporates the role of the prescriber, nurse, pharmacist, and patient in a typical inpatient environment. It also depicts the role of the organization's pharmacy and therapeutics committee and quality improvement functions, which will be discussed later in this chapter. The decision to treat a patient in a hospital or extended care facility typically adds a nurse or other healthcare provider (respiratory therapist, etc.) to the trio described in the ambulatory care setting. Every time that individual has to read, interpret, decide, or act is yet another opportunity for a mistake to occur. Each of the steps in the medication use process provides an opportunity for correct or incorrect interpretation and implementation of the tactics that support the therapeutic plan. With this many opportunities for medication misadventures to occur, it is easy to understand why tracking and improving quality are important aspects of medication use.

Philips and colleagues (12) found a 236% increase in medication-error-related deaths for hospitalized patients between 1983 and 1993. The same study showed an increase of over 800% for outpatient medication error deaths. The reported growth in medication error deaths may be partially attributed to more accurate reporting, but clearly represents a growth in the problem of medication errors from potent drugs. A 1999 study by the American Society of Health-System Pharmacists concluded that five of the top eight concerns of patients regarding hospitalization were related to medication use or medication error (13). A study by Bates et al. (14) determined that the 56% of

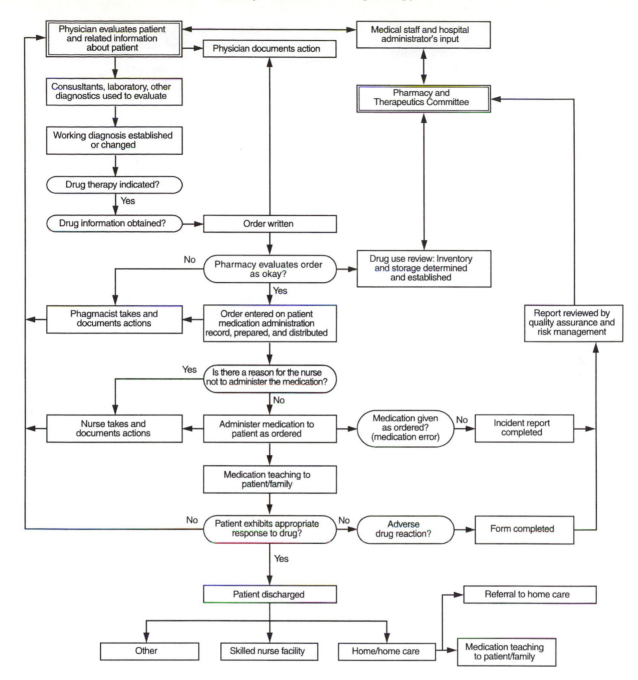

FIGURE 26.2 Flowchart of the inpatient medication use process showing the start and endpoints (*double-boxed rectangles*), intervening actions (*rectangles*), and decision-making steps (*ovals*) required for appropriate, safe, effective, and efficient medication use. (Reproduced with permission from Atkinson AJ Jr, Nadzam DM, Schaff RL. Clin Pharmacol Ther 1991;50:125–8.)

medication errors in a hospital setting were associated with the ordering process, 6% with transcription of written orders, 4% with pharmacy dispensing, and 34% with administration of medications. Based on these findings, it is easily concluded that there is room for improvement in how medications are used in the inpatient and outpatient setting.

Improving the Quality of Medication Use

There are multiple facets to the quality assessment of medication use. Among them are monitoring of adverse medication events and medication use evaluation programs. To improve medication use, Berwick (15) has applied the industrial principles of continuous

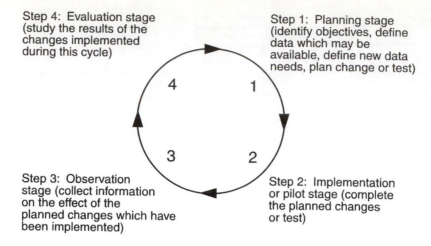

Step 4: Evaluation stage (study the results of the changes implemented during this cycle)

Step 1: Planning stage (identify objectives, define data which may be available, define new data needs, plan change or test)

Step 3: Observation stage (collect information on the effect of the planned changes which have been implemented)

Step 2: Implementation or pilot stage (complete the planned changes or test)

FIGURE 26.3 The Shewhart cycle. The cycle is repeated with desired improvements implemented with each iteration and the measured results used to guide the design of the next cycle. (Reproduced with permission from Deming WE. Out of the crisis. Cambridge, MA: MIT Press; 2000. p. 87–9.)

quality improvement to the healthcare setting. The critical elements of this approach are collection and use of data with a system focus. Deming (16) has championed the use of the Shewhart Cycle in continuous quality improvement. As shown in Figure 26.3, the Shewhart Cycle is an approach for implementing systematic change based on data collection and evaluation with each iteration of the cycle. Each time the work cycle is completed there is an obligation to evaluate the impact of any process modification on the result. Modifications that improve the result are permanently incorporated into the process. Changes with no impact or a negative result will be deleted in the next iteration. Deming's message is that ongoing process and system change, along with measurement of the result, provide the feedback loop to support continuous improvement of the product or service.

ORGANIZATIONAL INFLUENCES ON MEDICATION USE QUALITY

Several external organizations and internal elements of the healthcare system have an interest in optimizing medication use. These include the hospital or health system, the medical staff, the group purchasing organization with which the hospital participates for the contractual purchase of drugs, and external regulatory or accreditation organizations (e.g., Joint Commission on Accreditation of Healthcare Organizations; Health Care Financing Agency, state and local public health agencies, etc.) There is interest in what drugs are used, when and how they are used, the economic impact of drug selection, and outcomes that result in safe and effective use of medications.

The Joint Commission on Accreditation of Healthcare Organizations (JCAHO) is the organization that accredits most hospitals, health systems, and home care agencies. A significant element of the overall JCAHO review of patient care involves medication use quality and medication system safety. Accreditation standards for medication-related activities are applied to practice in the organization. Hospitals are expected to present evidence that ordering, dispensing, administering, and monitoring of medications, are overseen by the medical staff. The organization must be able to demonstrate that policies for safe medication use practices are in place. Evidence of ongoing medication use evaluation, adverse medication event investigation, and medication use performance improvement are required to meet the standards. Analogous accrediting organizations are often used for accrediting managed care organizations. State professional boards (medicine, nursing, or pharmacy) provide oversight of specialized domains such as prescribing, dispensing, and administering of medications. Most healthcare facilities are also regulated by local or state health departments that often have local regulations on medication-related issues.

It is the responsibility of the medical staff in a healthcare organization to oversee medication use activities. This includes development of medication use policies, selection of drug products that are appropriate to the needs of the patient population being served, and oversight of the quality of medication use.

The pharmacy and therapeutics committee is the normal focal point for medication related activities within the organization. The pharmacy and therapeutics committee develops policies for managing drug use and administration, develops and supervises the formulary, and evaluates the clinical use of drugs (17).

The exact structure of the pharmacy and therapeutics committee may vary to meet the unique needs and structure of the organization. It routinely reports to the medical staff executive committee or other leadership group within the medical staff organization. The committee is made up of representatives from the principal medication using services (internal medicine, surgery, pediatrics, etc.) within the organization, plus representatives from the nursing services, pharmacy services, quality improvement program, and hospital administration. The chair of the committee is most frequently a clinician with experience in systemwide activities and, most important, an interest in quality use of medications. It is customary for the director of the pharmacy department to serve as the executive secretary for the committee to assure a working link between pharmacy department and committee activities.

Pharmacy and therapeutics committees usually meet six to 12 times per year. The schedule is dependent on the traditions of the organization and the amount of work included during the full committee meeting. The agenda should be prepared under the supervision of the committee chair and distributed well in advance of the meeting to allow all participants to read formulary drug monographs and drug use reports before the meeting. Ongoing elements of many committees are special standing subcommittees or focused task force workgroups. Typical standing subcommittees focus on antimicrobial agents and medication use evaluation. Standing subcommittees are appropriate for providing ongoing special expertise on matters that can be referred back to the full committee for action. The task force workgroup is used to address special limited-scope issues, such as *ad hoc* evaluations of agents within a given therapeutic drug class.

Medication Policy Issues

The pharmacy and therapeutics committee is expected to oversee important policies and procedures associated with the use of medications. Medication policy includes a wide range of issues, from who may prescribe or administer drugs, to what prescribing direction and guidance are appropriate to assure safe and appropriate use of high-risk, high-volume, high-cost, or problem-prone drugs. Policies are often needed to identify who may prescribe or administer medications, to assure consistent supply or quality of drug products, or to allocate drugs in times of shortage. Responsibility for developing policies to address special circumstances or issues is often delegated to the pharmacy and therapeutics committee by the organization. Examples of this type of policy are special drug class restriction, (e.g., antimicrobial agents) and use of agents for sedation during medical procedures.

Formulary Management

The objective of an active formulary program is to direct medication use to preferred agents, which offer a therapeutic or safety benefit or an economic advantage for use. A statement of principles of a sound drug formulary system was developed in 2000 by a consortium composed of the U.S. Pharmacopoeia, the Department of Veterans Affairs, the American Society of Health-System Pharmacists, the Academy of Managed Care Pharmacists, and the National Business Coalition on Health (18). In this statement, a formulary is defined as "a continuously updated list of medications and related information, representing the clinical judgment of physicians, pharmacists, and other experts in the diagnosis and or treatment of disease and promotion of health." A specific formulary is intended for use in a defined population. That defined population may be patients in a single hospital, patients seen within a group practice, a managed care patient population (local, regional or national), or even an entire community.

Historically, formulary drug inclusion or exclusion has been used as an administrative hurdle to discourage prescribers from using less desirable drugs. The historical approach to formulary decision making was based on a simple "on formulary" or "not-on formulary" approach. Formulary drugs were available immediately with no special requirements. Often a formulary drug was selected by the prescriber to avoid a prolonged waiting period for the nonformulary item to be ordered and made available for the patient. This approach was more effective when the array of effective drug choices was somewhat limited, and the principal cost and quality management need was to reduce the number of "me-too" products.

With the advent of many of the newest generation of products, including monoclonal antibodies and cytokine agents, it is not logical to simply limit the formulary availability of these novel agents. Accordingly, the standard for most institutions has been to include these novel drugs with committee-approved restrictions and guidelines for use. In the future, genomics and genetic diversity, which can influence toxicity and effectiveness, will play an important role in formulary

338 Principles of Clinical Pharmacology

drug management. The ability to better customize patient-specific drug response will require a more sophisticated approach in selecting the most appropriate drug.

Drug Selection Process

Effective formulary development is based on the scientific evaluation of drug safety, clinical effectiveness, and cost impact (18). That information is used by the committee to determine the specific value and risk of the drug for the patient population to whom the drug will be administered. The committee evaluates a given drug relative to the disease states typically treated in this population. For instance, the presence or absence of certain tropical diseases may impact on the need to include some antimicrobial agents in the formulary. The evaluation of a drug should include discussion of what doses and duration of therapy might be most appropriate in order to establish guidelines for measuring prescribing quality. In some cases, it may be necessary to determine which healthcare professionals are appropriately trained or qualified to prescribe a particular drug. The committee may elect to restrict the use of a drug to certain specialists (e.g., board-trained cardiologists for high-risk antiarrhythmic agents) or the drug may be restricted by the manufacturer of FDA to those prescribers who have received some drug-specific training and been approved by the supplier (e.g., thalidomide).

Economic evaluation of medications is a routine element of formulary development. The development of many effective but expensive drugs, which are likely to cost thousands of dollars for a single short course of therapy or tens of thousands for long-term therapy, has placed financial impact at center stage in product selection. The availability of these high-cost agents has created a new specialty discipline called pharmacoeconomics. A growing list of academic medical centers have established units that focus research and practice efforts on outcomes measurement of drug therapy. These programs often provide sophisticated evaluations of the economic or quality-of-life elements of drug use.

It is important to understand that drug costs, and their impact, are perceived differently from different perspectives in the healthcare system. Each component of the healthcare system (hospital, home care, ambulatory provider) may have a different perspective on the cost of therapy. Hospitals are usually responsible for all drug-related costs (drug, medication administration, laboratory monitoring, etc.) for the finite period of time that a patient is hospitalized.

A stand-alone outpatient drug benefit manager might only worry about the drug cost for the nonhospitalized portion of the therapy. The overall health system may be at financial risk for all elements of outpatient and inpatient care. Because each element of the system may be responsible for a different component of the total cost of care, the cost-impact of a given drug product selection may be different for each of them. The "societal perspective" often represents yet another view of drug costs in that it incorporates nonhealthcare costs and the value of lost days of work and disability. Formulary inclusion is not routinely based on that level of evaluation, but public policy may be influenced by that information.

The cost-impact analysis of two hypothetical drug choices shown in Figure 26.4 demonstrates the role of cost perspective in the formulary selection process. Both regimens offer the same long-term clinical result and adverse reaction profile. This analysis shows that the decision as to which drug is the lower-cost option will vary with the perspective of the organization that is responsible for the different inpatient and outpatient components of care. This dilemma is a regular element of the formulary selection process in many institutions. The puzzle becomes more complex when one is trying to decide what elements of cost should be included (e.g., laboratory tests or other monitoring activities). Despite this lack of clarity, the cost impact of drug therapy, to all stakeholders, requires that this issue be considered in the decision process.

Most hospitals and healthcare organizations participate in a purchasing group to leverage volume-driven price advantages. The makeup and operations of these groups vary widely, but the price agreements and changing landscape of drug pricing add an additional dimension to the drug price factor. A specific drug may be the lowest price option for a given contract period, after which the choice may change. In another variation, a package of prices for bundled items may cause the price for a given item to change depending on the use of yet another item. How this influences formulary decisions is a function of the drug and many other factors.

Formulary Tactics

In addition to drug selection, the pharmacy and therapeutics committee is responsible for considering formulary tactics to support the overall goal of optimal medication use. Several of these tactics have been used successfully to direct drug use toward preferred agents. The most obvious tactic to direct use away from a given agent is to exclude it from the formulary. The use of nonformulary agents usually triggers some

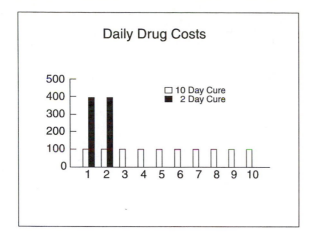
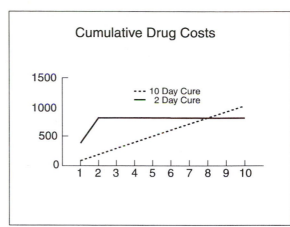

Financial Responsibility at Discharge

	Daily Cost	10 Day Total	Total at Hospital Discharge
2 Day Cure	$400	$800	$800
10 Day Cure	$100	$1000	$300

Perspective Based Financial Responsibility

	2 Day Cure	10 Day Cure
Hospital	$800	$300
Outpatient Payer	$ 0	$700
Total	$800	$1000

FIGURE 26.4   Financial perspective in formulary decision making. Comparison of two treatment options: 2-day cure at $400 per day versus 10-day cure at $100 per day, with an anticipated hospital stay of 3 days.

required override or *post hoc* review of use by the committee or designated individual. A second tactic involves a global management of medication use by therapeutic class. This tactic can be employed to minimize the use of drugs with a less clear profile of therapeutic efficacy or safety. A decision to limit the number of agents from a given drug class can also provide some advantages in price contracting, if formulary inclusion is effective in directing medication use to lower cost agents.

Limiting prescribing rights for some specific drugs to a subset of prescribers who possess special expertise that qualifies them to use these drugs can improve the quality of their use. In many cases, drug restriction is managed by one or more gatekeepers whose approval is required prior to beginning therapy with the drug (e.g., infectious disease approval prior to start of a specified antibiotic). In some cases, direct financial incentives have been used to encourage use of a given drug or group of drugs. These formulary tactics have

been used to influence decision making by prescribers, pharmacists, and patients.

Analysis and Prevention of Medication Errors

Reason (19) has described a model for looking at human error that portrays a battle between the sources of error and the system-based defenses against them. This model is often referred to as the "Swiss cheese model" because the defenses against error are displayed as thin layers with holes that are described as latent error in the system. Figure 26.5 demonstrates the model as applied to medication error. Each opportunity for error is defended by the prescriber, pharmacist, nurse, and patient. When a potential error is identified and corrected (e.g., dose error, route of administration error, etc.) the event becomes a "near miss" rather than an ADE. In those cases in which the holes in the Swiss cheese line up, a

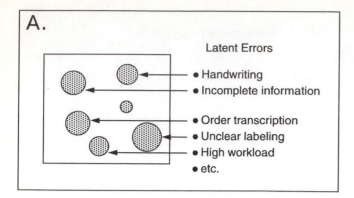
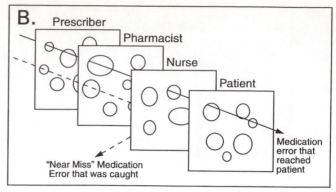

FIGURE 26.5 Latent medication system errors (*Panel A*) and defensive layers against error (*Panel B*) in the medication system.

preventable medication error occurs. The Swiss cheese model provides an interesting framework for research in this field.

The latent errors in the medication use system have been described in several studies. Major contributors to errors in medication use were found to be: knowledge gap related to drug therapy (30%); knowledge gap related to patient factors (30%); errors in dose calculations, placement of decimal points, and dosage units (18%); nomenclature failures such as wrong drug name, misinterpreted abbreviation, and so on (13%) (20). Cohen (21) describes six common causes of medication error based on his review of events reported to public reporting databases. These causes of errors include failed communication, poor drug distribution practices (including verbal orders), dose miscalculations, drug and device related problems (such as name confusion, labeling, or poor design), and lack of patient education on the drugs that are prescribed for their use. Leape et al. (22) identified 13 proximal causes of medication errors in an academic medical center. They are detailed in Table 26.1.

Medication Error Data

The rate and nature of medication errors have been studied by several authors. Nightingale et al. (23) found a medication error rate of 0.7% in a British National Health Service general hospital. Lesar et al. (20) describe the results of a review of 2103 clinically significant medication errors in an academic medical center. It was determined that 0.4% of medication orders were in error: 42% of the errors were overdosage, and 13% were the result of drug allergies that were not accounted for prior to prescribing. This work showed that medication errors result most frequently from failure to alter dose or drug after changes in renal or hepatic status, missed allergies, wrong drug name, wrong dosage form (e.g., IV for IM), use of abbreviations, or incorrect calculation of a drug dose. They concluded that an improved organizational focus on technological risk management and training should reduce errors and patient risk of ADEs.

Given the latent errors associated with some elements of human performance, it seems likely that

TABLE 26.1   **Proximal Causes of Medication Errors**[a]

Lack of knowledge of the drug	Faulty dose checking
Lack of information about the patient	Infusion pump and parenteral delivery problems
Violation of rules	Inadequate monitoring
Slips and memory lapses	Drug stocking and delivery problems
Transcription errors	Preparation errors
Faulty checking of identification	Lack of standardization
Faulty interaction with other services	

[a] Adapted from Leape LL, et al. Systems analysis of adverse drug events. JAMA 1995;274:35–43.

automation may reduce error. Several studies have demonstrated the value of computer assistance in the medication order entry process. Rules-based physician order systems have been shown to identify and reduce the chances of adverse medication events due to drug duplication, calculation errors, and drug-drug interactions (23, 24–27).

Some therapeutic categories of medications might be predicted to be prone to error due to narrow therapeutic index, complexity of therapy, or other factors. Phillips et al. (12) found that analgesics, central nervous system agents, and nontranquilizer psychotropic drugs were most frequently associated with deaths due to medication errors. Lesar et al. (20) found antimicrobials, and cardiovascular drugs to be the most error-prone therapeutic categories in an academic medical center. The JCAHO has identified a list of drugs and drug practices that are associated with high risk for significant error, and the Institute for Safe Medication Practices also has identified drugs that should generate a high-alert due to risk for medication errors (28, 29). Lambert and colleagues (30, 31) have described a series of experiments that test the likelihood of drug name confusion based on fixed similarity patterns. This theoretical concept is providing the basis for selecting drug names that minimize the chance of sound-alike errors (32).

Research methods on medication error data are not standardized. Therefore, they are subject to some limitations in generalizability. Because widespread interest in developing scientific approaches for reducing medication error is relatively recent, there are few well-established methods for conducting research in this field. However, funding for research in safe medication use and error reduction is available from several public and private sources, including the Agency for Healthcare Research and Quality.

Medication error data collection and analysis for clinical use and quality improvement is also a complex activity. Observational data, *post hoc* review of medical records, and self-reporting have all have been used with varying degrees of success for research and functional applications. Each offers strengths and weaknesses, and the appropriate method for data collection is in large part a function of its intended use and the resources available to collect it.

Most hospitals collect internal medication error data through a voluntary reporting mechanism. This system is used as the backbone of error reporting because it requires minimal resources for data collection and is supported by organizational risk management programs. Voluntary reporting is presumed to underreport total errors. It is widely believed that most significant errors are reported when they are

identified, but many mistakes are never recognized. Many other errors are determined to be insignificant and, therefore, not formally reported. For these reasons, it is difficult to determine in the hospital setting if changes in a given series of numbers represent a real change or simply a different level of reporting.

Figure 26.6 illustrates a typical presentation of aggregated or high-level medication error data in an institutional setting. This presentation allows for general trends in total numbers to be plotted and tracked over time. Review of high-level data shows trends and provides a framework for the first level of error analysis. Major changes can be seen that may trigger more intense analysis. However, this high-level data does not provide any detail to the analyst regarding the subcomponents of the composition of the reported errors. As a result, there are pitfalls in drawing conclusions from aggregated high level data that can make these conclusions problematic. For instance, one might presume that administration of medication to the wrong patient is generally more serious than administration of a medication at the wrong time. However, an increase of five "wrong patient" errors and a decrease

A.

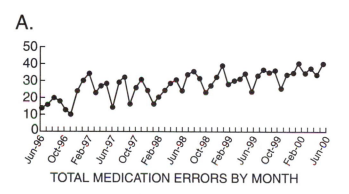

TOTAL MEDICATION ERRORS BY MONTH

B.

	Jun-97	Sep-97	Dec-97	Mar-98	Jun-98	Sep-98	Dec-98	Mar-99	Jun-99	Sep-99	Dec-99	Mar-00	Mean
Wrong Drug	5	3	6	2	10	2	4	5	4	8	2	2	4.4
Wrong Dose	11	17	8	13	6	12	18	17	21	15	22	14	14.5
Duplicate Dose	10	4	3	8	2	16	4	11	9	11	6	17	8.4
Wrong Route	3	2	4	0	2	1	1	5	3	0	3	1	2.1
Wrong Time	15	25	12	33	15	19	27	31	17	26	10	29	21.6
Wrong Fluid	6	7	4	10	3	8	7	5	8	2	3	2	5.4
Wrong Rate	16	20	12	17	21	8	24	8	11	19	23	14	16.1
Wrong Device	2	0	0	1	3	1	4	2	0	1	2	2	1.5
IV Infiltration	0	2	1	0	3	2	0	0	4	0	2	0	1.2
Total	68	80	50	84	65	69	89	84	77	82	73	81	**75.2**

MEDICATION ERRORS BY QUARTER

FIGURE 26.6 Typical presentation of medication error data in aggregate form by month (*Panel A*) or categorized by error type on a quarterly basis (*Panel B*).

of five "wrong time" errors for a specific time period will register as a zero change for that period if only aggregated data is used. In fact, it may represent a serious degradation in some element of the medication system that will not be seen through this level of error analysis.

Classification and analysis of medication error data by error type are recommended as a method to spot potentially important changes in system performance. The National Coordinating Council for Medication Error Reporting and Prevention system for classifying medication errors may be used (6). Commercial systems for cataloging and analyzing medication errors are available. A potentially valuable element of some programs is the ability to share anonymous data with other hospitals for comparison with similar institutions (33). Regardless of the system used to classify and analyze medication error data, clear and consistent classification must be made to avoid confounding conclusions regarding underlying problems.

Reducing Medication Errors

Collection and use of medication error data at the hospital level are challenging but important functions. A key organizational principle in quality improvement is to make reporting errors a nonpunitive process. This usually increases the number of errors that will be reported, but not the number occuring. Making errors visible is an important step in the process of finding and fixing system-related problems (34). The ongoing monitoring of adverse drug event data (both medication error and adverse drug reactions) is an important responsibility of the pharmacy and therapeutics committee. This committee is the organization's only point at which all the medication related issues converge. This convergence allows for a full review of the medication use process for system adjustments.

To identify opportunities for reduction of medication errors it is important that each error be carefully reviewed by a limited number of individuals to gain intimate knowledge of each reported incident. Collection and classification of error data must be followed by use of a careful epidemiological approach to problem solving at the system level. Narrative data, which may not be seen by looking at the categorical data alone, can be used to provide important details about proximal causes and latent error that may have contributed to the event. Success in this type of error reduction requires the reviewers to read between the lines, look for common threads between reports, and link multiple errors that are the result of system weaknesses.

There is still work to be done in understanding errors in the medication use process. However, available information provides suggestions on how to reduce medication errors. Bates's (35) ongoing studies of medication errors lead to eight specific error prevention strategies: 1) unit-dose medication dispensing; 2) targeted physician education on optimal medication use; 3) inclusion of the clinical pharmacist in decision-making patient activities; 4) computerized medication checking; 5) computerized order entry by the prescriber; 6) standardized processes and equipment; 7) automate medication dispensing systems; 8) bar-code medications for dispensing and administration. Other authors have reached similar conclusions.

The more complex a patient's drug therapy, the greater the likelihood of adverse medication events. Cullen et al. (36) determined that the rate of preventable and potential adverse drug events was twice as high in intensive care units compared to nonintensive care units. This is attributed to the higher number of drugs used in the ICU. Lesar et al. (37) reviewed medication prescribing errors over a nine-year period and concluded that the incidence of prescribing error increased as intensity of care increased and new drugs became available. Koechler et al. (38) reported than greater than five concurrent medications, 12 or more doses per day, or medication regimen changes four or more times in a year were all predictors for drug therapy problems in ambulatory patients. Gray et al. (39) determined that the occurrence of an ADE was positively related to the number of new medications received at hospital discharge. The knowledge that some patients are at higher risk for ADEs suggests possible high-return intervention targets. When selecting improvement opportunities, it is wise to look for those areas most likely to yield results.

Examples of system improvements to reduce medication errors have been reported in several projects. Leape et al. (40) reduced medication errors in an intensive care unit by inclusion of a pharmacist on the clinical rounding team. Flynn et al. (41) identified interruptions (telephone calls, conversations, etc.) during critical phases of pharmacist drug preparation activities as significant contributors to errors in medication preparation. Comprehensive efforts to prevent medication errors include the four-pronged medication error analysis program from the Institute for Safe Medication Practices. This four-pronged approach includes evaluation of specific medication errors, evaluation of aggregated error data and "near miss" data for the hospital, as well as evaluation of error reports from other hospitals (42). In addition, effective medication error prevention includes ongoing monitoring of drug therapy trends, changes in medication use patterns, information from the hospital quality improvement or risk management program, and general hospital programmatic information.

Monitoring institutional trends in medication use can provide clues to possible high-risk or error-prone therapies. Increased use of drugs with a history of medication errors, such as patient-controlled analgesia, should alert organizations to develop safeguards to protect against errors before rather than after they become problems. Cohen and Kilo (43) describe a framework for improving the use of high-alert drugs, which is based on reducing or eliminating the possibility of error, making errors visible, and minimizing the consequences of errors. Table 26.2 presents change concepts for safeguarding when using high-risk drugs.

Medication error prevention opportunities also may present themselves in unusual hospital programmatic information from sources not routinely applied to medication safety. For instance, reports of laboratory-related incidents, or hospital information system problems may be indicators that medication-related problems can be expected. Thoughtful use of this information may prevent medication-related errors attributed to supplemental systems that are critical to safe and appropriate medication use. Reports of staff shortages within an institution (e.g., critical care nursing, nurse anesthetist) can be used to identify potential problem areas prior to medication error reports. Reports of planned construction or information system conversions may also be an indicator that routines will be interrupted. This can be used to help provide safe alternatives before errors occur. Use of hospital program information in a prospective way can help avoid medication errors.

System improvements may improve the quality of prescribing by standardizing to an expert level. Morris (44) describes the development, testing, and use of computerized protocols for management of intravenous fluid and hemodynamic factors in patients with acute respiratory distress syndrome. Evans et al. (45) used a computerized antiinfectives management program to improve the quality of medication use and reduce costs. In consideration of all that is currently known, Leape (46) provides a simple set of recommendations to reduce medical error: Reduce reliance on memory; improve access to information; error-proof critical tasks; standardize processes; and instruct healthcare providers on possible errors in

TABLE 26.2   Safeguarding against Errors in High-Risk Drugs[a]

Concept	Example
Build-in system redundancies	Independent calculation of pediatric doses by more than one person (e.g., prescriber and pharmacist)
Use fail-safes	IV pumps with clamps that automatically shut off flow during power outage
Reduce options	Use of a single concentration of heparin for infusion (e.g., 25,000 units in 250 ml of saline)
Use forcing functions	Preprinted order forms for chemotherapy drugs that require patient height and weight information before preparation and dispensing
Externalize or centralize error-prone processes	Prepare IV admixtures in the pharmacy instead of on nursing units
Use differentialization	Supplemental labels for dosage forms that are not appropriate for intravenous use without dilution
Store medications appropriately	Store dopamine and dobutamine in separate locations
Screen new products	Review new formulary requests for labeling, packaging and medication use issues that may be error prone
Standardize and simplify order communication	Avoid use of verbal orders
Limit access	Restrict access to the pharmacy during "non-staffed" hours and follow up on all medications removed from the pharmacy during this time
Use constraints	Require approval before beginning therapy (e.g., attending signature on chemotherapy orders)
Use reminders	Place special labels on products when they are dispensed by the pharmacy to remind of special procedures for use (e.g., doublecheck rate calculation of insulin infusions)
Standardize dosing procedures	Develop standardized dose and rate charts for products such as vasoactive drugs (e.g., infusion rate expressed as micrograms per kilogram per minute)

[a] Adapted from Cohen MR, Kilo CM. High-alert medications: safeguarding against errors. In: Cohen MR, editor. Medication errors. Washington, DC: American Pharmaceutical Association; 1999. p. 5.3–5.11.

		SPENT FY 95	SPENT FY 96	SPENT FY 97	SPENT FY 98	SPENT FY 99	SPENT FY 00
40000	ANTIHISTAMINE TOTAL	$17,564	$21,175	$28,185	$41,918	$54,237	$64,221
80000	ANTI-INFECTIVE AGENTS						
80400	AMEBICIDES	$0	$1,522	$332	$884	$1,321	$746
80800	ANTHELMINTICS	$2,510	$996	$2,623	$1,231	$1,834	$2,702
81202	AMINOGLYCOSIDES	$9,457	$13,457	$10,351	$35,468	$47,014	$35,272
81204	ANTIFUNGAL ANTIBIOTICS	$256,806	$320,884	$357,206	$946,657	$1,082,165	$1,056,544
81206	CEPHALOSPORINS	$221,196	$197,231	$162,850	$180,186	$188,435	$146,069
81207	β-LACTAMS	$59,322	$77,722	$77,703	$90,073	$112,235	$81,442
81208	CHLORAMPHENICOLS	$626	$204	$172	$771	$1,331	$34
81212	ERYTHROMYCINS	$52,106	$69,377	$89,793	$112,984	$109,499	$92,816
81216	PENICILLINS	$50,569	$41,427	$65,243	$46,314	$61,153	$89,200
81224	TETRACYCLINES	$16,872	$4,427	$4,788	$4,569	$8,820	$5,962
81228	MISCELLANEOUS ANTIBIOTICS	$38,577	$35,347	$35,261	$37,811	$41,473	$80,727
81600	ANTITUBERCULOSIS AGENTS	$33,141	$27,937	$42,335	$53,318	$46,223	$39,438
81800	ANTIVIRALS	$658,157	$1,399,246	$2,472,982	$3,251,543	$3,417,004	$3,775,675
82000	ANTIMALARIAL AGENTS	$82,141	$60,942	$20,848	$19,051	$20,577	$17,524
82200	QUINOLONES	$82,319	$113,064	$94,705	$117,380	$116,301	$119,356
82400	SULFONAMIDES	$7,053	$6,730	$3,425	$3,660	$2,770	$4,579
82600	SULFONES	$5,207	$4,839	$4,651	$4,972	$5,366	$3,735
83200	ANTITRICHOMONAL AGENTS	$1,493	$3,923	$677	$924	$1,454	$1,627
83600	URINARY ANTI-INFECTIVES	$5,974	$2,009	$2,142	$1,632	$2,836	$763
84000	MISCELLANEOUS ANTI-INFECTIVES	$28,489	$34,661	$30,211	$27,401	$19,394	$23,766
	ANTI-INFECTIVE AGENTS TOTAL	$1,612,016	$2,415,944	$3,478,297	$4,936,828	$5,287,206	$5,577,978
160000	BLOOD DERIVATIVES TOTAL	$212,109	$188,350	$204,843	$236,087	$348,825	$11,095
200000	BLOOD FORMATION AND COAGULATION						
200404	IRON PREPARATIONS	$2,867	$2,687	$2,402	$2,240	$2,012	$6,150
201204	ANTICOAGULANTS	$41,207	$66,851	$75,294	$114,764	$179,357	$146,496
201208	ANTIHEPARIN AGENTS	$141	$237	$83	$182	$156	$52,186
201216	HEMOSTATICS	$56,030	$21,246	$27,266	$48,408	$75,817	$65,886
201600	HEMATOPOIETIC AGENTS	$1,228,251	$1,526,711	$1,471,910	$1,515,326	$2,027,767	$1,406,002
202400	HEMORRHEOLOGIC AGENTS	$3,179	$2,717	$2,046	$3,014	$6,683	$1,109
204000	THROMBOLYTIC AGENTS	$47,054	$72,684	$58,657	$87,678	$72,382	$51,789
	BLOOD FORMATION AND COAG. TOTAL	$1,378,728	$1,693,133	$1,637,657	$1,771,613	$2,142,912	$1,729,616
240000	CARDIOVASCULAR DRUGS						
240400	CARDIAC DRUGS	$168,786	$185,225	$179,912	$197,914	$258,000	$264,424
240600	ANTILIPEMIC AGENTS	$237,143	$237,827	$298,091	$269,520	$298,957	$333,476
240800	HYPOTENSIVE AGENTS	$97,583	$89,871	$106,383	$112,858	$122,181	$117,703
241200	VASODILATING AGENTS	$20,063	$21,023	$28,385	$39,040	$26,947	$25,841
241600	SCLEROSING AGENTS	$0	$0	$0	$0	$0	$220
	CARDIOVASCULAR DRUGS TOTAL	$523,575	$533,946	$612,771	$619,332	$706,085	$741,664

FIGURE 26.7 Sample therapeutic category drug monitoring report based on therapeutic classifications used by the American Hospital Formulary Service (48).

processes. These simple but thoughtful recommendations are an important concept to reduction in medication errors.

Medication Use Evaluation

Medication use evaluation (also referred to as drug use evaluation or DUE) is a required component of the medication use quality improvement process. It is a performance improvement method with the goal of optimizing patient outcomes (47). The first element of drug use tracking is global monitoring of organizational drug use. This can be completed by routine evaluation of totals and changes in drug use within a therapeutic drug category. The American Hospital Formulary Service has created a comprehensive therapeutic classification system that is often used for drug use monitoring, but other commercial medication databases are also available (48).

Figure 26.7 is an example of a global drug use report that may be used to look for trends and variations in medication use. This report should be examined for changes that represent increases or decreases in comparison to previous reporting periods. A change in any specific category or group of drugs may be important and worthy of specific follow-up. Smaller changes that support a trend over time can demonstrate ongoing changes in drug use patterns. Changes seen in global level monitoring may trigger a focused evaluation to assure quality of medication use.

Medication use evaluation has historically been categorized with regard to how and when data collection or intervention occurs. Table 26.3 describes retrospective, concurrent, and prospective activities based on the use and timing of intervention as part of the process that is used for screening and incorporation of data.

Focused Medication Use Evaluation

Focused or targeted medication use evaluation follows a reasonably well-established cycle: identification of a potential problem in the use of a specific drug or therapy, collection and comparison of data, determination of compliance with a preestablished guideline/expectation, and action as needed to improve discrepancies between expected and measured results. This type of medication use evaluation provides an excellent opportunity to apply the Shewhart cycle for continuous quality improvement (Figure 26.3). Focused medication use projects are typically selected for a specific reason. Table 26.4 lists reasons to consider drugs for focused evaluation projects.

TABLE 26.3   Drug Use Review Categories

Review category	Data collection model (s)	Typical application	Comments
Retrospective	Data is collected for a fixed period that may be archival or accumulates new patients for a fixed period of time	Data archive search for prescribing patterns of patients on seratonin antagonist antiemetic drugs	Supports large-scale epidemiologic approach No active intervention to change medication use patterns occurs due to the *post hoc* data collection process
Concurrent	Each new order generates an automatic review of previously approved criteria for use within a specified period of the initiation of therapy	Review of naloxone to investigate possible nosocomial adverse medication event	
	Laboratory or other monitoring criteria are reported for all patients on the drug	Digoxin monitoring based on daily review of digoxin serum levels (49).	
	Abnormal laboratory or other monitoring criteria are reported for all patients on the drug on a regular basis	Regular review of serum creatinine for patients on aminoglycosides	
Prospective	Each new order for the drug is evaluated for compliance with previously approved criteria for use. Variance to the criteria require intervention prior to initiation of therapy	Medication use guidelines (ketorolac) (50) Restricted antibiotics	

TABLE 26.4   Selection of Targets for Focused Medication Use Review[a]

Medication is known or suspected to cause adverse reactions or drug interactions	Medication is used in patients at high risk for adverse reactions
Medication-use process affects large number of patients or medication is frequently prescribed	Medication or process is a critical component of care for a specific disease, condition, or procedure
Medication is potentially toxic or causes discomfort at normal doses	Medication is most effective when used in a specific way
Medication is under consideration for formulary retention, addition, or deletion	Medication or process is one for which suboptimal use would have a negative effect on patient outcomes or system costs
Medication is expensive	

[a] Adapted from American Society of Health-System Pharmacists. ASHP guidelines on medication-use evaluation. Am J Health-Syst Pharm 1996;53:1953–5.

Concurrent or Prospective Focused Medication Use Review

Concurrent or prospective focused medication use review activities can be used to prevent medication-related adverse events and improve the quality of medication use. Information system support has been demonstrated to enhance response to changes in predefined laboratory values. Notice of abnormalities in coagulation, renal function, blood glucose, and electrolytes are all potential indicators of medication use problems in individual patients. When laboratory test results are reported along with specific drugs, it is possible to respond to potential medication-related problems before serious negative outcomes are seen. Kuperman et al. (51) concluded that incorporation of an automatic alerting system in the laboratory data system resulted in a 38% shorter response to appropriate treatment following alert to a critical value.

Strategies for Improving Medication Use

One approach to improving the quality of drug use is the development and implementation of medication use guidelines. This evidential approach to the use of medications is designed to rely on the best available clinical evidence for developing a treatment plan for a specific illness or use of a specific drug or drugs. Simple medication use guidelines can be developed based on literature and the best judgment of in-house experts. Development of more formal clinical practice guidelines is a complex process that relies on well-defined methods to combine the results of multiple studies to draw statistical conclusions. These sophisticated products are often addressed by professional or governmental organizations.

The use of "counter-detailing" by designated hospital staff to offset the impact of pharmaceutical sales forces has been an effective strategy for improving

medication use (52). The objective of this category of quality improvement program is to educate prescribers regarding the organization's approved and preferred medication use guidelines. This has been implemented by providing literature and prescriber contact from a pharmacist or other staff member to support the desired medication use objective.

Several approaches have been described for improving medication use through dosing service teams. Demonstrated enhancements in the quality of medication use have been reported for anticoagulants, antimicrobials, anticonvulsants, and other drugs. The common method of these programs is the use of expert oversight (physicians or pharmacists) to manage therapy with the targeted drug. Therapeutic management may rely on algorithms, pharmacokinetic models, or preapproved collaborative plans (53–63).

Use of standardized medication order forms has been demonstrated to increase quality and effectiveness in medications that are prone to error (64,65). Chemotherapy, patient-controlled analgesia, and antimicrobial drug therapy are likely candidates for order standardization. Yet another approach to improved medication use is implementation of alert systems for sudden, unexpected actions, such as medication stop orders, or use of antidote-type drugs, such as diphenhydramine, hydrocortisone, or naloxone. A computerized application of this method was described by Classen et al. (66).

SUMMARY

The medication use process is a complex system intended to optimize patient outcomes within organizational constraints. Quality medication use involves selection of the optimal drug, avoidance of adverse medication events, and completion of the therapeutic objective. Safe medication practices focus on the avoidance of medication errors. Medication use review and ongoing medication monitoring activities focus on optimizing medication selection and use. These two approaches are important means of assessing and optimizing the quality of medication use.

References

1. Hussar DA. New drugs of 1999. J Am Pharm Assoc 2000;40: 181–221.
2. Johnson JA, Bootman JL. Drug-related morbidity and mortality. Arch Intern Med. 1995;158:1641–7.
3. Committee on Quality of Health Care in America. To err is human: Building a safer health system. In: Kohn LT, Corrigan JM, Donaldson MS, editors. Washington, DC: National Academy Press; 1999. p. 223.
4. Leape LL, Brennan TA, Laird N, Lawthers AG, Localio AR, Barnes BA, et al. The nature of adverse events in hospitalized patients. Results of the Harvard Medical Practice Study II. N Engl J Med 1991;324:377–84.
5. Thomas EJ, Brennan TA. Incidence and types of preventable adverse events in elderly patients: Population based review of medical records. BMJ 2000;320:741–4.
6. National Coordinating Council for Medication Error Reporting and Prevention. Rockville, MD: U.S. Pharmacopoeia; 1999. (Internet at http://www.nccmerp.org.)
7. American Society of Health-System Pharmacists. Suggested definitions and relationships among medication misadventures, medication errors, adverse drug events, and adverse drug reactions. Am J Health-Syst Pharm 1998;55:165–6.
8. Bates DW, Boyle DL, Vander Vliet MB, Schneider J, Leape L. Relationship between medication errors and adverse drug events. J Gen Intern Med 1995;10:199–205.
9. Bates DW, Spell N, Cullen DJ, Burdick E, Laird N, Petersen LA, et al. The costs of adverse drug events in hospitalized patients. JAMA 1997;277:307–11.
10. Nadzam DM. A systems approach to medication use. In: Cousins DD, editor. Medication use: A systems approach to reducing errors. Oakbrook Terrace, IL: Joint Commission on Accreditation of Healthcare Organizations; 1998. p. 5–17.
11. Atkinson AJ Jr, Nadzam DM, Schaff RL. An indicator-based program for improving medication use in acute care hospitals. Clin Pharmacol Ther 1991;50:125–8.
12. Phillips DP, Christenfeld N, Glynn LM. Increase in U.S. medication-error deaths between 1983 and 1993. Lancet 1998;351:643–4.
13. ASHP survey gauges consumer concerns upon entering hospital. Am Soc Hosp Pharm Newsletter, 1999;32(10):1–7.
14. Bates DW, Cullen DJ, Laird N, Petersen LA, Small SD, Servi D, et al. Incidence of adverse drug events and potential adverse drug events. Implications for prevention. JAMA 1995;274:29–34.
15. Berwick DM. Continuous improvement as an ideal in health care. N Engl J Med 1989;320:53–6.
16. Deming WE. Out of the crisis. Cambridge, MA: MIT Press; 2000. p. 87–9.
17. American Society of Health-System Pharmacists. ASHP statement on the pharmacy and therapeutics committee. Am J Hosp Pharm 1992;49:2008–9.
18. Coalition Working Group. Principles of a sound drug formulary system. Rockville, MD: U.S. Pharmacopoeia; October 2000. p 5. (Internet at http://www.usp.org.)
19. Reason JT. Human error. New York: Cambridge University Press; 1990.
20. Lesar TS, Briceland L, Stein DS. Factors related to errors in medication prescribing. JAMA 1997;77:312–7.
21. Cohen MR. Causes of medication errors. In: Cohen MR, editor. Medication errors. Washington, DC: American Pharmaceutical Association; 1999. p. 1.2–1.7.
22. Leape LL, Bates DW, Cullen DJ, Cooper J, Demonaco HJ, Gallivan T, et al. Systems analysis of adverse drug events. JAMA 1995;274:35–43.
23. Nightingale PG, Adu D, Richards NT, Peters M. Implementation of rules based computerised bedside prescribing and administration: intervention study. BMJ 2000;320:750–3.
24. Bates DW, Leape LL, Cullen DJ, Laird N, Petersen NA, Teich JM, et al. Effect of computerized physician order entry and a team intervention on prevention of serious medication errors. JAMA 1998;280:1311–6.
25. Bates DW, Teich JM, Lee J, Seger D, Kuperman GJ, Ma'Luf N, et al. The impact of computerized physician order entry on medication error prevention. J Am Med Inform Assoc 1999;6:313–21.
26. Pestotnik SL, Classen DC, Evan RS, Burke JP. Implementing antibiotic practice guidelines through computer-assisted decision support: clinical and financial outcomes. Ann Intern Med 1996;124:884–90.
27. Raschke RA, Gollihare B, Wunderlich TA, Guidry JR, Leibowitz AI, Peirce JC, et al. A computer alert system to prevent injury from adverse drug events: Development and evaluation in a community teaching hospital. JAMA 1998;280:1317–20.
28. High-alert medications and patient safety. Sentinel Event Alert 11(Nov 19):1999.
29. Cohen MR, Kilo CM. High-alert medications: safeguarding against errors. In: Cohen MR, editor. Medication errors. Washington, DC: American Pharmaceutical Association; 1999. p. 5.11–5.39.
30. Lambert BL. Predicting look-alike and sound-alike medication errors. Am J Health-Syst Pharm 1997;54:1161–71.
31. Lambert BL, Lin SJ, Chang KY, Gandhi SK. Similarity as a risk factor in drug-name confusion errors: The look-alike (orthographic) and sound-alike (phonetic) model. Med Care 1999;37:1214–25.
32. Draft Guidance on Evaluating Proprietary Names. FDA, Rockville, MD. (In Preparation).
33. MedMARx™. Rockville, MD: U.S. Pharmacopoeia; 2000.
34. Nolan TW. System changes to improve patient safety. BMJ 2000;320:771–3.
35. Bates DW. Medication errors. How common are they and what can be done to prevent them? Drug Saf 1996;15:303–10.
36. Cullen DJ, Sweitzer BJ, Bates DW, Burdick E, Edmonson A, Leape LL. Preventable adverse drug events in hospitalized patients: A comparative study of intensive care and general care units. Crit Care Med 1997;25:1289–97.
37. Lesar TS, Lomaestro BM, Pohl H. Medication-prescribing errors in a teaching hospital. A 9-year experience. Arch Intern Med 1997;157:1569–76.
38. Koecheler JA, Abramowitz PW, Swim SE, Daniels CE. Indicators for the selection of ambulatory patients who warrant pharmacist monitoring. Am J Hosp Pharm 1989;46:729–32.
39. Gray SL, Mahoney JE, Blough DK. Adverse drug events in elderly patients receiving home health services following hospital discharge. Ann Pharmacother 1999;33:1147–53.
40. Leape LL, Cullen DJ, Clapp MD, Burdick E, Demonaco HJ, Erickson JI, et al. Pharmacist participation on physician rounds and adverse drug events in the intensive care unit. JAMA 1999;282:267–70.
41. Flynn EA, Barker KN, Gibson JT, Pearson RE, Berger BA, Smith LA. Impact of interruptions and distractions on dispensing errors in an ambulatory care pharmacy. Am J Health-Syst Pharm 1999;56:1319–25.
42. Four-pronged medication error evaluation. ISMP Medication Safety Alert. 1999;4(19):2.

43. Cohen MR, Kilo CM. High-alert medications: safeguarding against errors. In Cohen MR, editor. Medication errors. Washington, DC: American Pharmaceutical Association. 1999. p. 5.2–5.3.

44. Morris AH. Developing and implementing computerized protocols for standardization of clinical decisions. Ann Intern Med 2000;132:373–83.

45. Evans RS, Pestotnik SL, Classen DC, Clemmer TP, Weaver LK, Orme JF, et al. A computer-assisted management program for antibiotics and other antiinfective agents. N Engl J Med 1998;338:232–8.

46. Leape LL. Error in medicine. JAMA 1994;272:1851–7.

47. American Society of Health-System Pharmacists. ASHP guidelines on medication-use evaluation. Am J Health-Syst Pharm 1996;53:1953–5.

48. American Hospital Formulary Service. Drug information 2000. Bethesda, MD: American Society of Hospital Pharmacists; 2000. p. ix–xi.

49. Piergies AA, Worwag EM, Atkinson AJ Jr. A concurrent audit of high digoxin plasma levels. Clin Pharmacol Ther 1994;55:353–8.

50. Krstenansky PM. Ketorolac injection use in a university hospital. Am J Hosp Pharm 1993;50:99–102.

51. Kuperman GJ, Teich JM, Tanasijevic MJ, Ma'Luf N, Rittenberg E, Jha A, et al. Improving response to critical laboratory results with automation: results of a randomized controlled trial. J Am Med Inform Assoc 1999;6:512–22.

52. Soumerai SB, Avorn J. Predictors of physician prescribing change in an educational experiment to improve medication use. Med Care 1987;25:210–21.

53. Ellis RF, Stephens MA, Sharp GB. Evaluation of a pharmacy-managed warfarin-monitoring service to coordinate inpatient and outpatient therapy. Am J Hosp Pharm 1992;49:387–94.

54. Dager WE, Branch JM, King JH, White RH, Quan RS, Musallam NA, et al. Optimization of inpatient warfarin therapy: Impact of daily consultation by a pharmacist-managed anticoagulation service. Ann Pharmacother 2000;34:567–72.

55. Destache CJ, Meyer SK, Bittner MJ, Hermann KG. Impact of a clinical pharmacokinetic service on patients treated with amino-glycosides: A cost-benefit analysis. Ther Drug Monit 1990;12:419–26.

56. Cimino MA, Rotstein CM, Moser JE. Assessment of cost-effective antibiotic therapy in the management of infections in cancer patients. Ann Pharmacother 1994;28:105–11.

57. Okpara AU, Van Duyn OM, Cate TR, Cheung LK, Galley MA. Concurrent ceftazidime DUE with clinical pharmacy intervention. Hosp Formul 1994;29:392–4, 399, 402–4.

58. Kershaw B, White RH, Mungall D, Van Houten J, Brettfeld S. Computer-assisted dosing of heparin. Management with a pharmacy-based anticoagulation service. Arch Intern Med. 1994;154:1005–11.

59. De Santis G, Harvey KJ, Howard D, Mashford ML, Moulds RF. Improving the quality of antibiotic prescription patterns in general practice. The role of educational intervention. Med J Aust 1994;160:502–5.

60. Donahue T, Dotter J, Alexander G, Sadaj JM. Pharmacist-based i.v. theophylline therapy. Hosp Pharm 1989;24:440, 442–8, 460.

61. Ambrose PJ, Smith WE, Palarea ER. A decade of experience with a clinical pharmacokinetics service. Am J Hosp Pharm 1988;45:1879–86.

62. Li SC, Ioannides-Demos LL, Spicer WJ, Spelman DW, Tong N, McLean AJ. Prospective audit of an aminoglycoside consultative service in a general hospital. Med J Aust 1992;157:308–11.

63. McCall LJ, Dierks DR. Pharmacy-managed patient-controlled analgesia service. Am J Hosp Pharm 1990;47:2706–10.

64. Lipsy RJ, Smith GH, Maloney ME. Design, implementation, and use of a new antimicrobial order form: A descriptive report. Ann Pharmacother 1993;27:856–61.

65. Frighetto L, Marra CA, Stiver HG, Bryce EA, Jewesson PJ. Economic impact of standardized orders for antimicrobial prophylaxis program. Ann Pharmacother 2000;34:154–60.

66. Classen DC, Pestotnik SL, Evans RS, Burke JP. Description of a computerized adverse drug event monitor using a hospital information system. Hosp Pharm 1992;27:774, 776–9, 783.

DRUG DISCOVERY AND DEVELOPMENT

27

Portfolio and Project Planning and Management in the Drug Discovery, Development, and Review Process

CHARLES GRUDZINSKAS

Drug Development Consultant, Annapolis, Maryland

INTRODUCTION

Drug discovery, development, and regulatory review is a complex, lengthy, and costly process that involves in excess of 10,000 activities. To manage and optimize the returns of this process, the biopharmaceutical industry has embraced the two disciplines of 1) portfolio design, planning, and management (PDPM) and 2) contemporary project planning and management (PPM). The obvious benefits of good portfolio and project planning and management are shown in Table 27.1.

The beneficial use of these two tools by both the industry and the Food and Drug Administration (FDA) is evidenced by prioritized resource allocations and significant decreases in both drug development times and FDA review times. We are now entering an era in which the time from FIH (first in human) trial to submission of a New Drug Application (NDA) is, dependent on the therapeutic claim(s), expected to range from 3 to 4 years, rather than the 5 to 7 years that traditionally have been required. Likewise, as a result of the use of project management techniques, we have seen FDA review times for regular NDAs reduced from the 1988 average of 34.1 months to an average of 14.6 months in 1999 (1). Review times have been shortened even further for priority NDAs. Indeed, one NDA was reviewed within 18 days of the NDA submission (2). In 1999, 28 priority NDAs were reviewed with a mean review time of 6.1 months, and the antivi-

ral division has recently reviewed several HIV treatment NDAs in under 3 months (3).

What Is a Portfolio?

A *well-planned and managed* pharmaceutical research and development (R&D) portfolio can be defined as: "The combination of *all* R&D projects, that based on past company and industry performance, *will predictably yield* valuable new products at the *rate needed* to support the planned growth of the organization." Portfolio design, planning, and management are the processes that the industry uses to ensure a well-balanced and value-optimized portfolio. Likewise, the FDA and other regulatory agencies have a portfolio of projects that includes review of Investigational New Drug Applications (INDs), review of IND annual reports, meetings with sponsors, NDA reviews and advisory committee meetings, as well as legislated initiatives and reporting obligations.

What Is Project Planning and Management?

Project planning is an integral part of project management, which is defined in the Project Management Institute's *Guide to the Project Management Body of Knowledge* (4) as "the application of knowledge, skills, tools, and techniques to project activities in order to meet or exceed stakeholder needs and expectations

351

TABLE 27.1   Benefits of Good Portfolio and Project Planning and Management

The organization is able to do more with less

The organization is able to optimize the value of a portfolio of projects

Better planning

Better decision making

Projects finish on time

Projects finish within budget

from a project." For an excellent text on the application of project management principles, the reader is referred to *Practical Project Management* by Dobson (5). An excellent resource for those who would like to become actively involved in biopharmaceutical project management is the Drug Information Association's (DIA) Project Management Special Interest Advisory Committee (PM SIAC). Information on how to join the DIA PM SIAC can be found on the DIA website (6).

PORTFOLIO DESIGN, PLANNING, AND MANAGEMENT

Portfolio management is the term used to describe the overall process of program and franchise management. This process actually includes the three dimensions of portfolio design, portfolio planning, and portfolio management. Each of these three dimensions will be described. The five components needed for the successful use of portfolio design, planning, and management (PDPM) are identified in Table 27.2. If any one (or more) of the five components is missing or not fully operational, then the likelihood of successful PDPM will be limited.

Most large organizations have now adopted the portfolio management team (PMT) concept. PMT membership consists of the senior management of the organization, and the mission of the PMT is to oversee the successful design, planning, and management of the organization's portfolio. The PMT usually has several working groups that focus on specific therapeutic

TABLE 27.2   The Five Components of Successful Portfolio Design, Planning, and Management

Portfolio design

Portfolio planning

Portfolio management

Portfolio management teams (PMTs)

Portfolio optimization using sensitivity analysis

areas. The ultimate responsibility of the PMT is to ensure that the portfolio has been optimized to maximize its potential expected value.

Maximizing Portfolio Value

Portfolio value is maximized by appropriately prioritizing the projects within the portfolio based on the future potential financial value of each project multiplied by its probability of success. The future value of each development project is based on a calculation of its net present value *(NPV)*. In this calculation, the anticipated financial return from the project is compared with that of an alternative investment of an equivalent amount of capital (7). The general equation for calculating *NPV* is:

$$NPV = I_0 + \frac{I_1}{1+r} + \frac{I_2}{(1+r)^2} + \cdots + \frac{I_n}{(1+r)^n} \quad (27.1)$$

where the *I*s are given a negative sign for annual net cash outflow and a positive sign for projected net annual income. The subscripts and exponents correspond to the number of years of projected development and marketing time, and *r*, termed the *discount rate*, is the rate of return of an alternate investment, such as U.S. Treasury Bills. An *NPV* analysis using a 5% discount rate is summarized for a hypothetical drug in Table 27.3. It is assumed that the drug will be developed within 4 years at a total cost of $500 million. Because this investment is spread over 4 years, development funds budgeted for this project that are unexpended after year zero are assumed to be earning 5% interest until spent, and are discounted accordingly. Marketing begins in year 4 but income is similarly discounted as shown in Equation 27.1 and is assumed to be negligible when patent protection expires after year 7. The *NPV* for the project is the sum of the discounted cash inflows and outflows over the life of the product, and in this case is $31.3 million. The *NPV* is far less than the $150 million difference between total income and expenditures for the project because this latter difference makes no allowance for potential alternative use of the money. The *internal rate of return* is another metric that may be helpful in evaluating different projects in a portfolio (7). The internal rate of return is defined simply as the discount rate needed to yield an *NPV* of zero, and would be 6.78% for the hypothetical project shown in Table 27.3.

The probability of success is the product of the probability of technical success, the probability of regulatory success, and the probability of commercial success. The criteria for these probabilities of success need to be clearly defined and characterized so that future

TABLE 27.3 Discounted Cash Flows for a Hypothetical Drug Development Project[a]

	Year	0	1	2	3
Development	Expense	($25)	($75)	($200)	($200)
	Discounted expense	($25)	($71.4)	($181.4)	($172.8)
	Year	4	5	6	7
Marketing	Income	$50	$100	$200	$300
	Discounted income	$41.1	$78.4	$149.2	$213.2

[a] Dollar amounts are in millions. In this case, NPV (sum of discounted cash flows) equals $31.3 million.

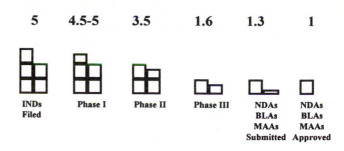

FIGURE 27.1 Attrition of pharmaceutical and biological candidate products during clinical development and regulatory review. For every five compounds entering clinical development, only one is eventually approved. Abbreviations: IND = Investigational New Drug Application, NDA = New Drug Application, BLA = Biologics License Application, MAA = Manufacturing Authorization Application (European Union equivalent of the NDA).

PMTs can translate the impact of project progress and decisions on the value of the projects in the portfolio (see the section on portfolio optimization using sensitivity analysis).

It is easy to see that projects that are at the FDA (or other worldwide regulatory review bodies) for review will most commonly have the highest probability of success. Therefore, they are likely to have the highest overall financial value in the portfolio (overall value equals possible future value times the probability of success), whereas projects that are in the discovery stage will have the lowest overall value in the portfolio (but are the lifeblood of the organization 4 to 5 years in the future). It is the role of the PMT to develop a "balanced portfolio" that supports both the near-term, mid-term, and long-term needs of the organization. The R&D senior management team needs to ensure that organizational resources are properly allocated according to the agreed upon prioritization.

Portfolio Design

It is not an overstatement to say that the near-term and long-term future of a biopharmaceutical company depends on the size and likelihood of success of its pipeline. The pipeline is the totality of a company's portfolio, consisting of projects ranging from very early discovery to marketed products that are ending their current life cycle and will need a line extension (new formulation or expanded indications) to remain competitive. A pharmaceutical R&D portfolio begins with a vision of the intended growth rate of the organization. Based on the envisioned growth rate, a portfolio can be developed that is based on what the future pipeline will need to look like at each stage of the drug development process. The size of the pipeline needed at each stage of drug development is estimated from both past industry and regulatory experiences. It is generally agreed that only one compound reaches the market for every five that enter the clinical development process. The odds of success for the phases of drug development are shown in Figure 27.1.

Therefore, as shown in the portfolio pyramid in Figure 27.2, a company that wants to have one new product (NDA or BLA) approved each year would have to submit five new INDs each year, initiate three to four new Phase 2 projects per year, and begin at least one or two new Phase 3 projects each year. Naturally, if a company wanted to develop two or three new NDAs/BLAs each year, it would have to have a pipeline that is respectively two or three times as large as that illustrated in Figure 27.1.

Portfolio Planning

Once the portfolio vision and design have been defined, the organization can focus on how to build that portfolio. As projects mature from one stage to the next, or are terminated for lack of success, additional projects will need to be added to the various stages of the portfolio to ensure a portfolio of adequate size at each stage. To maintain an aggressive portfolio, companies have acknowledged that it is nearly impossible to fill the pipeline by being dependent only on home-grown research. There are many sources for new products in addition to the organization's own discovery program. For example, companies can fill out their portfolios by entering into joint ventures and alliances with both established and start-up organizations. Additional sources of new products include licensing

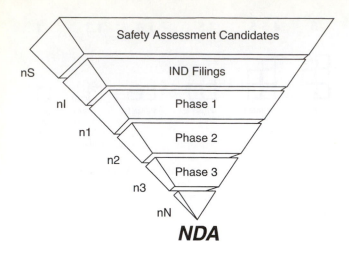

FIGURE 27.2 Size of the drug development portfolio needed to support an NDA pipeline. (nS = number of compounds that will need to be screened each year, nI = number of INDs that will need to be submitted each year, n1 = number of Phase 1 projects that will need to be initiated each year, n2 = number of Phase 2 projects that will need to be initiated each year, n3 = number of Phase 3 projects that will need to be initiated each year, and nN = number of NDAs that will to be submitted each year.

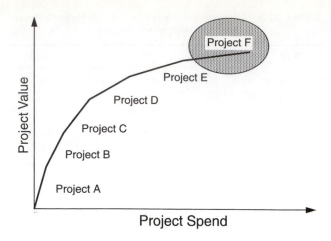

FIGURE 27.3 Relationship between project value and R&D funds invested in their clinical development (project spend). The value of this hypothetical portfolio would be the cumulative value of its constituent projects. The project in the oval clearly has the lowest expected value per project spend. These low-value projects are usually considered candidates for termination. In addition to termination as a possibility, effective companies evaluate the low expected value projects to identify the drivers that would lead to a significant increase in the project's expected value (see Portfolio Optimization Using Sensitivity Analysis and Figure 27.5).

early stage research from the NIH, universities and foundations (e.g., the Red Cross). Thus, the planning process includes both the identification and successful in-licensing of the products needed to populate the stages of the drug development process that we saw in Figure 27.2.

Portfolio Management

Portfolio management is primarily focused on the prioritization of projects within the portfolio. Several consulting groups and software programs are available to aid in the management of an existing portfolio. These same tools can be used to explore "what-if" scenarios to determine how the addition or deletion of projects to the portfolio either increases or decreases the portfolio's overall value. As with most processes of this nature, the most important consideration is the quality of the information regarding the potential value and probability of success of each project. Precise evaluations of the commercial, regulatory and technical probabilities need to come from those in the organization who have sufficient experience to be able to make educated and reliable estimates of both expected values and probabilities.

As illustrated in Figure 27.3, organizations can graph the value that is expected to be gained vs. the cost of the R&D needed to achieve the overall value that is calculated for each project. Organizations can

then make decisions as to how to allocate resources based on the "steepness" of the slope of each project, keeping in mind that projects closest to the market, which have the highest probability of success, will likely have the steepest slope. In the next section we examine how to avoid the pitfall of assuming that projects, such as the one identified in the oval, necessarily need to be terminated because they have less than acceptable expected value vs. cost slopes. Indeed, we will see how to determine how to increase the expected value of low-value projects.

Obviously, organizations will want to populate their portfolio with projects that balance potential value and probability of success, as illustrated in Figure 27.4. Clearly the most desirable projects are in Quadrant I (high value with a high probability of success). Projects in Quadrant IV, with low value and low probability of success, should be examined for ways to increase the expected project value or the probability of success, or recommended for termination. Unfortunately, few projects fall into Quadrant I, so a typical portfolio is composed of projects mostly from Quadrants II and III (most organizations try to avoid Quadrant IV type projects). Several analogies are used to describe the four quadrants that constitute Figure 27.4, of which my favorites are shown in Table 27.4.

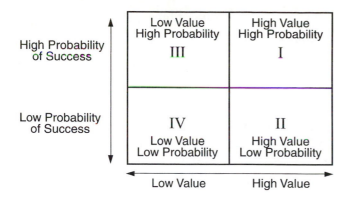

FIGURE 27.4 Four quadrant table used for portfolio analysis in which projects are evaluated on the basis of their potential financial return (value) and probability of development success.

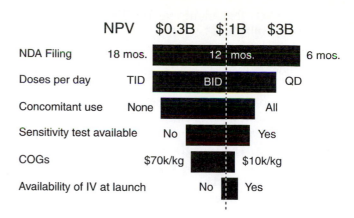

FIGURE 27.5 Tornado chart illustrating a sensitivity analysis for the development of a hypothetical antibiotic. Abbreviation: COGs = cost of goods.

Portfolio Optimization Using Sensitivity Analysis

Sensitivity analysis is used to identify and quantify project characteristics that are major factors in the expected value of a project, and is one of the most powerful tools of modern portfolio management. Sensitivity analyses serve two goals. The first goal is to identify the project characteristics that were used to determine the project value, the so-called value drivers, and ensure that the project plan developed by the project team solidly supports these value drivers. For example, a value driver for a potential sedative hypnotic might be that it has no potentiation or interaction with alcohol. Because much of the value of this project depends on this product characteristic, the project team will plan to assess this expected value driver as early as possible in the development cycle.

The second goal is to identify characteristics that, *if added* to the project characteristics, would significantly increase the expected value of the project. This type of sensitivity analysis is important for all projects in the portfolio, but is critically important for those that are in danger of being terminated from the portfolio for lack of adequate value. The results of a sensitivity analysis are plotted with ranges of value for each criterion and are called tornado charts because their shape resembles that of the meteorological phenomenon. Using as an example the project plan shown in Figure 27.5 for a hypothetical oral antibiotic, we see that the portfolio analysis has determined that the "as planned" NPV for the project is one billion dollars (represented by the dotted axis on the tornado chart). The stipulation of "as planned" underscores an important caveat, for the value determined was based on the project goals shown in Table 27.5.

What one can learn from this sensitivity analysis is that the scenario with the highest probability of occurring ("most likely") is the one that incorporates the following:

- The NDA will be filed in 12-months.
- Twice-a-day dosing will be established.
- The product can be administered concomitantly with many, but not all of the drugs that might be expected to be used by this patient population.
- A diagnostic kit for antibiotic sensitivity will not be widely available at the time that product marketing is launched.
- The cost of goods will be in the range of $25,000 per kg.

TABLE 27.4 The Four Portfolio Quadrants

Quadrant I	A diamond mine
Quadrant II	Betting the ranch
Quadrant III	A sure bet
Quadrant IV	A turkey ranch

TABLE 27.5 Example of "As Planned" Goals for a Hypothetical Oral Antibiotic

NDA filing	In 12 months
Dose regimen	Twice a day
Concomitant use	With some, but not all drugs likely to be used by this population
Laboratory kit	Available at launch
Cost of goods	~ $ 25,000/kg
IV formulation	Not available at launch

- It is unlikely that an intravenous form of the drug will be available at launch.

This "most likely" scenario values the oral antibiotic at one billion dollars. The bars for each of the critical goals indicate that product value would be increased by two billion dollars if the NDA could be filed in 6 months. Likewise, the value would be reduced to $300,000,000 if the time required for NDA filing slips to 18 months. The sensitivity analysis also indicates that the product could have an increased value of 2.5 billion if a once-a-day formulation could be developed. Although other changes would also increase the *NPV* of the product, the first two (a NDA within 6 months and a once-a-day formulation) provide the greatest increase in value. Clearly the PMT and the senior management board would focus the project resources on these two high-value areas. If there were limited resources, then the project team would be asked which of the two increased value goals (NDA or once-a-day formulation) would be the most likely to be achieved.

Once the portfolio has been designed, planned, and managed for optimization, it is the project team's job to make it happen.

PROJECT PLANNING AND MANAGEMENT

Project planning and management for the biopharmaceutical industry began in the early 1980s and became an integral part of the R&D organization by the mid-1980s. The paper entitled *Change + Communication = Challenge—Management of New Drug Development* provides a review of the tools that are still used in biopharmaceutical project management (8). Project planning and management have progressed to the point that there are now six dimensions of project planning and management that are routinely used to plan and manage biopharmaceutical projects (Table 27.6). An overview of each of these dimensions will be provided.

TABLE 27.6   Project Management Dimensions in the Biopharmaceutical Industry

Project planning

Project scheduling

Team management

Resource allocation

Decision making

Process leadership and benchmarking

Project Planning

Defining a Project

Biopharmaceutical projects, like all projects, consist of three components that must be planned and managed. These three components are *project specifications*, *project resources*, and *project timing*. These components can be thought of as "the what?," "the how?," and "the when?" of a project, respectively. Once these three components have been defined and agreed on, the resulting project components are known as the *baseline specifications*, the *baseline resources* and the *baseline timing*.

Project specifications (The What?) includes 1) the projected efficacy, safety, and especially the differentiation criteria of a project, 2) formulations (e.g., oral, parenteral, transdermal, controlled release, etc.), and 3) package styles (e.g., bottles, ampoules, and blister packs).

Project resources (The How?) includes funding, staff (both internal and external), subjects, beds, clinical supplies, bulk drug, animals, cages, and facilities.

Project timing (The When?) consists of the timing for both the overall project and the subproject goals.

Time can also be thought of as a resource. However, time is the one resource that cannot be replaced. An organization can provide additional staff, funds, animals, subjects, and so on, but it cannot recapture time once it has been consumed. Project timing can be established by three processes. The first process of establishing project timing is by the forward planning process based on project specifications and available (sometimes limited) resources. The second process for establishing project timing is by an impending deadline, which the organization uses to define the balance between 1) project specifications that can be accomplished within the specified project time frame and 2) the available project resources. The third process for establishing project timing is to set the deadline, define what must be accomplished, and then resource accordingly to ensure that the defined project can be completed by the deadline.

It needs to be noted that project planning and project scheduling are two separate, but interdependent dimensions. The ideal way to develop a drug development program is to first define the goals of the project (see label driven-question based development planning in Chapter 33). Once the goals are defined, a core project team is established. It is the role of the core team to: 1) develop a strategic and tactical plan that defines and supports the major project objectives, 2) define the project go/no-go decisions with prespecified decision criteria, as far as possible, 3) identify the individual activities and supporting tasks that will be needed to accomplish the project objectives, and 4) identify the order in which these tasks need to be carried out and any interdependencies between activities.

There are at least two approaches for defining the order of the activities. The first is the "plan for success" approach in which as many activities as possible are conducted in parallel to provide the shortest time path to the go/no-go decisions and to the project completion. The second approach is used when there are very scarce resources or when there is a low probability of project success. This second approach defers expensive activities until a "proof of concept" (POC) has been achieved for the project. Once the POC has been achieved, then a "plan for success" development plan for the project will be developed and implemented. One can also stage development of lower prioritized projects in a portfolio if resources are limited, or if the risk is still high and the project needs to be managed more conservatively by the organization.

An Example of a Project Definition

An example of a project definition in the biopharmaceutical industry would be the development of a new chemical entity for the indication of treating mild to severe congestive heart failure (CHF), with both an oral and an intravenous formulation being developed, and with a projected development time of 3 years to NDA submission and a budget of $75,000,000. A subproject would be to complete a clinical proof of concept (POC) for the severe CHF indication for the intravenous formulation in 1 year with a budget of $9,000,000.

The Project Management Triangle

Project components can be represented as the three sides of a triangle as illustrated in Figure 27.6. This representation is quite useful, since once the project components have been established, the length of each side (component) of the project management triangle can be locked-in. As usually happens with any project, changes constantly occur. If a project is changed by expanding the number of indications or formulations, then we realize from our geometric analogy that one or both of the other two components needs to change. Either the project resource component must be increased to adhere to the original schedule, or the project timing component must be lengthened to maintain the project resource component as originally defined, or a balance needs to occur, involving a change in both the project timing and project resource components.

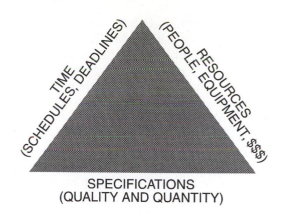

FIGURE 27.6 The project management triangle. A change in one side of the triangle necessitates changes to one or more of the other sides.

The Project Cycle

As illustrated in Figure 27.7, the project cycle consists of six stages (9). The first stage of a project, the *initiation stage*, encompasses the planning stage, which includes the definition of the three project components (specifications, resources, and timing), even in a preliminary fashion. The project initiation stage includes creation of a project team composed of individuals representing the many disciplines needed to complete the project. This stage usually begins with a kick-off meeting in which the project goals and project components are presented, team members are introduced to each other, and agreement is reached regarding operating procedures for the project team. The second stage of a project is called the *implementation stage*. During this stage, project planning, project scheduling, and resource allocation actually start. For a drug development project these first efforts will probably

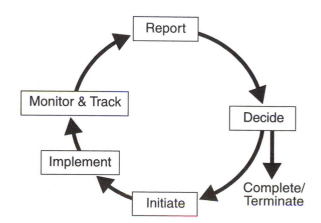

FIGURE 27.7 The project cycle. (Adapted from Szakonyi R. How to successfully keep R & D projects on track. Mt. Airy, MD: Lomond Publications, Inc.; 1988.)

focus on the preparation of bulk active compound for formulation screening and animal safety studies, and the start of these animal studies (e.g., see Chapter 29). The third stage of a project is called the *monitoring and tracking stage*. The critically important point to be made regarding monitoring and tracking is to focus and limit attention on what is tracked so that linkage is established to the major milestones that will determine whether forward motion on the project is being made. The fourth stage is the *reporting stage*. The decision on what needs to be reported and to whom the information needs to be reported should be based on what decisions will be made and by whom. Clearly, the level of detail reported to a project team member is more than the level needed by senior management to make major decisions. The next stage is the *decision-making stage*. A key point to remember regarding the decision-making stage is that a useful definition of a decision is "an allocation of resources." When a decision is made, resources must be either added to a project, taken away from it, or maintained. The next project stage is the *completion/termination stage*. This stage is reached for each project cycle and is determined by either achieving or not achieving the project goals and objectives of that cycle.

PROJECT PLANNING AND MANAGEMENT TOOLS

Several tools that are useful in the planning and management of biopharmaceutical projects are identified in Table 27.7. Definitions can be found in the PMI *A Guide to the Project Management Body of Knowledge* (4) and within the tutorial and help sections of Microsoft Project®. It is important to point out that these tools are useful only after the project objectives, goals, go/no-go decisions, decision criteria, and the operating assumptions have been established. The project planning management tools are presented in Table 27.7 in the order in which they would be introduced in a project planning process.

TABLE 27.7   Project Planning and Management Tools

Decision trees
Milestone charts
PERT charts
Gantt charts
Work breakdown structures (WBS)
Financial tracking

Decision Trees

The use of decision trees became more frequent during the mid-1990s as companies realized that drug development programs could indeed be completed in under 48 months. An example of the decision tree that was developed by CDER for the IND review process is shown in Figure 27.8. This example was obtained from the CDER Handbook website (10). For each of the boxes shown in this figure, the website includes a narrative that can be accessed by clicking on the respective box. The website contains a similarly informative decision tree for the NDA review process. The industry uses similar decision trees with prespecified criteria for success at each decision point. Decision points for a specific biopharmaceutical project should focus on technical hurdles such as those shown in Table 27.8.

Milestone Charts

Milestone charts consist of a tabulation of major drug development milestones. Whereas the go/no-go decisions previously discussed are very project specific, development milestones are much more generic and can usually be applied to a wide variety of projects. Typical milestones for pharmaceutical development are shown in Table 27.9.

PERT/CPM Charts

PERT (Performance Evaluation, Review, and Tracking) and CPM (Critical Path Method) charts (flowcharts) show the flow and connectivity and the interdependency of project tasks, activities, and goals. A PERT chart (Figure 27.9) depicts the activities in the order that they will need to be carried out, either in series or in parallel. These charts also identify which activities need to be completed (or initiated) before the next activity, which is dependent on it, can be initiated.

CPM is the methodology used to identify the longest or *critical path* from project initiation to project completion. In Figure 27.9, the critical path is Path 3 since this path is the longest path from "A" to "H." The significance of the critical path is two-fold. The first is that if any activity on the critical path is delayed by 1 day, the whole project will be delayed by 1 day. The second point is that once the critical path activities have been identified, the project team has three jobs to focus on. The first is to find a way to shorten the critical path. The second job is to track critical path activities very closely to ensure that there is no slippage. The third is to track all the activ-

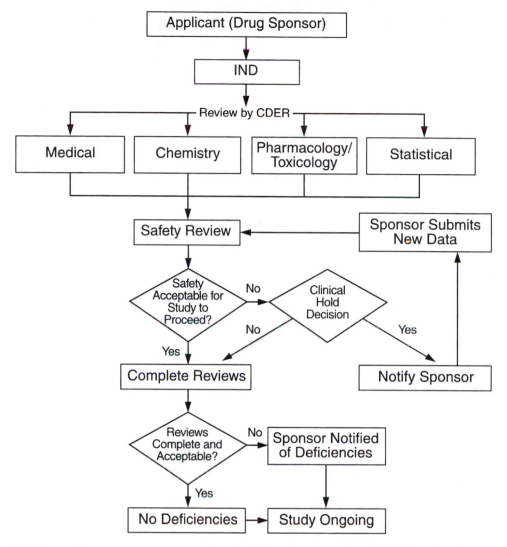

FIGURE 27.8 The decision tree used for the IND review process by CDER. (Reproduced from Internet at http://www.cder.fda.gov/cder/handbook/).

TABLE 27.8   Specific Project Go/No-Go Decisions

The serious toxicity observed in dogs will not be observed in primates

A stable IV formulation has now been identified

An effective dose and dosing regimen have been characterized

A process to reduce the high cost of goods has been achieved

The human safety observed is as predicted

Clinical activity is observed at 1/20th the highest no adverse effect human dose

Synergy is demonstrated with the new combination product

Highest survival ever observed is reported with this test medication

TABLE 27.9   Typical Project Milestones

Chemical lead identified

Clinical candidate selected

First in human (FIH) trial initiated

Effective dose and dose regimen characterized

Phase 3 trials initiated

Phase 3 trials completed

NDA/BLA submitted

NDA/BLA approved

Product launched

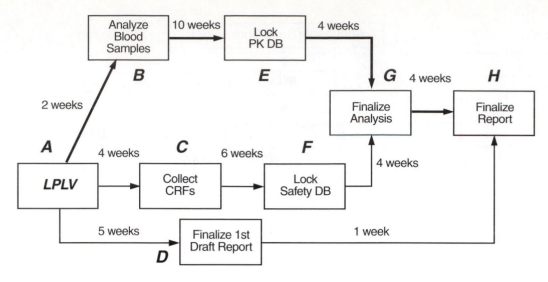

FIGURE 27.9 A PERT chart showing three paths. Path 1 (A + D + H) will require 6 weeks. Path 2 (A + C + F + G + H) will require 18 weeks. Path 3 (A + B + E + G + H) is the longest, requiring 20 weeks and is the critical path designated by the thick arrows. (Abbreviations: LPLV = Last Patient Last Visit, CRFs = case report forms, DB = data base).

ities that could possibly negatively impact the critical path to ensure that these "subcritical path activities" are initiated and completed as scheduled.

Gantt Charts

Horizontal bar charts (Figure 27.10) are used to view 1) the length (duration) of each task, activity, and objective, 2) the temporal relationship between various activities, and 3) the actual progress versus the original plan that has been made on each task, activity, and objective. A number of project-tracking software systems are available, and one has the ability to view the whole project as well as just the high-level objectives (milestones and decisions).

Project progress is shown in a number of ways,—for example, by shading part of the activity bar to indicate the proportion of the activity that has been completed (e.g., 75% shaded to represent that 75% of the subjects needed for a clinical trial have been enrolled). A particularly effective way to track both project progress and identify key activities that are lagging behind the agreed on schedule is to set up a comparison bar chart that includes the current bar chart schedule, the previous bar chart schedule, and the bar chart schedule that was originally planned.

Work Breakdown Structures (WBS)

A WBS can be thought of as an organizational chart of tasks and activities needed to achieve the project objectives. The project WBS can arranged either by deliverables (e.g., formulations, clinical trials, etc.) or by resource (formulation chemist, clinical trial monitor, etc.). A common way of illustrating these different approaches is by analogy with the construction of a new house. One part of the construction WBS would include plumbing and might be sorted by either house level or by room. A second option would be to sort the construction WBS by rooms, with each room having as part of its WBS items such as: framing, pluming, wiring, flooring, drywall, painting, and so on.

Financial Tracking

The financial tracking of individual projects has become an increasingly important role for biopharmaceutical project teams. In some organizations, a member of the R&D comptroller's office is a member of the project team. In other cases, individuals from this office are available to support the project team. The project team is asked on an annual basis to project the funds needed for the project over the next 36 months for the project to meet the approved goals. The team is also asked to help track the project costs on a real-time basis and to make quarterly projections as to the spend rate over the next 12 months. Although some organizations have developed financial tracking tools internally, a number of project-driven financial tracking tools are now commercially available (e.g., MS Project®, SAP).

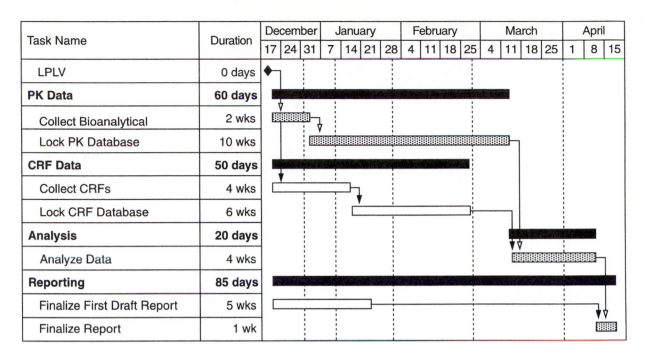

Task Name	Duration	December 17	24	31	January 7	14	21	28	February 4	11	18	25	March 4	11	18	25	April 1	8	15
LPLV	0 days																		
PK Data	**60 days**																		
Collect Bioanalytical	2 wks																		
Lock PK Database	10 wks																		
CRF Data	**50 days**																		
Collect CRFs	4 wks																		
Lock CRF Database	6 wks																		
Analysis	**20 days**																		
Analyze Data	4 wks																		
Reporting	**85 days**																		
Finalize First Draft Report	5 wks																		
Finalize Report	1 wk																		

FIGURE 27.10 A Gantt chart (bar chart) with the critical path indicated by the stippled bars and arrows. (Abbreviations: LPLV = Last Patient Last Visit, CRF = case report form.)

Project Scheduling

As mentioned earlier, the project schedule is a product of the scope of the project objectives, project resources, and time requirements. Projects can either be scheduled to complete "no later than...," in which case an appropriate balance of objectives and resources has to be determined. In other cases, the project objects are established, the resources that are available for the project are allocated, and the project team uses project management software to predict when the project is likely to be completed given the limitations of the allocated resources. Clearly, allocation of more resources to a resource-limited project could accelerate the project significantly.

PROJECT TEAM MANAGEMENT AND DECISION MAKING

Core Project Teams

In the pharmaceutical industry, the formal use of core project teams to accelerate drug development began in the early 1970s. Rather than review the attributes and value of the team concept here, the reader is referred to an excellent text on the subject by Katzenbach and Smith (11). The current standard for biopharmaceutical project team structure is the matrix team, which is made up of core-team members from relevant functional organizations that are needed for the development of a new drug (i.e., toxicology, discovery, analytical, formulations, clinical, and regulatory) and a project team leader and a project manager. It is the project manager's role to ensure that current project information has been incorporated into the various project planning and management tools that the organization is using. Using project management tools, the project manager develops various project scenarios for use at project decision-making meetings. Each core-team member represents the combined functions of his or her department and is supported by his or her own set of team members back in that department. Each core-team member is also the team leader of his or her respective functions for the project, which may be called subteams (e.g., clinical subteam, regulatory subteam).

The term *matrix* refers to the fact that project team members have a dual reporting relationship and therefore are known as multiply supervised employees (MSEs). The traditional matrix team concept has performed adequately. But, as initially conceived, the performance evaluation of team members was conducted only by their departmental management, so that the focus of team members was usually centered on their functional department. However, this evaluation structure was modified in the early 1990s by having each team member's performance evaluated, at least in part, by his or her project team leader. This change has greatly increased the effectiveness of the matrix team approach.

In the mid-1980s, Abbott Pharmaceuticals introduced the concept of the "project venture team" in which those who worked on a particular project reported to a project department head. In the mid-1990s, Lilly introduced the concept of "heavyweight teams." Heavyweight teams are formed at the end of Phase 2 and members of these teams devote their entire time to the advancement of a single project to NDA submission, approval, and launch. Most recently, both matrix and heavyweight teams are adopting the concept of co-location or a project "village." Although the core-team team members are formally part of a functional department, their "project offices" are all within a few feet of each other. This village concept has been particularly successful because it fosters rapid and frequent communication among the core-team members. Several large biopharmaceutical companies are now building new facilities just to house "villages" for the co-location of project teams.

Project Team Leadership and Project Support

Project teams are led and supported in a number of ways as identified in Table 27.10.

FDA Project Teams

With the advent of the Prescription Drug User Fee Act (PDUFA), which legislated new timelines for NDA reviews, the FDA introduced the project team concept for both IND and NDA reviews. For INDs, a FDA project team is established upon IND submission. When an NDA is received, an important responsibility of the NDA review team is to determine whether the submission is adequate for review by the FDA. Within 45 days of the NDA submission, the NDA review team will either accept the NDA for review or return the submission to the sponsor along with the reasons why it was not acceptable for review (Refuse to File). The role of Center Project Manager has been created in both CDER and CBER. An FDA medical officer generally leads the technical review and a project manager, sometimes called a regulatory manager, oversees the process.

Effective Project Meetings

The ability to manage a meeting effectively is a skill that is most highly regarded in all types of organizations. Effective meetings rarely occur without good preparation and effective meeting management. A well-developed agenda is the most effective tool for holding a successful meeting. Indeed, in some organizations the mantra is becoming "no agenda, no attenda." Having the right people attend the meeting is as important as having an effective agenda. This means that the team leader, the project manager, and all the team members have a special responsibility to ensure

TABLE 27.10   Team Leadership and Project Support Alternatives

Team leadership	Advantages	Disadvantages
Dual leadership Technical Process	Provides both strong technical *and* process leadership	Two bosses, mixed signals
Technical (usually clinical)	Strong technical leadership	Limited management of process Usually a part-time role in a full-time job
Full-time team leader	Team leader is dedicated to project	Might not have strong technical knowledge of the project Might be leading multiple projects

Team support	Advantages	Disadvantages
Dedicated project manager	Provides both strong process and project planning *and* management support	None
None	None	Places excess burden on the project team leader to both lead and provide process and project planning and management support

that those who are needed at the meeting do indeed attend. With modern day video capabilities and conference calling, many meetings can be very effective and productive even when not all the participants can be at the same physical site. It is important for one person to be responsible for ensuring that all the remote-site participants receive meeting materials in advance of the meeting, either electronically or by fax or mail. It is not acceptable to delay a meeting for 15 minutes while everyone is waiting for a fax to be sent to participants at a remote site. Most organizations have multimedia tools in their libraries to help their staff develop effective meeting management skills.

Resource Allocation

Resource allocation has become more important with the advent of prioritized portfolios. Once a portfolio is prioritized by the PMT, and the core project team has been informed of their project's priority, the core project team will allocate the available resources for their project in a manner that will provide for the most progress to be made over a given budget period, usually 12 months. For those who manage a department, resource allocation takes on an added dimension, for although a department head may have adequate resources for all of the approved projects, the need for the resources might not be evenly spaced over the next 12 months. For example, the portfolio of projects might need 75% of the department's annual resources in the first 6 months and the remaining 25% in the second 6 months. Ideally, project team leaders, project managers, and department staff will help to resolve this mismatch by meeting and developing several alternative scenarios for senior management review and approval. For the decisions to be soundly based, management will ask each team to identify the impact of each alternative scenario on the project objectives and milestones.

Effective Project Decision-Making

Decision Trees

An excellent example of a decision tree is shown in Figure 27.8. This example outlines the IND regulatory review and approval process. Similar decision trees are developed by project teams within the biopharmaceutical industry. Project teams are now being asked not only to construct decision trees, but to develop contingency plans based on "what-if" scenarios far in advance of the next decision points. The goal is to ensure that the project will not lose forward motion in the event of a "no" decision that requires

rework or another loop through the project cycle, or a decision by the PMT that resources for a particular project are more urgently needed for another project.

Prespecified Decision Criteria

To facilitate the decision-making process, project teams should develop prespecified criteria for each decision point or contingency. These criteria provide the critical targets for the project and speed up the decision-making process. An example of clinical go/no-go decision criteria for a potential antihypertensive drug might be: "lowers diastolic blood pressure by at least 10 mmHg for at least 6-months in at least 80% of the subjects treated with the middle of three doses, with a side-effect profile no worse that that observed for the active control." One can only imagine the debate that will occur if the blood pressure lowering observed at 6 months is 8 mmHg. Finally, effective decision making must include an assessment of resource allocation because, as previously emphasized decision making is in reality the allocation of resources.

Process Leadership and Benchmarking

It is appropriate to conclude this chapter with some comments about process leadership and benchmarking. The ability to understand how all the complex pieces of drug development come together can only be learned through hands-on experience as a team leader or project manager. Corporate management in the biopharmaceutical industry is now counting on individuals with this experience to identify ways in which the drug development process can be shortened even further than we have seen in the recent past.

Benchmarking has become an important tool that is being used to identify ways in which an organization can quantify, then exceed, industry standards for the time, cost, and quality of the R&D activities that are needed to discover and bring a new drug to market. Benchmarks can be as broad as "How long should it take from FIH to NDA submission?" to "How long should it take to design an approvable clinical protocol and case report form for a one-site clinical study?" The Centre for Medicines Research (CMR) has been formally conducting benchmarking studies for the industry and additional information can be found on their website (12).

The emphasis on both process leadership and benchmarking in the project planning and management (PPM) domain of biopharmaceutical R&D truly illustrates the level of maturity and sophistication that the discipline of PPM has achieved.

References

1. FDA/CDER. Approval times (in months) for NDAs and NMEs approved fiscal years 1988–2000 (Updated 11/21/2000). (Internet at http://www.fda.gov/cder/rdmt/fy00ndaap.htm.)
2. Grudzinskas CV, Wright C. Reshaping the drug development and review process—A case study of an 18-day approval. Pharmaceutical Executive, October 1994;14:74–80.
3. FDA/CDER. 1999 Report to the Nation. (Internet at http://www.fda.gov/cder/reports/rtn99.pdf.)
4. PMI Standards Committee. Guide to the project management body of knowledge, (A PMBOK® Guide). Newtown Square, PA: Project Management Institute; 2000.
5. Dobson M. Practical project management. Mission, KS: SkillPath Publications; 1996. p. 288.
6. See Internet at www.diahome.org.
7. Baker SL. Perils of the internal rate of return. (Internet at http://hadm.sph.sc.edu/Courses/Econ/invest/invest.html.)
8. Grudzinskas C. Change + Communication = Challenge—Management of new drug development, Clinical Research Practices and Drug Regulatory Affairs, 1988;6:87–111.
9. Szakonyi R. How to successfully keep R & D projects on track. Mt. Airy, MD: Lomond Publications Inc.; 1988. p. 103.
10. FDA/CDER. (Internet at http://www.cder.fda.gov/cder/handbook/.)
11. Katzenbach C, Smith D. The wisdom of teams: Creating the high-performance organization. New York: Harperbusiness; 1994. p. 336.
12. See Internet at www.cmr.org/metrics.html.

28

Drug Discovery

ROBERT R. GORMAN

Saguaro Consulting, Scottsdale, Arizona

INTRODUCTION

It would be beyond the breadth and scope of this chapter to try to outline and put into perspective the gradual growth and maturation of pharmaceutical discovery research over the past 100 years. I would refer the reader to an article by Jurgen Drews (1) that projects an excellent overview of the history and development of the modern pharmaceutical industry. This chapter will concentrate on what I view as a renaissance in drug discovery research that is revolutionizing the entire industry. This renaissance was brought about by a series of seemingly unrelated factors.

1. In the early 1990s, economic forces were working against the pharmaceutical industry. There were tremendous pressures (and still are) to control rising drug costs. Despite this fact, the cost of delivering one new drug to the market was skyrocketing from approximately 200 million dollars per drug in 1990 to about 500 million today (2).

2. The emergence of the generic drug industry significantly reduced the effective marketing life of a drug once the patent expired. Historically, pharmaceutical companies could continue to sell their products with excellent financial return and almost no competition for several years after a patent expired. Today, it is not unusual for over one-half of total sales to be lost during the first year after patent expiration.

These changes in the economic realties of the pharmaceutical industry led some to question whether the industry could sustain, or even should sustain, large research and development expenditures in view of the market constraints that had emerged.

3. It was at this time in the late 1980s and early 1990s that new enabling technologies began to emerge. These technologies included modern cellular and molecular biology, high-throughput screening, combinatorial chemistry, genomics, proteomics, computer-assisted drug design, transgenic animal models of disease, and the bioinformatics that are needed to integrate the large volumes of data that result from these new technologies. It is the integration of these new technologies with the existing infrastructure that has invigorated the modern pharmaceutical industry.

These new tools and technologies afforded pharmaceutical companies an opportunity to improve their level of innovation and the speed and efficiency of their drug discovery and development programs. These improvements have encouraged companies to continue to invest large sums in research and development, two to three billion dollars per year for the largest multinational companies today. This optimism was spurred by analyses of potential time savings associated with the use of new technologies. Savings in time equate directly to cost savings in drug development, as well as increased years of patent exclusivity due to a faster time to market. For example, one paradigm shows that if the time it took for a molecule to go through the drug discovery process into development was reduced by 40%, the cost per development candidate would drop approximately 50%. These types of improvements are being realized by some companies, but the real savings will come if the new technologies deliver molecules to development that have a higher success rate.

Historically, only one of five drugs that enter clinical development actually ends up as an approved and marketed drug. It is too early to tell if the new technologies will have a significant impact on this important statistic. However, if this ratio could be changed to only two of five, there would be a tremendous reduction in the cost of pharmaceutical research and development. Meanwhile, the belief that technology will improve the ratio of successful to unsuccessful candidates has spurred large increases in spending on research and development, and the renaissance that we will discuss in this chapter.

THE DRUG DISCOVERY PROCESS

The modern drug discovery process is graphically displayed in Figure 28.1. It is a multidisciplinary approach that begins by identifying a specific unmet medical need, such as treatment for AIDS. This is followed by the search for a drug that can interdict the disease in a predictable manner, based on a new or emerging biological hypothesis (e.g., inhibition of the HIV protease enzyme in AIDS patients).

This hypothesis is then used to identify a specific molecular target, and large libraries or collections of molecules are screened against the target to find a

potential new regulatory molecule or drug. The screening is an interactive process that can involve secondary and tertiary screens to validate the specificity of the molecule. Ideally, at least one of the secondary screens would be a validated animal model of the targeted disease (e.g., blood glucose normalization in genetically diabetic mice), but truly reliable animal models are seldom available. This is becoming even more problematic as molecular biology and genomics make more and more molecular targets available. Today, many new drugs move into early clinical development with only the knowledge that they activate or block a molecular target that is thought to be involved in a disease process. This is particularly true in diseases of the central nervous system in which truly validated animal models are rare.

Once the lead molecules are identified, classical medicinal chemistry approaches, as well as newer computer-assisted drug design, are used to further "fine tune" the molecule. This fine tuning may involve attempts to improve the intrinsic potency of the molecule; the selectivity of the molecule for the molecular target (e.g., inhibition of cyclooxygenase-2 but not cyclooxygenase-1 in anti-inflammatory molecules), the bioavailability of the molecule, and often its stability and formulation properties.

Once a molecule is identified as a true lead, the refined or advanced leads are further evaluated for bioavailability and other pharmacokinetic properties, and finally undergo preclinical safety evaluation. Today, drug discovery extends well into the phases of human clinical testing. But since these aspects are covered in subsequent chapters, we will focus the discussion here on the discovery process up to the point of lead compound identification.

ENABLING TECHNOLOGIES

To understand their potential impact, it is important that we discuss each of the enabling technologies so that the reader has a clearer understanding of their potential influence on the drug discovery process.

High-throughput Screening

High-throughput screening has been defined as the collection of technologies that enable the rapid assay of compounds for therapeutic potential (3). Historically, screening was viewed as a necessary but laborious aspect of drug discovery in the pharmaceutical industry. It was usually done by a few people who could screen (or evaluate for activity) a few hundred compounds per week, and a complete screen of an

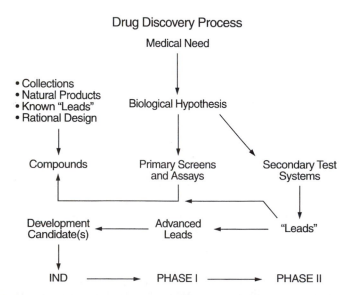

FIGURE 28.1 Drug discovery process—the modern drug discovery process is an iterative procedure that is directed toward the discovery and development of new medicines.

entire library of compounds might take 6 months to a year to complete.

New automated technology has allowed companies to completely robotize the screening process. Robots weigh out the compounds, dissolve the compounds in an appropriate solvent, and complete the screen, including data entry, often in a completely automated manner. This automation, combined with new detection and analysis techniques, has completely revolutionized the screening process. In a matter of weeks, literally hundreds of thousands of molecules can be screened against a variety of targets that include receptors, ion channels, and cell lines (4).

The advances in assay automation and format and data analysis have enabled scientists to screen against more targets more quickly and to rapidly move into lead optimization with interesting molecules. In purely pragmatic terms, the increased efficiencies and sensitivities of the new screening techniques also preserve valuable compounds within the collection, some of which may have been synthesized or collected decades earlier. This also allows for the rapid evaluation of large collections of new compounds that can be generated using combinatorial chemistry.

Combinatorial Chemistry

There are many different combinatorial schemes, but all the approaches attempt to assemble every possible permutation of a group of distinct chemical building blocks. One of the most often used schemes is the so-called "split-and-mix" or "split-and-pool" technique (5). This process involves starting with a single chemical building block and attaching it with a corresponding chemical identification tag to a large pool of polymer beads. These beads are split into, say, 10 batches, and a different building block and tag combination is then added to each of the 10 batches. All the beads and their 10 molecular pairs are then mixed together and subdivided into 10 groups, so each group now contains all 10 pairs. As additional chemical building blocks are added, the number of different combinations grows exponentially.

Combinatorial chemistry was originally envisioned as a way to synthesize collections of macromolecules, such as peptides, that were tethered to tiny polymer beads. The power of the combinatorial approach is demonstrated in Figure 28.2. In this example, the chemist starts with 20 discrete synthons (e.g., 20 natural amino acids). If the 20 synthons are taken through three synthetic steps, 8.0×10^3 new combinations of molecules are possible. Five discrete synthetic steps can drive the number to 3.2×10^6 new molecules. Obviously, the size of combinatorial libraries can

Size of Combinatorial Libraries

No. Synthons (Step 1) x No. Synthons (Step II x ... No. Synthons (Step n) = No. Members

	Steps	Members
20 Synthons (e.g. natural amino acids)	3	$20^3 = 8.0 \times 10^3$
	4	$20^4 = 1.6 \times 10^5$
	5	$20^5 = 3.2 \times 10^6$
100 Synthons	3	$100^3 = 1 \times 10^6$
	4	$100^4 = 1 \times 10^8$
	5	$100^5 = 1 \times 10^{10}$

FIGURE 28.2 Combinatorial chemistry—using combinatorial chemistry, scientists can expand a pool of new molecules exponentially in a very short period of time.

become huge. Thus, the strengths of combinatorial chemistry are 1) the size of the libraries, 2) the large number of nonbiased structural entities that are made, and 3) the fact that the libraries are based on a common "parent" template. The weaknesses of combinatorial chemistry are: 1) the difficulties associated with dereplicating or identifying individual molecules; 2) the challenge of purifying the hits from the combinatorial mixture; 3) the lack of overall structural diversity within a particular combinatorial library; and 4) the fact that not all molecules are amenable to combinatorial approaches. However, many chemical and analytical approaches have been developed that are beginning to overcome these potential drawbacks (6).

Combinatorial chemistry is now being done entirely in solution without solid supports. Solution approaches also have drawbacks, but new chemical and analytical approaches are rapidly making combinatorial chemistry the preferred approach for many medicinal chemistry problems (7).

Similarity-Dissimilarity Testing

One of the most useful of the new enabling technologies combines classical chemical structure and physical chemical information together in a relational database. These data can be "searched" for both similar and dissimilar characteristics (5). These databases are generated so that companies can track the hundreds of thousands of molecules that are held in their compound libraries. Using a predetermined set of parameters such as chemical structure, solubility, melting point, previous screening data, and even such biological data as oral bioavailability, compounds are entered into the chemical database. Using the computer, it is possible to select the 10,000 compounds that are most dissimilar from a library of perhaps 500,000 discrete compounds. Another way to conceptualize this is to consider the process as the selection of the 10,000 compounds that present the maximum diversity within the entire collection. It is often this collection of dissimilar compounds that are first screened using high-throughput methods. If a hit is found in these first 10,000 compounds, the computer is then queried for the 500 compounds within the collection that are most similar to the original hit. Using this technique, it is possible to quickly identify the best lead molecule that will serve as the basis for subsequent lead optimization and rational drug design.

Genomics

No other area of technological change has had or will have a greater impact on modern drug discovery than genomics (8). The term *genomics* really encompasses a whole series of sophisticated technologies and data management systems that are all pointed toward developing a new series of medicines that treat the cause of the disease, not just the symptoms. These techniques include: 1) the brute force sequencing of DNA in humans and other organisms that has led to the first complete map of the human genome; 2) cDNA microarray technology that analyzes gene expression in various disease states; and 3) positional cloning and family history analyses that are used to identify disease-causing mutations in specific genes. Often, genetic information and analysis will elucidate a gene target, but the actual activity or function of the gene product is not known. In some cases, transgenic or knockout mice can give a clue to the function of a gene product, but these experiments are fraught with difficulties. To address this problem, the field of functional genomics has been established. This technique establishes actual gene function in humans by extrapolating genetic information from other species where genetics are more easily done, such as fruit flies, nematodes, yeast, bacteria, and mice.

One impact of genomic data is the realization that, almost certainly, not all patients with a particular disease will react in exactly the same manner to a particular drug therapy. As scientists discover more sophisticated measurements of genetic variation, physicians will be able to correlate genetic patterns with particular responses or nonresponse to drug therapy. This will have a huge impact on the drug discovery process. Clinical trials will only be done on those patients who could potentially benefit from the treatment, and the size of the patient population tested will be smaller. This specificity should improve the proportion of drug candidates entering clinical trials that actually become successful drugs.

Although not usually discussed, the information systems and super computers needed to manage the genetic information are nearly as important as the genetic information itself. Without the growth of bioinformatics, there would be no renaissance in drug discovery today. Ideally, all the concentration on these new enabling technologies will soon lead us to where we all want to go: the discovery and development of more specific and efficacious drugs.

DISCOVERY OF A DRUG—A CASE HISTORY

For the remainder of the chapter, we will demonstrate how many of the enabling technologies were used to discovery an actual molecule, tipranavir (PNU-140690)[1], that is in clinical development as an HIV protease inhibitor (9).

The HIV protease inhibitors initially brought to market (ritonavir, indinavir, and saquinavir) were all peptidomimetics based on a similar chemical backbone (9). Because they are peptidomimetics, they are expensive to manufacture and, because they are structurally similar, considerable cross-resistance has been a problem. In other words, once an AIDS patient becomes resistant to one peptide-based HIV protease inhibitor, a substantial degree of resistance is also encountered with the other inhibitors. Because of this, pharmaceutical companies began to search for non-peptide-based inhibitors of the HIV protease.

Similarity-Dissimilarity Screening

The first step in the drug discovery process is to screen a so-called similarity-dissimilarity (sim-disim) collection of molecules against the active recombinant human HIV protease. Figure 28.3 shows a representative large and structurally diverse collection of molecules. Within the collection, there may be a number of active compounds, but we do not know which ones they are. The collection of dissimilar compounds is quickly screened and an active molecule is found. Then the search is expanded from the small (10,000 compound) dissimilar collection to the entire compound database (500,000 compounds), looking for compounds that are most similar in structure and activity to the initial hit from the dissimilar collection (Figure 28.4).

---

[1] PNU-140690 is the library designation number for N-(3)(1R)-1-[(6R)-4-hydroxy-2-oxo-6-phenethyl-6-propyl-5,6-dihydro-2H-pyran-3-1] (propylphenyl)-5-(trifluoromethyl)-2-pyridine sulfonamide.

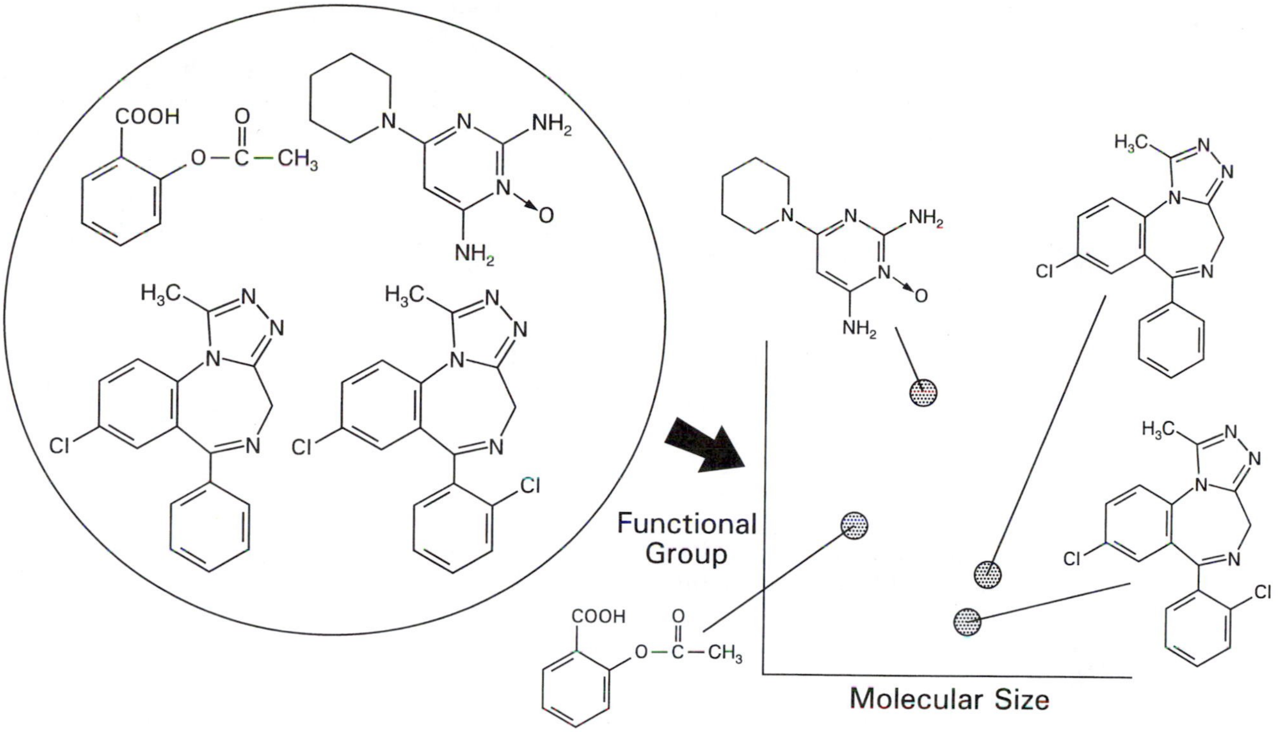

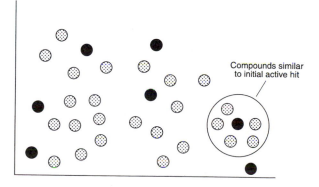

FIGURE 28.3 Dissimilarity screening—pharmaceutical companies have large collections of molecules. By testing structurally diverse molecules first, the efficiency of the screening process is enhanced.

This screening process was followed in searching for a nonpeptide inhibitor of HIV protease (9, 10). The most potent HIV protease inhibitor within the sim collection of molecules proved to be phenprocoumon[2]. This coumarin analog is a competitive inhibitor ($K_i \sim 1$ μM) of both the HIV-1 and the HIV-2 protease, and effectively blocks HIV replication in human peripheral blood leukocytes (ED_{50} 100–300 μM).

Structure-based Design

Phenprocoumon could be readily incorporated into and studied within the crystal structure of the HIV-1 protease. This ability to visualize the molecule within the crystal structure of the protease allowed for the use of an iterative structure-based design paradigm to design even more potent analogs. In the simplest sense, one can view the interaction of the coumarin analogs with the active site of the protease as a classical lock-and-key interaction of a drug with a receptor

molecule. After this interaction was visualized, new molecules were designed and synthesized and tested as inhibitors of the protease. As more active molecules were found, these were again visualized within the crystal structure and the process was repeated through multiple steps.

Similarity-Based Compound Selection

Compounds similar
to initial active hit

FIGURE 28.4 Similarity-based screening—once an active molecule is found through dissimilar screening, molecules that are structurally similar to the "hit" can be quickly identified and studied.

[2] Phenprocoumin is the trivial name for 4-hydroxy-3-(1-phenyl-propyl)-2H-chromen-2-one.

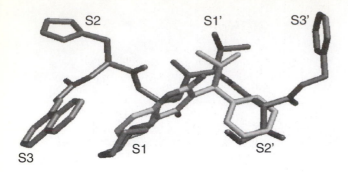

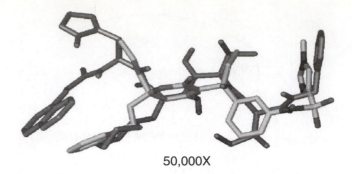

50,000X

FIGURE 28.5 Structure-based drug design—computer-generated overlay of phenprocouman (*light structure*) and a peptide-based HIV protease inhibitor (*dark structure*) within the crystal structure of the enzyme.

FIGURE 28.6 Structure-based drug design—computer-generated overlay of the newly designed coumarin analog, tipranavir (PNU-140690, *light structure*), and a peptide-based HIV protease inhibitor (*dark structure*) within the crystal structure of the enzyme. The new coumarin analog is 50,000 times more potent than the original lead.

Figure 28.5 shows a computer-generated overlay of both phenprocouman and a highly potent peptide mimetic inhibitor ($K_I < 1nM$) within the active site of the HIV protease. Chemists used this information to "build" highly active peptide mimetic molecules that filled the same binding pocket and interacted with particular amino acid residues. Within a period of 4 months, the iterative process generated a new molecule that was 50,000 times more potent than the original phenprocouman molecule. As can be seen in Figure 28.6, an overlay of the highly potent tipranavir molecule against the peptide mimetic shows great similarity between the two when visualized within the structure of the HIV protease. Based on this high intrinsic potency, favorable data from secondary screens, and importantly, the finding that the molecule could inhibit viral replication of ritonovir resistant

HIV, tipranavir was taken into clinical development (10, 11).

THE DRUG DISCOVERY FUNNEL

This chapter can be summarized by Figure 28.7. The entire drug discovery process can be thought of as a funnel. Movement through the funnel depends on an understanding of the disease, the selection of an appropriate molecular target, the construction of a high-throughput screen, the identification of a hit, the optimization of the hit through the use of modern enabling technologies, and finally the selection of the best lead(s). Statistically, perhaps only five molecules

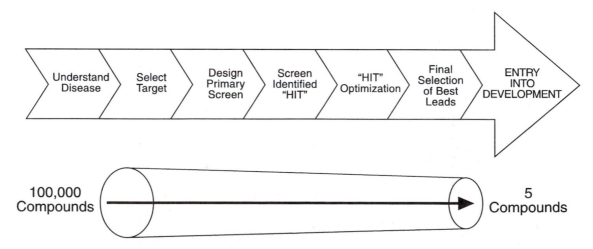

FIGURE 28.7 Drug discovery funnel—drug discovery can be viewed as a funnel in which hundreds of thousands of molecules enter the funnel, but only five out of 100,000 compounds actually enter into drug development

in 100,000 are considered for actual development. Once the lead(s) are chosen for development, a myriad of preclinical and clinical programs are initiated. These steps will be the subject of subsequent chapters.

This type of funnel could have been drawn 20 years ago. What has changed is the science that drives the process. Genomics allows for a much fuller understanding of the molecular basis of disease. This improves target selection, and the enabling technologies that we have discussed have greatly accelerated the discovery process and increased the number of molecules entering into clinical development. Only time will tell if this increase in knowledge also reduces the number of drug development failures and generates the types of innovative medicines that the new technologies promise.

References

1. Drews J. Drug discovery: A historical perspective. Science 2000;287:1960–4.
2. Agnew B. When pharma merges, R & D is the dowry. Science 2000;287:1952–3.
3. Persidis A. High-throughput screening. Nat Biotechnol 1998;16:488–9.
4. Kenny BA, Bushfield M, Parry-Smith DJ, Fogarty S, Treherne JM. The application of high-throughput screening to novel lead discovery. Prog Drug Res 1998;51:245–69.
5. Schreiber SL. Target-oriented and diversity-oriented organic synthesis in drug discovery. Science 2000;287:1964–9.
6. Houghten RA, Pinilla C, Blondelle SE, Appel JR, Dooley CT, Cuervo JH. Generation and use of synthetic peptide combinatorial libraries for basic research and drug discovery. Nature 1991;354:84–6.
7. Jung G. Combinatorial chemistry: Synthesis, analysis, screening. Weinheim, Germany: Wiley-VCH; 1999. p. 480.
8. Housman D, Ledley FD. Why pharmacogenomics? Why now? Nat Biotechnol 1998;18(suppl):2–3.
9. Tomasselli AG, Heinrikson RL. Targeting the HIV-protease in AIDS therapy: A current clinical perspective. Biochim Biophys Acta 2000;1477:189–214.
10. Thaisrivongs S, Strohbach JW. Structure-based discovery of tipranavir disodium (PNU-14069E): A potent, orally bioavailable, nonpeptidic HIV protease inhibitor. Biopolymers 1999;51:51–8.
11. Poppe SM, Slade DE, Chong KT, Hinshaw RR, Pagano PJ, Markowitz M, Ho DD, Mo H, Gorman RR 3rd, Dueweke TJ, Thaisrivongs S, Tarpley WG. Antiviral activity of the dihydropyrone PNU-140690, a new nonpeptidic human immunodeficiency virus protease inhibitor. Antimicrob Agents Chemother 1997;41:1058–63.

29

Preclinical Drug Development

CHRIS H. TAKIMOTO* AND SAMIR N. KHLEIF†

*Division of Medical Oncology, Department of Medicine, University of Texas Health Science Center, San Antonio, Texas
†Developmental Therapeutics Department, Medicine Branch, National Cancer Institute,
National Institutes of Health, Bethesda, Maryland,

INTRODUCTION

From the time a promising molecule is first identified in a drug discovery and screening program to the time it enters a Phase I clinical trial, an enormous amount of scientific work and evaluation must be performed. Preclinical development, as defined in this chapter, encompasses all the activities that must take place before a new chemical entity can be administered to humans. As such, it spans the gap between drug discovery and clinical testing.

This chapter describes the general processes and concepts involved in the preclinical development of oncologic agents with specific examples taken from the current program for developmental therapeutics as established by the National Cancer Institute (NCI) of the National Institutes of Health. The details of the preclinical development programs for other types of agents that are under industry sponsorship are frequently regarded as proprietary information, whereas those of the NCI are open and accessible to the public. For this reason, this chapter will focus on the U.S. federal government's approach to preclinical drug development to provide specific examples of how these programs are integrated into the greater overall effort of developing new and clinically useful drugs for the treatment of human disease.

COMPONENTS OF PRECLINICAL DEVELOPMENT

The components of preclinical drug development can be divided into four general areas that include: 1) *in vitro* studies defining a new agent's pharmacologic properties, 2) drug supply and manufacturing, 3) drug formulation, and, finally, 4) *in vivo* studies in animal models demonstrating a potential for clinical efficacy and proof of therapeutic principle.

In Vitro Studies

Preliminary *in vitro* studies of a new pharmacologic agent are often closely related to drug discovery and screening efforts. *In vitro* systems can be used to identify new agents or classes of agents with novel pharmacologic properties, such as the ability to inhibit a specific enzyme or to block receptor-ligand interactions. Laboratory studies can help to characterize a drug's molecular mechanism of action and to identify specific drug targets. Understanding the molecular pharmacology of a drug at this stage of development is also important for identifying determinants of drug response and for characterizing a drug's pharmacodynamic effects. These studies can also provide insight into potential mechanisms of drug resistance. With the recent advent of molecular target-based drug screening programs, as discussed in Chapter 28, the molecular pharmacology of promising compounds will already have been extensively studied at a relatively early stage in preclinical development.

In vitro assessment of new drugs can be performed in intact cell lines or in cell-free systems. Examples of cell-free systems include assays that measure enzyme inhibition, receptor binding, or protein-small molecule interactions. These types of tests may form the basis for high-throughput screening assays employed in large-scale drug discovery or combinatorial chemistry efforts designed to identify new agents with specific molecular properties. For example, the ability of small molecules to stabilize topoisomerase I-DNA cleavable complex formation was recently assessed using a novel scintillation proximity assay (SPA) (1). The synthesis of microsphere SPA beads containing a fluorescence scintillant embedded within their matrix allowed for the emission of a fluorescence signal when the beads were in close proximity to a beta-emitting radioisotope, such as tritium. Coating of the SPA beads with recombinant human topoisomerase I protein followed by incubation with tritium-labeled DNA permitted rapid high-throughput screening of compounds for camptothecin-like activity that stabilized the [3H]-DNA-topoisomerase I protein-cleavable complex. In the presence of a camptothecin topoisomerase I poison, stabilization of the [3H]-DNA bound to the topoisomerase I-SPA bead resulted in the emission of a fluorescence signal. This method rapidly detected agents that promoted the stabilization of DNA-topoisomerase I cleavable complexes in 96-well microtiter plates. Furthermore, it could easily be generalized to screen for compounds that promote any specific DNA-protein binding interaction of interest (1).

Another novel approach to preclinical *in vitro* drug testing is to use genetically defined cell lines to assess drug effects against cells containing known specific DNA mutations. For example, the NCI has been studying the use of genetically defined yeast strains as a screening tool for the *in vitro* testing of potential anticancer agents (2). The identification of drugs that selectively kill yeast cells containing the same molecular mutations that are commonly found in human cancers, such as *p53* or *ras* gene mutations, could lead to the discovery of entirely new classes of drugs with selective activity against cancer cells. Obviously, this approach depends on a detailed understanding of the specific molecular abnormalities that exist in human cancers and on the ability to characterize and grow yeast strains containing defined mutations analogous to those found in human tumors.

The most common *in vitro* screen used to identify potential anticancer agents has been the demonstration of growth inhibitory or cytotoxicity potency in cultured murine or human tumor cell lines. Although the demonstration of anticancer effects *in vitro* is quite far removed from anticancer activity in clinical studies, it does provide predictive information about the potential for anticancer activity. Cell-line studies performed *in vitro* also provide the opportunity to study the biochemical and molecular effects of a new agent on various cell processes, such as macromolecule synthesis of RNA, DNA, or proteins. Effects on tumor cell growth, cell cycle distribution, cell differentiation, or the induction of apoptosis can also be readily measured at this stage of drug development. Growth inhibitory activity against human tumor cell lines growing in culture forms the basis for the 60 human tumor cell-line screen, which is the principle anticancer screening instrument used by the NCI (3). Finally, the relative cytotoxic potency against cell lines derived from specific human tumors can also provide a preliminary assessment of the likely spectrum of antitumor activity of a new agent.

In vitro cell-line studies are also useful for analyzing specific mechanisms of drug resistance. Well-characterized sublines have been developed that differ from parental wild-type cells in their expression of specific drug resistance mechanisms. Common examples include cell lines that express the P-glycoprotein-mediated, multidrug resistance (MDR) phenotype, or the multidrug resistance protein (MRP), both of which confer drug resistance to a wide variety of natural product anticancer agents. Assessment of the relative antitumor activity in an MDR-expressing cell line compared to the nonresistant, parental wild-type cells can provide information regarding the potential importance of this particular mechanism of drug resistance for a new anticancer agent (4).

In vitro methods for predicting important pharmacokinetic parameters, such as oral absorption and hepatic metabolism, have also been developed. For example, oral bioavailability can be predicted by measuring drug transport across a monolayer of Caco-2 human colon carcinoma cells, as discussed in Chapter 4 (5, 6). Furthermore, there is now a growing body of literature on predicting the extent of *in vivo* drug metabolism based on *in vitro* metabolism experiments (7). It is now common to use human liver microsomes or commercially available recombinant human P450 systems to study *in vitro* drug metabolism and identify potentially serious drug interactions during preclinical drug development (see Guidance for industry: Drug metabolism/drug interaction studies in the drug development process: studies *in vitro*, available on the Internet at http://www.fda.gov/cder.)

Drug Supply and Formulation

Prior to entering clinical trials, adequate drug supplies of pharmaceutical grade material must be available. This may require the development of bulk chemical synthesis protocols or, in the case of natural product isolation, adequate amounts of raw materials for the extraction of either a drug or its synthetic precursors. Manufacturing of pharmaceutical products for clinical testing in the United States must be conducted under current Good Manufacturing Practice (cGMP) guidelines that have been specifically defined by the U.S. Food and Drug Administration (FDA). An extensive discussion of these regulations is beyond the scope of this text, but the current regulations have been published in the U.S. Code of Federal Regulations and are available over the Internet at the U.S. FDA website at http://www.fda.gov/cder.

Drug supply problems initially delayed the development of paclitaxel, a natural product antitumor agent with activity against ovarian, breast, and lung cancer (8). Paclitaxel is found in the bark of the Pacific yew tree, *Taxus brevifolia* (9). Poor yields (0.01%) of paclitaxel from harvested tree bark meant that very large amounts of the plant product were necessary to sustain the clinical development of this agent (10). As a consequence, its availability during the early clinical testing program was limited (11). However, pharmaceutical scientists have now found that more favorable yields of paclitaxel precursors can be isolated from the yew tree needles, which represent a renewable source material (12). Semisynthetic production of paclitaxel from these precursors has helped to improve the supply of this active anticancer agent.

Formulation of drugs for clinical use may also present major difficulties in developing new agents. This is particularly true for drugs that require special routes or methods of administration, such as transdermal, inhalational, or topical therapies, or for agents that are given as timed-released formulations. However, even routine intravenous administration can sometimes be challenging for drug formulation scientists. For example, paclitaxel is poorly soluble in standard aqueous intravenous solutions. Clinical development of this agent could not proceed until a suitable intravenous formulation in Cremophore EL (polyoxyethylated castor oil) was developed (8). However, use of complex vehicles such as Cremophore EL can have substantial clinical consequences. The high incidence of potentially life-threatening hypersensitivity reactions seen during short infusions of paclitaxel has been attributed to the intravenous administration of Cremophore EL (13–15). Another example of a formulation problem that delayed the clinical development involved 9-aminocamptothecin (9-AC), an insoluble camptothecin derivative. Clinical development of 9-AC was given a high priority by the National Cancer Institute in 1989; however, clinical trials of this natural product derivative did not begin until 1993. This delay represented the time required to develop a suitable formulation of the drug in dimethylacetamide, polyethylene glycol and phosphoric acid (16, 17).

In Vivo Studies—Efficacy Testing in Animal Models

Although animal models were used for screening promising anticancer agents in the past, they are generally considered too cumbersome and expensive for large-scale high-throughput screening of drugs in the current era. Consequently, *in vivo* animal models of drug activity are now generally employed for later testing after promising agents have been identified in preliminary drug screening and discovery programs. Nonetheless, studies in animal models are extremely important for demonstrating potential clinical efficacy and establishing proof of therapeutic principle. Preclinical animal studies are also the first opportunity to define the toxicity profile of a new agent and to perform detailed single-dose and multiple-dose toxicology studies. Practical issues that can also be addressed in animal models include the initial assessment of drug pharmacokinetics and pharmacodynamics as well as the determination of a safe starting dose and schedule of treatment for the initial Phase I clinical trials in humans (see Chapter 31).

In the field of cancer drug development, there are many properties that distinguish a malignant from a normal cell, including uncontrolled growth, metastasis, de-differentiation, genetic plasticity, and drug resistance. However, only uncontrolled growth has been extensively studied as a target for cancer chemotherapy. Newer therapeutic strategies now in clinical testing include interfering with the metastatic cascade, inducing differentiation, interrupting autocrine or paracrine growth loops, blocking tumor angiogenesis pathways, inhibiting cell cycle and growth signaling cascades, enhancing tumor immunogenicity, and reversing drug resistance. However, despite substantial advances in *in vitro* laboratory models, many of these approaches can only be adequately assessed in *in vivo* animal model systems.

A number of animal model systems have been developed to provide tumor microenvironments that mimic the clinical situation. However, there are no perfect animal models for drug development. The adequacy of any specific animal model depends on its validity, selectivity, predictability, and reproducibility (18). In cancer chemotherapy, animal models are selected to simultaneously demonstrate antitumor efficacy and systemic toxicity in an intact organism. Ideally, the tumor system under study in the animal model should be genetically stable with homogeneous biologic characteristics over time.

Spontaneous Tumors

The tumors used in animal models arise either spontaneously or are artificially transplanted into the animal. Spontaneous tumors can be idiopathic, or they can be induced by the application of carcinogenic stimuli (19, 20). Although spontaneous tumors can highly resemble the human clinical situation, a number of factors make these tumors poorly reproducible in controlled settings. These include difficulties in adequately staging the tumors, variations in their natural history, and the low yield of animals that actually develop tumors. Consequently, spontaneous tumors have greater utility in the study of carcinogenesis or chemoprevention, and are somewhat less useful as routine models for the treatment of established tumors.

Transplanted Tumors

In contrast, transplanted animal or human tumor xenograft models are some of the most widely used tools for studying experimental therapeutics in cancer. Established transplantable murine tumors have been extensively characterized and demonstrate excellent homogeneity and reproducibility (21). Examples of murine tumors commonly used in preclinical screening of antitumor agents include Lewis lung carcinoma, melanoma B16, sarcoma 180, L1210 leukemia, and P388 leukemia. A major advantage of these transplantable murine tumors is that the animals under study have intact immune systems.

An important advance in preclinical models for anticancer agents was the development of immunosuppressed mouse strains that allowed for the reproducible implantation and growth of human tumor cells *in vivo*. The first xenograft of a human colon cancer cell line into immunocompromised "nude" mice was reported in 1969 by Rygaard and Povlsen (22). These mouse strains contained an autosomal recessive mutation in the *nu* (for nude) gene on chromosome 11. Homozygous mutations in the *nu* gene resulted in the absence of hair, poor growth, decreased fertility, an absent thymus gland, and a shortened life span (22–24). These animals exhibited a severe T-cell immunologic defect that impaired

their ability to reject tissue transplants (25). Consequently, these animals could tolerate the implantation and growth of human tumor cell xenografts. This discovery has led to a revolution in experimental therapeutics in cancer research (26–29). Currently, xenograft tumors have been established for virtually all common human solid tumors. A high degree of correlation has been observed between the sensitivity of disease-specific human xenografts and complete clinical response rates in the same tumor type (30, 31).

In NCI screening studies, simplicity and ease of access make subcutaneous implantation the most common approach for growing human tumor xenografts in mice (18). Injection of human tumor cell suspensions into the animal's flank leads to implantation and growth over a period of days to weeks. Human tumor xenografts can also be implanted in other sites. Implantation in the renal subcapsule has the advantage of requiring relatively short inoculation time prior to drug treatment, making it particularly useful for short-term *in vivo* assays. Tumors are implanted as a small tissue fragment under the kidney capsule of the nude mouse (32). Because the renal subcapsule is a relatively immunopriviliged site, human tumor xenograft implantation has also been employed successfully in immunocompetent mice (32–34). Renal subcapsule implanted tumors maintain much of the same morphology and growth characteristics as the original tumor from which they were derived (33, 35). In most cases, cell-cell contact is preserved and cells maintain the spatial relationships found in the original tumor. Thus, renal subcapsule implants may be a much more representative model for metastatic human tumors than subcutaneous xenografts. Renal subcapsular tumor responses can be assessed in a variety of ways, including the measurement of subcapsular renal size, clonogenic assay of surgically removed tumors following *in vivo* treatment, or overall animal survival (36).

Orthotopic xenograft models involve implanting tumors into defined sites within the animal to mimic metastases to specific organs. This concept is based on the premise that tumor metastases are not random, but occur because of a specific tropism or affinity of various tumors to grow in specific sites (37). This is based on the familiar seed and soil hypothesis originally proposed in 1889 by Paget (38). Orthotopic xenograft models have been developed for a number of different tumors, including renal cell carcinoma (39), central nervous system tumors (40), and pancreatic, prostate, colon, and lung cancers (37). However, because of its expense and technical difficulties, orthotopic xenograft models have not been routinely used by the NCI.

Despite their popularity, xenograft models still have limitations (41). For example, subcutaneous xenograft implants metastasize infrequently and are rarely invasive. Therefore, animal survival is not an ideal endpoint for subcutaneous xenograft studies because death usually results from gross tumor bulk (18). In addition, xenograft growth in the subcutaneous space obviously differs from most clinical human tumors, with shorter tumor doubling times, better tumor vasculature, and less overall necrosis (42). Finally, xenograft studies are expensive and require special antiseptic facilities. Rigorous attention to maintaining a sterile laboratory environment is essential because infections in immunocompromised nude mice are common.

The most recent addition to the NCI screening program has been the implementation of the hollow fiber *in vivo* assay (43, 44). This technique involves the insertion of human tumor cells into polyvinylidene fluoride biocompatible hollow fibers that can be implanted intraperitoneally or subcutaneously into immunocompetent mice. The hollow fibers prevent lymphocytes from infiltrating the human tumor cells, but systemically administered drug can still penetrate into the growing tumor mass. An additional advantage of this system is that more than one xenograft cell line can be implanted into a single animal. Recent data also suggest that neovascularization can arise from extended incubation of subcutaneously implanted tumor cell lines growing in hollow fibers (45). Thus, this model may also prove useful in screening for antiangiogenic agents.

Newer Animal Models

An exciting area of ongoing research is the increasing use of genetically engineered animals for preclinical drug testing. Transgenic and knockout mice are genetically altered species that can provide a versatile environment for testing novel experimental therapies. Advantages of these newer systems include the spontaneous development of tumors in the endogenous target organ, more natural growth rates and patterns of growth, and, most significantly, the use of immunocompetent animals (46, 47).

Transgenic mice arise from the introduction of a foreign gene into the pronucleus of a fertilized egg. This can be accomplished by either microinjection (46, 47), retroviral infection (48), or embryonal stem cell transfer (49, 50). This latter technique involves the transfer of genetic material into embryonal stem cells that can then be transplanted into blastocysts to ultimately create a chimeric mouse. If the germ cells in the chimeric animal are derived from the embryonal stem cells, then the offspring of the animal will be transgenic and will express the inserted gene of interest. The capability of introducing and expressing a specific gene of interest in an intact organism provides a powerful means for manipulating the genetic milieu of an experimental animal.

Insertion of known oncogenes, such as *ras* (47, 51), or N-*myc* (52), can generate transgenic animals that develop spontaneous tumors in a predictable fashion. For example, transgenic mice expressing a mutated *ras* gene frequently develop mammary tumors and can be used to screen for agents active in breast cancer (51). This model is also useful for testing novel agents that specific target abnormalities in the *ras* signaling pathway, such as farnesyl transferase inhibitors (53). Use of organ specific promoters can further enhance the power of these systems. For example, the association of the human *c-myc* oncogene with an immunoglobulin promoter can lead to the development of pre-B-cell lymphomas (54), while its association with a mouse mammary tumor virus promoter can result in mammary gland tumors (55). Tumor resistance genes, such as the multiple drug resistance gene *(mdr)* have also been inserted and expressed in transgenic animals (56). These animals are highly resistant to a variety of different natural product antitumor agents and are able to tolerate otherwise lethal doses of drugs in this class. Such animals may be useful as screens for agents that can reverse the multidrug resistant phenotype.

Knockout mice are animals that have been genetically altered to remove both alleles of a specific gene (57). This is accomplished by homologous recombination techniques that insert the defective gene into embryonic stem cells that are then isolated and injected into a blastocyst to generate heterozygous mice. Further inbreeding will generate homozygous "knockout" animals (57). Knockout animals can be developed that are similar to transgenic animals in that they lack the function of a specific tumor suppressor gene, such as *p53*, and have a very high incidence of spontaneous tumor development (58, 59). Currently, these models are being extensively used in the study of carcinogenesis and chemoprevention; however, their application in testing therapeutic agents is growing.

In Vivo Studies—Preclinical Pharmacokinetic and Pharmacodynamic Testing

Animal experiments also provide the first opportunity to study drug pharmacokinetics and pharmacodynamics. Assessment of pharmacodynamic drug effects in animal target tissues is often of key importance because similar measurements in specific target organs or in actual tumors are difficult to perform in human studies. The development and validation of the analytical methods for measuring drug concentrations in biologic matrices and the implementation of these assays can also begin during this phase of preclinical development. Ideally, the same formulation of drug planned for clinical use should be tested in a preclinical animal model. This can provide essential information about drug kinetics that will help define the initial starting dose and schedule of drug administration for the initial Phase I clinical trials in humans.

In Vivo Studies—Preclinical Toxicology

The major goals of preclinical toxicology assessments are to determine a safe starting dose for Phase I studies and to assess the drug's toxicity profile after both acute and chronic administration. In the 1970s, the NCI performed its preclinical toxicology studies in dogs and monkeys. Starting doses for clinical studies were calculated as one-third the lowest toxic dose for the most sensitive animal species, either monkey or dog (60). In 1979, FDA guidelines recommended that one-tenth the dose that causes lethality in 10% of the treated mice (LD_{10}) could be selected as the starting dose for clinical trials. The NCI adopted this policy, but also added additional toxicology studies in dogs to its routine preclinical testing guidelines (60). Currently, all agents targeted for clinical development at the NCI have single and multidose toxicity studies performed in at least two species, typically mice and beagle dogs (61).

In 1980, the NCI Division of Cancer Treatment adopted the following general guidelines for preclinical toxicity for anticancer agents (61). Murine single dose and multidose (daily $\times$ 5) studies are performed to determine the doses that result in 10%, 50%, and 90% lethality (LD_{10}, LD_{50}, and LD_{90}, respectively). The mouse equivalent LD_{10} ($MELD_{10}$) in mg/m² is converted to the $MELD_{10}$ dose for dogs using the following formula for scaling from species to species:

$$MELD_{10} \ (mg/m^2) \text{ in dogs} = (Km \ dog/Km \ mouse) \times MELD_{10} \ (mg/m^2) \text{ in mice}$$

where Km (species) is the surface-to-weight ratio for each species (62). The Km values are 3 for mice, 6 for rats, 20 for dogs, whereas corresponding values for humans are 25 for children and 37 for adults (62). One-tenth of the calculated $MELD_{10}$ in dogs is then administered to beagle dogs and, if no toxicity is seen, the dose is escalated until minimal reversible toxicity is observed. This dose, defined as the toxic dose low (TDL), is the lowest dose that produces drug-induced

pathologic changes in either hematological, chemical, clinical, or morphological parameters in the test animals. In addition, double the TDL must not produce any lethality in the test species. The human equivalent of one-third the TDL in dogs is then recommended as the starting Phase I dose in humans (61). Further details regarding allometry and animal scale-up issues are discussed in Chapter 30.

In 1980, the European Organization for Research and Treatment of Cancer (EORTC) adopted more streamlined guidelines for the assessment of preclinical toxicology in animals (63). Use of rodent-only toxicology was instituted with full histopathologic studies conducted only in mice and more limited studies performed in rats. One-tenth the mouse LD_{10} was used as the clinical Phase I starting dose. A recent review of the EORTC's use of these guidelines in the testing of over 50 different new agents in human clinical studies found no ethical or safety problems leading to the conclusion that preclinical rodent-only toxicology allowed for a considerable savings in cost and time (63).

In the United States, the FDA has issued guidelines that make specific recommendations for the nonclinical pharmacology and toxicology sections of an investigational new drug application (IND). These guidelines have not materially changed since 1987 [see Guidance for industry: Guideline for the format and content of the nonclinical pharmacology/toxicology section of an application (available at http://www.fda.gov/cder/guidance/index.htm.)] Specific sections that must be included in an IND submission are: pharmacology, acute toxicity, multidose toxicity, special toxicity, reproductive toxicity, mutagenicity, and pharmacokinetics.

According to the FDA guidelines, the pharmacology sections should include pharmacodynamic information regarding the pharmacodynamic effect dose in 50% of subjects (ED_{50}). Drug effects related to the therapeutic indication should be described in detail followed by a discussion of effects related to possible adverse reactions. Identification of possible interactions with other drugs should also be listed. Acute toxicity studies should specify the condition and age of the test animals, dose, vehicle, and dosage volume utilized, as well as the type and severity of toxic effects. Lethal dose data is also required. Subchronic, chronic, and carcinogenicity studies should be organized by the species studied, and gross and histopathologic toxicity data should also be included. Special toxicity studies such as skin or eye irritation, acute hemolysis, or other studies should be included if relevant to a particular formulation or route of drug administration. Mutagenicity studies describing both *in vitro* and *in vivo* experiments should be included, if available. Finally, pharmacokinetic information should be organized into subtopics consisting of absorption, distribution, metabolism, and excretion. Protein binding, tissue distribution, accumulation, enzyme induction or inhibition, metabolism, and drug excretion patterns should be included.

DRUG DEVELOPMENT PROGRAMS AT THE NCI

History

Systematic drug screening began at the NCI in 1955 with the establishment of the Cancer Chemotherapy National Service Center (NSC) screening program (64). Even today, all screened compounds are given an NSC number to aid in their identification. However, until the 1980s, most screening was performed *in vivo* using murine P388 or L1210 leukemia cell lines (65). These hematologic murine tumors were employed because they were generally inexpensive, stable, reproducible, and easily handled. However, these *in vivo* screening efforts also had substantial limitations. Screening with rapidly growing leukemic cells was biased toward identifying compounds with activity against rapidly growing tumors with high growth fractions. The relative lack of success during this period in identifying agents with activity against common human solid tumors was thought to be due, at least in part, to the lack of more appropriate screening models.

Because of these limitations, the NCI in 1989 changed to a rationally designed "disease-oriented" screening panel incorporating 60 cell lines derived from a variety of different human solid tumors (66). Currently, this cell-line screen is a key component of a comprehensive *in vitro* and *in vivo* preclinical screening and drug development program that is overseen by the NCI's Developmental Therapeutics Program in the Division of Cancer Treatment and Diagnosis. An overview of this program is available at http://dtp.nci.nih.gov.

Three Cell-line Prescreen and 60 Cell-line Screen

Because over 85% of the compounds submitted for screening are found to have no antiproliferative activity, the NCI adopted a three cell-line prescreen in 1999. All compounds submitted to the NCI are now prescreened *in vitro* against a panel of three highly sensitive human tumor lines that include the MCF-7 breast, NCI-H640 lung, and the SF-268 glioma cell lines. Demonstration of growth inhibitory activity is required in this prescreen panel before a compound can proceed to advanced testing in the full 60 cell-line screen.

Originally, the NCI 60 cell-line screening panel was composed of lines derived from seven different human histologic tumor types including brain, colon, leukemia, lung, melanoma, ovarian, and renal cancers (66). Later, breast, and prostate cancer cell lines were also added. An automated sulforhodamine blue cytotoxicity assay is used to assess the relative potency of a compound against all 60 cell lines using five different drug concentrations incubated for a standard 48 hours. Endpoint parameters that are calculated for each individual cell line include the GI_{50}, which is defined as the drug concentration that inhibits growth by 50%; the TGI, which is the lowest drug concentration that totally inhibits cell growth; and the LC_{50}, which is the lowest concentration that kills 50% of cells.

These data are then analyzed by the COMPARE algorithm, which is a software program that categorizes and compares different groups of agents based on their patterns of cytotoxic activity in the 60 cell-line screen (Figure 29.1) (67). This powerful program can identify similar classes of anticancer agents, such as platinum analogs, microtubule agents, or topoisomerase I inhibitors, based purely on their cytotoxicity patterns (68). Thus, hypotheses can be generated about the potential mechanisms of action of completely new anticancer agents using data generated in the 60 cell-line screening panel. New and exciting agents with a novel mechanism of action may be identified by the screen if they demonstrate a unique pattern of antitumor activity. Thus, the COMPARE program has converted a relatively simple test of growth inhibition into a sensitive probe for studying drug pharmacology.

Recent efforts have made the 60 cell-line screen an even more powerful tool for analyzing drug effects at the molecular level. This new approach involves the characterization of the relative expression of specific molecular targets important for drug sensitivity in each of the cell lines contained in the 60 cell-line screen (Figure 29.2). For example, this diverse group of targets can include oncogenic proteins such as RAS, N–myc, p53, RB protein, or key metabolic enzymes, such as thymidylate synthase, dihydrofolate reductase, or topoisomerase I and II. Relative expression of drug resistance proteins, such as P-glycoprotein or MRP, are other examples. Characterization of these molecular targets in each of the 60 cell lines allows for the screening data to be analyzed from an entirely new perspective. The relative pattern of drug sensitivity in each cell line can now be correlated with the relative expression of hundreds or more different specific molecular targets (Figure 29.2). This generates a much

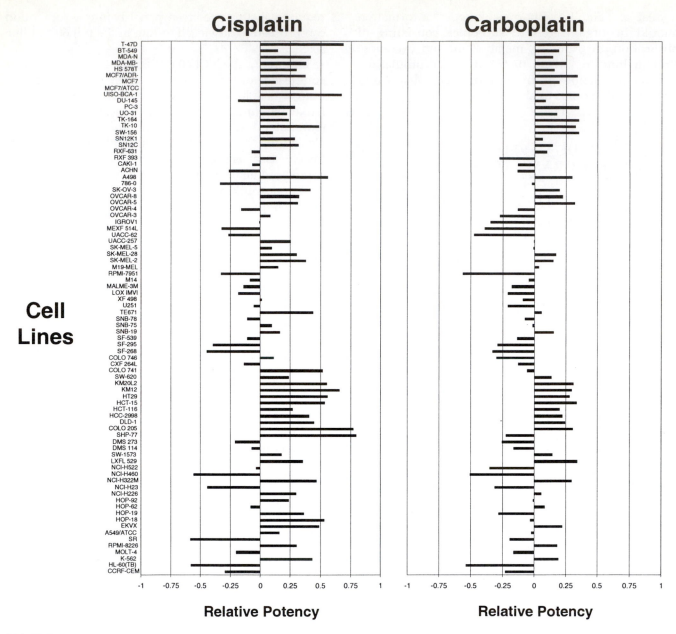

FIGURE 29.1 COMPARE program algorithm output. Plots of the mean relative sensitivity of various cell lines used in the NCI drug screening panel for cisplatin and carboplatin. The zero value represents the mean concentration required to inhibit 50% growth for all the cell lines (GI_{50}). The horizontal bars represent the relative difference in the GI_{50} value for a particular cell line from the mean value using a logarithmic scale. Cell lines with a bar extending to the right have a GI_{50} greater than the mean and are more resistant, while those that extend to the left have a GI_{50} lower than the mean and are more sensitive. A very similar pattern of growth inhibitory potency is demonstrated for these two platinum analogues. (Data obtained from the NCI website at http://dtp.nci.nih.gov.)

more data rich screening tool for analyzing new compounds. Because of the complexity and wealth of information generated, it also creates a major bioinformatics challenge. However, pioneering work by Weinstein et al. (69) in analyzing this type of data-rich information has enabled correlations to be made between patterns of drug sensitivity in the cell lines and the relative expression of these molecular targets.

This is an extremely powerful approach for identifying novel new anticancer agents based on their activity in cell lines expressing different molecular targets relevant to drug action. In addition, it is rapidly becoming possible to characterize the relative expression of thousands of different specific molecular targets at the mRNA level in the 60 cell lines using cDNA microarray chip technology (70). This flood of additional

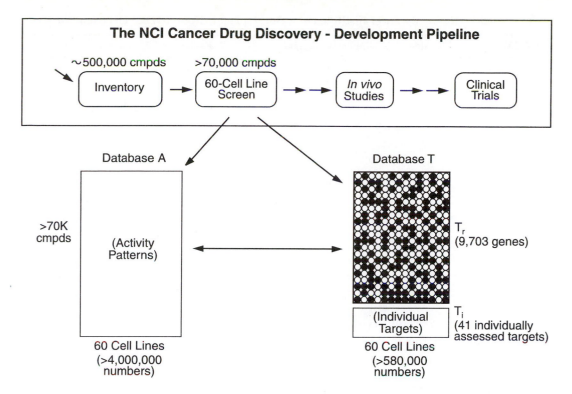

FIGURE 29.2   Molecular target expression in the NCI screening program. A schematic representation of the database generation or molecular target gene expression in the NCI drug discovery development program. Each row of the activity database (A) represents the pattern of cytotoxic activity of a specific compound across the 60 cell lines, and each column represents the pattern of sensitivities of a particular cell line to the compounds tested. The gene-expression database (Tr) contains fluorescence hybridization ratio values from two-color cDNA microarray measurements on the 60 cell lines. Microarray experimental data provide information on the relative expression of literally thousands of different potentially important molecular targets that may be related to drug efficacy. Also added to the target database is the relative expression of 40 additional individually measured molecular targets (Ti) that is the product of many experiments in different laboratories, as compiled at the NCI's DTP Internet site located at http://dtp.nci.nih.gov. The sum of Tr and Ti constitute an overall database (T) of molecular targets. Analysis of the relationships between database A (cytotoxic activity) and database T (relative molecular target expression) can potentially identify novel and new agents being screened that have cytotoxic activity against defined patterns of gene expression common to various types of human tumors. (Reproduced by permission from Scherf U, et al. Nat Genet 2000;24:236–44. Additional information may be found on the Internet at http://discover.nci.nih.gov.)

information will further increase the power of this approach.

Although the utility of this method of anticancer drug screening and discovery must still be proven, its potential is great. Conceptually, it is important because it extends the "disease-oriented" approach originally envisioned when the 60 cell-line screen was created to a more comprehensive drug discovery approach that is based on molecular targets. Thus, the 60 cell lines no longer represent a simple collection of cell lines arising from nine different human histologic tumor types; instead, they have been transformed into a panel of thousands of different molecular targets, each of which is expressed at 60 different levels. Each individual target can then be individually correlated with

drug sensitivity for any new or novel anticancer agent that is screened (71). This correlation has enormous potential for identifying new molecular target-based agents for further clinical development.

NCI Drug Development Group Decision Network

At the NCI, a series of decision stages and reviews has been established by the Developmental Therapeutics Program to guide compounds through the current drug screening and development process (Table 29.1). Currently, over 70,000 compounds have been screened since the system was established in 1990. The Drug Development Group (DDG) Decision Net-

TABLE 29.1   National Cancer Institute Drug Development Group (DDG) Decision Process

DDG stage	Timing in development program	Review and decision activities
Stage I	Compound screening	3 cell line *in vitro* prescreen
		60 cell line *in vitro* screen
		Preliminary *in vivo* testing
Stage IIA	Early preclinical development	Review of *in vivo* data
		Drug procurement
		Analytical assay development
Stage IIB	Late preclinical development	cGMP manufacturing
		Drug formulation
		Animal toxicology and pharmacokinetics
Stage III	Inception of clinical trials	Initiation of Phase I trials
		Further clinical development plan

work Stage I (screening) process involves several different committees that oversee the initial screening process. The process begins when a compound or agent submitted to the NCI is approved for preliminary *in vitro* screening by the Acquisitions and Input Committee (AIC). The AIC is a small group of chemists that selects and prioritizes new compounds for screening and ensures that the agent has a unique chemical structure. Results of the 3 cell-line screen and 60 cell-line screen for a particular compound are then reviewed by the Screening Data Review Committee (SDRC) that selects compounds for further *in vivo* testing in animals. Specific factors used to select agents for further testing include significant potency in a variety of cell lines, a novel pattern of activity in the COMPARE program algorithm, or a special interest in an agent because of its chemical structure or biologic activity. Animal studies are initially conducted at the NCI with 12 different human cell lines using the previously described hollow fiber assay. The initial *in vivo* data are then reviewed by the Biological Evaluation Committee for Cancer (BEC/C) and active agents are selected for more extensive human xenograft studies in nude mice using tumors selected for prior sensitivity in earlier *in vitro* tests. At the NCI, human xenografts are implanted subcutaneously and the drugs are administered intraperitoneally. A relative difference in the tumor weight ratio of treated to control animals of less than 0.5 is considered promising for further development.

Agents with activity in the *in vivo* screen are then reviewed at a DDG Stage IIA (early preclinical) meeting at which recommendations are made for further preclinical studies. These include studies designed to determine an acceptable clinical formulation and

select the optimal dose, route, and schedule of administration. Procurement of sufficient drug for further preclinical and clinical studies is planned, and drug assay development for pharmacokinetic studies is also initiated. If no additional problems arise and the compound remains promising, then the agent progresses to the DDG Stage IIB (late preclinical) meeting. At this juncture, a major commitment of research resources is required to further develop the agent. This includes contracting for cGMP drug manufacturing, the initiation of preclinical toxicology studies in two different species with histopathological correlation, and animal pharmacokinetic and toxicokinetic studies. Toxicology, manufacturing, and formulation frequently represent the most costly steps in preclinical drug development. If a compound appears likely to be safe in humans, then a final DDG Stage III (inception of clinical trials) meeting is convened to discuss issues related to the initiation of NCI-sponsored Phase I clinical trials, such as the recommendation of a safe starting dose and appropriate laboratory and clinical endpoints. At this time, an NCI-sponsored IND application will also be filed with the FDA. A substantial commitment is also made by the NCI to conduct an appropriate Phase I and Phase II clinical research program. Guidelines have been established for structuring partnership agreements between the NCI and drug sponsors in industry or academia in such a way that the sponsor's intellectual property rights are protected (72). Further information about these programs is available at http://dtp.nci.nih.gov.

Clearly, the NCI efforts in anticancer drug development are extensive and will continue to grow and change as the science of drug discovery and development evolves. The tremendous advances now occurring in our understanding of the molecular basis of human cancer and the identification of new molecular targets for developmental therapeutics ensure that this will be an active and exciting program for the foreseeable future.

THE CHALLENGE—INTRACELLULAR PHARMACODYNAMICS AND NEW PARADIGMS FOR CLINICAL TRIALS

Clinical pharmacologists involved in preclinical and early clinical drug development will face a number of new challenges as we begin the new millennium. The greatest immediate challenge will be to determine how to best incorporate our extensive preclinical understanding of drug pharmacology into the design of early clinical trials (73). In the area of cancer chemotherapy, advances in drug screening and discovery will ensure that all new compounds entering clinical studies will have well-defined theoretical molecular mechanisms of action. Therefore, new paradigms for Phase I and II clinical trials will be necessary to determine if mechanisms of drug action defined in preclinical studies are relevant to the clinical use of these agents.

One area requiring further study is the relationship between intracellular molecular drug effects and clinical outcomes, an area that Martin and Kemeny (74) have defined as *intracellular pharmacodynamics*. Incorporation of extensive biochemical and molecular endpoints in the design of clinical trials is predicated on an understanding of this relationship and requires thorough elucidation of the mechanism of drug action. These trials are technically difficult to perform in cancer patients because they require sampling tumor or organ tissues targeted by the drug. However, this approach is particularly relevant for anticancer drugs because only a small percentage of the large number of compounds entering into Phase I clinical trials will successfully be developed into therapeutically useful agents. It is not clear why the vast majority of agents fail during clinical testing due to either severe toxicity or lack of efficacy because, by definition, all these agents are active in preclinical models. An increased understanding of how these agents behave in patients is thus needed to provide important information for screening and designing more successful agents in the future.

As scientists devoted to the study of developmental therapeutics in humans, clinical pharmacologists are in an ideal position to span the interface between preclinical and clinical drug development studies. The preclinical experiments described in this chapter provide a wealth of information regarding a new agent's

toxicology, determinants of response, and mechanisms of drug action. Furthermore, developing new technologies and model systems will allow us to better define drug absorption, metabolism, and drug safety and efficacy prior to the initiation of Phase I trials. Although optimally using this information to rationally design early clinical trials remains a daunting challenge, successfully meeting this challenge offers the best opportunity for improving our therapeutic options for the treatment of human disease.

References

1. Lerner CG, Saiki AYC. Scintillation proximity assay for human DNA topoisomerase I using recombinant biotinyl-fusion protein produced in baculovirus-infected insect cells. Anal Biochem 1996;240:185–96.
2. Hartwell LH, Szankasi P, Roberts CJ, Murray AW, Friend SH. Integrating genetic approaches into the discovery of anticancer drugs. Science 1997;278:1064–8.
3. Monks A, Scudiero D, Skehan P, et al. Feasibility of a high-flux anticancer drug screen using a diverse panel of cultured human tumor cell lines. J Natl Cancer Inst 1991;83:757–66.
4. Jansen WJ, Hulscher TM, van Ark-Otte J, Giaccone G, Pinedo HM, Boven E. CPT-11 sensitivity in relation to the expression of P170-glycoprotein and multidrug resistance-associated protein. Br J Cancer 1998;77:359–65.
5. Meunier V, Bourrie M, Berger Y, Fabre G. The human intestinal epithelial cell line Caco-2; pharmacological and pharmacokinetic applications. Cell Biol Toxicol 1995;11:187–94.
6. Wilson G. Cell culture techniques for the study of drug transport. Eur J Drug Metab Pharmacokinet 1990;15:159–63.
7. Iwatsubo T, Hirota N, Ooie T, et al. Prediction of *in vivo* drug metabolism in the human liver from *in vitro* metabolism data. Pharmacol Ther 1997;73:147–71.
8. Rowinsky EK, Donehower RC. Paclitaxel (taxol). N Engl J Med 1995;332:1004–14.
9. Wani MC, Taylor HL, Wall ME, Coggon P, McPhail AT. Plant antitumor agents. VI. The isolation and structure of taxol, a novel antileukemic and antitumor agent from Taxus brevifolia. J Am Chem Soc 1971;93:2325–7.
10. Rao KV, Hanuman JB, Alvarez C, et al. A new large-scale process for taxol and related taxanes from Taxus brevifolia. Pharm Res 1995;12:1003–10.
11. Cragg GM, Boyd MR, Cardellina JH, et al. The search for new pharmaceutical crops: Drug discovery and development at the National Cancer Institute. In: Janick J, Simon JE, editors. New crops. New York: Wiley; 1993. p. 161–7.
12. Witherup KM, Look SA, Stasko MW, Ghiorzi TJ, Muschik GM, Cragg GM. Taxus spp. needles contain amounts of taxol comparable to the bark of Taxus brevifolia: Analysis and isolation. J Nat Prod 1990;53:1249–55.
13. Lorenz W, Schmal A, Schult H, et al. Histamine release and hypotensive reactions in dogs by solubilizing agents and fatty acids: Analysis of various components in cremophor E1 and development of a compound with reduced toxicity. Agents Actions 1982;12:64–80.
14. Liebmann J, Cook JA, Mitchell JB. Cremophor EL, solvent for paclitaxel, and toxicity [letter; comment]. Lancet 1993;342:1428.
15. Theis JG, Liau-Chu M, Chan HS, Doyle J, Greenberg ML, Koren G. Anaphylactoid reactions in children receiving high-dose

intravenous cyclosporine for reversal of tumor resistance: The causative role of improper dissolution of Cremophor EL. J Clin Oncol 1995;13:2508–16.

16. Dahut W, Harold N, Takimoto C, et al. Phase I and pharmacologic study of 9-aminocamptothecin given by 72-hour infusion in adult cancer patients. J Clin Oncol 1996;14:1236–44.

17. Rubin E, Wood V, Bharti A, et al. A phase I and pharmacokinetic study of a new camptothecin derivative, 9-aminocamptothecin. Clin Cancer Res 1995;1:269–76.

18. Khleif SN, Curt GA. Animal models in drug development. In: Holland JF, Bast BR Jr, Morton DL, Frei E III, Kufe DW, Weischelbaum RR, editors. Cancer medicine. 4th ed. Baltimore: Williams & Wilkins; 1997. p. 855–68.

19. Corbett TH, Griswold DP, Jr., Roberts BJ, Peckham JC, Schabel FM, Jr. Tumor induction relationships in development of transplantable cancers of the colon in mice for chemotherapy assays, with a note on carcinogen structure. Cancer Res 1975;35:2434–9.

20. Corbett TH, Roberts BJ, Leopold WR, et al. Induction and chemotherapeutic response of two transplantable ductal adenocarcinomas of the pancreas in C57BL/6 mice. Cancer Res 1984;44:717–26.

21. Rockwell S. In vivo-in vitro tumour cell lines: Characteristics and limitations as models for human cancer. Br J Cancer 1980;41(suppl 4):118–22.

22. Rygaard J, Povlsen CO. Heterotransplantation of a human malignant tumour to "Nude" mice. Acta Pathol Microbiol Scand 1969;77:758–60.

23. Flanagan SP. 'Nude', a new hairless gene with pleiotropic effects in the mouse. Genet Res 1966;8:295–309.

24. Pantelouris EM. Absence of thymus in a mouse mutant. Nature 1968;217:370–1.

25. Raff MC, Wortis HH. Thymus dependence of theta-bearing cells in the peripheral lymphoid tissues of mice. Immunology 1970;18:931–42.

26. Neely JE, Ballard ET, Britt AL, Workman L. Characteristics of 85 pediatric tumors heterotransplanted into nude mice. Exp Cell Biol 1983;51:217–27.

27. Houghton JA, Taylor DM. Growth characteristics of human colorectal tumours during serial passage in immune-deprived mice. Br J Cancer 1978;37:213–23.

28. Houghton JA, Taylor DM. Maintenance of biological and biochemical characteristics of human colorectal tumours during serial passage in immune-deprived mice. Br J Cancer 1978;37:199–212.

29. Gazdar AF, Carney DN, Sims HL, Simmons A. Heterotransplantation of small-cell carcinoma of the lung into nude mice: Comparison of intracranial and subcutaneous routes. Int J Cancer 1981;28:777–83.

30. Nowak K, Peckham MJ, Steel GG. Variation in response of xenografts of colo-rectal carcinoma to chemotherapy. Br J Cancer 1978;37:576–84.

31. Giovanella BC, Stehlin JS Jr., Shepard RC, Williams LJ Jr. Correlation between response to chemotherapy of human tumors in patients and in nude mice. Cancer 1983;52:1146–52.

32. Bogden AE, Cobb WR, Lepage DJ, et al. Chemotherapy responsiveness of human tumors as first transplant generation xenografts in the normal mouse: Six-day subrenal capsule assay. Cancer 1981;48:10–20.

33. Aamdal S, Fodstad O, Nesland JM, Pihl A. Characteristics of human tumor xenografts transplanted under the renal capsule of immunocompetent mice. Br J Cancer 1985;51:347–56.

34. Suonio E, Lipponen P, Maenpaa J, Syrjanen K, Kangas L, Tuomisto L. Mitotic index in the subrenal capsule assay as an indicator of the chemosensitivity of ovarian cancer. Cancer Chemother Pharmacol 1997;41:15–21.

35. Aamdal S, Fodstad O, Pihl A. Human tumor xenografts transplanted under the renal capsule of conventional mice. Growth rates and host immune response. Int J Cancer 1984;34:725–30.

36. Edelstein MB, Smink T, Ruiter DJ, Visser W, van Putten LM. Improvements and limitations of the subrenal capsule assay for determining tumour sensitivity to cytostatic drugs. Eur J Cancer Clin Oncol 1984;20:1549–56.

37. Hoffman RM. Fertile seed and rich soil: The development of clinically relevant models of human cancer by surgical orthotopic implantation of intact tissue. In: Teicher B, editor. Anticancer drug development guide: Preclinical screening, clinical trials and approval. Totowa, NJ: Humana Press; 1997. p. 127–44.

38. Paget S. The distribution of secondary growth in cancer of the breast. Lancet 1889;1:571.

39. Fidler IJ. Rationale and methods for the use of nude mice to study the biology and therapy of human cancer metastasis. Cancer Metastasis Rev 1986;5:29–49.

40. Shapiro WR, Basler GA, Chernik NL, Posner JB. Human brain tumor transplantation into nude mice. J Natl Cancer Inst 1979;62:447–53.

41. Gura T. Systems for identifying new drugs are often faulty [news]. Science 1997;278:1041–2.

42. Steel GG, Courtenay VD, Peckham MJ. The response to chemotherapy of a variety of human tumour xenografts. Br J Cancer 1983;47:1–13.

43. Hollingshead MG, Alley MC, Camalier RF, et al. In vivo cultivation of tumor cells in hollow fibers. Life Sci 1995;57:131–41.

44. Plowman J, Dykes DJ, Hollingshead M, Simpson-Herren L, Alley MC. Human tumor xenograft models in NCI drug development. In: Teicher B, editor. Anticancer drug development guide: Preclinical screening, clinical trials, and approval. Totowa, NJ: Humana Press; 1997. p. 101–25.

45. Phillips RM, Pearce J, Loadman PM, et al. Angiogenesis in the hollow fiber tumor model influences drug delivery to tumor cells: Implications for anticancer drug screening programs. Cancer Res 1998;58:5263–6.

46. Rosenberg MP, Bortner D. Why transgenic and knockout animal models should be used (for drug efficacy studies in cancer). Cancer Metastasis Rev 1998;17:295–9.

47. Thomas H, Balkwill F. Assessing new anti-tumour agents and strategies in oncogene transgenic mice. Cancer Metastasis Rev 1995;14:91–5.

48. Jaenisch R. Retroviruses and embryogenesis: microinjection of Moloney leukemia virus into midgestation mouse embryos. Cell 1980;19:181–8.

49. Kuehn MR, Bradley A, Robertson EJ, Evans MJ. A potential animal model for Lesch-Nyhan syndrome through introduction of HPRT mutations into mice. Nature 1987;326:295–8.

50. Hooper M, Hardy K, Handyside A, Hunter S, Monk M. HPRT-deficient (Lesch-Nyhan) mouse embryos derived from germline colonization by cultured cells. Nature 1987;326:292–5.

51. Dexter DL, Diamond M, Creveling J, Chen SF. Chemotherapy of mammary carcinomas arising in ras transgenic mice. Invest New Drugs 1993;11:161–8.

52. Sheppard RD, Samant SA, Rosenberg M, Silver LM, Cole MD. Transgenic N-myc mouse model for indolent B cell lymphoma: tumor characterization and analysis of genetic alterations in spontaneous and retrovirally accelerated tumours. Oncogene 1998;17:2073–85.

53. Mangues R, Corral T, Kohl NE, et al. Antitumor effect of a farnesyl protein transferase inhibitor in mammary and lymphoid tumors overexpressing N-ras in transgenic mice. Cancer Res 1998;58:1253–9.

54. Schmidt EV, Pattengale PK, Weir L, Leder P. Transgenic mice bearing the human c-myc gene activated by an immunoglobulin

enhancer: A pre-B-cell lymphoma model. Proc Natl Acad Sci USA 1988;85:6047–51.

55. Weaver ZA, McCormack SJ, Liyanage M, et al. A recurring pattern of chromosomal aberrations in mammary gland tumors of MMTV-*c-myc* transgenic mice. Genes Chromosomes Cancer 1999;25:251–60.

56. Dell'Acqua G, Polishchuck R, Fallon JT, Gordon JW. Cardiac resistance to adriamycin in transgenic mice expressing a rat alpha-cardiac myosin heavy chain/human multiple drug resistance 1 fusion gene. Hum Gene Ther 1999;10:1269–79.

57. Majzoub JA, Muglia LJ. Knockout mice. N Engl J Med 1996;334:904–7.

58. Donehower LA. The *p53*-deficient mouse: a model for basic and applied cancer studies. Semin Cancer Biol 1996;7:269–78.

59. Attardi LD, Jacks T. The role of *p53* in tumour suppression: Lessons from mouse models. Cell Mol Life Sci 1999;55:48–63.

60. Grieshaber CK, Marsoni S. Relation of preclinical toxicology to findings in early clinical trials. Cancer Treat Rep 1986;70:65–72.

61. Toppmeyer DL. Phase I trial design and methodology. In: Teicher B, editor. Anticancer drug development guide: Preclinical screening, clinical trials, and approval. Totowa, NJ: Humana Press; 1997. p. 227–47.

62. Freireich EJ, Gehan EA, Rall DP, Schmidt LH, Skipper HE. Quantitative comparison of toxicity of anticancer agents in mouse, rat, hamster, dog, monkey, and man. Cancer Chemother Rep 1966;50:219–44.

63. Connors TA, Pinedo HM. Drug development in Europe. In: Teicher B, editor. Anticancer drug development guide: Preclinical screening, clinical trials, and approval. Totowa, NJ: Humana Press; 1997. p. 271–88.

64. Zubrod CG. The national program for cancer chemotherapy. JAMA 1972;222:1161–2.

65. Waud WR. Murine L1210 and P388 leukemia. In: Teicher B, editor. Anticancer drug development guide: Preclinical screening, clinical trials, and approval. Totowa, NJ: Humana Press; 1997. p. 59–74.

66. Boyd MR. The NCI *in vitro* anticancer drug discovery screen: Concept, implementation, and operation, 1985–1995. In: Teicher B, editor. Anticancer drug development guide: Preclinical screening, clincal trials, and approval. Totowa, NJ: Humana Press; 1997. p. 23–42.

67. Paull KD, Shoemaker RH, Hodes L, et al. Display and analysis of patterns of differential activity of drugs against human tumor cell lines: Development of mean graph and COMPARE algorithm. J Natl Cancer Inst 1989;81:1088–92.

68. Rixe O, Ortuzar W, Alvarez M, et al. Oxaliplatin, tetraplatin, cisplatin, and carboplatin: Spectrum of activity in drug-resistant cell lines and in the cell lines of the National Cancer Institute's Anticancer Drug Screen panel. Biochem Pharmacol 1996;52:1855–65.

69. Weinstein JN, Myers TG, O'Connor PM, et al. An information-intensive approach to the molecular pharmacology of cancer. Science. 1997;275:343–9.

70. Scherf U, Ross DT, Waltham M, et al. A gene expression database for the molecular pharmacology of cancer [comments]. Nat Genet 2000;24:236–44.

71. Shi LM, Myers TG, Fan Y, et al. Mining the National Cancer Institute Anticancer Drug Discovery Database: Cluster analysis of ellipticine analogs with p53-inverse and central nervous system-selective patterns of activity. Mol Pharmacol 1998;53:241–51.

72. Sausville EA. Working with the National Cancer Institute. In: Teicher B, editor. Anticancer drug development guide: Preclinical screening, clinical trials, and approval. Totowa, NJ: Humana Press; 1997. p. 217–26.

73. Gelmon KA, Eisenhauer EA, Harris AL, Ratain MJ, Workman P. Anticancer agents targeting signaling molecules and cancer cell environment: Challenges for drug development? J Natl Cancer Inst 1999;91:1281–7.

74. Martin DS, Kemeny NE. Modulation of fluorouracil by N-(phosphonacetyl)-L-asparate: a review. Semin Oncol 1992;19(suppl 3):49–55.

30

Animal Scale-up

ROBERT L. DEDRICK

Division of Bioengineering and Physical Science, Office of Research Services, National Institutes of Health, Bethesda, Maryland

INTRODUCTION

The title of this chapter was derived from a talk presented to a chemical engineering audience. It was meant as a play on words by analogy to the design and scale-up of chemical plants. The title of the field has stuck, but the play has been lost. To most of those interested in clinical pharmacology, "plant scale-up" probably conveys quite a different idea. The science and technology of chemical engineering have proven to be a powerful methodology for addressing a variety of problems in pharmacokinetics such as extrapolation from one biological system to another. The experimental systems include *in vitro* cultures and isolated organ perfusions as well as animals.

Despite the influence of allometry on the development of biology and an underlying belief that experimental systems provide useful information about humans, disproportionate emphasis has been placed on species differences. This would appear to derive from the culture of biology because differences among species have often been more interesting than similarities and because these differences can provide important information on the development of species. We recognize that no other animal is the same as a human in any general biological sense and that insistence on "sameness" in a model system is illusory. I would propose that we adopt more of an engineering-design view when we develop experimental systems in pharmacokinetics and attempt to use data from these systems for predictive purposes. If we do this, it is

axiomatic in biology as in engineering that the model system is *never* the same as the prototype. Interpretation is always required. In some simple systems, concepts of similitude place design on a sound theoretical basis. But in more complex situations rigorous similitude may not be attainable. In these cases it is often possible to model parts of a complex system and use model-dependent information in a design process that incorporates sound theoretical principles, but often contains judgment and experience as well. The approach is illustrated by a discussion of the extrapolation of data from one biological system to another.

This chapter contains a brief discussion of allometry, physiological pharmacokinetics, and the use of *in vitro* systems to predict drug metabolism in experimental animals and human subjects.

THE ALLOMETRIC EQUATION

It has been observed that many physiological processes and organ sizes show a relatively simple power-law relationship with body weight when these are compared among mammals (1). The well-known allometric equation is

$$P = a(BW)^m \tag{30.1}$$

where P = physiological property or anatomic size
a = empirical coefficient
BW = body weight
m = allometric exponent

Note that a is not dimensionless; its value depends on the units in which P and BW are measured, while the exponent, m, is independent of the system of units. Note further that if $m = 1$, then P is proportional to BW. If $m < 1$, P increases less rapidly than BW. If $m > 1$, P increases more rapidly that BW.

Dividing both sides of Equation 30.1 by BW shows that

$$\frac{P}{BW} = a(BW)^{m-1} \qquad (30.2)$$

Thus, if the allometric exponent is less than unity, as observed for many measures of physiologic function such as basal oxygen consumption and creatinine clearance, the function per unit of body weight *decreases* as body weight increases.

These concepts are illustrated in Figure 30.1, which shows a plot of an illustrative physiologic property versus body weight, both in arbitrary dimensionless terms, on a log-log plot. Equation 30.1 is linearized in this form with a slope equal to the allometric exponent, a. If the property were proportional to body weight, increasing the body weight from 1 to 100 would result in a concomitant increase in the property. If the allometric exponent were 0.7, then increasing the body weight from 1 to 100 would result in an increase in the property from 1 to 25 and a value of the property per unit body weight only one-fourth as large.

In more concrete terms, if $m = 0.7$ for the renal clearance of a particular drug, the clearance per unit body weight in a 20-gm mouse would expected to be $[(70{,}000)/(20)]^{0.3} = 12$ times that in a 70-kg human. If the volume of distribution is similar on a L/kg basis between the two species (such as body water) and the drug is cleared only by the kidney, then, as a rough approximation, the elimination half-life would be 12 times shorter in the mouse. Thus, 1 hour in a mouse would be pharmacokinetically equivalent to 12 hours in a human. Such considerations are important in the design of drug studies because pharmacokinetic time scales vary greatly among species.

Allometric principles may be used to answer a variety of questions relevant to the design of preclinical pharmacokinetic studies. For example, antineoplastic drugs have been given intraperitoneally in large volume to treat the serosal spread of malignancies such as ovarian and gastrointestinal cancer. Key issues include both the kinetics of absorption of the drug from the peritoneal cavity and the depth of penetration of the drug into tumor nodules. The rate of absorption of the drug from the peritoneal cavity is equal to $PA(C_{PC} - C_{Pl})$, where PA is the peritoneal permeability-area product, C is the concentration of the drug, and the subscripts PC and Pl refer, respectively, to peritoneal cavity and plasma.

Figure 30.2 shows the variation of PA, which is approximately equivalent to peritoneal clearance if $C_{PC} \gg C_{PL}$, for urea and inulin in rat, rabbit, dog, and human (2). The slope of the urea line is 0.74; the slope of the inulin line is 0.62. The average of these is 0.68 or approximately two-thirds, as might be expected for peritoneal surface area. This would imply that the intrinsic membrane permeability, P, is similar among the species. That this is plausible is supported by a spatially distributed model devised to examine the penetration of drug into tissue (2). If the drug does not react with the tissue, then the peritoneal permeability may be shown to be $P = [D(ps)]^{1/2}$, where D is the diffusivity of the drug in the tissue, p is the capillary per-

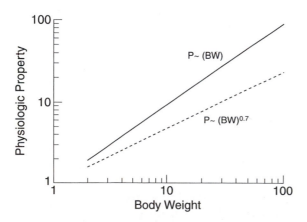

FIGURE 30.1 Illustrative allometric chart. The physiologic property and body weight are in arbitrary dimensionless units.

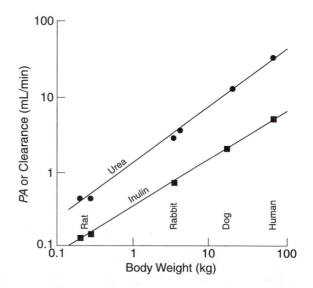

FIGURE 30.2 Peritoneal permeability-area product or clearance vs. body weight across four species for urea (●) and inulin (■). (Reproduced from Dedrick RL, et al. ASAIO J 1982;5:1–8.)

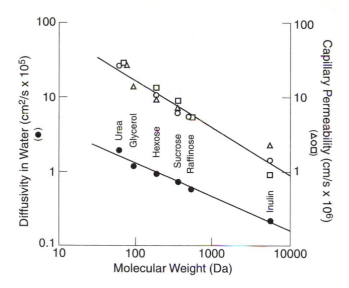

FIGURE 30.3 Aqueous diffusivity (●) and capillary permeability in cat leg (○), human forearm (□), and dog heart (△) of hydrophilic solutes vs. molecular weight. (Reproduced from Dedrick RL, et al. ASAIO J 1982;5:1–8.)

is possible to describe these processes and interactions in mathematical terms and, if sufficient data are available, to predict the time course of drug and metabolite(s) in specific anatomic sites. A physiological pharmacokinetic model was developed to predict the deamination of cytosine arabinoside (Ara-C) in humans from enzyme parameters determined from homogenates of human tissue (3). Ara-C is converted to its inactive metabolite, uracil arabinoside (Ara-U) by cytidine deaminase, the activity of which varies substantially among tissues.

The basis of a physiological pharmacokinetic model is a flow diagram showing the anatomic relationships among the various organs and tissues. Figure 30.4 was employed to incorporate both principles of drug distribution within the body and saturable enzyme kinetics. The accumulation of a drug within a compartment is described by an appropriate mass-balance equation. As an illustration, we consider the accumulation of a drug in the kidney, which is assumed both to metabolize the drug by a saturable process and to clear it by filtration and possibly secretion. It is further assumed

meability, and s is the capillary surface area per unit volume of tissue. Perhaps surprisingly, the permeability of continuous capillaries appears to be very similar among mammals as shown for a number of solutes in cat leg, human forearm and dog heart (Figure 30.3). As discussed in Chapter 3, the diffusivity of these compounds in tissue may be taken proportional to their diffusivity in water. These observations support the similarity of P among mammalian species.

During the design of preclinical studies of intraperitoneal drug administration, consideration must be given to the fact that PA is relatively larger in small laboratory animals than it is in humans. The time constant for drug absorption from the peritoneal cavity is V_{PC}/PA, where V_{PC} is the intraperitoneal volume. Since PA varies approximately as the 0.7 power of body weight, the pharmacokinetic time scales in the peritoneal cavity can be duplicated among species if the volume that is given to the laboratory animals also varies as the 0.7 power of body weight. Then, to stimulate the time course of peritoneal drug concentration in a 70-kg human patient receiving 2 liters (29 mL/kg) of drug-containing solution, a 200-gm rat would have to be given $(200/70,000)^{0.7} (2,000) = 33$ mL.

PHYSIOLOGICAL PHARMACOKINETICS

The distribution and disposition of a drug in the body result from a complex set of physiological processes and biochemical interactions. In principle, it

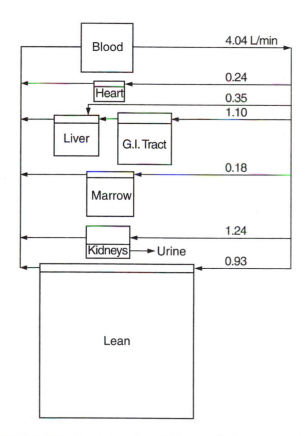

FIGURE 30.4 Physiological model for Ara-C pharmacokinetics. (Reproduced from Dedrick RL, et al. Biochem Pharmacol 1972;21:1–16.)

that the concentration within the compartment is uniform and equal to that of venous blood.

$$V_K \frac{dC_K}{dt} = Q_K C_B - Q_K C_K - CL_K C_B - \left[\frac{V_{max,K} C_K}{K_{m,K} + C_K}\right] V_K \quad (30.3)$$

where V = compartment volume, mL

$\quad\quad C$ = drug concentration, µg/mL

$\quad\quad t$ = time, min

$\quad\quad Q$ = blood flow rate, mL/min

$\quad V_{max}$ = maximum rate of metabolism, µg/(min.mL)

$\quad\quad K_m$ = Michaelis constant, µg/mL

$\quad\quad CL$ = nonmetabolic clearance, mL/min

and the subscripts K and B refer to kidney and arterial blood, respectively.

Similar equations can be written for all relevant compartments. If parameters are chosen, the resulting set of nonlinear ordinary differential equations can be solved numerically to yield predictions of the concentration of the drug and metabolite(s) in each of the compartments as a function of time. Of course, the previous simplifying assumptions can be relaxed to include much more detail concerning plasma and tissue binding, transport at the level of the blood capillary and cell membrane, and spatial nonuniformity—but at the cost of increasing complexity and the requirement for more parameters.

Figure 30.5 shows a prediction of the plasma concentration of Ara-C and total radioactivity (Ara-C plus Ara-U) following administration of two separate bolus intravenous injections of 1.2 mg/kg to a 70-kg woman. All compartment sizes and blood flow rates were estimated *a priori,* and all enzyme kinetic parameters were determined from published *in vitro* studies. None of the parameters was selected specifically for this patient; only the dose per body weight was used in the simulation. The prediction has the correct general shape and magnitude. It can be made quantitative by relatively minor changes in model parameters with no requirement to adjust the parameters describing metabolism.

Examination of Equation 30.3 or its counterpart for any drug-metabolizing organ shows that blood flow and organ metabolism interact (see Chapter 7). The chemical reaction occurs at a concentration equal to the concentration in the organ, which has been assumed in this example to equal the concentration in the venous blood draining that organ. Because the organ cannot metabolize more drug than reaches it by flow, the absolute upper limit on the organ's contribution to metabolism is QC_B. This is known as *flow limitation.* Whenever the intrinsic clearance is large compared with the blood flow, attenuation of the effects of enzyme induction or inhibition should be

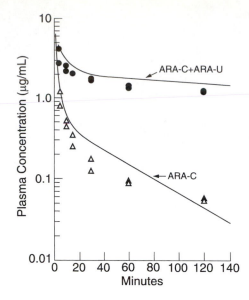

FIGURE 30.5 Predicted *(solid lines)* and observed *(symbols)* concentrations of Ara-C and total radioactivity (Ara-C + Ara-U) in the plasma of a 70-kg female patient following two separate intravenous injections of 1.2 mg/kg. (Reproduced from Dedrick RL, et al. Biochem Pharmacol 1972;21:1–16.)

expected. In fact, analysis of pharmacokinetics *in vivo* may require knowledge of the size and blood flow of all compartments including those that do not directly play a major role in drug metabolism.

Cytidine deaminase had been reported to vary greatly among mammalian species, both in its kinetic characteristics and its dominant location (4). In humans, the highest levels (µg Ara-C/min · gm) were found in the liver with smaller amounts in the kidney and heart. By comparison, the highest levels in the mouse were found in the kidney while the dog had very low enzyme activities and the monkey had high levels in liver, heart, kidney, and lean tissue. The Michaelis constant was found to vary by a factor of seven from the human to the mouse. We simulated plasma and tissue concentrations in these species to verify the participation of the tissues in the distribution process and to further validate the pharmacokinetic model. The model is quite general and can be applied to any mammalian species with the proper choice of blood flows, organ sizes, kidney clearance, and enzyme kinetic parameters. The model was quite successful in simulating Ara-C distribution and deamination in the several species with the expected result that the drug is eliminated very rapidly by the monkey, less rapidly by the human and mouse, and very slowly by the dog.

Although the interspecies variability in metabolism precludes the possibility of a simple allometric relationship for the plasma kinetics of Ara-C, the non-metabolic clearance by the kidney does exhibit a power-law relationship with body weight. Figure 30.6 shows the kidney clearance of Ara-C (and its deaminated product Ara-U) on a log-log plot as a function of body weight for mice, monkeys, dogs, and humans. The slope is 0.80, which is essentially the same as the value of 0.77 for inulin (1).

Like Ara-C, 5-fluorouracil (5-FU) is extensively and variably metabolized among species. The principal catabolic enzyme is dihydropyrimidine dehydrogenase (DPD). Khor et al. (5) examined 5-FU plasma kinetics of mice, rats, and dogs that had been rendered functionally deficient in the enzyme by administration of an inhibitor. They compared these data with plasma levels in a human subject who was genetically deficient in DPD. The data are shown in Figure 30.7. The ordinate has been made comparable among the studies by division of the plasma concentration (ng/mL) by the dose (mg/kg). Examination of the curves shows that the mouse clears 5-FU most rapidly followed by the rat, dog, and human. As discussed in the section on allometry, the natural pharmacokinetic time scale is the volume of distribution divided by the clearance. If the volume of distribution is proportional to BW and the kidney clearance is proportional to $(BW)^m$, then the times can be normalized by dividing the clock time by the pharmacokinetic time scale which would be proportional to $(BW)^{1-m}$. This normalization is shown in Figure 30.8. In the figure the exponent on body weight was calculated on both the concentration and time scales. It was found to be 0.995 and 0.26, respectively. These exponents agree with the values of one and one-quarter that we had observed for methotrexate (6).

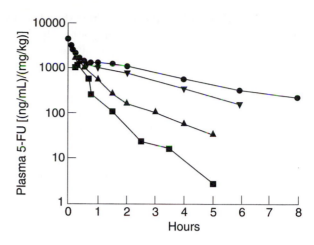

FIGURE 30.7 Dose-normalized 5-FU concentrations in plasma of experimental animals [mouse (■), rat (▲), dog (▼)] and a human subject (●), both lacking dihydropyrimidine dehydrogenase activity. (Reproduced with permission from Khor SP, et al. Cancer Chemother Pharmacol 1997;39:233–8.)

IN VITRO-IN VIVO CORRELATION OF HEPATIC METABOLISM

The liver has been the focus of most drug metabolism studies. Although there is extrahepatic metabolism of some drugs, which may be extensive in some cases, the liver is generally considered the dominant organ in drug metabolism. Since liver tissue can be obtained from most species including humans, study of hepatic metabolism has been an active and productive field of investigation. Studies have been con-

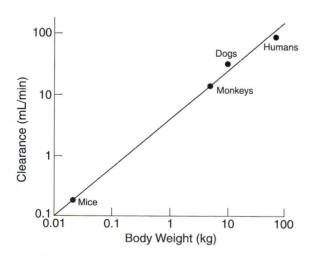

FIGURE 30.6 Kidney clearance of Ara-C and Ara-U vs. body weight for mice, monkeys, dogs, and humans. (Reproduced from Dedrick RL, et al. Biochem Pharmacol 1973;22:2405–17.)

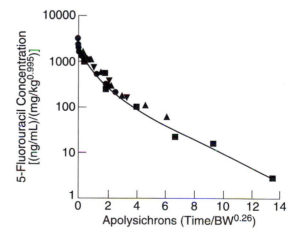

FIGURE 30.8 Complex Dedrick plot of data from Figure 30.7. Symbols are the same as in Figure 30.7. (Reproduced with permission from Khor SP, et al. Cancer Chemother Pharmacol 1997;39:233–8.)

ducted on microsomal preparations, hepatocytes, and liver slices. Interpretation is required for extrapolating *in vitro* results to the pharmacokinetically relevant rate of metabolism by the liver in the body. Issues such as drug binding in the culture medium and in plasma, distribution between plasma and red blood cells, and penetration into liver slices must be considered. Further, stability and intraspecies variability of liver specimens are important considerations.

Houston (7) has reviewed the prediction of *in vivo* intrinsic clearance of cytochrome P450 substrates in the rat from studies using microsomal preparations and isolated hepatocytes. The results are reproduced in Figures 30.9 and 30.10. In the calculation he normalized to a standard rat weight (SRW) of 250 gm with an 11-gm liver containing 1.9×10^9 hepatocytes and yielding 500 mg of microsomal protein. Liver blood flow of 20 mL/min was assumed. Nineteen drugs were summarized for the microsomal predictions; 17 drugs are included in the hepatocyte calculations. In Figures 30.9 and 30.10 the solid symbols represent metabolite formation during *in vitro* studies while the open symbols represent substrate loss. By reference to the liver blood flow of 20 mL/min, it is apparent that drugs exhibiting both relatively low and high extraction ratios were included. The diagonal line is the line of identity on which the observations would fall if the prediction were exact. It is clear that the predictions from hepatocytes are generally better than those from microsomes,

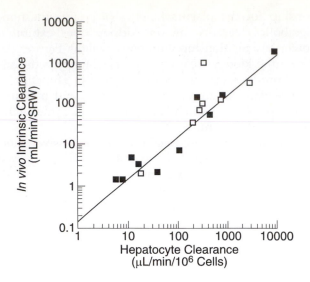

FIGURE 30.10   Intrinsic clearance *in vivo* versus hepatocyte clearance of 17 drugs metabolized by cytochromes P-450 in the rat. The line represents the predicted correlation. Hepatocyte clearance was measured either by substrate loss (□) or metabolite formation (■). Intrinsic clearance was normalized to a standard rat weight (SRW) of 250 gm. (Reproduced with permission from Houston JB. Biochem Pharmacol 1994;47:1469–79.)

and only one of the 17 data points predicted from hepatocytes is very far from the expected value. The microsomal predictions are fairly good at low clearances, but there is frequently an underprediction at higher values. The observation may reflect the fact that local environment and probably the configuration of the cytochrome P450 isoform in microsomal preparations differ significantly from those in hepatocytes.

Similar predictions of *in vivo* intrinsic clearance in the human from *in vitro* data have been produced by Ito et al. (8). The results are shown in Figure 30.11. The liver blood flow of about 1 mL/min · gm places the intrinsic clearances in perspective. These correlations show considerably more variability than those for the rat. This reflects both methodologic difficulties and probably a large variability of enzyme activities within the human population. Also, there seems to be a systematic underprediction for low-clearance drugs. This may reflect difficulties in measuring these low rates *in vitro* and/or extrahepatic metabolism.

Thummel et al. (9) avoided the intrinsic variability of enzyme activity in the human population by predicting *in vivo* clearances from *in vitro* kinetic data in liver transplant patients. They were interested in using midazolam (MDZ) as a probe of CYP3A isoforms in the liver. Because biopsies were performed for the medical management of the transplant patients, the authors had the ethical opportunity to study enzyme

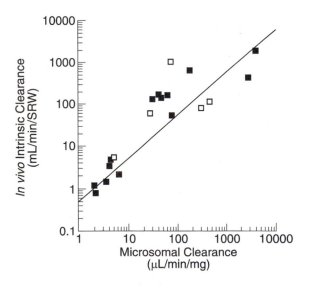

FIGURE 30.9   Intrinsic clearance *in vivo* versus hepatic microsomal clearance of 19 drugs metabolized by cytochromes P450 in the rat. The line represents the predicted correlation. *In vitro* clearance was measured either by substrate loss (□) or metabolite formation (■). Intrinsic clearance was normalized to a standard rat weight (SRW) of 250 gm. (Reproduced with permission from Houston JB. Biochem Pharmacol 1994;47:1469–79.)

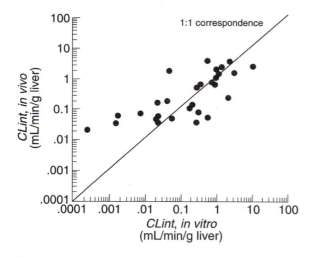

FIGURE 30.11 Observed versus predicted intrinsic metabolic clearance of 29 drugs in humans. (Reproduced with permission from Ito K, et al. Annu Rev Pharmacol Toxicol 1988;38:461–99.)

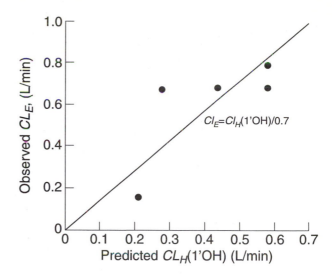

FIGURE 30.12 Observed total elimination clearance (CL_E) of midazolam (MDZ) in liver transplant patients versus hepatic clearance (CL_H) of 1'OH MDZ predicted from biopsy specimens. The line is the predicted hepatic clearance of MDZ if the 1'-hydroxylation pathway accounts for 70% of the substrate loss. (Data from Thummel KE, et al. J Pharmacol Exp Ther 1994;271:549–56.)

activity in biopsies from human livers following transplantation. In addition, MDZ pharmacokinetics were studied in the recipients of the same transplanted livers. Five of the liver recipients provided sufficient tissue for the determination of V_{max} and K_m for MDZ 1'-hydroxylation. V_{max} determined for each biopsy sample was then scaled to the estimated total liver mass and intrinsic clearance estimated as total liver V_{max}/K_m. Hepatic clearance then was predicted from Equation 7.6. Figure 30.12 compares the observed total elimination clearance with predicted hepatic clearance based on the assumption that the 1'-hydroxylation pathway accounts for 70% of the substrate loss. The prediction is quite good. The average absolute deviation between the five observed data points and their predicted values is only 28%, and the differences are uniformly distributed.

References

1. Adolph E F. Quantitative relations in the physiological constitutions of mammals. Science 1949;109:579–85.
2. Dedrick RL, Flessner MF, Collins JM, Schultz JS. Is the peritoneum a membrane? Am Soc Artific Intern Organs J 1982;5:1–8.
3. Dedrick RL, Forrester DD, Ho DHW. *In vitro-in vivo* correlation of drug metabolism—Deamination of 1-β-D-arabinofuranosylcytosine. Biochem Pharmacol 1972;21:1–16.
4. Dedrick RL, Forrester DD, Cannon JN, El Dareer S M, Mellett LB. (1973). Pharmacokinetics of 1-β-D-arabinofuranosylcytosine (Ara-C) deamination in several species. Biochem Pharmacol 1973;22:2405–17.
5. Khor SP, Amyx H, Davis ST, Nelson D, Baccanari DP, Spector T. Dihydropyrimidine dehydrogenase inactivation and 5-fluorouracil pharmacokinetics: Allometric scaling of animal data, pharmacokinetics and toxicodynamics of 5-fluorouracil in humans. Cancer Chemother Pharmacol 1997;39:233–8.
6. Dedrick RL, Bischof KB, Zaharko DS. Interspecies correlation of plasma concentration history of methotrexate (NSC-740). Cancer Chemother Rep 1970;54:95–101.
7. Houston JB. Utility of *in vitro* metabolism data in predicting *in vivo* metabolic clearance. Biochem Pharmacol 1994;47:1469–79.
8. Ito K, Iwatsubo T, Kanamitsu S, Nakajima Y, Sugiyama Y. Quantitative prediction of in vivo drug clearance and drug interactions from in vitro data on metabolism, together with binding and transport. Annu Rev Pharmacol Toxicol 1998;38:461–99.
9. Thummel KE, Shen DD, Podoll TD, Kunze KL, Trager WF, Hartwell PS, et al. Use of midazolam as a human cytochrome P-450 3A probe: I. *In vitro-in vivo* correlations in liver transplant patients. J Pharmacol Exp Ther 1994;271:549–56.

31

Phase 1 Clinical Studies

JERRY M. COLLINS

Laboratory of Clinical Pharmacology, Center for Drug Evaluation and Research, Food and Drug Administration, Rockville, Maryland

INTRODUCTION

In the drug development pipeline, Phase 1 clinical studies sit at the interface between the end of preclinical testing and the start of human exploration (Figure 5.1). Somewhat surprisingly, this stage of drug development does not generally attract much attention. For clinical pharmacologists as well as other practitioners of drug development, the entry of a novel molecular entity into human beings for the first time is unquestionably a very exciting event.

Some features of a Phase 1 study are invariant; others have changed considerably over time. On a periodic basis, a set of new investigators enters the field and almost everyone is inclined to reinvent the design features of Phase 1 studies. First-in-human studies are an extraordinary opportunity to integrate pharmacokinetics, pharmacodynamics, and toxicology information while launching the new molecule on a path for rational clinical development (1). Above all, it's a major domain for application of the principles of clinical pharmacology.

At present, the reengineering of the entire drug development process places additional scrutiny on Phase 1. Drug discovery and high-throughput screening have created a bulge in the pipeline as it heads toward the clinic. It is essential that truly useful medicines are not lost in the sheer numbers of compounds under evaluation, and it is just as essential that marginal candidates be eliminated as expeditiously as pos-

sible. Although the science generated via the discovery and development process can be dazzling, the "art" of Phase 1 trials requires continual focus on safety and probability of therapeutic effect (2).

DISEASE-SPECIFIC CONSIDERATIONS

There is a large amount of conceptual similarity in the approach to Phase 1 trial design, regardless of the therapeutic area; however, there are some important differences. One major consideration is the selection of the population of human subjects for the Phase 1 study. For most therapeutic indications, healthy volunteers are the subjects. They are compensated for the inconveniences of participating in the study, but aren't in a position to receive medical benefit. The use of healthy volunteers substantially limits the ability to observe the desired therapeutic goal. For example, if an agent is intended to correct metabolic deficiencies or lower elevated blood pressure, there may be no detectable changes in healthy subjects.

In several therapeutic areas, patients with the disease are the subjects in Phase 1 studies, rather than healthy volunteers. This tradition is strongest in oncology, because many cytotoxic agents cause damage to DNA. For similar reasons, many anti-AIDS drugs are not tested initially in healthy persons. In neuropharmacology, some categories of drugs have an acclimatization or tolerance aspect, which makes them difficult to study in healthy persons (3). On the other hand, as oncology drugs have shifted toward different targets and with milder side effect profiles, more first-in-human trials are being conducted in healthy populations.

The primary goal of Phase 1 studies is always to evaluate safety in humans. When patients are the subjects, there is an additional element of therapeutic intent. In the determination of human safety, there has been an emphasis on defining the maximum tolerated dose (MTD) as an endpoint of the study. Whereas determination of the MTD is important from the standpoint of clinical toxicology, the MTD has been selected in many cases as the dose for subsequent clinical trials, resulting in the registration and initial marketing of drug doses that are inappropriately high for some clinical conditions (4). However, because the therapeutic index for anticancer drugs is so narrow, and because the disease is life-threatening, the concept of MTD has played a central role in Phase 1 studies of these drugs. A large portion of my own experience with Phase 1 trials has been in the area of anticancer drugs; thus, my examples will be taken from oncology.

STARTING DOSE AND DOSE ESCALATION

Regardless of the details for Phase 1 trial design, the two essential elements are the starting dose and the dose escalation scheme.

For a first-in-human study, selection of the starting dose is caught in a conflict between a desire for safety (leading to a cautious choice) versus an interest in efficiency. When patients are the subjects in a Phase 1 trial, efficiency is also tied to a desire to provide therapeutic benefit, and can stimulate a more aggressive choice of starting dose.

The same conflicts exist for the escalation scheme. Once the current dose level has been demonstrated to be safe, the move to the next higher level is clouded by uncertainty about the steepness of the dose-toxic response curve. Recently, there has been an appreciation of the linkage between choices for starting dose and escalation rate. In particular, the combination of a cautious starting dose with a very conservative escalation rate can lead to trials that are so lengthy that no one's interests are served.

Modified Fibonacci Escalation Scheme

Some version of the modified Fibonacci escalation scheme is probably the most frequently used escala-

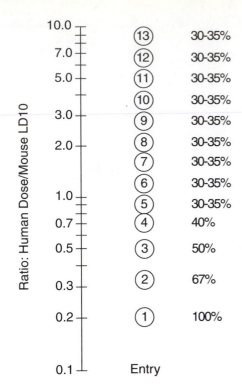

FIGURE 31.1 Modified Fibonacci dose escalation procedure, expressed as a ratio of the human dose to a reference dose in mice (e.g., the LD10). Human studies typically start at one-tenth the murine dose, expressed on the basis of body surface area. If tolerated, the next dose is initially doubled, then the percentage change at each escalation step decreases. (Reproduced from Collins JM, Zaharko DS, Dedrick RL, Chabner BA. Cancer Treat Rep 1986;70:73–80.)

tion scheme, particularly in oncologic Phase 1 studies. However, its preeminence is fading. The sequence of escalation steps for a typical scheme is shown in Figure 31.1. Implicit in the design of this scheme is an attempt to balance caution and aggressiveness. Rapid increases in dose are prescribed at early stages of the trial (i.e., starting with a doubling of the dose), when the chance of using a nontoxic dose is highest. The incremental changes in dose become more conservative at later stages (e.g., 30%) when the probability of side effects has increased. When a modified Fibonacci design is submitted to the local review board and regulatory authorities for approval, the escalation rate is completely determined in advance, at least until toxicity intervenes.

Many variations of the Fibonacci scheme have arisen, driven by statistical and/or pharmacologic principles (5). From the perspective of clinical pharmacology, a particularly attractive goal is to integrate whatever is known about the properties of the drug into an adaptive design. One type of adaptive design modulates the

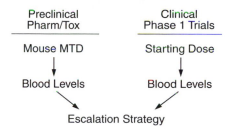

Bridges Between Preclinical and Clinical Development

FIGURE 31.2 Pharmacologically guided dose escalation. As an alternative to the fixed procedure for increasing doses (e.g., Figure 31.1), the size of each dose escalation step is based on current concentrations of drug in human blood, along with target concentrations defined in preclinical studies.

rate of dose escalation based on plasma concentrations of the drug, as described in the next section.

Pharmacologically Guided Dose Escalation (PGDE)

The PGDE design is based on a straightforward PK-PD hypothesis: When comparing animal and human doses, expect equal toxicity for equal drug exposure (6, 7). A fundamental principle of clinical pharmacology is that drug effects are caused by circulating concentrations of the unbound ("free") drug molecule, and are less tightly linked to the administered dose (Figure 2.1). The advantage of PGDE is that it minimizes the numbers of patients at risk and pays more attention to the individual patient's risk of receiving too low a dose. A series of Phase 1 studies were found to be excessively lengthy because a starting dose was chosen that was too low, thus pushing the major portion of the trial into the conservative portion of the modified Fibonacci design.

As illustrated in Figure 31.2, for PGDE, there is a continual evaluation of plasma concentrations as the trial is under way. Thus, unlike a modified Fibonacci design, the escalation rate is adapted throughout the procedure. Although the decisions are expressed in terms of pharmacokinetics (plasma concentrations of the drug), the design is named pharmacologic because it is intended to permit adjustments in the target plasma concentration, based on pharmacodynamic information, such as species differences in IC90 for bone marrow or tumor cells.

A retrospective survey was conducted prior to embarking on "real-time" use of PGDE. The results shown in Figure 31.3 permit a comparison of limiting doses in humans versus mice. The doses used for this comparison were normalized for body surface area (e.g., 100 mg/m^2), which is very exceptional for any other therapeutic class. There are two major conclusions from an evaluation of the data in Figure 31.3:

1. There is enormous scatter in the ratio of human:murine tolerable doses. Thus, while murine doses may seem to give reasonable predictions for acceptable human doses on the average, there is no predictive consistency that could be relied on for any specific drug about to enter Phase 1 study.

2. The drug exposure (AUC) ratio at approximately equitoxic doses has much less variability, indicating that pharmacokinetic differences account for almost all the differences observed for toxic doses between humans and mice.

What is the underlying cause for these interspecies differences? For equal doses, differences in plasma AUC values simply indicate differences in total body clearance. Renal and metabolic elimination are the major contributors to total body clearance. When allometric scaling is used as described in Chapter 30, renal clearance tends to exhibit only small differences across species, whereas there are many examples of

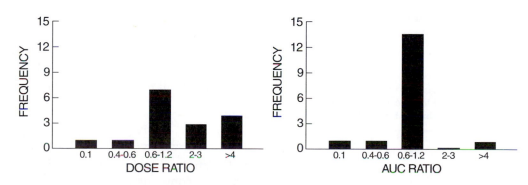

FIGURE 31.3 Survey of acute toxicity of anticancer drugs in humans versus mice. Comparisons based on dose *(left panel)* exhibit more scatter than those based on drug exposure (AUC) *(right panel)*.

interspecies differences in metabolism. Further, across many drug categories, metabolism is quantitatively more important than renal elimination. Therefore, more emphasis on interspecies differences in drug metabolism could improve Phase 1 studies. The next two sections provide specific examples of the impact of monitoring metabolism during early human studies.

Interspecies Differences in Drug Metabolism

The data in Table 31.1 for iododeoxydoxorubicin (I-Dox) were obtained during first-in-human studies conducted by Gianni et al. (8). There was greater exposure to the parent drug in mice, and to the hydroxylated metabolite (I-Dox-ol) in humans. Overall, there was a 50-fold difference in the relative AUC exposure ratios (metabolite:parent drug) for humans and mice. Because I-Dox and I-Dox-ol are approximately equiactive and equitoxic, these exposure comparisons are also indicative of pharmacologic response. This extreme example of an interspecies difference in drug metabolism was comparable to studying one molecule (the parent) in mice and then (unintentionally) studying a different molecule (the metabolite) in humans.

Figure 31.4 illustrates an interspecies difference in paclitaxel metabolism (9). The principal metabolite formed in humans was not produced by rat microsomes. This example illustrates the potential of *in vitro* studies to discover interspecies differences in metabolism. In most cases, it is no longer necessary (or advisable) to wait for *in vivo* Phase 1 studies to discover such differences.

Active Metabolites

During first-in-human studies with the investigational anticancer drug penclomedine, it was discovered that exposure to parent drug concentrations was less than 1% of the exposure to its metabolite, demethylpenclomedine (10). As shown in Figure 31.5, exposure to the parent drug is very brief, while the

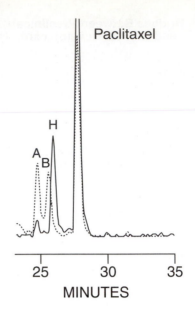

FIGURE 31.4 Comparison of *in vitro* paclitaxel metabolism by hepatic microsomes from rats and humans. The major human peak ("H"), was not formed by rats. (Adapted from Jamis-Dow CA, Klecker RW, Katki AG, Collins JM. Cancer Chemother Pharmacol 1995;6:107–14.)

metabolite accumulates during the course of a 5-day treatment cycle. Since the toxicity of the parent molecule limits the amount of tolerable exposure to the metabolite, which provides the antitumor effect, the penclomedine case clearly demonstrates the danger of not knowing which molecules are circulating in the body. If this type of information is determined early enough in drug development, the metabolite can be selected to replace the parent molecule as the lead development candidate.

There is stunning similarity of the penclomedine story to the history of terfenadine (Seldane), a highly successful antihistamine product that was withdrawn from marketing. In early clinical studies, it was not appreciated that the major source of clinical benefit was its metabolite, fexofenadine (Allegra, see structures in Figure 1.1). It became obvious that the metabolite should have been the lead compound only after cardiotoxicity was subsequently discovered for the parent drug but not the metabolite.

BEYOND TOXICITY

The study of toxicity without consideration of efficacy is inherently unsatisfying. Indeed, when patients are the subjects in Phase 1 trials, there is always therapeutic intent. Realistically, there is only a

TABLE 31.1 AUC Values in Plasma for Iododeoxydoxorubicin (I-Dox) and Its Metabolite (I-Dox-ol) in Mouse and Human Equitoxic Doses[a]

Compound	Mouse (μM · hr)	Human (μM · hr)
I-Dox	5.0	0.3
I-Dox-ol	1.2	4.0

[a] Data from Gianni L, et al. J Natl Cancer Inst 1990;82:469–77.

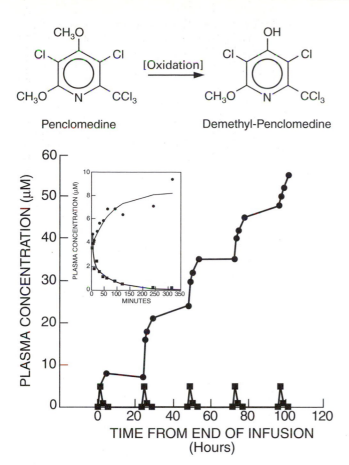

FIGURE 31.5 The investigational anticancer drug, penclomedine, was administered to patients once a day for 5 consecutive days. The parent drug disappeared rapidly from plasma, whereas the metabolite, demethylpenclomedine, accumulated over the course of therapy. (Adapted from Hartman NR, O'Reilly S, Rowinsky EK, Collins JM, Strong JM. Clin Cancer Res 1996;2:953–62.)

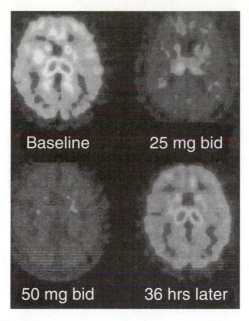

FIGURE 31.6 PET scans showing dose dependency and time dependency of lazabemide inhibition of monoamine oxidase, type B in human brain. (Reproduced with permission from Fowler JS, Volkow ND, Wang G-J, Dewey SL. J Nucl Med 1999;40:1154–63.)

low probability of success in many settings, but our obligation is to maximize that chance. As it becomes more common to seek "proof-of-concept" or mechanistic evaluations during Phase 1, an increased emphasis on demonstrating therapeutic activity, the usual domain for Phase 2 study, looms on the horizon. By monitoring a target biomarker, both proof-of-concept and dose determination might be achieved simultaneously. Further, by enrolling in the trial patients who have favorable expression profiles of the target, an "enriched" population is obtained with a higher likelihood of response, if the therapeutic concept has merit.

For "accessible" targets such as blood pressure or heart rate, these concepts are not new. The techniques of external, noninvasive imaging now permit real-time monitoring of targets such as *in situ* regions of the human brain that were previously considered inaccessible. Fowler et al. (11) reported a study of the inhibition of monoamine oxidase, type B (MAO-B) by lazabemide (Figure 31.6). A dose of 25 mg twice a day inhibited most MAO-B activity in subjects, and doubling the dose to 50 mg abolished all detectable activity. Also, brain activity for MAO-B had returned to baseline values within 36 hours of the last dose of lazabemide.

This example of MAO-B inhibition demonstrates the successful investigation in early human studies of three areas of fundamental interest in developing drug therapy (Table 31.2): monitoring impact at the desired target, evaluating the dose-response realtionship (dose-ranging), and determining an appropriate dose interval from recovery of enzyme activity. This blurring of the traditional lines of demarcation between clinical phases of drug development has its pitfalls and disorienting aspects, but also presents exciting new opportunities for clinical pharmacologists and other stakeholders in drug development.

TABLE 31.2 Therapeutic Issues for Drug Development

Does treatment impact the desired target?
What is the minimum/maximum dose?
What dose (therapeutic course) interval is appropriate?

References

1. Peck CC, Barr WH, Benet LZ, Collins J, Desjardins RE, Furst DE, et al. Opportunities for integration of pharmacokinetics, pharmacodynamics, and toxicokinetics in rational drug development. Clin Pharmacol Ther 1992;51:465–73.
2. Peck CC, Collins JM. First time in man studies: A regulatory perspective—art and science of Phase I trials. J Clin Pharmacol 1990;30:218–22.
3. Cutler NR, Stramek JJ. Scientific and ethical concerns in clinical trials in Alzheimer's patients: The bridging study. Eur J Clin Pharmacol 1995;48:421–8.
4. Rolan P. The contribution of clinical pharmacology surrogates and models to drug development—A critical appraisal. Br J Clin Pharmacol 1997;44:219–25.
5. Simon R, Freidlin B, Rubinstein L, Arbuck SG, Collins J, Christian MC. Accelerated titration designs for Phase I clinical trials in oncology. J Natl Cancer Inst 1997;89:1138–47.
6. Collins JM, Zaharko DS, Dedrick RL, Chabner BA. Potential roles for preclinical pharmacology in Phase I trials. Cancer Treat Rep 1986;70:73–80.
7. Collins JM, Grieshaber CK, Chabner BA. Pharmacologically-guided Phase I trials based upon preclinical development. J Natl Cancer Inst. 1990;82:1321–6.
8. Gianni L, Vigano L, Surbone A, Ballinari D, Casali P, Tarella C, Collins JM, Bonadonna G. Pharmacology and clinical toxicity of 4'-iodo-4'-deoxydoxorubicin: An example of successful application of pharmacokinetics to dose escalation in Phase I trials. J Natl Cancer Inst. 1990;82:469–77.
9. Jamis-Dow CA, Klecker RW, Katki AG, Collins JM. Metabolism of taxol by human and rat liver in vitro: A screen for drug interactions and interspecies differences. Cancer Chemother Pharmacol 1995; 6:107–14.
10. Hartman NR, O'Reilly S, Rowinsky EK, Collins JM, Strong JM. Murine and human in vivo penclomedine metabolism. Clin Cancer Res 1996;2:953–62.
11. Fowler JS, Volkow ND, Wang G-J, Dewey SL. PET and drug research and development. J Nucl Med 1999;40:1154–63.

Pharmacokinetic and Pharmacodynamic Considerations in the Development of Biotechnology Products and Large Molecules

PAMELA D. GARZONE

Clinical Pharmacology and Preclinical Studies, Cell Therapeutics, Inc., Seatlle, Washington

INTRODUCTION

In 1998, the FDA approved 13 biotechnology products. Of these, one was a humanized monoclonal antibody (Herceptin), one was a soluble receptor (Enbrel); one was the first in the class of the matrix metalloproteinase enzyme inhibitors (Periostat), one was a combination product (Rebetron Combination Therapy containing interferon alpha-2b as an injection), and one was a diagnostic for thyroid cancer (Thyrogen) (1). The remaining approved products were either new indications for older medications (e.g., cyclosporine oral solution) or chemically synthesized new molecules (e.g., Provigil). As of this writing, over 250 biotechnology compounds were in late stage development, and, of these, 40 are macromolecules. These statistics emphasize how important it is to understand how macromolecules behave in the body, and the special considerations required of researchers and clinicians working with these compounds. For the purpose of this chapter, the definition of macromolecule is a large molecule, with a molecular weight in kilodaltons (kDa), such as a protein, built up from small chemical structures. (Protein will be used interchangeably with macromolecule in this chapter.)

This chapter will focus only on macromolecules and not on monoclonal antibodies. The reader is referred to a separate review article on this topic (2). Well-known macromolecules that have been approved and are currently marketed are listed in Table 32.1. This chapter will discuss methodology used to assay macromolecules, interspecies scaling of macromolecules, pharmacokinetic (PK) characteristics of macromolecules, and pharmacodynamics (PD) of macromolecules.

Assay of Macromolecules

The most common types of assays employed to quantitate protein concentrations in biological matrices are listed in Table 32.2. Because immunoassays measure immunoreactivity, they also detect macromolecule fragments, (i.e., peptides), but they do not provide information on whether or not the fragment is biologically active.

Enzyme-linked immunosorbent assays (ELISAs), radioimmunoassays (RIAs), and immunoradiometric assays (IRMAs) require protein-specific antibodies, labeled proteins or labeled antibodies as reagents, and are generally competitive inhibition assays. Radioimmunoassays measure concentrations by displacing ligands from cell-bound receptors. The most common assay, the ELISA, is based on antibody recognition of an antigenic epitope (i.e., a molecular region on the surface of a molecule capable of bind-

TABLE 32.1   Examples of Currently Marketed
              Macromolecules

Macromolecule	Abbreviation	Trade name
Erythropoietin	Epo	Epogen
Growth hormone	GH	Nutropin
Granulocyte colony stimulating factor	G-CSF	Neupogen
Granulocyte-macrophage colony stimulating factor	GM-CSF	Leukine
Interleukin-2	IL-2	Proleukin
Interleukin-11	IL-11	Neumega
Factor IX	FIX	BeneFIX
Recombinant tissue plasminogen activator	rt-PA	Activase

ing to the specific antibody). The general steps involved in a sandwich ELISA are shown in Table 32.3. Most ELISAs are performed in the solid phase, such as microtiter plate wells, but ELISAs can be altered, customized, or automated to meet the specific needs of the investigator. For example, the assay can be changed to detect antibodies, termed an "indirect antibody" capture assay. Also, there are several choices of the enzyme label that can be used depending on the assay application. The most common of these is horseradish peroxidase.

These assays have only a limited ability to quantify proteins. Their limitations include lack of sensitivity of the antibody reagents such that the level of quantitation is near the lower limit of the assay's sensitivity. In addition, the assays do not reveal anything about biological activity. In some cases, the peptide fragment containing the epitope is captured but interpreted as total protein.

Other currently evolving technologies may be useful to look at the structural characteristics of intact and proteolytic proteins. An example is matrix-assisted laser desorption time of flight mass spectrometry or MALDI-TOF MS. MALDI-TOF MS is already employed in peptide fingerprinting and high-throughput analyses for

TABLE 32.2   Examples of Immunoassays Used to
              Quantitate Macromolecules

Assay acronym	Assay description
ELISA	Enzyme-linked immunosorbent assay
RIA	Radioimmunoassay
IRMA	Immunoradiometric assay
RRA	Radioreceptor assay

TABLE 32.3   General Steps in Sandwich ELISA

Step	Activity
1	Adsorb primary antibody to solid phase to "capture" target antigen
2	Wash away excess antibody
3	Apply biological matrix (e.g., serum)
4	Wash unbound substances away
5	Add second enzyme-labeled antibody
6	Add chromogenic substrate to identify complex bound to solid phase
7	Quantitate amount of colored products (proportional to amount of targeted product)

genomics research. Combined with ELISAs, MALDI-TOF MS may be a powerful and sensitive tool to identify "metabolites" or proteolytic fragments of exogenously administered proteins, an area in which research has not been extensive.

Interspecies Scaling of Macromolecules: Predictions in Humans

As discussed in Chapter 30 and elsewhere (3), interspecies scaling is based on allometry (an empirical approach) or physiology. Pharmacokinetic parameters for proteins such as volume of distribution (V_d), elimination half-life $(t_{1/2})$, and elimination clearance (CL) have been scaled across species using the standard allometric equation (4):

$$Y = aW^b \qquad (32.1)$$

In this equation, Y is the parameter of interest, the coefficient a is the value of the parameter at one unit of body weight, W is body weight, and b is the allometric exponent. For convenience, this equation is linearized to:

$$\log Y = \log a + b \log W \qquad (32.2)$$

In this form, $\log a$ is the y-intercept and b is the slope of the line. In Figure 32.1, representative linearized plots of CL and initial volume of distribution (V_1) are shown for recombinant growth hormone (GH) across four species.

Allometric equations for V_1 and CL for some representative macromolecules are depicted in Table 32.4. The theoretical exponent approximations for V_1 (mL) and CL (mL/min) are $aW^{0.8}$ to $aW^{1.0}$ and $aW^{0.6}$ to $aW^{0.8}$, respectively. Parameter estimates can be normalized for body weight simply by subtracting 1.0 from the exponent.

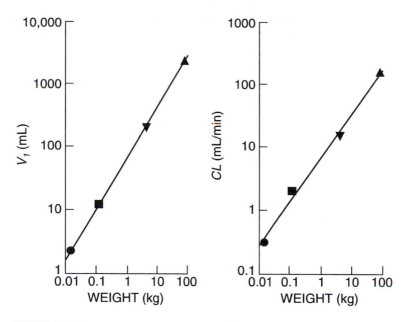

FIGURE 32.1 Log-log plots of V_1 and CL versus body weight for rhGH: mouse (●), rat (■), cynomolgous monkey (▼), human (▲). (Reproduced with permission from Mordenti J, et al. Pharm Res 1991;8:1351–9.)

In Table 32.5 the predicted parameter estimates derived from the allometric equations in Table 32.4 are compared with the corresponding parameter estimates reported in humans. The observed values of V_1 for the macromolecules listed fall within the expected range of observed results. However, the observed clearances of FIX and IL-12 were not predicted from allometry. Factors such as species specificity in the endothelial binding of FIX (5) or saturation of clearance mechanisms may account for the inability to predict these parameters in humans.

Factors to be considered in deciding whether interspecies scaling would be predictive of human PK parameter estimates include: 1) binding characteristics; 2) receptor density; 3) size and charge of molecule; 4) end-terminal carbohydrate characteristics; 5) degree of sialylation; and 6) saturation of elimination pathways. These factors are known to influence clearance and distribution volumes, as will be discussed in subsequent sections. For example, clearance may involve several mechanisms including immune-mediated clearance that results in nonconstant clearance rates. The interspecies predictability of clearance in this situation would be questionable.

Despite the limitations, interspecies scaling can be used to relate dosages across species in toxicology

TABLE 32.4 Allometric Equations for Representative Macromolecules

	Allometric equations		
Macromolecule	V_1 (mL)	CL (mL/hr)	Ref.
Factor IX (FIX)[a]	87 $W^{1.26}$	14 $W^{0.68}$	6,7[b]
Factor VIII[a]	44 $W^{1.04}$	10 $W^{0.69}$	8
Interleukin-12 (IL-12)[a]	65 $W^{0.85}$	8 $W^{0.62}$	9,10[b]
Growth hormone (GH)[c]	68 $W^{0.83}$	7 $W^{0.71}$	4
Tissue plasminogen activator (rt-PA)[c]	91 $W^{0.93}$	17 $W^{0.84}$	4

[a] Based on parameter estimates in at least two species.

[b] Allometric equations determined from pharmacokinetic parameter estimates reported in published literature.

[c] Based on parameter estimates in at least four species.

TABLE 32.5   Prediction of Human Pharmacokinetic Parameters Based on Allometric Scaling

Macromolecule	V_1			CL			
	Predicted (mL)	Observed (mL)	Expected range[a] (mL/kg)	Predicted (mL/hr)	Observed (mL/hr)	Expected range[a] (mL/hr)	Ref.
FIX	18,380	10,150[b]	9,190–27,570	248	434[b]	124–372	11
Factor VIII	3,617	3,030	1,809–5,426	195	174	98–293	8
IL-12	2,406	3,360	1,203–3,609	113	406	57–170	12
GH	2,243	2,432	1,122–3,365	148	175	74–222	4
rt-PA	5,814	4,450	2,907–8,721	646	620	323–969	4

[a] For comparison with observed results, an expected range is chosen that is 0.5 to 1.5 times the predicted value.

[b] Calculated from Figure 1 of referenced article.

studies, to predict human PK parameter estimates for macromolecules, and, as discussed in Chapters 30 and 31, to guide dose selection in Phase 1 clinical trials. An understanding of the characteristics of the macromolecule is important for the interpretation and application of these results.

PHARMACOKINETIC CHARACTERISTICS OF MACROMOLECULES

Endogenous Concentrations

Unlike chemically synthesized molecules, many of the macromolecules currently marketed or under investigation are naturally occurring substances in the body. This presents some unique challenges for estimating pharmacokinetic parameters. Most commercially available ELISAs used to quantitate exogenously administered proteins do not distinguish between the native protein in the body and the exogenously administered protein. Clearly, concentrations of endogenous proteins, which can fluctuate because of stimulation or feedback control [e.g., insulin growth factor (IGF-1)], can result in erroneous parameter estimates. There are several approaches to deal with the problem posed by detectable endogenous protein concentrations.

In a study by Cheung et al. (13), the investigators administered erythropoietin subcutaneously to 30 healthy subjects. Blood sampling times included a predose sample and samples collected multiple times post-administration. Erythropoietin was detected in all subjects in the predose sample. In general, all detected concentrations were in the physiological range (<7 to 30 IU/mL) with one exception: a subject whose baseline erythropoietin concentration was 48 IU/mL, exceeding the normal physiologic range. Prior to estimating PK parameters, the investigators subtracted

each predose concentration from all concentrations detected post-administration. The underlying assumption for this approach was that the low endogenous concentrations remained relatively stable over the post-administration times. However, data were not presented to confirm or refute this assumption.

Another approach for dealing with this problem is that proposed by Veldhuis and colleagues (14) for GH. A deconvolution method is employed to minimize the influence of circulating endogenous GH on PK parameter estimates derived from exogenously administered growth hormone. In this method, the 24-hour secretory rate of GH is estimated by approximating endogenous plasma GH concentration data with cubic spline smoothing controlled by setting a maximum limit for the weighted residual square sum (15). Patient-specific parameters can be estimated from individual endogenous hormone concentrations or from group means. An example of this kind of analysis is shown in Figure 32.2.

Another option is to estimate PK parameters from the sum of exogenous and endogenous protein concentrations detected after the exogenous administration of the protein. The basic assumption is that the PK parameter estimates are not significantly altered by the presence of endogenous protein concentrations. This generally is true in the very early part of the concentration vs. time profile when the endogenous concentration may represent less than 10% of the total concentration. However, in the example depicted in Figure 32.3, endogenous concentrations are oscillating and pulsatile, reaching peaks during the sampling period that are greater than 100-fold the initial basal values. This illustrates how changes in endogenous protein concentrations over the sampling period can influence model fits and confound PK parameter estimation.

Finally, a crossover study design can be employed such that subjects are randomized to placebo or treat-

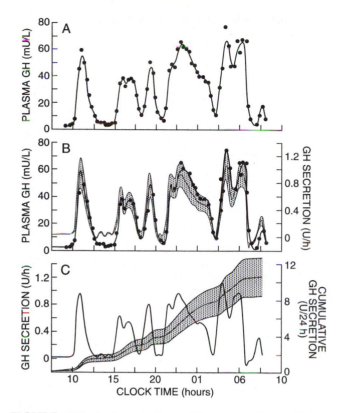

FIGURE 32.2 Analysis of plasma GH-concentration profile by a model-based deconvolution technique. *Panel A:* observed concentrations (●) fitted by a spline approximation curve. *Panel B:* plasma GH concentrations (●) and calculated GH secretory rate with 95% confidence limits *(line and stippled area)*. *Panel C:* GH secretion *(thin line)* and cumulative secretion with 95% confidence limits *(line and stippled area)*. (Reproduced with permission from Albertsson-Wikland K, et al. Am J Physiol 1989;257:E809–14.)

ment on one occasion and the alternate regimen on a second occassion, assuring an adequate washout period between the two occasions. The endogenous concentrations determined in the same subjects after placebo administration can be subtracted from the matching sample collected after treatment administration. This design accommodates the intrasubject variability and variations in endogenous concentrations due to pulsatile secretion, but assumes that the two separate study days are similar.

Thus, it is important to recognize that current analytical methods cannot distinguish endogenous protein concentrations from exogenous concentrations. Administering radiolabeled proteins would allow for exogenous and endogenous proteins to be distinguished, but there are experimental limitations to the use of radiolabeled proteins. Although the accuracy of PK parameter estimation may be impacted by the presence of endogenous concentrations, study designs and data analysis methods can be employed that take endogenous concentration into consideration.

Absorption

The absolute bioavailability of macromolecules following extravascular administration is shown in Table 32.6. It is apparent that bioavailability is variable with the different molecules and with different routes of administration, reflecting individual molecule characteristics. In addition, in one report the bioavailability after subcutaneous (SC) or intramuscular (IM) administration was greater than 100% relative to an intravenous (IV) bolus injection (20). This implausible result may reflect the inability of the immunoradiometric assay to distinguish proteolytic fragments of

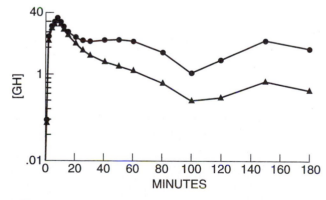

FIGURE 32.3 Simulated effects of increasing basal GH concentrations on measured total GH concentrations at various times during and after an 8-minute infusion of rhGH using basal concentrations 10 times (▲) and 100 times (●) the observed pre-infusion value of 0.042 ng/mL. (Reproduced with permission from Bright GM, et al. J Clin Endocrinol Metab 1999;84:3301–5.)

TABLE 32.6   Bioavailability of Macromolecules after Extravascular Routes of Administration

	Route of administration			
Macromolecule	SC[a]	IP[a]	Other	Ref.
Erythropoietin	22.0%	2.9%	—	17
Granulocyte macrophage colony stimulating factor (GM-CSF)	83.0%	—	—	18
GH	49.5%	—	7.8–9.9%[b]	19
Interferon-alpha (IFN-α-2b)	> 100%	42.0%	> 100%[c]	20, 21
Interleukin-11 (IL-11)	65%	—	—	22

[a] SC = subcutaneous, IP = intraperitoneal.
[b] Nasal administration.
[c] Intramuscular administration.

TABLE 32.7   Absorption and Apparent Elimination Rates of Macromolecules after SC and IV Administration

Macromolecule	Route of administration	k_a (hr^{-1})	Apparent k_e (hr^{-1})	Ref.
GH	SC	0.23 ± 0.04	0.43 ± 0.05	23
	IV	—	2.58	16
IFN-α-2b	SC	0.24	0.13	20
	IV	—	0.42	
Erythropoietin	SC	0.0403 ± 0.002	0.206 ± 0.004	24
	IV	—	0.077	25

interferon-α (IFN-α) from the intact molecule, the slow absorption phase of either the SC or IM routes, or a saturable elimination process. The authors did not elucidate which of these factors might have contributed to their observation.

Flip-flop Pharmacokinetics of Macromolecules

When the absorption rate constant, k_a, is greater than the elimination rate constant, k_e, elimination of the molecule from the body is the rate-limiting step and the terminal portion of the concentration-time curve is primarily determined by the elimination rate. However, as discussed in Chapter 4, if k_a is less than k_e, absorption is rate limiting and the terminal slope of the curve reflects the absorption rate. This phenomenon is illustrated for several molecules in Table 32.7.

In the absence of concentration-time profiles after IV administration, it is impossible to estimate the actual elimination rate constant, and the interpretation of absorption and elimination rates after SC administration of macromolecules must be done cautiously. It is for this reason surprising that so few published pharmacokinetic studies include IV administration to assess whether the macromolecule follows flip-flop pharmacokinetics.

Factors Affecting Absorption from Subcutaneous Sites

Two very important principles on the absorption of macromolecules after SC administration were elucidated by Supersaxo et al. (26). First, in the range of the molecular weight of the various molecules tested (246–19,000 Da), there was a linear relationship between molecular weight and absorption by the lymphatic system (Figure 32.4). Second, the authors concluded that molecules with a molecular weight greater than 16 kDa are absorbed mainly by the lymphatic system that drains the SC site of injection, whereas molecules with a molecular weight of less than 1000 are absorbed almost entirely by blood cap-

illaries. The authors hypothesized that macromolecules are absorbed preferentially by lymphatic rather than blood capillaries because lymphatic capillaries lack the subendothelial basement membrane present in continuous blood capillaries, and also may have 20- to 100-nm gaps between adjacent endothelial cells.

In addition to molecular weight, injection site may influence the absorption of macromolecules after SC administration. For example, the absorption half-life was significantly longer, 14.9 vs. 12.3 hours, after injection of recombinant human erythropoeitin (RhEPO) into the thigh than after injection into the abdomen (27). Also, the concentration vs. time profile displayed a double peak after injection into the thigh that was more pronounced than after the abdominal injection (Figure 32.5). No statistically significant differences were observed in area under the curve [AUC (5684 vs.

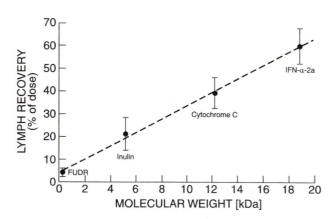

FIGURE 32.4 Correlation between molecular weight (MW) and cumulative recovery of IFN-α-2a (MW 19,000), cytochrome c (MW 12,300), inulin (MW 5200), and 5-fluoro-2′-deoxyuridine (FUDR—MW 246.2) in the efferent lymph from the right popliteal lymph node following SC administration into the lower part of the right hind leg of sheep. Each point and bar show the mean and standard deviation of three experiments performed in three separate sheep. The line drawn represents a least-squares fit of the data ($r = 0.988$, $P < 0.01$). (Reproduced with permission from Supersaxo A, et al. Pharm Res 1990;7:167–9.)

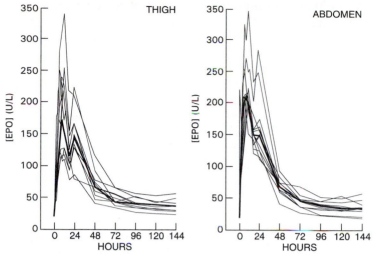

FIGURE 32.5 Serum erythropoietin concentrations as a function of time after SC injection of 100 U/kg of recombinant human erythropoietin in the thigh and abdomen of 11 healthy volunteers. The bold curve represents the median. (Reproduced with permission from Jensen JD, et al. Eur J Clin Pharmacol 1994;46:333–7.)

6185 U·hr/L)], maximum concentration [C_{max} (175 vs. 212 U/L)], or time of maximum concentration (t_{max} = 10 hrs) for thigh vs. abdomen, respectively.

In another study, recombinant human GH was absorbed faster after SC injection into the abdomen compared with the absorption after SC injection into the thigh (28). C_{max} was higher (29.7 ± 4.8 mU/L) and t_{max} was faster (4.3 ± 0.5 hr) after injection into the abdomen than after injection into the thigh (23.2 ± 3.9 mU/L and 5.9 ± 0.4 hr, respectively). However, mean IGF-1 and insulin growth factor-binding protein 1 (IGFBP-1) concentrations, a pharmacodynamic marker of GH, were unaffected by the site of injection. Other effects independent of injection site were blood glucose, and serum insulin and glucagon levels. Thus, absorption differences may be related to lymphatic drainage of the two injection sites and may depend on differences in lymph flow. However, for both recombinant erythropoeitin and GH, site of injection is clinically irrelevant.

In summary, molecular weight and site of injection are two factors that may affect the absorption characteristics of macromolecules and should be considered both in clinical trials and when treating patients.

Distribution

As discussed in Chapter 3, proteins and other macromolecules distribute initially into the plasma volume and then more slowly into the interstitial fluid space. It can be seen from Table 32.8 that the initial distribution volume of interleukin-2 (IL-2) IL-12, G-CSF and rt-PA approximates that of plasma volume. In contrast, the initial distribution volume of FIX is approxi-

TABLE 32.8   Distribution Volume of Representative Macromolecules

Macromolecule	MW (kDa)	V_1 (mL/kg)	$V_{d(ss)}$ (mL/kg)	Ref.
Inulin	5.2	55	164	29
FIX	57	136[a]	271[a]	11
IL-2	15.5	60	112	30, 31
IL-12	53	52	59	12
Granulocyte colony stimulating factor (G-CSF)	20	44	60	32, 33
rt-PA	65	59	106	34

[a] Calculated from Figure 1 of referenced article.

mately twice that of plasma volume. On the other hand, the volume of distribution at steady state ($V_{d(ss)}$) for IL-12, granulocyte colony stimulating factor (G-CSF), and recombinant tissue plasminogen activator (rt-PA) are considerably smaller than the $V_{d(ss)}$ of inulin, a marker for extracellular fluid volume (ECF)

When distribution volume estimates are much less than expected values for ECF, this could reflect the slow transport of large molecules across membranes and the fact that either assay sensitivity or sampling times have been inadequate to characterize the true elimination phase of the compound.

Binding to Alpha₂-macroglobulin

Alpha₂-macroglobulin, one of the major proteins in the serum, is highly conserved across species and can bind many molecules, such as cytokines, enzymes, lipopolysaccharide (LPS), and ions such as zinc and nickel (35). Alpha₂-macroglobulin is found in extravascular secretions, such as lymph. It exists in two forms, a slow native form, and a fast form, an alpha₂-macroglobulin-protease complex that results in a conformational change that increases electrophoretic mobility. This conformational change results in exposure of a hydrophobic region that can bind to cell surface receptors such as those on hepatocytes.

There is a growing body of evidence suggesting that alpha₂-macroglobulin plays an important role in human immune function. Specifically, studies have shown that the fast form can inhibit antibody dependent cellular toxicity and natural killer (NK) cell-mediated cytolysis (36), as well as superoxide production by activated macrophages (37).

As shown in Table 32.9, alpha₂-macroglobulin can bind to exogenously administered proteins. Three different mechanisms for this binding have been identified (38). The binding can be non-covalent and reversible. An example of this type of binding is seen with growth factors such as tissue growth factor-β (TGF-β). The binding to alpha₂-macroglobulin can be covalent, and the third mechanism involves covalent linkages with proteinase reactions. Subsequent to the binding, the pharmacokinetics and pharmacodynamic properties of the macromolecule may be altered. The binding of alpha₂-macroglobulin is associated with variable results: the alpha₂-macroglobulin-cytokine complex may interfere with bioassay results (e.g., nerve growth factor) (39); serve as a carrier (e.g., TGF-β) (38); prevent proteolytic degradation (e.g., IL-2) (40); or enhance removal of the protein from the circulation (e.g., tissue necrosis factor-α) (41).

Binding to Other Proteins

Insulin-like growth factor-1 (IGF-1) is produced by many tissues in the body and has approximately 50% structural homology with insulin. In plasma, IGF-1 exists as "free" IGF-1 and "bound" IGF-1. Its physiology is very complex as depicted in Figure 32.6 (42) and discussed further in the section on pharmacodynamics. To date, eight binding proteins (designated IGFBP-1 through 8) have been identified, with IGFBP-3 the most abundant. The binding proteins vary in molecular weight, distribution, concentration in biological fluids, and binding affinity (43). It is important to note that the interactions between the binding proteins and their physiologic role are poorly understood, but probably serve to modulate the clearance of IGF-1.

Metabolism

Table 32.10 summarizes the effects of various cytokines on the cytochrome P-450 (P450) mixed function oxidase system. With the exception of IL-2, these cytokines depress the activity of P450 enzymes. Data on cytokine-mediated depression of drug-metabolizing ability has been obtained primarily in rodents under conditions of inflammation or infection (44). The reduction in drug biotransformation capacity parallels a decrease in total P450 content and enzyme activity, and is due primarily to a down-regulation of P450 gene transcription, but modulation of RNA and enzyme inhibition may also be involved (45, 46).

As shown in Table 32.10, the expression of CYP2C11 and CYP2D isoenzymes is frequently suppressed by cytokines. These two P450 gene families are constitutively expressed in male and female rats. In the rat,

TABLE 32.9   Binding of Macromolecules to Alpha₂-macroglobulin

Macromolecule	Physiological effect	Relevance of binding
Nerve growth factor (NGF)	Stimulates nerve growth	Interferes with assay
Interleukin-2 (IL-1)	Regulates proliferation of thymocytes	Regulates cell activity
Interleukin-2 (IL-2)	Impairs proliferation of T-cells	Inactivates cytokine
Tissue growth factor (TGF-β)	Stimulates growth of kidney fibroblasts	Functions as carrier and accelerates clearance

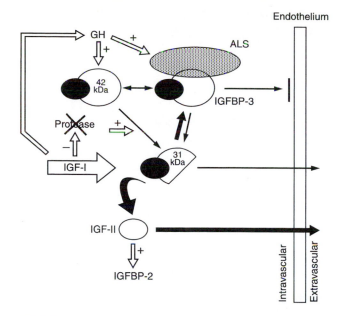

FIGURE 32.6 Hypothetical model of the effects of IGF-1. Open arrows show regulating influences. Plasma IGF-1 consists of free and bound IGF-1. IFGBP-3 exists in two forms, a 42 kDa complete form or a 31 kDa fragment. IGF-1 drives the reaction toward binding with the acid labile subunit (ALS) to form a ternary complex that is retained in the intravascular space. IFG-1 also suppresses GH secretion, decreasing the synthesis of IGFBP-3. (Reproduced with permission from Blum WF, et al. Acta Paediatr Suppl 1993;82(suppl 391):15–9.)

CYP2C is under developmental and pituitary hormone regulation. Although there is approximately 70% c DNA-deduced amino acid sequence homology with the human CYP2C, caution is needed in extrapolating these observations on CYP2C regulation in rats to humans (47). In both rats and humans, there is polymorphic expression of the CYP2D and CYP2D1 isoenzymes that exhibit debrisoquine 4-hydroxylase activity. However, this gene family has evolved differently in rats than in humans. Specifically, the rat has four genes that are approximately 73 to 80% similar while the human has three genes that are 89 to 95%

similar. Thus, results in rat studies may not be predictive of results in humans because of the difference in number of genes, their regulation, and their complexity (47).

In vitro study results have been consistent with those obtained *in vivo*. For example, in primary rat hepatocyte cultures IL-1, tumor necrosis factor (TNF) and interleukin-6 (IL-6) concentrations ranging from 0.5 to 10.0 ng/mL suppressed the expression of CYP2C11 mRNA. (46). It is interesting to note that in rat liver microsomes, IL-2 increased both the amount of immunoreactive CYP2D protein and its mRNA (48). In human primary hepatocytes, IL-1β, IL-6, and TNF-α caused a decrease in all mRNAs and P450 isoenzyme activities. Moreover, interferon γ (IFNγ) was shown to decrease CYP1D2 and CYP2E1 mRNA, but had no effect or CYP2C or CYP3A mRNAs (44).

The clinical significance of the aforementioned findings is unknown. A report by Khakoo et al. (49) did not demonstrate a pharmacokinetic interaction between IFN-α-2b and ribavirin or an additive effect of the combination therapy on safety assessments. In another study, administration of IFN-α prior to the administration of cyclophosphamide significantly impaired the metabolism of cyclophosphamide and 4-hydroxycyclophosphamide. In contrast, the administration of IFN-α after cyclophosphamide resulted in higher 4-hydroxycyclophosphamide concentrations and produced a significant decrease in leukocyte count (50).

Finally, the interaction between IL-2 and doxorubicin was explored in patients with advanced solid tumors (51). Doxorubicin was given alone, then three weeks later patients received the combination of rhIL-2 (18 mIU/m^2 given SC on days 1 to 5) and doxorubicin. Doxorubicin pharmacokinetics were assessed for 48 hours after each administration period. SC injections of rhIL-2 did not affect doxorubicin PK. Doxorubicin, given before IL-2, prevented IL-2-induced lymphocyte rebounds, but not did not qualitatively alter nonmajor histocompatibility complex-restricted cytotoxicity.

TABLE 32.10   Effect of Various Macromolecules on P450 Isoenzymes

Macromolecule	Isoenzyme	Effects
Interferon α (IFN-α)	CYP2C11	Decreased mRNA and enzyme levels
Interleukin-1 (IL-1)	CYP2C11	Decreased mRNA and enzyme levels
	CYP2D	Decreased mRNA and enzyme levels
Interleukin-2 (IL2)	CYP2D1	Increased mRNA and enzyme levels
Interleukin-6 (IL-6)	CYP2C11	Decreased mRNA and enzyme levels
Tumor necrosis factor (TNF)	CYP2C11	Decreased enzyme levels

In summary, various cytokines have been shown to affect P450 protein content, mRNA, and enzyme activities. However, there are few reports that evaluate the extent and clinical significance of corresponding PK or PD changes when used in combination with other drugs.

Excretion

Little is known regarding the catabolism of macromolecules that are either currently marketed or under investigation. The absence of suitable biological assays or other analytical methods for identifying and quantitating macromolecule degradation products obviously limits evaluation of this catabolism.

The renal excretion of proteins is size dependent and glomerular filtration is rate limiting. It has been suggested that the renal clearance rate of macromolecules, relative to the glomerular filtration rate of inulin, decreases with increasing molecular radius (52). The following general conclusions are based on studies using indirect methods to estimate the glomerular sieving coefficients. Small proteins (<25 kDa) cross the glomerular barrier, and filtration accounts for most of their plasma clearance; the degree of sieving is independent of biologic activity; and the filtered load of protein is directly related to plasma concentration. The effect of molecular charge is negligible for these small proteins, whereas charge retards glomerular filtration of anionic proteins as large as albumin (approximately 70 kDa). Subsequent to glomerular filtration, macromolecules may undergo hydrolysis and tubular reabsorption, mainly in endocytotic vesicles located in the apical regions of renal tubular cells (53).

In addition to physical characteristics, the clearance of rt-PA and other glycoproteins is mediated by cell surface receptors for specific terminal carbohy-

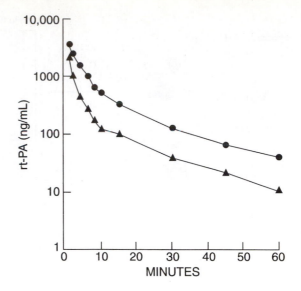

FIGURE 32.7 Clearance of different forms of rt-PA in rabbits after administration of rt-PA by itself (▲) or in combination with *p*-aminophenyl-α-D-mannoside BSA (BSA-Man) (●). (Reproduced with permission from Lucore CL, et al. Circulation 1988;77:906–14.)

drates and monosaccharides (Table 32.11). There are at least eight such receptors, the most well known of these being the Ashwell or asialoglycoprotein receptor (54). Once the glycoprotein ligand binds to its receptor, it is internalized by endocytosis and degraded. The degree of glycosylation, sialylation, or fucosylation are all factors determining the clearance of these glycoproteins.

Clearance of rt-PA appears to mediated by the mannose/*N*-acetylglucosamine specific receptor on hepatic reticuloendothelial cells. To confirm that the mannose receptor is involved, Lucore et al. (55) evaluated the clearance of rt-PA from rabbits' circulation. Analysis of sequential blood samples by fibrin autography indicated that circulating free t-PA (approximately 55 kDa) was predominant, but that minimal amounts of higher molecular weight complexes of approximately 110 and 170 kDa were also present. Competition experiments were conducted to determine the effect of glycosylation on rt-PA clearance. As shown in Figure 32.7, co-administration of rt-PA with *p*-aminophenyl-α-D-mannopyranoside-BSA (BSA-Man) prolonged both the α-phase and β-phase half-lives of rt-PA. The fact that BSA-Man inhibits the clearance of rt-PA suggests that the Man-GlcNAc specific glycoprotein receptor contributes to its clearance. In contrast, co-administration of rt-PA with asialofetuin did not alter rt-PA the α-phase and β-phase half-lives, suggesting that the galactose receptor does not mediate clearance. This study demonstrates that the nature and extent of the glyco-

TABLE 32.11   Cell Surface Receptors for the Clearance of Carbohydrates and Monosaccharides

Specificity[a]	Cell type
Gal/Gal/NAc	Liver parencymal cells (asialoglycoprotein receptor)
Gal/GalNAc	Liver Kupfer and endothelial cells, peritoneal macrophages
Man/GlcNAc	Liver Kupfer and endothelial cells, peritoneal macrophages
Fuc	Liver Kupfer cells

[a] Abbreviations: Gal = D-galactose, NAc = *N*-Acetylglucosamine, Glc = D-glucose, Man = D-mannose, Fuc = Fucose.

sylation have a direct effect on the clearance of rt-PA and its interaction with the mannose receptors in the liver.

Production of recombinant proteins using Chinese hamster ovary (CHO) cells, or other mammalian cells, results in a glycosylation pattern that differs from that of recombinant proteins produced by bacteria such as *E. coli* in that CHO-produced proteins are heavily glycosylated whereas those produced by bacteria are not glycosylated. Figure 32.8 depicts the results of an experiment comparing the plasma concentration vs. time profile of granulocyte macrophage colony stimulating factor (GM-CSF) produced by CHO cells with that produced by *E. coli* (56). After intravenous administration, the *E. coli* produced GM-CSF had a significantly shorter α-phase half-life than CHO produced GM-CSF, but there was no significant difference in the terminal half-life. The AUC of the glycosylated GM-CSF was approximately four to five times higher (6.3 μg · min/mL) than the AUC of the nonglycosylated product (1.27 μg · min/mL). However, since no difference in neutrophil counts was observed, the choice of one product over the other may only be a theoretical concern.

Similar to GM-CSF, G-CSF is available as either the glycosylated or nonglycosylated form of the protein. *In vitro* studies suggest that the glycosylated form is more stable and of a higher potency than the nongly-

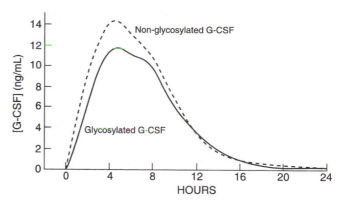

FIGURE 32.9 Comparison of serum concentration vs. time profiles in healthy subjects after SC administration of glycosylated G-CSF (——) and nonglycosylated G-CSF (– – –). (Reproduced with permission from Watts MJ, et al. Eur J Haematol 1997;98:474–9.)

cosylated form (57, 58). The pharmacokinetics of these two forms of G-CSF were evaluated in 20 healthy volunteers (59). As shown in Figure 32.9, the nonglycosylated form was more rapidly absorbed after SC administration and produced a higher C_{max} (14.23 vs. 11.85 pg/mL), but there was little difference in the elimination-phase half-life (2.75 vs. 2.95 hr, respectively). The AUC for the nonglycosylated form was approximately 1.2 times higher than that of the glycosylated form. However, despite these pharmacokinetic differences, the progenitor cell count was significantly higher with the glycosylated product, confirming the *in vitro* potency results.

The results with G-CSF are dissimilar from those produced after IV administration of GM-CSF, where it was found that the C_{max} was higher and the α-half life was longer for the glycosylated than for the nonglycosylated form. The reason for these differences is unknown, but it is apparent that the comparison and subsequent interpretation of study results are dependent on knowing the production source of the protein and the structural features that may influence the potency, PK, and/or PD of individual proteins.

Finally, clearance may change over time for macromolecules whose clearance is mediated by cell surface receptors. This is illustrated by an experiment in three patients with metastatic breast cancer who received G-CSF for two consecutive days as a continuous infusion (33). Absolute neutrophil counts were obtained every morning and there was a very strong positive correlation between neutrophil count and G-CSF clearance (Figure 32.10). Clearance on day 2 was 4.6 mL/hr/kg, increasing to 8.3 mL/hr/kg on day 9. Thus, neutrophil production may mediate the clearance of G-CSF.

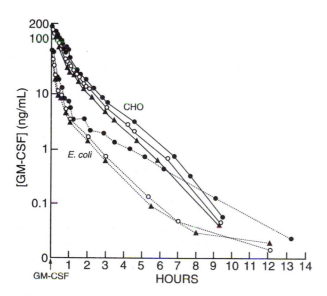

FIGURE 32.8 GM-CSF serum concentration vs. time profiles for three patients after IV bolus injection of 8 μg/kg CHO-produced GM-CSF (*solid lines*), and for three patients who received *E. coli*-produced GM-CSF (*dotted lines*) (one patient received 5.5 μg/kg and two patients received 3 μg/kg). (Reproduced with permission from Hovgaard D, et al. Eur J Haematol 1993;50:36–6.)

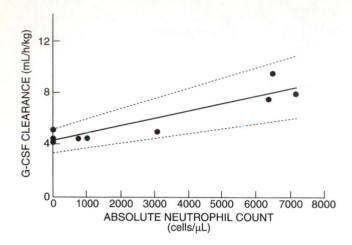

FIGURE 32.10 Relationship between G-CSF clearance and absolute neutrophil count ($r = 0.85$, $P = 0.00025$). The dotted lines represent the 95% confidence intervals of the regression. (Reproduced with permission from Ericson SG, et al. Exp Hematol 1997;25:1313–25.)

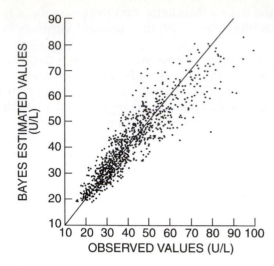

FIGURE 32.11 Correlation between observed and predicted erythropoietin concentration values analyzing sparse sampling data with a population pharmacokinetic model (no r value given). (Reproduced with permission from Hayashi W, et al. Br J Clin Pharmacol 1998;46:11–9.)

In summary, there are multiple characteristics of proteins that influence their PK; some of these are listed in Table 32.12.

Application of Sparse Sampling and Population Kinetic Methods

Finally, there have been attempts to study the pharmacokinetics of macromolecules by applying the sparse sampling strategy and population kinetic methods described in Chapter 10 (24, 60). In one study, erythropoietin was administered SC to 48 healthy adult male Japanese volunteers (24). The analysis estimated the population mean values of k_a, k_e, V_d and the endogenous erythropoietin production rate to be 0.043 hr^{-1}, 0.206 hr^{-1}, 3.14 L, and 15.7 IU hr^{-1}, respectively. The good correlation between predicted and observed concentration values shown in Figure 32.11 supports

the choice of model, as does the fact that the values for k_e and V_d determined by this analysis were similar to those reported for intravenous erythropoietin with the standard two-step method of determining PK parameters. However, given the flip-flop PK characteristics of erythropoietin (Table 32.7), the comparison to the IV parameter estimates may be misleading. In fact, the values for k_e estimated by the population kinetics are dissimilar to those obtained by other authors after SC administration of erythropoietin (13).

Population pharmacokinetic methods also were used to analyze the concentration vs. time profiles of IFN-α in 27 patients with chronic hepatitis C virus infection who received an SC injection of this macromolecule (60). The investigators reported that the absorption rate was best described by two processes: an initial zero-order process, accounting for 24% of net absorption, followed by a first-order process that had a rate constant of 0.18 hr^{-1}. The authors noted that this value for k_a is consistent with the result of 0.13 hr^{-1} reported by Radwanski et al. (20). Both results confirm that IFN-α is slowly absorbed after SC administration.

PHARMACODYNAMICS

The relationship between circulating protein concentrations following exogenous administration and pharmacodynamic endpoints, either for efficacy or for safety, has been explored for a number of molecules such as growth hormone, IGF-1, recombinant Factor

TABLE 32.12　Characteristics That Affect the Pharmacokinetics of Macromolecules

Physical characteristics	Size, structure, net charge
Post-translational modifications	Degree of glycosylation, sialyation, fucosylation
Protein binding	Plasma proteins, induced proteins
Route of administration	Transient peaks and troughs, sustained concentrations
Duration of administration	Time-dependent changes in elimination clearance
Frequency of administration	Up- or down-regulation of receptors

VIII, and interleukins (IL-2, IL-12). Several conclusions emerge from the currently published data: these relationships are complex and not easily explained by a simple E_{max} model; the endpoints are not clear cut (except for those macromolecules intended to substitute for endogenous proteins that are deficient); and there is a high likelihood of regimen dependency.

Models

Several of the PK/PD models described in Chapter 19 have been employed to explore the relationship between circulating protein concentrations and pharmacodynamic endpoints. For example, a dog model of hemophilia (61) was used to study the activity of recombinant FIX (6). Activity was determined in a bioassay, a modified one stage-partial thromboplastin time assay with pooled human plasma as the internal standard. As shown in Figure 32.12, the relationship between activity and recombinant FIX (BeneFIX) concentration was linear ($r^2 = 0.86$), suggesting that for every 34.5 ng/mL of FIX, there would be a corresponding 1% increase in FIX activity. In 11 males with hemophilia B, it was necessary to use a sigmoid E_{max} model to describe the relationship between FIX activity and concentration (unpublished observations). In this study, a FIX serum concentration of approximately 46 ng/mL was necessary to obtain a 1% increase in FIX activity. This translates into a 20% increase in the dosage of recombinant FIX necessary to achieve the same efficacy.

Figure 32.13 represents a theoretical model of IGF-1 and IGFBPs after intravenous infusion (62). The IGF-

BPs have a significant role in controlling circulating IGF-1. As shown in Figure 32.6 and Table 32.13, there are three components to the IGFBP complex: α (acid labile); β (binding); and γ (growth factor) subunits (63). In addition, GH is involved in regulating IGF-1 (64). The major circulating IGF-1 binding protein, IGFBP3, combines with a glycoprotein known as the acid-labile subunit (ALS) to form a ternary complex of approximately 150 kDa. This complex is retained within the intravascular space, which in turn decreases the clearance of IGFBP-3. IGF-1 also decreases GH secretion thereby reducing the synthesis of IGFBP-3 and the ALS.

Fourteen differential equations were needed to describe the PK and PD interactions of IGF-1 and its binding proteins that are depicted in Figure 32.13. The assumptions were as follows: 1) all IGFBPs exhibit first-order elimination kinetics; 2) binding to the receptor is a first-order process; 3) IGFBPs act as reservoirs for the retention of IGF-1 in the vascular compartment; 4) IGF-1 bound to IGFBPs is excluded from the interstitial fluid space; and 5) the production rates of the IGBPs are invariant over time. There was fairly good agreement between the predicted and observed concentrations of free and bound IGF-1 in plasma. However, there was not good agreement between the predicted and observed concentrations of total IGFBPs in either the 150 kDa or 50 kDa plasma fractions. This disagreement probably is the result of two wrong assumptions: that IGFBPs exhibit first-order elimination kinetics and that IGBP production rates do not vary over time, which would only be the case if IGF-1 did not alter the production rates or if the influence of growth hormone secretion on the production rate of IGFBP-3 was negligible.

To establish the relationship between free IGF-1, binding proteins and insulin sensitivity, 11 healthy subjects were given IV glucose (0.3 gm/kg) and insulin (0.05 U/kg) at two times with each administration separated by 20 minutes (65). Blood samples for measurement of free IGF-1, total IGF-1, IGFBP-1, and IGFBP-3 were collected over 3 hours. Free IGF-1 decreased by 20% 20 minutes after the first insulin administration and by 35% 20 minutes after the second administration. IFGBP-3 increased to 20% above the basal level, mirroring the decline in free IFG-1. Insulin sensitivity was positively correlated with free IGF-1 ($r = 0.52$, $P < 0.005$) and inversely correlated with IGFBP-1 ($r = -0.65$; $P < 0.001$) and glucose ($r = 0.51$, $P < 0.005$).

Other investigators have reported that the exogenous administration of IGF-1 increased IGFBP-2 concentrations, but had no effects on IGFBP-1 and IGFBP-3 concentrations in patients with Type 1 diabetes mellitus (66) or in adolescent patients with GH

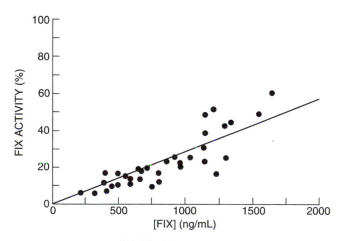

FIGURE 32.12 The relationship between Factor IX (FIX) activity (determined by a modified one-stage partial thromboplastin assay) and FIX concentration in hemophilia B dogs after an infusion of 50 μg/kg FIX over 10 minutes. (Reproduced with permission from Schaub R, et al. Semin Hematol 1998;35(suppl 2):28–32.)

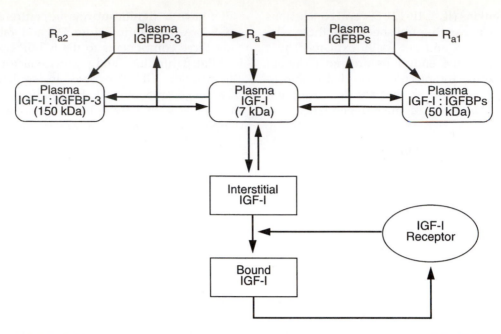

FIGURE 32.13 Theoretical model of IGF-1 pharmacokinetics. Abbreviations: $R_{a,1}$ = IGFBPs, 50 kDa production rate, $R_{a,2}$ = IGFBPs, 150 kDa production rate, R_a = IGF-1 production rate. The 150-kD compartment represents bound IGF-1/IGFBP3 in a tenary complex with ALS. The 50-kD compartment includes fractions of IGF-1 bound to IGFBP 1 through 6. IGF-1 and IGFBPs are the substrates for their degradation—that is, the binding proteins inhibit the transfer of IGF-1 to their tissue sites of action. (Reproduced with permission from Boroujerdi MA, et al. Am J Physiol 1997;273:E438–47.)

receptor deficiency (67). In contrast, Cheetham et al. (68) showed that IGF-1 administered as a single 40 µg/kg SC dose increased IGFBP-3 concentrations.

During the administration of GH to GH deficient children, IGFBP-3 increased 76%, IGFBP-2 decreased by 56% and ALS increased by 41% (69). The response to GH therapy was correlated with the percent change in total IGFBP-3 ($r = 0.72$), intact IGFBP-3 ($r = 0.845$), and proteolyzed IGFBP-3 ($r = 0.703$), and ALS ($r = 0.813$). There was a significant percentage increase of

TABLE 32.13   Role of Different Molecules in the Hypothetical Model of IGF-1 Physiology

Molecule	Role
IGFBP-3	Exists in a 42 kDa "complete" form and a 31 kDa "fragment"
IGF-1	Displaces IGF-2 from IGFBP-3
	Drives reaction toward forming a ternary complex with ALS
	Formed complex is retained within the intravascular space
	Suppresses GH secretion
IGF-2	Induces IGFBP-2
GH	Increases synthesis of IGFBP-3 and ALS

IGF-1 in the ternary complex and a significant percentage decrease in uncomplexed IGF-1.

In contrast to the aforementioned direct relationships, the indirect response model shown in Figure 32.14 was used to describe the relationship between the administration of GH and IGF-1 in nonhuman primates (70). It was assumed in this model that the production of IGF-1 varied over time, a reasonable assumption. As shown in Figure 32.15, the indirect model provided a reasonable characterization of the induction of IGF-1 after both single and multiple GH doses. However, one limitation to this simple model is its inability to account for the role of the IGFBPs in both GH and IGF-1 responses.

Taken together, these observations suggest a complex, internal, multiple-level control of glucose metabolism, insulin sensitivity, and growth. The binding proteins may not only alter the PK of exogenously administered IGF-1, but ultimately its efficacy and/or safety in patients.

Regimen Dependency

Regimen dependency was first shown for the antitumor efficacy of IL-2. Mice given 12 injections of a 1500-unit dose of this cytokine showed greater tumor

Model of rhGH Pharmacokinetics

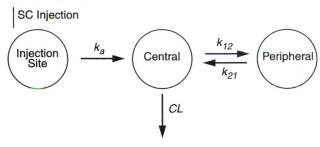

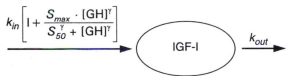

Indirect Response Model of IGF-I Induction by rhGH

$$k_{in}\left[1+\frac{S_{max}\cdot[GH]^{\gamma}}{S_{50}^{\gamma}+[GH]^{\gamma}}\right]$$

FIGURE 32.14 Pharmacokinetic model for rhGH coupled with an indirect response model for IGF-1 induction by rhGH. The Hill equation was used to model IGF-1 induction by rhGH. Abbreviations: k_a = absorption rate of rhGH after SC injection, CL = elimination clearance of rhGH, k_{12} and k_{21} = intercompartmental transfer rates of rhGH, IGF-1 = total IGF concentration, and k_{in} = basal formation rate of IGF-1. Stimulation of IGF-1 production is modeled by the Hill function shown in brackets, where S_{max} = maximum IGF stimulation of k_{in} by rhGH, S_{50} = rhGH concentration for 50% maximal stimulation of k_{in}, [GH] = rhGH concentration, γ = the Hill coefficient, and k_{out} = elimination rate of IGF-1. (Modified from Sun YN, et al. J Pharmacol Exp Ther 1999;289:1523–32.)

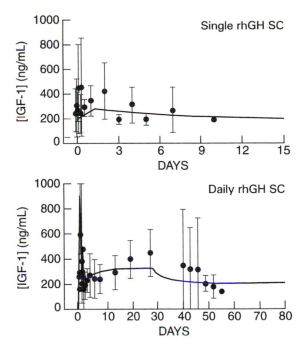

FIGURE 32.15 Total IGF-1 concentrations resulting from single (*upper panel*) and daily (*lower panel*) SC injections of rhGH. Data points and bars represent the mean and standard deviation of results from four monkeys. Solid lines are the values that were simulated from the model shown in Figure 32.14. (Reproduced with permission from Sun YN, et al. J Pharmacol Exp Ther 1999;289:1523–32.)

inhibition than those that received two doses of 9000 units (71). Similar results were obtained in a Phase 1 clinical trial in which patients with renal cell carcinoma were given one of three schedules of IL-2 at an IV dosage of either 1.0 or 3.0×10^6 U/m²/day: a 24-hour continuous infusion; a single daily bolus injection; and a combination of one-half of the dosage by bolus and the remaining one-half by 24-hour infusion (72). At least three patients received each schedule. Two of the 23 patients with renal cell carcinoma had a partial response and acceptable toxicity with the combined bolus and continuous infusion regimen of 3.0×10^6 U/m²/day. On the other hand, the patients who received 3.0×10^6 U/m²/day as a daily bolus injection had progressive disease.

Regimen dependency has also been described for IL-12 given IV (73) and SC (74). For example, Motzer and colleagues (74) treated patients with renal cell carcinoma with IL-12, administered on days 1, 8, and 15 either as a fixed dose of 1.0 µg/kg or as a series of escalating doses. As shown in Figure 32.16, IL-12 concentrations and IFN-γ response were greater after patients received their initial 1.0 µg/kg dose on the fixed dose

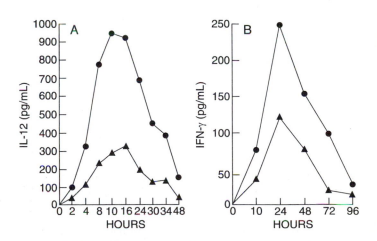

FIGURE 32.16 Regimen dependency of IL-12 pharmacokinetics and IFN-γ stimulating effects. In the *left panel*, IL-12 serum concentrations are compared in patients who received an SC dose of 1.0 g/ml IL-12 on day 1 of their therapy (●) with levels obtained in other patients who received the same dose on day 15 of an escalating dose scheme (▲). In the *right panel*, the IFN-γ responses of these two patient groups are compared. (Reproduced with permission from Motzer RJ, et al. Clin Cancer Res 1998;4:1183–91.)

regimen than after they received the same dose on day 15 as part of the dose-escalation scheme. However, more severe toxicity was encountered with the single, fixed dose regimen and the maximum tolerated dose was lower (1.0 µg/kg) than that achievable with the escalation scheme (1.5 µg/kg). As a result, Phase 2 trials with this cytokine were begun with a regimen in which doses were escalated to 1.25 µg/kg.

References

1. Whidden B, editor. FDA wraps up 1998 with 13 biotech approvals. Bioworld Phase III Report. 1999;4:1–52.

2. Colcher D, Pavlinkova G, Beresford G, Booth BJ, Choudhury A, Batra SK. Pharmacokinetics and biodistribution of genetically engineered antibodies. Quart J Nucl Med 1998;42:225–41.

3. Chappell WR, Mordenti J. Extrapolation of toxicological and pharmacological data from animals to humans. In: Testa B, editor. Advances in drug research. New York: Academic Press; 1991;20:1–116.

4. Mordenti J, Chen SA, Moore JA, Ferraiolo BL, Green JD. Interspecies scaling of clearance and volume of distribution data for five therapeutic proteins. Pharm Res 1991;8:1351–9.

5. Wolberg AS, Stafford DW, Erie DA. Human factor IX binds to specific sites on the collagenous domain of collagen IV. J Biol Chem 1997;272:16717–20.

6. Schaub R, Garzone P, Bouchard P, Rup B, Keith J, Brinkhous K, et al. Preclinical studies of recombinant factor IX. Semin Hematol 1998;35(suppl 2):28–32.

7. Brinkhouse KM, Sigman JL, Read MS, Stewart PF, McCarthy KP, Timony GA, et al. Recombinant human factor IX: Replacement therapy, prophylaxis, and pharmacokinetics in canine hemophilia B. Blood 1996;88:2603–10.

8. Mordenti J, Osaka G, Garcia K, Thomsen K, Licko V, Meng G. Pharmacokinetics and interspecies scaling of recombinant human factor VIII. Toxicol Appl Pharmacol 1996;136:75–8.

9. Nadeau RR, Ostrowski C, Ni-Wu G, Liberator DJ. Pharmacokinetics and pharmacodynamics of recombinant human interleukin-12 in male rhesus monkeys. J Pharmacol Exp Ther 1995;274:78–83.

10. Rakhit A, Yeon MM, Ferrante J, Fettner S, Nadeau R, Motzer R, et al. Down-regulation of the pharmacokinetic-pharmacodynamic response to interleukin-12 during long-term administration to patients with renal cell carcinoma and evaluation of the mechanism of this "adaptive response" in mice. Clin Pharmacol Ther 1999;65:615–29.

11. White G, Shapiro A, Ragni M, Garzone P, Goodfellow J, Tubridy K, et al. Clinical evaluation of recombinant factor IX. Semin Hematol 1998;35(suppl 2):33–8.

12. Atkins MB, Robertson MJ, Gordon M, Lotze MT, DeCoste M, DuBois JS, et al. Phase 1 evaluation of intravenous recombinant human interleukin 12 (rhIL-12) in patients with advanced malignancies. Clin Cancer Res 1997;3:409–17.

13. Cheung WK, Goon BL, Guilfoyle MC, Wacholtz MC. Pharmacokinetics and pharmacodynamics of recombinant human erythropoietin after single and multiple subcutaneous doses to healthy subjects. Clin Pharmacol Ther 1998;64:412–23.

14. Veldhuis JD, Evans WS, Johnson ML. Complicating effects of highly correlated model variables on nonlinear least-squares estimates of unique parameter values and their statistical confidence intervals: estimating basal secretion and neurohormone half-life by deconvolution analysis. Methods Neurosci 1995;28:130–8.

15. Albertsson-Wikland K, Rosberg S, Libre E, Lundberg LO, Groth T. Growth hormone secretory rates in children as estimated by deconvolution analysis of 24-h plasma concentration profiles. Am J Physiol 1989;20:E809–14.

16. Bright GM, Veldhuis JD, Iranmanesh A, Baumann G, Maheshwari H, Lima J. Appraisal of growth hormone (GH) secretion: Evaluation of a composite pharmacokinetic model that discriminates multiple components of GH input. J Clin Endocrinol Metab 1999;84:3301–8.

17. Macdougall IC, Roberts DE, Neubert P, Dharmasena AD, Coles GA, Williams JD. Pharmacokinetics of intravenous, intraperitoneal, and subcutaneous recombinant erythropoietin in patients on CAPD. A rationale for treatment. Contrib Nephrol 1989;76:112–21.

18. Cetron JS, Bury RW, Lieschke GJ, Morstyn G. The effects of dose and route of administration on the pharmacokinetics of granulocyte-macrophage colony stimulating factor. Eur J Cancer 1990;26:1064–9.

19. Lauresen T, Grardjean B, Jørgensen JOL, Christiansen JS. Bioavailability and bioactivity of three different doses of nasal growth hormone (GH) administered to GH-deficient patients: Comparison with intravenous and subcutaneous administration. Eur J Endocrinol 1996;135:309–15.

20. Radwanski E, Perentisis G, Jacobs S, Oden E, Affrime M, Symchowicz S, et al. Pharmacokinetics of interferon alpha-2b in healthy volunteers. J Clin Pharmacol 1987;27:432–5.

21. Schuller J, Czejka MJ, Schernthaner G, Wirth M, Bosse C, Jager W, et al. Pharmacokinetics of interferon-alfa-2b after intrahepatic or intraperitoneal administration. Semin Oncol 1992;19(suppl 3):98–104.

22. Aoyama K, UchidaT, Takanuki F, Usui T, Watanabe T, Higuchi S, et al. Pharmacokinetics of recombinant human interleukin-11 (rhIL-11) in healthy male subjects. Br J Clin Pharmacol 1997;43:571–8.

23. Kearns GL, Kemp SF, Frindik JP. Single and multiple dose pharmacokinetics of methionyl growth hormone in children with idiopathic growth hormone deficiency. J Clin Endocrin Metabol 1991;72:1148–56.

24. Hayashi W, Kinoshita H, Yukawa E, Higuchi S. Pharmacokinetic analysis of subcutaneous erythropoietin administration with non-linear mixed effect model including endogenous production. Br J Clin Pharmacol 1998;46:11–9.

25. Kindler J, Eckardt KU, Ehmer B, Jandeleit K, Kurtz A, Schreiber A, et al. Single-dose pharmacokinetics of recombinant human erythropoietin in patients with various degrees of renal failure. Nephrol Dial Transplant 1989;4:345–9.

26. Supersaxo A, Hein WR, Steffen H. Effect of molecular weight on the lymphatic absorption of water-soluble compounds following subcutaneous administration. Pharm Res 1990;7:167–9.

27. Jensen JD, Jensen LW and Madsen JK. The pharmacokinetics of recombinant human erythropoietin after subcutaneous injection at different sites. Eur J Clin Pharmacol 1994;46:333–7.

28. Laursen T, Jørgensen JOL, Christiansen JS. Pharmacokinetics and metabolic effects of growth hormone injected subcutaneously in growth hormone deficient patients: Thigh versus abdomen. Clin Endocrinol 1994;40:373–8.

29. Odeh YK, Wang Z, Ruo TI, Wang T, Frederiksen MC, Pospisil PA, et al. Simultaneous analysis of inulin and $^{15}N_2$-urea kinetics in humans. Clin Pharmacol Ther 1993;53:419–25.

30. Sculier JP, Body JJ, Donnadieu N, Nejai S, Glibert F, Raymakers N, et al. Pharmacokinetics of repeated i.v. bolus administration of high doses of r-met-Hu interleukin-2 in advanced cancer patients. Cancer Chemother Pharmacol 1990;26:355–8.

31. Konrad MW, Hemstreet G, Hersch EM, Mansell PW, Mertelsmann R, Kolitz JE, et al. Pharmacokinetics of recombinant interleukin-2 in humans. Cancer Res 1990;50:2009–17.

32. Watari K, Ozawa K, Takahashi S, Tojo A, Tani K, Kamachi S, et al. Pharmacokinetic studies of intravenous glycosylated recombinant human granulocyte colony-stimulating factor in various hematological disorders: Inverse correlation between the half-life and bone marrow myeloid cell pool. Int J Hematol 1997;66:57–67.

33. Ericson SG, Gao H, Gericke GH, Lewis LD. The role of PMNs in clearance of granulocyte colony-stimulating factor (G-CSF) *in vivo* and *in vitro*. Exp Hematol 1997;25:1313–25.

34. Tanswell P, Seifried E, Su PCAF, Feuerer W, Rijken DC. Pharmacokinetics and systemic effects of tissue-type plasminogen activator in normal subjects. Clin Pharmacol Ther 1989;46:155–62.

35. James K. Interactions between cytokines and alpha-2 macroglobulin. Immunol Today 1990;11:163–6.

36. Dickinson AM, Shenton BK, Alomran AH, Donnelly PK, Proctor SJ. Inhibition of natural killing and antibody-dependent cell-mediated cytotoxicity by the plasma protease inhibitor alpha 2-macroglobulin (alpha 2M) and alpha 2M protease complexes. Clin Immunol Immunopathol 1985;36:259–65.

37. Hoffman M, Feldman SR, Pizzo SV. α_2-macroglobulin 'fast' forms inhibit superoxide production by activated macrophages. Biochim Biophys Acta 1983;760:421–3.

38. Feige JJ, Negoescu A, Keramidas M, Souchelnitskiy S, Chambaz EM. Alpha 2-macroglobulin: A binding protein for transforming growth factor-beta and various cytokines. Horm Res 1996;45:227–32.

39. Huang JS, Huang SS, Deuel TF. Specific covalent binding of platelet-derived growth factor to human plasma alpha 2-macroglobulin. Proc Natl Acad Sci USA 1984;81:342–6.

40. Legrès LG, Pochon F, Barray M, Gay F, Chouaib S, Delain E. Evidence for the binding of a biologically active interleukin-2 to human alpha 2-macroglobulin. J Biol Chem 1995;8381–4.

41. LaMarre J, Wollenberg GK, Gonias SL, Hayes MA. Cytokine binding and clearance properties of proteinase-activated alpha 2-macroglobulin. Lab Invest 1991;65:3–14.

42. Blum WF, Hall K, Ranke MB, Wilton P. Growth hormone insensitivity syndromes: A preliminary report on changes in insulin-like growth factors and their binding proteins during treatment with recombinant insulin-like growth factor I. Kabi Pharmacia Study Group on Insulin-like Growth Factor I Treatment in Growth Hormone Insensitivity Syndromes. Acta Paediatr Suppl 1993;82(suppl 391):15–9.

43. Kostecka Y, Blahovec J. Insulin-like growth factor binding proteins and their functions. Endocr Regul 1999;33:90–4.

44. Abdel-Razzak ZA, Loyer P, Fautrel A, Gautier JC, Corcos L, Turlin B, et al. Cytokines down-regulate expression of major cytochrome P-450 enzymes in adult human hepatocytes in primary culture. Mol Pharmacol 1993;44:707–15.

45. Morgan ET. Regulation of cytochrome P450 during inflammation and infection. Drug Metab Rev 1997;9:1129–88.

46. Chen JQ, Ström A, Gustafsson JA, Morgan ET. Suppression of the constitutive expression of cytochrome P-450 2C11 by cytokines and interferons in primary cultures of rat hepatocytes: comparison with induction of acute-phase genes and demonstration that CYP2C11 promoter sequences are involved in the suppressive response to interleukins 1 and 6. Mol Pharmacol 1995;47:940–7.

47. Gonzalez FJ. Molecular biology of cytochrome P450s. Pharmacol Rev 1989;40:243–87.

48. Kurokohchi K, Matsuo Y, Yoneyama H, Nishioka M, Ichikawa Y. Interleukin-2 induction of cytochrome P450-linked monooxygenase systems of rat liver microsomes. Biochem Pharmacol 1993;45:585–92.

49. Khakoo S, Glue P, Grellier L, Wells B, Bell A, Dash C, et al. Ribavirin and interferon alfa-2b in chronic hepatitis C: Assessment of possible pharmacokinetic and pharmacodynamic interactions. Br J Clin Pharmacol 1998;46:563–70.

50. Hassan M, Nilsson C, Olsson H, Lundin J, Osterborg A. The influence of interferon-alpha on the pharmacokinetics of cyclophosphamide and its 4-hydroxy metabolite in patients with multiple myeloma. Eur J Haematol 1999;63:163–70.

51. Le Cesne A, Vassal G, Farace F, Spielmann M, Le Chevalier T, Angevin E, et al. Combination interleukin-2 and doxorubicin in advanced adult solid tumors: Circumvention of doxorubicin resistance in soft-tissue sarcoma? J Immunother 1999;22:268–77.

52. Venkatachalam MA, Rennke HG. The structural and molecular basis of glomerular filtration. Circ Res 1978;43:337–47.

53. Maack T, Johnson V, Kau ST, Figueiredo J, Sigulem D. Renal filtration, transport, and metabolism of low-molecular-weight proteins: A review. Kidney Int 1979;16:251–70.

54. Ashwell G, Harford J. Carbohydrate-specific receptors of the liver. Annu Rev Biochem 1982;51:531–54.

55. Lucore CL, Fry ETA, Nachowiak DA, Sobel BE. Biochemical determinants of clearance of tissue-type plasminogen activator from the circulation. Circulation 1988;77:906–14.

56. Hovgaard D, Mortensen BT, Schifter S, Nissen NI. Comparative pharmacokinetics of single dose administration of mammalian and bacterially-derived recombinant human granulocyte-macrophage colony stimulating factor. Eur J Haematol 1993;50:32–6.

57. Moonen P, Mermod JJ, Ernst JF, Hirschi M, DeLamarter JF. Increased biological activity of deglycosylated recombinant human granulocyte-macrophage colony stimulating factor produced by yeast or animal cells. Proc Natl Acad Sci USA 1987;84:4428–31.

58. Kauskansky K. Role of carbohydrate in the function of human granulocyte-macrophage colony stimulating factor. Biochemistry 1987;26:4861–7.

59. Watts MJ, Addison L, Long SG, Hartley S, Warrington S, Boyce M, et al. Crossover study of the haematological effects and pharmacokinetics of glycosylated and non-glycosylated G-CSF in healthy volunteers. Br J Haematol 1997;98:474–9.

60. Chatelut E, Rostaing L, Grégoire N, Payen JL, Pujol A, Izopet J, et al. A pharmacokinetic model for alpha interferon administered subcutaneously. Br J Clin Pharmacol 1999;47:365–7.

61. Evans JP, Brinkhouse KM, Brayer GD, Reisner HM, High KA. Canine hemophilia B resulting from a point mutation with unusual consequences. Proc Natl Acad Sci USA 1989;86:10095–9.

62. Boroujerdi MA, Jones RH, Sönkesen PH, Russell-Jones DL. Simulation of IGF-1 pharmacokinetics after infusion of recombinant IGF-1 in human subjects. Am J Physiol 1997;273:E438–47.

63. Baxter RC. Insulin-like growth factor (IGF) binding proteins: The role of serum IGFBPs in regulating IGF availability. Acta Paediatr Scand Suppl 1991;372:107–14.

64. Hartman ML, Clayton PE, Johnson ML, Celniker A, Perlman AJ, Alberti KG, et al. A low dose euglycemic infusion of recombinant human insulin-like growth factor 1 rapidly suppresses fasting-enhanced pulsatile growth hormone secretion in humans. J Clin Invest 1993;91:2453–62.

65. Nyomba BL, Berard L, Murphy LJ. Free insulin-like growth factor I (IGF-I) in healthy subjects: Relationship with IGF-binding proteins and insulin sensitivity. J Clin Endocrinol Metab 1997;82:2177–81.

66. Carroll PV, Umpleby M, Alexander EL, Egel VA, Callison KV, Sönkesen PH, et al. Recombinant human insulin-like growth factor-I (rhIGF-I) therapy in adults with type 1 diabetes mellitus: Effects on IGFs, IGF-binding proteins, glucose levels and insulin treatment. Clin Endocrinol 1998;49:739–46.

67. Wilson KF, Fielder PJ, Guevara-Aguirre J, Cohen P, Vasconez O, Martinez V, et al. Long-term effects of insulin-like growth factor

(IGF)-I treatment on serum IGFs and IGF binding proteins in adolescent patients with growth hormone receptor deficiency. Clin Endocrinol 1995;42:399–407.

68. Cheetham TD, Holly JM, Baxter RC, Meadows K, Jones J, Taylor AM, et al. The effects of recombinant human IGF-I administration on concentrations of acid labile subunit, IGF binding protein-3, IGF-I, IGF-II and proteolysis of IGF binding protein-3 in adolescents with insulin-dependent diabetes mellitus. J Endocrinol 1998;157:81–7.

69. Mandel SH, Moreland E, Rosenfeld RG, Gargosky SE. The effect of GH therapy on the immunoreactive forms and distribution of IGFBP-3, IGF-I, the acid-labile subunit, and growth rate in GH-deficient children. Endocrine 1997;7:351–60.

70. Sun YN, Lee JH, Almon RR, Jusko WJ. A pharmacokinetic/pharmacodynamic model for recombinant human growth hormone. Effects on induction of insulin-like growth factor 1 in monkeys. J Pharmacol Exp Ther 1999;89:1523–32.

71. Vaage J, Pauly JL, Harlos JP. Influence of the administration schedule on the therapeutic effect of interleukin-2. Int J Cancer 1987;39:530–3.

72. Sosman JA, Kohler PC, Hank J, Moore KH, Bechhofer R, Storer B, et al. Repetitive weekly cycles of recombinant human interleukin-2: responses of renal carcinoma with acceptable toxicity. J Natl Cancer Institute 1988;80:60–3.

73. Leonard JP, Sherman ML, Fisher GL, Buchanan LJ, Larsen G, Atkins MB, et al. Effects of single dose interleukin-12 exposure on interleukin-12-associated toxicity and interferon-gamma production. Blood 1997;90:2541–8.

74. Motzer RJ, Rakhit A, Schwartz LH, Olencki T, Malone TM, Sandstrom K, et al. Phase 1 trial of subcutaneous human interleukin-12 in patients with advanced renal cell carcinoma. Clin Cancer Res 1998;4:1183–91.

Design of Clinical Development Programs

CHARLES GRUDZINSKAS

Drug Development Consultant, Annapolis, Maryland

INTRODUCTION

This chapter provides an overview of the clinical drug development process, which includes the clinical proof of concept (POC), the characterization of clinical safety, the characterization of clinical activity, and the characterization of clinical efficacy (the confirmation of clinical activity). It is this understanding of the clinical effectiveness and safety of a new drug that provides the knowledge for informed decision making regarding the clinical development, approval, marketing, prescribing, and proper use of a new drug. The clinical development process consists of (a) clinical trials for scientific development, (b) clinical trials for scientific regulatory purposes, and (c) clinical trials that are pharmacoeconomically motivated (1). This chapter will cover the clinical drug development process with a focus on *critical decision points* and the use of a *label driven-question-based* approach to developing clinical development plans.

This chapter is intended to provide the reader with a strategic overview of the manner in which an effective and efficient contemporary clinical development program is created. It is beyond the scope of a single chapter to be able to adequately cover all aspects of a clinical development program. More comprehensive overviews of the operational aspects of clinical plans and clinical trial design are provided by texts written by Spilker (2) and Friedman (3). For a comprehensive overview of clinical trial design and analysis, the reader is referred to *Studying a Study and Testing a Test* by Riegelman and Hirsch (4). Information about the new drug review process and how it relates to new drug development is presented in Chapter 34 and at the CDER Handbook website (5). Another valuable resource for the design and conduct of clinical trials is a comprehensive glossary of clinical drug development terminology (6).

PHASES, SIZE, AND SCOPE OF CLINICAL DEVELOPMENT PROGRAMS

The FDA broadly defines *drugs* as those compounds that are synthesized and *biologics* as those that are produced by living organisms. However, for the purposes of this chapter, we will be using the term drug to represent both drugs and biologics.

Clinical Drug Development Phases

Traditionally, the clinical development process has been divided into the following four phases.

Phase 1

As described in Chapter 31, this phase includes first-in-human (FIH) trials to provide information about the safety (tolerability) and pharmacokinetics of a new drug. These trials are usually conducted in volunteers unless they involve certain drugs such those used in cancer and HIV treatments. It should be noted that Phase 1-type trials, such as those to study pharmacokinetics in special populations, can and do occur throughout the clinical drug development process (see Figure 5.1).

Phase 2

This phase consists of small trials in subjects with the illness to be treated (usually trials of 24 to 300 subjects). The goals of Phase 2 trials are to provide proof of the hypothesized therapeutic concept, identify the patient population(s) in which the new drug appears to work, and determine an appropriate dose regimen for subsequent large-scale trials.

Phase 3

Phase 3 trials are conducted to confirm the efficacy of a new drug in a broad patient population in order to establish clinical settings in which the drug works or doesn't work. These trials are also designed to provide an evaluation of adverse drug events that may be encountered in subsequent clinical use. These trials are large (250 to > 1000 patients) so as to provide information that reasonably can be extrapolated to the general population. After successful completion of Phase 3 trials that meet U.S. requirements, the sponsor of the development program generally files a New Drug Application (NDA) or Biologics License Application (BLA) with the Food and Drug Administration (FDA). FDA approval of these applications is required before the product can be marketed in the United States. Similar procedures are in place in other countries, but this chapter will focus primarily on U.S. requirements.

Phase 4

Phase 4 trials are conducted post-marketing to further evaluate the characteristics of the new drug with regard to safety, efficacy, new indications for additional patient populations, and new formulations. Phase 4 is generally used to characterize all post-NDA clinical development programs. However, some organizations use Phase 4 to describe only FDA requested clinical trials and Phase 5 to describe internally motivated market expansion trials.

It is noteworthy that in an attempt to better characterize the types of information and knowledge that each phase is developing, terms such as early-Phase 2 or late-Phase 3 (or Phase 2A and Phase 3B, respectively) have crept into the clinical development lexicon. Although the traditional four phases are helpful in broadly defining a clinical drug development pro-

gram, the use of these phases in a strict chronological sense or as milestones would be misleading. A strict chronological interpretation would infer that pharmacokinetic determinations are very limited and only occur in the early (Phase 1) part of the clinical drug development process, and that Phase 4 market expansion trials are started only after the new drug has been approved. Therefore, instead of thinking of drug development as a series of consecutive phases, it is preferable to regard the drug development process as a series of interactive knowledge building efforts like the expanding layers of an onion, that allow us to make cogent scientific drug development decisions.

Drug Development Time and Cost—A Changing Picture

Clinical drug development is a complex, expensive, and lengthy process that can be thought of as having several main objectives in support of the ultimate goal—marketing approval with the desired indications. The average cost of bringing one new medicine to market cited by PhRMA is $500 million (7, 8). This figure takes into consideration:

- The actual cost of the successful drug discovery and development programs.
- The cost of money (the financial return that would be realized if the money spent on research and development were invested in long-term notes).
- The cost of unsuccessful discovery and development projects "dry holes."

The actual "out-of-pocket" expense for a single new drug varies, depending on the number of indications, formulations, and subjects needed to obtain regulatory approval, but is probably in the neighborhood of $125 to more than $250 million. Estimates for the cost per subject in a clinical trial range from less than $1000 per subject for a short treatment to as much as $10,000 per subject for lengthy or complex treatments. In addition to clinical grants to investigators, the full clinical costs include development of the protocol and clinical investigators' brochure, clinical investigator meetings, monitoring and site visits, clinical data collection, data quality resolution, data management and analysis, and report preparation. If the clinical database needed to achieve approval requires 4000 to 8000 subjects, one can see how the cost of drug development can quickly exceed $100 million.

Clinical drug development requires the integration of many disciplines, including discovery research, nonclinical and clinical development, pharmacometrics, statistics and bioinformatics, regulatory science, and marketing to identify, evaluate, develop, and achieve regulatory approval for the successful marketing of new drugs.

In the recent past, the overall time from the initiation of a drug discovery program to regulatory approval was 10 to 15 years (7). Much of the time and expense of drug development is related to the large numbers of subjects who need to be studied in clinical trials. Clinical development programs with large numbers of subjects are required for therapies such as broad spectrum antibiotics that usually are developed for many indications. Similarly, large clinical programs are needed for a vaccine or flu treatment when the incidence of the disease is small and many subjects are needed to demonstrate a clinically significant difference in disease incidence between test-drug treated and placebo treated subjects. As a result, contemporary clinical development plans usually include a minimum of 1500 subjects and often exceed 6000.

Although the cost of drug development is likely to remain high, contemporary drug development technologies, the availability of high-quality contract research organizations (CROs) for the outsourcing of key efforts, and the emergence of on-line clinical trial management ("e-R&D") have reduced the average time from drug discovery to NDA submission to a new benchmark of 4 to 6 years. In addition, regulatory review procedures have been streamlined, further shortening the time required to bring new drugs to market.

The Impact of Regulation on Drug Development Programs

As described in Chapter 34, the Kefauver-Harris Drug Amendments (9) were passed by Congress in 1962 to ensure drug efficacy and greater drug safety. For the first time, drug manufacturers were required to prove to FDA the clinical effectiveness of their products before marketing them. This legislation led to the corresponding development at the FDA of a formalized process of regulatory review. This process is needed to determine whether there is adequate knowledge to be able to make an informed evaluation about the benefit-to-risk ratio of the new drug, and to then decide whether the proposed product should be approved for use by which segments of that nation's population. The regulatory review process requires the integration of many of the same disciplines required for drug development, including basic pharmacology, pharmacometrics, toxicology, chemistry, clinical medicine, statistics, and regulatory science. As will be emphasized subsequently, the ultimate "product" of the drug development and drug review process is the *package insert* (PI) or *label* that a pre-

scriber uses to decide what drug to prescribe for which patients, what dose and dose interval to prescribe, and for how long.

The statement that the proof of effectiveness would be derived from "well-controlled investigations" has been the cornerstone of the FDA's position for the requirement of two positive adequate and well-controlled clinical trials, both of which must demonstrate effectiveness at the $P < 0.05$ level (9). However, in practice, most clinical development plans include more than just two studies to document efficacy and evaluate safety. In a pilot study reported by Peck (1) of a cohort of 12 of the 51 NDAs that were approved by the FDA in 1994–1995, the total number of clinical trials in each submission ranged from 23 to 150. In those trials that were designed to establish efficacy and evaluate safety, the number of subjects ranged from 1000 to 13,000. Peck has pointed out that these NDAs probably reflect clinical plans that were designed in the mid-1980s.

A retrospective review of five recent NDAs and BLAs was conducted by research fellows at the Center for Drug Development Science (CDDS) using information found on the CDER and CBER websites (10). This review is summarized in Table 33.1 and indicates that the size of the clinical development plans for these five diverse products ranged from a total of 10 to 68 clinical trials and included between 1069 and 8528 subjects. The large number of subjects in some clinical development programs may reflect the intensity with which sponsors focus on demonstrating a clinically significant differentiation. For example, the sildenafil NDA for treating erectile dysfunction included population subgroups to demonstrate efficacy regardless of baseline severity, race, and etiology. Patient etiology subgroups included specific trials in patients whose erectile dysfunction was psychogenic, due to spinal cord injury or a result of diabetes (11). The rofecoxib NDA supported both an indication for osteoarthritis and an indication for pain management, requiring demonstration of effectiveness in three distinct pain models as well as the demonstration of differentiation in improved gastrointestinal safety when compared with multiple traditional nonsteroidal antiinflammatory drugs (NSAIDs). Similar retrospective analyses can be made for both NDAs (12) and BLAs (13) by downloading the reviews prepared by the FDA medical officers, chemists, pharmacologists, and clinical pharmacologists. These reviews provide an excellent starting place for understanding the design of a clinical drug development program.

In several of the clinical development programs analyzed in Table 33.1, there is a substantial reduction in the number of clinical trials from that reported in

TABLE 33.1 Retrospective Reviews of Recently Approved NDAs and BLAs[a]

Drug	Indication	FIH[b] to NDA Filing (years)	Phase 1 Trials[c]	Phase 1 Subjects	Phase 2 Trials	Phase 2 Subjects	Phase 3 Trials	Phase 3 Subjects	Total Trials[d]	Total Subjects[e]
Trastuzumab (Herceptin®)	Breast cancer	6–10	3	48	6	532	1	489	10	1,069
Etanercept (Enbrel®)	Rheumatoid arthritis	6–7	8	163	3	503	23	1,381	34	2,048
Zanamivir (Relenza®)	Treatment of influenza	4–5	18	446	7	3,275	3	1,588	28	5,309
Sildenafil (Viagra®)	Erectile dysfunction	5	42	905	13	498	13	4,679	68	6,082
Rofecoxib (Vioxx®)	Osteoarthritis, pain	4–5	31	940	2	1,855	13	5,733	46	8,528

[a]The assignment of trials and subjects was not always straightforward based on the source documents and should be used as only semi-quantitative estimates of the size of each phase. For instance, in the etanercept BLA there were 3 efficacy and 23 safety studies. We have categorized the efficacy studies as Phase 2 and the safety studies as Phase 3.

[b]Time of FIH trial for the approved indication was derived from sources in addition to those on the FDA web sites and in several cases represents an educated estimate.

[c]Phase 1 includes all of the clinical pharmacology studies that in many cases were conducted within 12 months of the NDA/BLA submission.

[d]The total number of trials indicated is the number of trials included in the NDA/BLA and might not include certain trials ongoing at the time of the NDA/BLA submission.

[e]The total number of subjects indicated is the number of subjects in the NDA/BLA and might not include subjects in certain trials ongoing at the time of the NDA/BLA submission.

the pilot study of 1994–1995 NDA approvals. This reduction is seen as a positive move in shortening the time and expense of drug development. Even more impressive speed records are being set for drug development that uses structure-based drug discovery approaches and effective and efficient clinical development programs based on critical label-driven, question-based decision making. The development of a protease inhibitor may hold the speed record with the following metrics (14):

- The first in human dose (FIH) was 18 weeks after the start of the nonclinical safety program.
- Phase 2 began 9.5 months after the start of the nonclinical safety program.
- The NDA was submitted 3.5 years after the discovery of the drug.

In the 1999 annual report from Monsanto, it was stated that the development and NDA submission of the COX-2 inhibitor celecoxib was completed in 39 months from the FIH dose. This is even more remarkable when one takes into account that the celecoxib NDA contained data from over 9000 patients with osteoarthritis, rheumatoid arthritis, and surgical pain. These data were used by the FDA to approve celecoxib for the indications of osteoarthritis and rheumatoid arthritis.

Another important development that may help reduce the time and cost of drug development is found in the May 1998 FDA "Guidance for Industry—Providing Clinical Evidence of Effectiveness for Humans Drug and Biological Products." This guidance points out that in section 115(a) of the FDA Modernization Act (FDAMA), Congress amended section 505(d) of the Food Drug and Cosmetic Act to indicate that the FDA may consider "data from one adequate and well-controlled clinical investigation and confirmatory evidence" to constitute substantial evidence if FDA determines that such data and evidence are sufficient to establish effectiveness (15). In making this clarification, Congress raised the possibility that fewer clinical trials may be needed than in the past. This appears to reflect the fact that contemporary multicenter clinical trials typically enroll more patients than single-center trials that were conducted in the past, as well as the substantial progress in drug development science that has resulted in higher quality clinical trial data.

GOAL AND OBJECTIVES OF CLINICAL DRUG DEVELOPMENT

The ultimate goal of the clinical drug development process is to achieve approval to market a new drug for the desired indications based on an effective and efficient clinical plan that fully characterizes the differentiating features of the new drug. This goal is met by achieving seven objectives that generate an understanding of the intrinsic and extrinsic characteristics of the new drug being developed:

Objective 1—Clinical Pharmacology

This objective of clinical development focuses on understanding the factors influencing the absorption, distribution, metabolism, and elimination (ADME) of a new drug, as well as the relationship between drug concentrations in various body fluids or organs and the observed pharmacological effects. This understanding includes how different and special patient populations handle the drug, the potential for drug-drug interactions, as well as how patients might handle the drug differently in short-term treatments vs. long-term-treatments. Clinical pharmacology underlies the entire clinical drug development process, but deserves particularly heavy emphasis at the beginning and the end of the clinical drug development program.

Objective 2—Safety

This objective entails the assessment of a new drug to determine what types of clinical side effects can be expected and in which patient populations, at what doses, for how long, and whether the side effects are reversible. This knowledge is summarized in the integrated summary of safety (ISS) portion of the NDA/BLA submission and is used to decide what should be included in the precautions or warnings sections of the drug label.

Objective 3—Activity

This objective is to characterize as early as possible the dose, dose frequency, and patient populations in which the new drug is active in order to be able to select the dose to be used in subsequent large confirmatory trials.

Objective 4—Efficacy

This objective is to confirm drug efficacy in large-scale clinical trials. The results of these trials are summarized in the integrated summary of efficacy (ISE) portion of the NDA/BLA submission and play an important role in determining appropriate dose regimens and benefit/risk ratios for various patient populations.

Objective 5—Differentiation

This objective is to provide evidence that the new drug will provide enhanced value to patients over other available drugs with regard to efficacy, safety, and compliance.

Objective 6—Preparation of a Successful NDA/BLA Submission

This objective centers on the preparation of a reviewer-friendly submission that regulatory authorities will use to determine whether to permit marketing of the new drug for the indications and dose regimens being sought.

Objective 7—Market Expansion and Post-Marketing Surveillance

This objective underscores the fact that clinical development efforts do not stop with the regulatory approval of an NDA or BLA, but continue throughout the life cycle of the product. Market expansion is accomplished by demonstrating effectiveness, safety, and value of the drug in new patient populations, by demonstrating its use in combination with another product, or by introducing new formulations to improve patient compliance or simply increase market share. Planning for this expansion process begins far in advance of the submission of the drug dossier to a regulatory agency for a review. Likewise, it is increasingly common for sponsors to initiate a post-marketing surveillance program to track the emergence and severity of any of adverse events that were or were not observed during the pre-NDA clinical development program.

CRITICAL DRUG DEVELOPMENT PARADIGMS

Six critical paradigms that have evolved within the last decade are valuable tools in ensuring the rapid and successful clinical development of new drugs.

The Label Driven-Question Based Clinical Development Plan Paradigm

It is appropriate that we begin with the question-based-label-driven focus, since the ultimate product that is "produced" from a clinical drug development program is the descriptive drug label that is approved by a regulatory agency. The label-driven-question-based paradigm is one in which the entire drug development program is designed with a focus on generating the knowledge about the new drug that is needed to be able to address the elements that make up the drug label or PI. The objective of a well-written PI of an approved drug is to provide prescribers with the information that is needed to make informed decisions regarding the clinical use of the drug.

Information in a PI includes: Who should receive this new drug? How much drug should be given? How frequently should the drug be given? For how long does the drug need to be given to be effective? And of course, the PI must include much additional important prescribing information regarding drug–drug interactions, the effect of the patient's age on the drug's activity, how to administer the drug, potential adverse effects of which the prescriber needs to be aware, and the contraindications, precautions, and warnings. One way to remember the "label-driven-question-based" drug development concept is to think:

"We sell only the package insert, we give away the product!"

An appropriate analogy is the purchase of a computer program on a compact disk (CD). The CD itself probably costs pennies to manufacture. What we purchase is the value of the knowledge that is on the CD and the effort that went into producing that knowledge. The costs of medicines are very much the same as the costs associated with software products. We are of course paying for the research and development costs associated with bringing the new product to the market, the manufacturing, advertising, and distribution costs of the medicine, but the majority of the costs are associated with the value of the product to our health.

The Differentiation Paradigm

Differentiation is the term used to describe how the new product being developed will be unique from the products currently marketed or under development. Differentiation could be based on:

- A better prevention-of-relapse profile such as a proton pump inhibitor for duodenal ulcers.
- A better gastrointestinal safety profile such as the COX-2 inhibitors vs. traditional NSAIDs.
- Better patient compliance such as a weekly transdermal patch.
- A formulation that is easier to use, such as oral or inhaled insulin vs. injected insulin.

Whatever the differentiating feature is, both the drug discovery and the clinical development programs need to be designed to demonstrate the specific differentiation(s) that can be incorporated in the drug label and in product advertising.

One of the most valuable educational tools in developing an understanding of differentiation for a clinical

trial program is to study the PIs and advertisements for approved drugs. Serious students of clinical drug development would be well advised to take a few minutes when they see a journal advertisement for a drug to read the entire PI, which is found on the back of the advertisement. Based on the information found in the PI, one can reasonably reconstruct the elements of a clinical development plan for that drug, or design a clinical drug development plan for a drug with similar indications.

Indeed, the starting point for the development of a clinical plan to demonstrate the differentiation of a new drug could be the creation of a spreadsheet with the rows consisting of all drugs (marketed and in development) for the same or similar indications. The spreadsheet columns might include: indications, special indications, dose, dose regimen, dose duration, warnings, precautions, contraindications, adverse events, serious adverse events, life-threatening events, drug–drug interactions, elimination half-life, C_{max}, t_{max}, V_d, CL, food effect, compatible drugs, noncompatible drugs, how supplied, and so on. This type of spreadsheet would be invaluable in identifying specific areas for differentiation.

The selected areas of differentiation become the points of focus in designing a clinical development plan that is able to demonstrate advantages of a new drug over existing and pending drugs. One precautionary note: It is never too early to develop a draft PI that incorporates the target elements. Indeed, the very best drug discovery programs use a *target PI* to define the criteria for the selection of promising clinical leads and to guide the selection and design of subsequent clinical trials. To facilitate this approach, the Pharmaceutical Research Manufacturers Association and the FDA's Office of Drug Evaluation IV have collaborated in drawing up a Targeted Product Information Template (16).

Of course, the contents of the target PI will evolve over time as knowledge about the new drug is generated. The target PI not only serves as an effective means of establishing initial consensus goals that are shared by all stakeholders in the drug development process (e.g., discovery, development, and marketing), but provides metrics to determine whether the development process is subsequently yielding the essential differentiating features that were the original basis for undertaking the project.

The Drug Action → Response → Outcome → Benefit Paradigm

The usefulness of a new drug is based on a cascade of pharmacological events, which result in both desired (efficacy) and undesired (side effects) pharmacological outcomes. As described by Holford et al. (17), we can think of this cascade as having four levels. The first level is the *action* of the drug at a pharmacologically active site in humans (e.g., binding to a receptor). The second level is the *effect* that the drug produces as a result of that binding (e.g., the up-regulation of a protein). The third level is the *patient response* observed (e.g., the lowering of blood pressure). And the fourth level is the resulting *clinical outcome* (e.g., a lowering in the risk of stroke due to elevated blood pressure).

What distinguishes contemporary clinical drug development from traditional approaches is the important role that pharmacometrics plays in our understanding of the relationships between drug action, drug effect, patient response, and clinical outcome. The value of this understanding is not just in the definitive nature of the specific knowledge gained, but rather in its predictive utility that allows us, as clinical drug developers, to use knowledge that we have just learned to enhance the effectiveness and efficiency of the overall clinical development program. An extension of this paradigm can be found in the paper by Shiener (18) that illustrates the usefulness of the "learn and confirm" paradigm in contemporary drug development.

The Learning vs. Confirming Paradigm

In 1997, Sheiner (18) proposed the formal use of the learning vs. confirming paradigm for clinical drug development. *Learning* trials address an essentially infinite set of quantitative questions concerning the functional relationship between prognostic variables, dosage, and outcomes. On the other hand, *confirming* trials must answer only a single yes/no question: Is the null hypothesis falsified or not? An important distinction is that detailed knowledge regarding protocol compliance is imperative if valid conclusions are to be drawn from learning trials. Clearly, the introduction of the learning vs. confirming paradigm into a clinical development program has the potential to provide for more efficient, effective, and rapid decision making.

The Decision-Marking Paradigm

Well-designed clinical development programs support effective decision making. In this context, a *decision* can be defined as a commitment of resources towards a prespecified target. Unfortunately, the resource portion of the definition is frequently missing in a clinical development plan. Many "decisions" are often made that involve the need for a resource

change, yet no resource change occurs. Therefore, these become "hollow decisions." The successful implementation of a decision in a clinical project may entail the following:

- Resources may need to be added.
- Resources may need to be taken away.
- There might be no need to change the resources allocated to a project.

A clinical development plan cannot be considered complete until the required resources (people, funds, equipment, sites, clinical supplies, etc.) are identified for each major objective.

For those who design, track, and make decisions regarding the progress of clinical development programs, the inclusion within the development plan of critical decision points, with prespecified go/no go criteria, provides a focus for the clinical development team. The key clinical drug development decisions are identified in Table 33.2, with the critical go/no go decisions being shown in boldface. These critical decisions will be expanded on later in this chapter. It is important to note that the driver for these decisions is our question-based-label-driven clinical development plan. Indeed, the creation of a label-driven-question-based clinical development plan not only increases the efficiency and speed of the clinical development process, but supports the question-based review by the FDA of an NDA as recently described by Lesko and Williams (19).

The Fail Early/Fail Cheaply Paradigm

A critically important point is that on average only one out of five compounds selected for clinical trials will make it to the market (7). Based on this average, most companies are adopting the "fail early/fail cheaply" paradigm. The intent here is to conduct "killer experiments" early in the drug development process to identify as soon as possible those projects that, by their intrinsic properties, have a low probability of success later in the clinical development process. Successful implementation of this paradigm entails identifying potential failures:

- Before the compound even gets into the pre-FIH development process
- Early in the clinical development process for those compounds that pass the preclinical screens

With an understanding of these six clinical development paradigms we are ready to move forward to the critical issues in clinical drug development.

TABLE 33.2   Label Driven-Question Based Clinical Development Decision Points[a]

1. **What is the intended clinical disease model (prevention, treatment, cure or diagnosis)?**

2. **Is animal safety and activity data adequate to justify human clinical trials?**

3. **What are the efficacy and safety differentiation targets and respective success criteria?**

4. What starting dose should be used for the first in humans trial?

5. What dose escalation scheme should be used for the early clinical safety trials?

6. Is there dose proportionality such that if the dose of the drug is doubled, the blood levels also will double?

7. What are the appropriate primary and secondary clinical outcome metrics for determination of drug effect?

8. What are the appropriate patient population subgroups for clinical determination of drug effect?

9. **Has "proof of concept" been achieved using either a biomarker or a clinical outcome?**

10. **Based on the safety and pharmacometric profile observed from the early clinical trials, what starting dose and dose escalation scheme is appropriate for patient population subgroups to be studied for the determination of drug effect?**

11. Is there a clinical advantage to using the new drug in combination with an already marketed drug?

12. Do the formulations being developed (oral, parenteral, transdermal, etc.) release the drug at the desired rate?

13. What dose adjustments are needed for special patient populations (age, sex, ethnicity, renal and hepatic impairments)?

14. For how long should one take the drug?

15. Should the same dose be used for different levels of disease progression?

16. What is the right time(s) of day for dosing?

17. What is the clinical significance of any observed food effect upon bioavailability?

18. What is the clinical significance of any observed drug-drug interactions?

19. What are the appropriate primary and secondary clinical outcome metrics for determination of clinical efficacy?

20. **Have the patient populations, dose and dose regimen, and benefit/safety ratio have been adequately characterized to support the conduct of the large trials that are needed to confirm efficacy and to achieve the intended clinical differentiation**

21. **Have the frequency and severity of any side effects been adequately characterized, and the reversibility established of any severe or life-threatening side effects**

22. Are there any patients who should not take this drug?

23. **Do some individuals metabolize the new drug differently such that those individuals could have serious and life-threatening adverse reactions?**

24. **Does the route of metabolism of this drug, or of an already marketed drug, pose a risk of important drug-drug interactions?**

25. Is the drug highly protein bound? Will medical conditions or other drugs compete and increase this drug's unbound blood levels or will this drug compete for plasma protein binding sites of another drug the patient is taking?

26. What happens when the patient suddenly stops taking the drug or misses a few doses? Is there a rebound?

27. Is the drug addictive? How addictive?

28. **Have adequate clinical efficacy and safety data been generated to support the proposed indications and labeling that will be submitted to a regulatory agency for marketing approval?**

29. **Have adequate clinical efficacy and safety data been generated to differentiate this drug from those that are already marketed?**

[a]Critical decisions are in bold type.

CRITICAL CLINICAL DRUG DEVELOPMENT DECISION POINTS

Once one recognizes that the end product of clinical drug development is the knowledge and the information needed to permit the informed peer review, approval, and use of our new drug, one can then establish prespecified criteria for the critical clinical drug decision points. The decision-making criteria, outlined as follows are guided by evolving clinical knowledge (the learning and confirming cycle) about the drug being developed and are supported by label-driven-question-based clinical development plan concepts.

Which Disease State?

At least four approaches can be targeted with regard to drug development:

- Dx = Diagnosis to identify potential drug responders
- Px = Prevention of the illness
- Tx = Treatment to relieve signs and symptoms of illness
- Cx = Treatment to arrest or cure the illness

Of course subsets exist within each of these four approaches. For example, within each category there can be subjects with mild, moderate, or severe disease states and symptoms. Although one drug may work well for patients with mild or moderate disease, that same drug might not be effective for patients with the most severe conditions.

Identification of Potential Drug Responders

The Human Genome Project has laid the foundation for not only finding both new Cx and Tx drugs, but also for new methods to be able to identify which patient subgroups will respond to which drugs. An excellent overview of the impact of the Human Genome Project can be found in the article entitled "The Genome Gold Rush" (20).

The results of the Human Genome Project will provide breakthroughs in three major areas.

1. The identification of differences between patients that explain why some respond in clinical trials, while others do not.
2. The development of new drugs that will be able to treat specific patient populations.
3. The identification of which patients are more prone to serious or life-threatening side effects from a particular drug so that the prescriber will avoid that drug in these vulnerable individuals.

In the past, the need to include a plan for the co-development of a corresponding diagnostic method to indicate whether a drug would be useful was mainly limited to the domain of antibiotics. With the advent of the powerful tools that the Human Genome Project has introduced, many of the future clinical development programs will need to include a companion development and validation component for an FDA-approved diagnostic kit. The future for the identification and clinical development of diagnostic tests to determine whether an individual will respond to a certain medication is already a reality with drugs like trastuzumab for first-line use in treating breast cancer in patients who over express HER2. Because approximately one-third of all breast cancer patients over express the HER2 protein (and likewise two-thirds do not over express the HER2 protein), it is important to be able to identify which patients over express HER2 before prescribing trastuzumab. It was reported recently that 90% of newly diagnosed stage IV metastatic breast cancer patients are being tested for HER2 and that 67% of metastatic breast cancer patients are aware of their HER2 status (21). It is noteworthy that the BLA clinical program for the approval of trastuzumab consisted of 10 clinical trials and 1069 subjects (see Table 33.1).

Another example of the clinical usefulness of genomics in the clinical development of both a Dx and a Tx product is the investigation of the contribution of IL-9 to the pathogenesis of asthma. It has been reported that expression of interleukin-9 was significantly increased ($P > 0.001$) in the airways of asthmatics compared to normal individuals or those with other lung diseases (22).

Preventive Therapy

The next great breakthough in new drugs will be those that can prevent or reduce the probability of the first occurrence, or of a relapse, of a serious and life-threatening disease. A recent example is the supplemental approval in December 1999 by the FDA for the use of the COX-2 inhibitor celecoxib to reduce the number of adenomatous colorectal polyps in patients with familial adenomatous polyposis (FAP). This is intended as an adjunct to usual care of these patients (e.g., endoscopic surveillance, surgery). Similarly, tamoxifen has been approved for the "reduction of risk" of breast cancer. A major portion of the September 1998 FDA Oncologic Advisory Committee meeting was dedicated to a discussion of how the general practitioner would be able to predict the benefit/risk ratio for various patient populations from the clinical data that made up the NDA.

A major challenge for clinicians will be the design of clinical development programs that can answer the benefit/risk questions for prevention and risk reduction drugs. Px drug development will require new animal models and a new way of thinking about the conduct of clinical trials, especially in cases in which the incidence of the disease to be prevented is low and the new drug might also produce undesirable side effects, albeit at a low rate.

Relief of Signs and Symptoms

Drugs that treat the signs and symptoms of an illness can range in diversity from sildenafil for erectile dysfunction to drugs that reduce blood pressure, lower cholesterol levels, help control diabetes, or relieve acute or chronic pain. These Tx drugs, by definition, provide relief from the signs and symptoms, but do not slow down or treat the underlying disease state. Outcomes in clinical development programs for Tx drugs can range from demonstrating a reduction in the signs and symptoms of the disease such as stiffness and swollen joints for an arthritis drug, to an improvement in exercise tolerance for a drug that treats congestive heart failure.

Treatment That Arrests or Cures Disease

Therapy for patients with rheumatoid arthritis provides an example of the distinction between Cx vs. Tx drugs. Tx treatment drugs like the traditional

NSAIDs and COX-2 inhibitors relieve the signs and symptoms of pain and stiffness, but do little or nothing to arrest the disease progression. However, Cx drugs like entanercept, leflunomide, and infliximab have been designed to actually arrest disease progression as demonstrated by serial radiographic assessment of a patient's joints. Additional examples of Cx drugs include antibiotics that eradicate bacteria, and drugs that restore bone density. In some cases, the "cure" might end if the subject no longer takes the drug. However, the future looks particularly bright for the development of drugs that not only correct presently untreatable diseases but do not have to be taken for the remainder of a patient's life. The challenge for those who design the clinical development programs for these drugs will be to demonstrate that disease progression has been arrested or ideally even reversed.

What Are the Differentiation Targets?

Differentiation targets and quantified metrics will need to be clearly defined for a new drug to be "first in class" or "best in class." This can be illustrated by examining the development of the COX-2 inhibitor celecoxib. The hoped-for differentiating features for this drug were to maintain the antiinflammatory effectiveness of the traditional NSAIDs, while at the same time significantly reducing potential for gastrointestinal bleeding, and avoid platelet aggregation inhibition and nephrotoxicity. The candidate compounds selected for clinical trials had to pass rigorous *in vitro* and *in vivo* preclinical tests to demonstrate a high probability that they would possess the desired differentiation when they were tested in humans. This was accomplished for gastrointestinal and platelet side effects, but there was no reduction in the potential for nephrotoxicity. It is noteworthy that at the FDA Advisory Committee meeting for celecoxib, the office director for antiinflammatory drugs at CDER pointed out that the sponsor could have demonstrated antiinflammatory activity by studying only 1500 subjects. But in order to demonstrate a lower potential for gastrointestinal adverse events, the sponsor needed to conduct a clinical development program that included more than 9000 subjects. This illustrates the point that clinical trials designed to demonstrate an enhanced safety profile compared to an already marketed product will have to be designed with more power that would normally be needed to demonstrate a statistically and clinically meaningful efficacy difference from placebo.

An additional cautionary note needs to be considered in planning a clinical program to differentiate a product on the basis of improved safety. Clinical trials in general have been sized to be able to demonstrate

either an increase in effectiveness vs. an active comparator or a placebo or to demonstrate being "no different than" an active comparator. To indicate that a new drug is safer than a comparator, the FDA has rightly established the precedent with oxybutynin that one must also demonstrate equivalent efficacy before being able to make a claim with regard to an enhanced safety profile (23).

Is the Drug "Reasonably Safe" for FIH Trials?

The topic of preclinical assessment of a clinical candidate has been reviewed in Chapter 29. It is mentioned here because the decision as whether it is safe to take a candidate drug into humans is ultimately a medical judgment that can only be made by individuals responsible for clinical drug development. Preclinical safety assessments are designed to provide the knowledge needed to decide whether it is reasonably safe to study a drug candidate in humans. The term *reasonably safe* is used in this context because that is what a FDA reviewer must answer when reviewing an IND application.

Two simple questions can be asked to help decide if a candidate drug is ready to be studied in Phase I FIH trials:

1. Based on the preclinical data we have, would I be willing to roll up my sleeve and be the first to receive this drug?
2. Would I be willing to let my son or daughter be the first to receive this drug?

If the answer is "yes" to both questions, the development team is ready to prepare an IND or a CTC, the European equivalent of an IND, to request permission to begin a clinical trial program.

Starting Dose for the FIH Trial

This topic has been covered in Chapters 30 and 31. Additional information regarding allometric scaling is available in "Man versus Beast: Pharmacometric Scaling in Mammals" (24).

Has a Clinical Proof of Concept (POC) Been Obtained?

Once the human safety and pharmacokinetic profiles are established, the focus shifts to the design and conduct of early clinical trials that will confirm the hypothesized mechanism of drug action and characterize the differentiating features of the drug. These trials to establish mechanism of action and differentiation profile are the "killer experiments" that must be conducted early in the program to provide the data to support a critically important go/no go decision. It is essential to have answered the following four questions before proceeding to more extensive clinical trials in patients with the illness to be treated:

1. What is the mechanism of action in humans?
2. Does the clinical activity profile meet the prespecified safety criteria?
3. Are the bioavailability, half-life, and other features of the pharmacokinetic profile within the prespecified criteria?
4. Can the new drug be administered safely together with expected concomitant medications?

Mechanism of Action

Typical mechanism-of-action POC questions are:

- Has the hypothesized mechanism of action been demonstrated in humans?
- Is the dose within the projected dose range using the intended route of administration?
- Is the size of the diseased patient population that is responding to the drug large enough to justify continued development?
- How many subjects were screened to find those who qualified for our trials? Does this indicate that there will be enough patients who meet the entry criteria to justify continuing this clinical program?

Safety

The following are typical safety questions:

- Is the safety adequate at the active dose? Was any unusual toxicity that was observed in animals either observed or ruled out in humans?
- What do we know about human safety at several times the therapeutically active dose?
- Have we "stressed" the conditions to ensure that toxicity observed with currently marketed products will not occur with our candidate?

Pharmacokinetics

Typical questions regarding drug absorption, distribution, metabolism, and excretion are:

- Does the drug have the bioavailability, elimination half-life, and other pharmacologic properties needed to support the desired dosing regimen?
- Will a special formulation be able to overcome any deficiencies in the pharmacokinetic profile?
- What are the sources of interindividual and intrasubject variability in pharmacokinetics?

Drug Interactions

Typical questions regarding interactions resulting from concurrent administration of other drugs are:

- If this drug is to be given in combination with another drug, have therapeutic activity and safety been demonstrated with combination dosing?
- Is the dose for combination therapy different (higher or lower) than the single agent dose?
- Have clinically significant CYP450 drug interactions (inhibition or induction) been identified or ruled out by *in vitro* or *in vivo* studies?

Have the Dose, Dose Regimen and Patient Population Been Characterized?

The goal of a Phase 2 program is to provide three essential pieces of information that are critical to the success of subsequent long-term confirmatory Phase 3 trials.

1. Dose: The dose needed for effectiveness of each of the various disease states (early, mid, and late stage disease).

2. Dose regimen: The regimen (frequency or interval) at which the dose needs to be given (once daily, twice a day, every other day, weekly?)

3. Patient population: The patient population that will respond to the drug:

- Mild, moderate, severe disease?
- Refractory to existing therapies?
- Old, young, male, female?

Because Phase 3 is in actuality the confirmation of Phase 2 observations, it is likely that the Phase 3 program will be successful only if the answers to these questions are known with a high degree of certainty. Many times when a Phase 3 program is not successful, the reason for failure is either that the patient population for Phase 3 was not the same as the Phase 2 population or that the dose and dose regimen were not appropriately characterized.

Within the last decade there has been significant interest in determining whether the use of clinical modeling and simulation software would increase the probability of conducting successful clinical trials (25). This approach incorporates the technique of pharmacokinetic-pharmacodynamic modeling that was discussed in Chapter 19 with the disease progression models described in Chapter 20. Although this type of a clinical development tool has considerable potential, the outcomes to date have been mixed. For example, this approach has identified the placebo-response rate for various disease states as an area requiring better understanding. If the placebo-response rate observed in a large clinical trial is significantly higher than what was projected in the preliminary simulations, the size of the actual trial might not be adequate to distinguish the new drug from placebo, even if the new drug is active at the doses tested.

Will the Product Grow in the Post-Market Environment?

To maximize the value of a new drug, project teams are charged with ensuring that there is a full life-cycle global development and regulatory plan that includes post-marketing growth. Clinical trials to support new indications and new formulation development must therefore begin even before the NDA/BLA is filed. In some cases, clinical trials that demonstrate synergism of the new drug in combination with other drugs can provide information that will aid in expanding the market. The exploration of this synergism has been the subject of several alliances between pharmaceutical manufacturers, such as the joint development by Merck and Schering of a combination of an asthma product, montelukast, with an allergy product, loratidine.

Will the Clinical Development Program Be Adequate for Regulatory Approval?

It is important to establish a global clinical development and regulatory strategy early in the development program. Most organizations require a draft of a global clinical development and regulatory strategy at the time of the clinical lead selection. The regulatory strategy, along with the label-driven-question-based development plan, establishes the framework for a comprehensive FIH-to-market-expansion clinical development program.

An important consideration is to determine whether the development program is global or regional. If the program is global, then a global clinical development plan will need to be drafted at the beginning of the development project. Most drug development conducted today is of a global nature designed to meet the regulatory requirements of the United States, Europe, and Asia. The task of achieving global drug approvals has been greatly simplified with the advent of International Conference on Harmonization (ICH) guidelines for the development and registration of new medicines (25). Critical global clinical development considerations include:

- Ensuring the inclusion of local populations with all the disease states that the package insert indications is to support.
- Ensuring the inclusion of subjects who are taking the types of concomitant drugs that these patient populations usually take in individual countries.

Until 1990, sponsors had to essentially conduct three parallel development programs in the United States, in Europe and in Asia. However, the ICH was started in 1990 with the goal of producing a common technical document that could be used by sponsors to file for marketing approval in any country in the world. The ICH is a joint initiative that involves both regulators and industry as equal partners in scientific and technical discussions of the testing procedures that are required to ensure and assess the safety, quality, and efficacy of medicines. Despite the progress that has been made by the ICH, it is critical to establish the intended filing strategy for Europe as early as possible since there still are multiple ways to proceed in this region. Until recently, drug develop programs in Japan generally ran considerably longer than their U.S./European counterparts. However, there have been recent regulatory changes in Japan that are intended to speed up the process. Nevertheless, Phase 1 and Phase 2 studies will need to be repeated in Japan before the Phase 3 trials can be started in that country.

An important development that is consonant with the presentation in this chapter is that the CDER Division of Cardio-Renal Drug Products announced in 1999 that they had launched a pilot program for working with sponsors to develop a label-driven drug development program. It is anticipated that this program will be extended to other FDA divisions. In addition, the following clinical/regulatory questions are representative of those that need to be considered in designing clinical development plan to meet U.S. regulatory requirements:

- *Does the drug qualify for accelerated approval?* Accelerated approval enables the FDA, under 21 CFR 314 (Subpart H), to provide marketing approval for a drug on the basis of efficacy based on a surrogate endpoint, with the understanding that the sponsor will continue trials to provide evidence of efficacy based on a clinical endpoint. Accelerated approval is usually granted for drugs, such as HIV antiretroviral agents, that address an unmet medical need.
- *Does the drug qualify for priority review?* Priority review is designated by the FDA shortly after the NDA/BLA is filed. Priority Reviews are to be reviewed within 6 months of the filing date.
- *Does the drug qualify for a rolling NDA/BLA review?* The rolling NDA/BLA describes a process in which the FDA works with the sponsor during the phases of clinical development and accepts for review parts of the NDA/BLA before a complete NDA can be filed. In 1993, the rolling NDA/BLA was pioneered by the FDA Pilot Drug Division and the Medications Development Division of NIDA/NIH for the NDA filing for L-alpha-acetylmethadol, an alternative to methadone for the treatment of heroin addiction. This process enabled the FDA to approve L-alpha-acetylmethadol 18 days after the complete NDA was

submitted (27). Subsequent rolling NDA/BLA approvals have been made for HIV antiretroviral drugs by CDER Anti-Viral Division.

- *Does the drug meet the FDA requirement to develop pediatric labeling?* As discussed in Chapter 23, sponsors are now required to develop pediatric dosing information or, if the drug is not expected to be used in pediatric populations, to seek a waiver of this requirement.

LEARNING CONTEMPORARY CLINICAL DRUG DEVELOPMENT

Drug development is as much an art as a science. We are trained in various professions such as biology, pharmacology, chemistry, medicine, biostatistics, computer science, and so on, but rarely does a university offer a course, yet alone a curriculum, in drug development.

Courses and Other Educational Opportunities

Courses, workshops, and meetings are offered by the Pharmaceutical Education and Research Institute (PERI) (28), Drug Information Association (DIA) (29), Georgetown University Center for Drug Development Science (CDDS) (30), Tufts University Center for the Study of Drug Development (CSDD) (31), the NIH (32), the FDA's Center for Drug Evaluation and Research (CDER) (33), and other organizations.

In addition to courses and workshops, instructive drug development case studies are provided by:

- Attending FDA Advisory Committee meetings, or viewing the videotapes, or reading the transcripts of these informative meetings (33, 34).
- Reading FDC Report "Pink Sheets" (34).
- Reading FDC Report "Pharmaceutical Approvals Monthly" (34).
- Attending the annual meetings of DIA (29), Regulatory Affairs Professionals Society (RAPS) (35), American Association of Pharmaceutical Scientists (AAPS) (36), American College of Clinical Pharmacology (ACCP) (37), American Society for Clinical Pharmacology and Therapeutics (ASCPT) (38), and other professional organizations associated with drug development.

Failed Clinical Drug Development Programs as Teaching Examples

One way to learn how to avoid the pitfalls of drug discovery and development is to examine examples of failed programs. We will examine three cases:

1. Tasosartan, which the sponsor withdrew from FDA review during the NDA/BLA review since it was likely not to be approved.
2. Cisapride, for which the FDA requested revised labeling, leading the sponsor to withdraw the drug from U.S. marketing.
3. Mibefradil, which was withdrawn from the marketplace.

Safety NDA Withdrawal During the NDA Review Process

On March 3, 1998, the tasosartan application was withdrawn from FDA consideration by the sponsor who stated that the "action was the result of an unresolved question [with FDA] regarding the safety profile" of the product (39). The product had been found to be associated with liver enzyme elevations during clinical trials. The sponsor is reanalyzing the safety data for this angiotensin II inhibitor in hopes of resubmitting the NDA.

Drug-Drug Internations—Revised Labeling and Removal from the Market

Cisapride underwent significant PI changes that reserved the drug for second-line use for patients with gastroesophageal reflux before it eventually was removed from the market in mid-2000 (41). Following reports of cardiac adverse events and deaths associated with cisapride use, the FDA instructed the sponsor to revise the labeling to include a "black box" warning that "serious cardiac arrhythmias including ventricular tachycardia, ventricular fibrillation, *torsades de pointes*, and QT prolongation have been reported" in patients taking cisapride with other drugs that inhibit CYP3A4. The new labeling contraindicated the use of cisapride with at least 20 different drugs, including antibiotics (erythromycin, clarithromycin, and troleandomycin), antifungals (fluconazole, itraconazole, and ketoconazole), protease inhibitors (indinavir and ritonavir), and the antidepressant nefazodone. Additional labeled contraindications were concomitant use of cisapride with certain medications known to prolong the QT interval: antiarrhythmics such as quinidine, procainamide, and sotalol, amitryptiline, maprotiline, and phenothiazines.

Safety NDA Removal from the Market

The calcium channel blocker mibefradil (Posicor®) was removed from the market in 1998. The headline for the Pink Sheets article describing this action was "Posicor® Withdrawal Reflects 'Complexity' of Interaction Profile" (42). Products identified as potentially dangerous in combination with mibefradil included cardiac drugs such as amiodarone, flecainide, and propafenone; oncologic products such as tamoxifen, cyclophosphamide, etoposide, ifosfamide, and vinblastine; and the immunosuppressant medications cyclosporine and tacrolimus. The sponsor's decision to withdraw mibefradil was based on the complexity of the drug interaction information that would have to be communicated to ensure safe usage.

References

1. Peck CC. Drug development: Improving the process. Food Drug Law J 1997;52:163–7.
2. Spilker B. Guide to clinical trials. Philadelphia: Lippincott-Raven; 1996. p.1156.
3. Friedman LM, Furberg C. Demets DL. Fundamentals of clinical trials. 3rd ed. New York: Springer Verlag; 1998. p. 384.
4. Riegelman RK, Hirsch RP. Studying a study and testing a test—How to read the medical literature (with CD-ROM for Windows & Macintosh). Boston: Little, Brown and Co.; 2000. p. 356.
5. Internet at http://www.fda.gov/cder/handbook/index.htm.
6. Clinical Research Terminology. Appl Clin Trials 1998;4:28–50.
7. PhRMA Annual Report 2000–2001. Washington, DC: Pharmaceutical Research and Manufacturers of America. (Internet at http://www.phrma.org/.)
8. The Pharmaceutical Industry's R&D Investment—The Rising Cost of R&D. PhRMA Annual Report 2000–2001. Washington, DC: Pharmaceutical Research and Manufacturers of America. (Internet at http://www.phrma.org/.)
9. Federal Register Title 21CRF310, Kefauver-Harris Drug Amendments of the Food, Drug and Cosmetic Act, 1962.
10. Personal communications from Rob Bies (sildenafil, Viagra®), Jianguo Li (zanamivir, Relenza®), Mike Staschen (trastuzumab, Herceptin®), Theo Jang (rofecoxib, Vioxx®), and Agnes Westelinck (etanercept, Enbrel®), Center for Drug Development Science, Georgetown University, Washington DC.
11. The Pink Sheet, March 30, 1998. Chevy Chase, MD: F-D-C Reports, Inc.; p. 4. (Internet at http//www.fdcreports.com/.)
12. Internet at http//www.fda.gov/cder/approval/index.htm.
13. Internet at http//www.fda.gov/cber/efoi/htm.
14. Clemento A. New and integrated approaches to successful accelerated drug development. Drug Inf J 1999;33:699–710.
15. CDER, CBER. Guidance for Industry: Providing clinical evidence of effectiveness for human drug and biological products. Rockville, MD: FDA;1998. (Internet at http://www.fda.gov/cder/guidance/index.htm.)
16. CDER. ODE IV Pilot Targeted Product Information. Rockville, MD:FDA;2000. (Internet at http://www.fda.gov/cder/tpi/default.htm.)
17. Holford NHG, Peck CC. Population pharmacodynamics and drug development. In: Van Boxtel C, Holford NHG, Danhof M, editors. The in vivo study of drug action. Amsterdam: Elsevier; 1992. p. 401–13.
18. Sheiner LB. Learning versus confirming in clinical drug development. Clin Pharmacol Ther 1997;61:275–91.
19. Lesko L, Williams R. Early clinical development: The question based review. Appl Clin Trials 1999;8:56–62.
20. Carey J. The genome gold rush. Business Week. June 13, 2000;147–58.
21. The Pink Sheet, January 31, 2000. Chevy Chase, MD: F-D-C Reports, Inc.; p. 30. (Internet at http//www.fdcreports.com/.)
22. Gounni AS. Nutku E. Koussih L, Aris F. Louahed J. Levitt RC. Nicolaides NC, Hamid Q. IL9 expression by human eosinophils: Regulation by IL-1 beta and TNF-alpha. J Allergy Clin Immunol 2000;106:460–6.
23. Pharmaceutical Approvals Monthly, April 1999, Chevy Chase, MD: F-D-C Reports, Inc.; p. 26–30. (Internet at http//www.fdcreports.com/.)
24. Mordenti J. Man versus beast: Pharmacokinetic scaling in mammals. J Pharm Sci 1986;75:1028–40.
25. Holford NHG, Kimko HC, Monteleone JPR, Peck, CC. Simulation of clinical trials. Annu Rev Pharmacol Toxicol 2000;40:209–34.
26. International Conference on Harmonisation of Technical Requirements for Registration of Pharmaceuticals for Human Use. (Internet at http://www.ifpma.org/ich1.html.)
27. Grudzinskas CV, Wright C. Reshaping the drug development and review process—A case study of an 18-day approval. Pharmaceutical Executive. October 1994;14:74–80.
28. Pharmaceutical Education and Research Institute. (Internet at http://www.peri.org.)
29. Drug Information Association. (Internet at http://www.dia-home.org.)
30. Center for Drug Development Science at Georgetown University Medical Center. (Internet at http://www.georgetown.edu/research/cdds/.)
31. Tufts Center for the Study of Drug Development. (Internet at http://www.tufts.edu/med/research/csdd/.)
32. NIH clinical pharmacology website. (Internet at http://www.cc.nih.gov/OD/clinprat/.)
33. CDER list of advisory committee meetings and workshops. (Internet at http://www.fda.gov/cder/calender/default.htm.)
34. Transcripts, videotapes, and subscriptions to the Pink Sheet can be obtained from the FDC Reports website. (Internet at http//www.fdcreports.com/.)
35. Regulatory Affairs Professionals Society. (Internet at http://www.raps.org/.)
36. American Association of Pharmaceutical Scientists. (Internet at http://www.aaps.org/.)
37. American College of Clinical Pharmacology. (Internet at http://www.accp1.org/.)
38. American Society for Clinical Pharmacology and Therapeutics. (Internet at http://www.ascpt.org/.)
39. The Pink Sheet, March 9, 1998. Chevy Chase, MD: F-D-C Reports, Inc.; p.22. (Internet at http//www.fdcreports.com/.)
40. The Pink Sheet, July 6, 1998. Chevy Chase, MD: F-D-C Reports, Inc.; p. 5. (Internet at http//www.fdcreports.com/.)
41. FDA Talk Paper T0014, March 23, 2000, Food and Drug Administration, U.S. Department of Health and Human Services, Public Health Service, Rockville, MD. (Internet at http://www.fda.gov/bbz/topics/answers/ans01007.html.)
42. The Pink Sheet, June 15, 1998. Chevy Chase, MD: F-D-C Reports, Inc.; p. 5. (Internet at http//www.fdcreports.com/.)

34

Role of the FDA in Guiding Drug Development

LAWRENCE J. LESKO

Office of Clinical Pharmacology and Biopharmaceutics, Center for Drug Evaluation and Research,
Food and Drug Administration, Rockville, Maryland

The drug development process is defined here as a process that includes the preclinical and clinical phases of drug development, along with the regulatory review phase leading to market authorization. As discussed in Chapter 33, this process is extensive and expensive. A typical new molecular entity (NME), if approved for marketing, has gone through a preclinical discovery, screening, and evaluation stage that lasts, on average, 5 to 7 years. Following the preclinical phase, the NME next goes through a clinical phase that lasts 6 to 7 years. With an average of 6 to 12 months for regulatory review, the entire process may take up to 15 years, with a cost that may exceed $500 million (1, 2). Given the current high failure rate of drugs that enter into clinical testing, the need for efficient and informative drug development is obvious.

A goal of the drug development process, which includes regulatory review, is to get effective drugs to patients as quickly as possible, and to manage the risks associated with these drugs in the best way possible. Another goal is to make sure that ineffective or unsafe drugs, or drugs for which risk management is a problem, do not get to the marketplace. To achieve these goals, there needs to be a transparent and accountable review process. The Food and Drug Administration (FDA) not only reviews the results of the sponsor in terms of a submitted New Drug Application (NDA) but plays a critical role in guiding drug development by providing advice, gleaned from institutional expertise and experience, to sponsors regarding the conduct

of drug development in conformance with applicable regulations. In either context, effective communication between the FDA and sponsors is essential to achieving the goals of the drug development process in an efficient and informative manner. Meetings are a key part of this communication, but domestic and international guidances, telephone conferences, FDA presentations at public meetings, and the FDA website combine to provide transparency and accountability that should facilitate the drug development and regulatory review process by enabling sponsors to learn about the FDA's thinking.

This chapter reviews the various ways that the FDA gets involved in guiding drug development and communicating with sponsors during the preapproval period and following NDA approval and market authorization. This chapter is written from the perspective of the manufactured NMEs that are the responsibility of the Center for Drug Evaluation and Research (CDER). However, similar considerations apply to the development of new biologic products.

WHY DOES THE FDA GET INVOLVED IN DRUG DEVELOPMENT?

According to 21 CFR 393, the FDA has a dual mission of promoting the public health by promptly and efficiently reviewing clinical research and taking appropriate action on the marketing of regulated

TABLE 34.1   Chronology of Pharmaceutical Legislation

1906—Food and Drugs Act

1938—Federal Food, Drug and Cosmetic Act (FD&C Act)

1962—Kefauver-Harris Amendments

1974—Dissolution Rate Testing Requirements

1992—Prescription Drug User Fee Act (PDUFA)

1997—FDA Modernization Act (FDAMA)

products in a timely way. In this regard, the FDA and the pharmaceutical industry have basically the same goals—namely, to promote public health by getting safe and effective drugs to patients as quickly as possible and to protect public health by assuring that drugs with inadequate benefit/risk attributes do not get into the marketplace. In addition, both the FDA and the industry maintain pharmacovigilance programs to monitor adverse drug reactions after a new drug is marketed.

The chronology of legislation regulating drug development is summarized in Table 34.1. Beginning with the Food and Drugs Act in 1906 that prohibited interstate commerce in misbranded and adulterated foods, drinks, and drugs, the FDA has had an important role in protecting the public health. Over the years, public health safety disasters have contributed to the evolution of drug regulations that currently impact the development of drugs. For example, the elixir of sulfanilamide disaster in 1937, in which the sulfanilamide was dissolved in the poisonous solvent diethylene glycol, killed 107 persons and dramatized the need to establish drug safety before marketing. The Federal Food, Drug and Cosmetic Act of 1938, which contained provisions to require sponsors to show that new drugs were safe before marketing, ushered in a new system of drug regulation. The thalidomide tragedy of 1962, in which the drug caused birth defects in thousands of babies, aroused public support for stronger drug regulations. As a result, the Kefauver-Harris Drug Amendments were passed to ensure drug efficacy and greater drug safety. The bioavailability problems with digoxin reported in 1974, which included substantial variability in bioavailability between different manufacturers and between different lots of the same manufacturer, led to a greater awareness of the need for better regulatory standards in manufacturing to assure high-quality drug products for the American public (3). Dissolution-rate testing requirements for digoxin tablets initiated by the FDA in 1974 improved the uniformity of performance of digoxin tablets from various manufacturers. More recently, drug regulations have focused on the individ-

ualization of drug therapy in patient subsets defined by age, sex, and race. With the pharmacogenomic advances in molecular biology, the next stage in the evolution of drug regulations may well focus on individualization of drug therapy.

WHEN DOES THE FDA GET INVOLVED IN DRUG DEVELOPMENT?

For over 25 years, the FDA has had a formal process for holding meetings with sponsors to discuss scientific and clinical issues related to drug development. These formal meetings are consistent with the FDA's goal of facilitating drug development by providing advice and assuring a transparent review process. Although these meetings are voluntary, they are quite common and generally helpful. The meetings are referred to by the time frame in which they occur during the drug development process, and meetings at different times have different purposes and goals. Examples are meetings held before submission of an Investigational New Drug Application (IND), end-of-Phase I or end-of-Phase II meetings, and pre-NDA meetings.

Each of these meetings can have a major impact on the drug development process, including regulatory review of an NDA. For example, pre-IND meetings that are held early in the drug development process are extremely valuable to both the FDA and the sponsor because they routinely focus on critical issues in the drug development program before the sponsor has expended substantial resources in the conduct of clinical trials. A major goal for sponsors also is to avoid, if at all possible, any issues that might lead to an FDA order to halt clinical trials, a *clinical hold*. During the clinical development phase, the end-of-Phase II meeting is critical to discuss product development, major safety parameters, and the efficiency and appropriateness of the design and endpoints of pivotal Phase III efficacy studies. They also play an important role in resolving any outstanding manufacturing issues, or questions regarding dose, dose regimen selection, or major modifications to the drug development plan that are contemplated prior to filing an NDA. Pre-NDA meetings are intended to focus on the content and format of the sponsor's marketing application, and to familiarize the reviewers from various disciplines with the NDA that will be submitted. Any issues that remain to be resolved, [e.g., chemistry, manufacturing, and control (CMC) problems or questions] may also be discussed at this meeting. Important interactions between a pharmaceutical company and the FDA occur at the end of the marketing application review process, when meetings and discussions take place about the content and language of the label and package insert. Following market authorization, the FDA continues to be involved with the development and approval of new uses or new dosage forms for an approved product and maintains the MedWatch post-marketing surveillance program of adverse drug reactions (4).

HOW DOES FDA GUIDE DRUG DEVELOPMENT?

As previously indicated, the FDA guides drug development in many different ways, such as by interpreting laws, rules, and regulations, disseminating policy statements, providing advice and sharing experiences and expertise in face-to-face meetings, via written agreements and letters, by domestic and international guidances, by planned telephone conferences and/or scheduled videoconferences, and on the FDA website (5). Communicating with the FDA is sometimes confusing for sponsors who may wonder about what to ask, whom to ask, and what to do with the answers. Conversely, communicating with sponsors is sometimes a challenge for the FDA, who has to balance its advice and guidance to sponsors with the need to remain objective when the sponsor's application is being reviewed later on. To help with these situations, there are regulatory requirements for the various types of meetings with the FDA. Policies and procedures for requesting, scheduling, and conducting formal meetings between CDER and a sponsor are described in the FDA Guidance for Industry entitled "Formal Meetings with Sponsors and Applicants for PDUFA Products" (6).

The FDA receives many meeting requests and must balance its review responsibility with its obligation to respond to meeting requests. In 1999, for example, the FDA had over 1200 formal meetings with sponsors, and, depending on the type of meeting, these meetings occur within 30 to 75 days following a meeting request. The FDA prepares official minutes for these meetings within 4 weeks after the meeting. According to the formal meeting guidance, sponsors have the option to contact the appropriate FDA project manager to arrange discussion of any differences of opinion expressed in the minutes of the meeting. There is also a formal pathway described in the guidance for dispute resolution if this is necessary.

One or more formal meetings with the FDA generally occur for every development plan for a new chemical entity. Given the relatively short time available for meetings, the quality of these meetings is an important determinant of their impact on the drug development process. Both sponsors and the FDA review division that is involved in the meeting share the responsibility for planning and conducting these meetings in an optimally productive way. To assure a high-quality meeting with substantive agreements or understanding about issues, the meetings should be focused, designed with a specific purpose in mind, and should have a defined agenda. Timing is important if the meeting involves a discussion of drug development plans. For example in planning a meeting to discuss a clinical trial protocol, the sponsor should allow sufficient time so that the meeting is held before the study is begun, otherwise the meeting and the sponsor's resources may be wasted. The pre-planning for these meetings on both the sponsor's and the FDA's part may entail substantial expenditure of time and money. Meetings that are expected to have a significant impact on drug development or approval are attended by many consultants or investigators representing the sponsor, and sponsors should request attendance by discipline-specific reviewers from the FDA review divisions that are appropriate for the agenda.

In the last 10 years, the FDA has implemented regulatory initiatives that have impacted the drug development process, and sponsors should be quite familiar with their regulatory options. As discussed in Chapter 33, these include fast-track drug development programs, accelerated approvals (21 CFR 314.500–560) and priority reviews. The Subpart E (21 CFR 312.80–88) and fast track regulations (21 CFR 356), respectively, have expedited the drug development process and market access for new drugs for severely debilitating and serious conditions or life-threatening diseases without approved alternative treatments. An additional requirement for fast-track status is that there is an unmet medical need. In these instances, multiple meetings between sponsors and the FDA early in the development process are recommended to gain agreement on the development plan, and it is imperative for the sponsor to stay in close contact with the responsible FDA review division. It is also possible under Subpart E to gain approval with less safety data than normal. The accelerated approval regulations were developed as a complementary program to the Subpart E initiative, and encourage the use of surrogate endpoints as a basis for accelerated approval. The Prescription Drug User Fee Act of 1992 (PDUFA) has allowed CDER to increase the number of reviewers, and CDER has made a commitment to schedule the planned meetings that sponsors request in a reasonable time, so that the drug development process can be advanced expeditiously (7).

The FDA also guides drug development by holding closed or open advisory committee meetings. These meetings facilitate the regulatory review and FDA approval process by bringing together external experts to assess data, recommend the need for new studies, and address specific questions formulated by the FDA to help resolve scientific or clinical problems related to the drug development process. Podium presentations by senior FDA personnel are another way that the FDA attempts to guide drug development. It is advantageous to sponsors to pay attention to these talks. These presentations, usually given at public conferences or workshops, often explain the current scientific thinking of the FDA on a given topic. Slides and handouts presented in these public meetings generally are available to anyone who requests them.

WHAT ARE FDA GUIDANCES?

Perhaps the most widespread, effective, and important way that the FDA communicates with sponsors and guides drug development is through guidances issued either by the FDA or the International Conference on Harmonization (ICH). Guidances represent a wealth of knowledge and experience, generally drawn collectively from academia, industry, and the FDA. The FDA published the first guidance to industry in 1949, which was related to procedures for the appraisal of the toxicity of chemicals in food. Information on over 340 final or draft guidances can be found on the Internet (8).

The development of guidances proceeds by a process known as Good Guidance Practices that is intended to ensure the appropriate level of meaningful public participation in the guidance development process (9, 10). Recent guidance development was motivated, in part, by the Food and Drug Administration Modernization Act of 1997 (FDAMA) that reauthorized the PDUFA of 1992 and mandated the most wide-ranging reforms in FDA practices since 1938 (11). Approximately 36% of final or drafts guidances on the FDA guidance website were published since 1997. For example, under FDAMA, Section 111, a guidance has been developed that deals with the important application of "bridging studies" for pediatric drug approval, in which a pharmacokinetic study can serve to bridge to children the efficacy and safety database that has been established in adults. Another key provision of FDAMA, Section 115, deals with clinical investigations in which data from *one* adequate and well-controlled clinical investigation, and *confirmatory evidence,* are sufficient to establish effectiveness. Much speculation has focused on the meaning of confirmatory evidence

(e.g., if a relevant and well-designed pharmacokinetic/pharmacodynamic study would serve as confirmatory evidence) and further discussion of this issue is needed in a public forum.

The FDA recognizes the value to sponsors of consistency and predictability in regulatory decision making, and guidances for industry are developed as good faith efforts to share with sponsors the current thinking on a scientific topic. Guidances are intended to provide sponsors with assurances that FDA staff will interpret statutes and regulations in a consistent manner across its various divisions. However, guidances, in contrast to regulations that are substantive and binding, do not legally bind the FDA or sponsors. Sponsors are not required to follow guidances, and with appropriate rationale may propose alternative approaches to an issue. Likewise, the FDA may not accept data that is generated by following a guidance if there is a valid scientific reason. Many more guidances are being planned by the FDA. However, maintenance and updating of existing guidances will be a challenge in the future.

Guidances cover a wide range of topics that focus on standards of quality, such as CMC, preclinical animal toxicology requirements, ethical standards for clinical trials, and documentary requirements for INDs, Abbreviated New Drug Applications (ANDAs), and NDAs. Other guidances focus on the clinical phase of drug development, including biopharmaceutics, clinical pharmacology, and clinical trial design. Many of the newer guidances issued by the FDA are based on the principles of clinical pharmacology. These include guidances related to *in vitro* and *in vivo* drug metabolism-drug interaction studies, to the design and conduct of pharmacokinetic studies in special populations (renal disease, hepatic disease and pediatrics), and to the use of clinical pharmacology tools in drug development (e.g., population pharmacokinetics). All the clinical pharmacology guidances are intended to provide sponsors with ways to streamline the drug development process and gather important information efficiently.

One of the most important guidances, issued by the FDA in 1998, is entitled "Providing Clinical Evidence of Effectiveness for Human Drug and Biological Products." This guidance puts forth advice and experience in drawing evidence of effectiveness from all clinical phases of drug development. In particular, it provides examples to demonstrate how exposure-response relationships may be used to provide the primary evidence of efficacy in drug development. Among these examples are recommendations regarding requests for approval of new formulations and new doses or dosing regimens of approved drug products.

In the area of biopharmaceutics, three newly issued guidances are noteworthy because they are the culmination of a decade of public discussion of scientific principles related to the documentation of product quality. The General Bioavailability (BA) and Bioequivalence (BE) Guidance provides advice on the design, analysis, and utility of BA and BE studies in new and generic drug development, including the use of replicate design studies. A companion statistical guidance provides aid on how to analyze BE studies using three statistical approaches: average, individual, and population methods. The so-called biopharmaceutical classification system (BCS) guidance offers advice on when BA and BE studies may be waived on sound scientific principles of drug absorption as it relates to the solubility and permeability of drug substances, and the dissolution of drug products (see Chapter 4). Together, these guidances, along with four or five other drafts of planned guidances, provide a framework for the biopharmaceutical development of new and generic drug dosage forms.

In short, the FDA attempts to communicate extensively with industry via guidances. The ultimate value of guidances may be related to the quality of the data and NDA and ANDA submissions provided by sponsors.

References

1. Internet at http://www.phrma.org/.
2. PhRMA 2005: An industrial revolution in R&D. London: PricewaterhouseCoopers; 1998. p. 11.
3. Lindenbaum J, Mellow MH, Blackstone MO, Butler VP Jr. Variation in biologic availability of digoxin from four preparations. N Engl J Med 1971;285:1344–7.
4. MedWatch: the FDA medical products reporting program.. (Internet at http://www.fda.gov/medwatch/.)
5. Internet at http://www.fda.cder.gov.
6. CDER, CBER. Formal meetings with sponsors and applicants for PDUFA products. Guidance for industry, Rockville, MD: FDA; 2000. (Internet at http://www.fda.gov/cder/guidance/index.htm.)
7. Prescription Drug User Fee Act of 1992. Public Law 102–571. In the US Code of Federal Regulations 21 CFR 379.106 Stat 4491; October 29, 1992.
8. Internet at http://www.fda.gov/cder/guidance/index.htm.
9. Good guidance practices (Notice): The FDA's development, issuance, and use of guidance documents. Federal Register 62 FR 8961; February 17, 1977.
10. Good guidance practices (Final Rule). Federal Register 65FR182; September 29, 2000.
11. Food and Drug Administration Modernization Act of 1997. Public Law 105–115. In the US Code of Federal Regulations 21 CFR 355a.111 Stat 2296, November 21, 1997. (Internet at http://www.fda.gov/cber/fdama.htm.)

I

Abbreviated Table
of Laplace Transforms

Table of Operations ($\mathcal{L}$)

Time Domain	Laplace Domain
$F(t)$	$f(s) = \int_0^\infty F(t)\, e^{-st}\, dt$
1	$1/s$
A	A/s
$F'(t)$	$sf(s) - F(0)$
$F''(t)$	$s^2 f(s) - sF(0) - F'(0)$

Table of Inverse Operations ($\mathcal{L}^{-1}$)

Laplace Domain	Time Domain
$\dfrac{1}{s}$	1
$\dfrac{1}{s-a}$	e^{at}
$\dfrac{1}{(s-a)^2}$	te^{at}
$\dfrac{1}{s(s-a)}$	$\dfrac{1}{a}(e^{at} - 1)$
$\dfrac{1}{(s-a)(s-b)} \quad a \neq b$	$\dfrac{1}{a-b}(e^{at} - e^{bt})$

II

Answers to Study Problems

ANSWERS TO STUDY PROBLEMS— CHAPTER 2

(Note how dimensional analysis has been performed by including units in the calculations.)

Problem 1:   Answer—E

$$V_d = \frac{\text{Dose}}{C_0} = \frac{80 \text{ mg}}{4 \text{ mg/L}} = 20 \text{ L}$$

Problem 2:   Answer—A

$$V_d = 2.0 \text{ L/kg} \cdot 80 \text{ kg} = 160 \text{ L} \qquad t_{1/2} = 3 \text{ hr}$$

Therefore,

$$CL_E = \frac{\ln 2 \cdot V_d}{t_{1/2}} = \frac{\ln 2 \cdot 160 \text{ L}}{3 \text{ hr}} = 37 \text{ L/hr}$$

and the infusion rate should be:

$$I = C_{SS} \cdot CL = 4 \text{ mg/L} \cdot 37 \text{ L/hr} = 148 \text{ mg/hr}$$
$$= 2.5 \text{ mg/min}$$

Problem 3:   Answer—C

The gentamicin plasma level fell to half of its previous value in the 5-hour interval between blood draws. Therefore: $t_{1/2} = 5$ hr and $k = \ln 2/t_{1/2} = 0.139$ hr^{-1}

$$CF = \frac{1}{(1 - e^{-k\tau})}$$

Since $\tau = 8$ hrs

$$CF = \frac{1}{(1 - e^{-1.11})} = \frac{1}{0.67} = 1.49$$

Therefore, the expected steady state peak level is:
$1.49 \cdot 10 \text{ μg/mL} = 14.9 \text{ μg/mL}$

Problem 4:   Answer—C

Target level of 12 μg/mL = $^1/_2$ toxic level of 24 μg/mL

Therefore, one should wait one half-life before restarting aminophylline.

$$t_{1/2} = \frac{0.693 \, V_d}{CL} \qquad V_d = 60 \text{ kg} \cdot 0.45 \text{ L/kg} = 27 \text{ L}$$

$$CL = \frac{I}{C_{SS}} = \frac{(0.5 \text{ mg/kg} \cdot \text{hr}) \cdot (60 \text{ kg})}{24 \text{ mg/L}} = 1.25 \text{ L/hr}$$

Therefore,

$$t_{1/2} = \frac{0.693 \cdot 27 \text{ L}}{1.25 \text{ L/hr}} = 15 \text{ hr}$$

Problem 5:   Answer—D

It requires 3.3 half-lives to reach 90% of the eventual steady-state level:

$$3.3 \cdot 7 \text{ days} = 23 \text{ days}$$

Problem 6: Answer—B

On admission the digoxin plasma level was 3.2 ng/mL and it fell to 2.7 ng/mL 24 hours later. Hence, the daily excretion fraction is 0.5/3.2 = 0.156 (the excretion fraction with normal renal function = 1/3). Therefore, levels can be expected to fall by 0.156 every 24 hours as follows:

Hospital day:	0	1	2	3	4
Digoxin level:	3.2 ng/mL	2.7 ng/mL	2.28 ng/mL	1.92 ng/mL	1.62 ng/mL
"More days":			1	2	3

We can see that levels can be expected to reach the 1.6 ng/mL target on the fourth hospital day, or *three more days after the level of 2.7 ng/mL was measured.*

Problem 7: Answer—E

Three half-lives are needed for plasma levels to fall from 8 μg/mL to 1 μg/mL:

Level:	8 μg/mL	→	4 μg/mL	→	2 μg/mL	→	1 μg/mL
Half-lives:	0		1		2		3

Since the elimination-phase half-life is given as 2 hours, three half-lives would require 6 hours. However, the question asks for a dosing interval that would allow peak levels *to exceed 8 μg/mL and fall below 1 μg/mL.* The only dosing interval offered that is longer than 6 hours is 8 hours.

Problem 8: Answer—D

Since:

$$Dose/\tau = \frac{V_{max}}{K_m + \overline{C}_{SS}} \cdot \overline{C}_{SS} \qquad (\text{II.1})$$

$$(Dose/\tau)K_m + (Dose/\tau)\overline{C}_{SS} = V_{max}\overline{C}_{SS}$$

Two simultaneous equations can be set up, one for the concentration measured at each previously administered dose.

$$300\,mg/day \cdot K_m + 300\,mg/day \cdot 5\,\mu g/mL = 5\,\mu g/mL \cdot V_{max} \quad (\text{II.2})$$

$$600\,mg/day \cdot K_m + 600\,mg/day \cdot 30\,\mu g/mL = 30\,\mu g/mL \cdot V_{max} \quad (\text{II.3})$$

These can be simplified to:

$$300\,mg/day \cdot K_m + 1,500\,mg^2/L \cdot day = 5\,mg/L \cdot V_{max} \quad (\text{II.4})$$

$$600\,mg/day \cdot K_m + 18,000\,mg^2/L \cdot day = 30\,mg/L \cdot V_{max} \quad (\text{II.5})$$

By multiplying Equation II.4 by 2 and subtracting it from Equation II.5 we obtain:

$$15,000\,mg^2/L \cdot day = 20\,mg/L \cdot V_{max}$$

Therefore:

$$V_{max} = 750\,mg/day$$

Substituting this value for V_{max} into Equation II.4 yields:

$$300\,mg/day \cdot K_m + 1,500\,mg^2/L \cdot day = 5\,mg/L \cdot 750\,mg/day$$
$$300\,mg/day \cdot K_m = 2,250\,mg^2/L \cdot day$$
$$K_m = 7.5\,mg/L$$

We can now substitute these parameters into Equation II.1 to estimate the dose that will provide a phenytoin level of 15 μg/mL.

$$Dose/\tau = \frac{750\,mg/day}{7.5\,mg/L + 15.0\,mg/L} \cdot 15\,mg/L$$
$$Dose/\tau = 500\,mg/day$$

ANSWERS TO STUDY PROBLEMS— CHAPTER 3

Problem 1

We are given that $CF_{obs} = 1.29$ and $\tau = 12$ hours. Since

$$k_{eff} = \frac{1}{\tau} \ln\left[\frac{CF_{obs}}{CF_{obs} - 1}\right]$$

$$k_{eff} = \frac{1}{12} \ln\left[\frac{1.29}{0.29}\right] = 0.124$$

Therefore,

$$t_{1/2\,eff} = \frac{\ln 2}{0.124} = 5.6\,hr$$

Problem 2

Part a

Although a number of software packages are available to facilitate analysis of this type of data, most of them require the kineticist to provide initial estimates of parameter values. The technique of "curve peeling" is widely used for this purpose, and also provides an initial evaluation of data quality.

The first step is to graph the experimental data as shown by ● in the semilog plot of drug concentration vs. time shown in Figure II.1. Then draw a line through the terminal exponential phase and back-extrapolate it to the y-axis. Read the y-intercept (B') and half-life of this line ($\beta_{t1/2}$) from the graph. Next, as shown in Table II.1, obtain the difference (alpha values

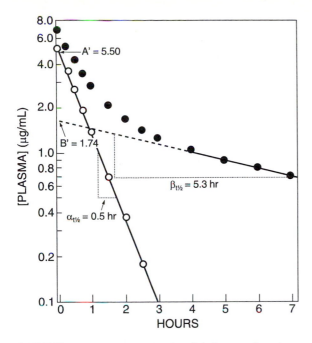

FIGURE II.1 Curve peel of the data (●) that are plotted on semi-logarithmic coordinates. The points for the α-curve (○) are obtained by subtracting back-extrapolated β-curve values from the experimental data as shown in Table II.1.

in the table) between the experimental data points lying above the back-extrapolated line and the corresponding values on the back-extrapolated line (beta values in the table).

The alpha values are then plotted on the graph (○) and used to draw an alpha line from which the y-intercept (A') and $\alpha_{t1/2}$ are obtained. Criteria that can be used to assess data quality at this point are: 1) the number of points that lie on each of the exponential lines, and 2) the scatter of the points about the alpha and beta lines.

The values for α and β are obtained from their half-life estimates as follows:

TABLE II.1   Results of Curve Peel

Time (hr)	[Plasma] (μg/mL)	Beta value (μg/mL)	Alpha value (μg/mL)
0.10	6.3	1.7	4.6
0.25	5.4	1.7	3.7
0.50	4.3	1.6	2.7
0.75	3.5	1.6	1.9
1.0	2.9	1.5	1.4
1.5	2.1	1.43	0.67
2.0	1.7	1.34	0.36
2.5	1.4	1.25	0.15

$$\alpha = \frac{\ln 2}{\alpha_{t1/2}} = \frac{\ln 2}{0.5 \text{ hr}} = 1.39 \text{ hr}^{-1}$$

$$\beta = \frac{\ln 2}{\beta_{t1/2}} = \frac{\ln 2}{5.3 \text{ hr}} = 0.131 \text{ hr}^{-1}$$

Please note: Although it might seem easier to calculate α and β directly from the graph as slopes, this is complicated by the fact that this semilogarithmic graph paper uses a $\log_{10}$ rather than natural log scale on the y-axis. A simple way to circumvent this difficulty is to calculate the values of α and β from their respective half-lives.

The intercept values of $A' = 5.50$ μg/mL and $B' = 1.74$ μg/mL are normalized as follows:

$$A = \frac{A'}{A' + B'} = \frac{5.50}{5.50 + 1.74} = 0.76$$

$$B = \frac{B'}{A' + B'} = \frac{1.74}{5.50 + 1.74} = 0.24$$

As shown here, normalization is a technique for converting the sum of A and B to 1 and is required because we have stipulated that the administered dose is 1 in our derivation of the equations for calculating the model parameters.

Part b

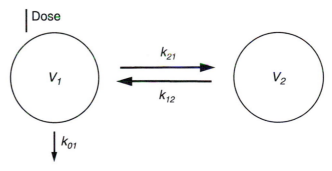

FIGURE II.2 Diagram of the two-compartment model used to analyze the experimental data.

From Equation 3.10:

$$k_{01} = \frac{1}{A/\alpha + B/\beta} = \frac{1}{\dfrac{0.76}{1.39} + \dfrac{0.24}{0.131}} = 0.42 \text{ hr}^{-1}$$

From Equation 3.13:

$$k_{12} = \beta A + \alpha B = (0.131)(0.76) + (1.39)(0.24) = 0.43 \text{ hr}^{-1}$$

From Equation 3.14:

$$k_{21} = \frac{AB(\alpha - \beta)^2}{k_{12}} = \frac{(0.76)(0.24)(1.39 - 0.13)^2}{0.43}$$

$$= 0.67 \text{ hr}^{-1}$$

Part c

$$V_1 = \frac{\text{Dose}}{A' + B'} = \frac{100 \text{ mg}}{(5.50 + 1.74) \text{ mg/L}} = 13.8 \text{ L}$$

The elimination clearance is:

$$CL_E = k_{01} \cdot V_1 = (0.42 \text{ hr}^{-1})(13.8 \text{ L}) = 5.8 \text{ L/hr}$$

Similarly,

$$CL_I = k_{21} \cdot V_1 = (0.67 \text{ hr}^{-1})(13.8 \text{ L}) = 9.25 \text{ L/hr}$$

Part d

$$V_2 = \frac{CL_I}{k_{12}} = \frac{9.25 \text{ L/hr}}{0.43 \text{ hr}^{-1}} = 21.5 \text{ L}$$

$$V_{d(SS)} = V_1 + V_2 = 13.8 \text{ L} + 21.5 \text{ L} = 35.3 \text{ L}$$

Compare this value with:

$$V_{d(area)} = \frac{CL_E \cdot t_{1/2\beta}}{\ln 2} = \frac{5.8 \text{ L/hr} \cdot 5.3 \text{ hr}}{\ln 2} = 44 \text{ L}$$

and

$$V_{d(extrap.)} = \frac{\text{Dose}}{B'} = \frac{100 \text{ mg}}{1.74 \text{ mg/L}} = 57.5 \text{ L}$$

The reason $V_{d(ss)}$ is smaller than either of these two estimates is that neither the half-life equation used to calculate $V_{d(area)}$ nor the single-compartment model implied in calculating $V_{d(extrap)}$ makes any provision for the contribution of intercompartmental clearance to the prolongation of the elimination-phase half-life. Therefore, these estimates must compensate for this by increasing distribution volume, which in these approaches is the only way that half-life can be prolonged without affecting elimination clearance.

ANSWERS TO STUDY PROBLEMS— CHAPTER 4

Problem 1

AUC after a Single Intravenous Drug Dose

We have shown that after a single drug dose (D):

$$F \cdot D = CL \cdot AUC$$

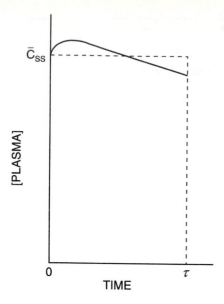

FIGURE II.3 Diagram of a plasma level-vs.-time curve during a dosing interval at steady state. $\overline{C}_{SS}$ is the average plasma concentration during the dosing interval τ. $AUC_{0-\tau}$ is equal to the area given by the product $\overline{C}_{SS} \cdot \tau$.

When the dose is administered intravenously it is completely absorbed, so $F = 1$, and:

$$AUC_{IV} = \frac{D_{IV}}{CL}$$

$AUC_{0 \to \tau}$ after an Oral Dose at Steady State

The mean steady state concentration ($\overline{C}_{SS}$) with oral dosing is:

$$\overline{C}_{SS} = \frac{F \cdot D_{oral} / \tau}{CL}$$

where the dose (D_{oral}) divided by the dosing interval (τ) is the dosing rate. As shown in Figure II.3, the area under the plasma-level-vs.-time curve during a steady state dosing interval is equivalent to the area of rectangle whose height equals $\overline{C}_{SS}$ and whose base equals τ. In other words:

$$AUC_{0 \to \tau(oral)} = \overline{C}_{SS} \cdot \tau$$

Substituting for $\overline{C}_{SS}$:

$$AUC_{0 \to \tau(oral)} = \frac{F \cdot D_{oral} / \tau}{CL} \cdot \tau = \frac{F \cdot D_{oral}}{CL}$$

Therefore, it can be seen by inspection that:

$$\frac{AUC_{0 \to \tau(oral)}}{D_{oral}} = F \cdot \frac{AUC_{IV}}{D_{IV}}$$

and that the extent of absorption of the oral dose formulation is:

$$\% \ Absorption = \frac{D_{IV} \cdot AUC_{0 \to \tau(oral)}}{D_{oral} \cdot AUC_{IV}} \times 100$$

Problem 2

We are asked to obtain $X(t)$ from the convolution of $G(t)$ and $H(t)$ where the input function $G(t)$ is a constant intravenous drug infusion:

$$X(t) = G(t) * H(t)$$

Since the operation of convolution in the time domain corresponds to multiplication in the domain of the subsidiary algebraic equation given by Laplace transformation, we can write the subsidiary equation as:

$$x(s) = g(s) \cdot h(s)$$

The intravenous infusion provides a constant rate of drug appearance in plasma (I), so:

$$G(t) = I$$

Since $\mathcal{L} \ 1 = 1/s$:

$$g(s) = \frac{I}{s}$$

We have shown on page 38 that the Laplace transform of the disposition function is:

$$h(s) = \frac{1}{s + k}$$

Therefore, the subsidiary equation for the output function is:

$$x(s) = \frac{I}{s} \cdot \frac{1}{s + k}$$

and $\mathcal{L}^{-1} \ x(s)$ is:

$$X(t) = \frac{I}{k} \left(1 - e^{-kt}\right)$$

Problem 3

Part a

From the equation derived above for $X(t)$, we see that steady state is only reached when $t = \infty$. At infinite time:

$$x_\infty = \frac{I}{k}$$

Since $C_{SS} = X_\infty / V_d$ and $k = CL_E / V_d$:

$$C_{SS} = \frac{I}{CL_E}$$

Note that this is Equation 2.2 that we presented in Chapter 2. In the problem that we are given, $I = 2$ mg/min, and $V_{d \ (area)} = 1.9$ L/kg $\cdot$ 70 kg = 133 L. Therefore,

$$C_E = \frac{0.693 \ V_{d(area)}}{t_{1/2}} = \frac{0.639 \cdot 133 \ \text{L}}{90 \ \text{min}} = 1.02 \ \text{L/min}$$

and:

$$C_{SS} = \frac{2 \ \text{mg/min}}{1.02 \ \text{L/min}} = 2.0 \ \mu g/mL$$

Note: Many nurses who work in cardiac intensive care units have learned that the expected steady state lidocaine level in $\mu g/mL$ equals the infusion rate in mg/min (usual therapeutic range: 2–5 $\mu g/mL$). Somewhat higher levels occur in patients with congestive heart failure or severe hepatic dysfunction.

Part b

Since:

$$X(t) = \frac{I}{k} \left(1 - e^{-kt}\right)$$

When $t = \infty$:

$$X_\infty = \frac{I}{k}$$

Therefore, for any fraction of the eventual steady state:

$$X(t) / X_\infty = (1 - e^{-kt})$$

When 90% of the eventual steady state level is reached:

$$0.90 = (1 - e^{-kt_{.90}})$$
$$e^{-kt_{.90}} = 0.10$$
$$kt_{.90} = \ln 10 = 2.30$$

Since:

$$k = \frac{\ln 2}{90 \ \text{min}} = 0.0077 \ \text{min}^{-1}$$

It follows that:

$$t_{.90} = \frac{2.30}{0.0077 \ \text{min}^{-1}} = 299 \ \text{min}$$

Note: Because it takes so long for an infusion to provide stable therapeutic drug concentrations, lidocaine therapy of life-threatening cardiac arrhythmias is usually begun by administering an intravenous loading dose together with an infusion.

Part c

Since $t_{1/2} = 90$ min, this corresponds to 3.3 half-lives.

Note: This result for a continuous intravenous infusion is equivalent to Equation 2.17 that was derived for intermittent dosing.

ANSWER TO STUDY PROBLEM— CHAPTER 5

Part a

$CL_E = 233$ mL/min $= 14.0$ L/hr; % Renal excretion $= 85.5\%$

$$CL_R = 0.855\, CL_E = 12.0\ \text{L/hr}$$
$$CL_{NR} = 0.145\, CL_E = 2.03\ \text{L/hr}$$
$$V_{d(area)} = \frac{CL_E \cdot t_{1/2}}{\ln 2} = \frac{(14.0\ \text{L/hr})(6.2\ \text{hr})}{\ln 2} = 125.2\ \text{L}$$

Therefore, if CL_{NR} is unchanged in functionally anephric patients, the expected elimination-phase half-life would be:

$$t_{1/2} = \frac{(\ln 2)V_{d(area)}}{CL_{NR}} = \frac{(\ln 2)(125.2\,\text{L})}{2.03\ \text{L/hr}} = 42.7\ \text{hr}$$

Note: The mean elimination half-life measured in six functionally anephric patients was 41.9 hr. (Stec GP, Atkinson AJ Jr, Nevin MJ, Thenot J-P, Ruo TI, Gibson TP, Ivanovich P, del Greco F: *N*-Acetylprocainamide pharmacokinetics in functionally anephric patients before and after perturbation by hemodialysis. Clin Pharmacol Ther 1979;26:618–28.)

Part b

From Figure II.4:

When $CL_{CR} = 50$ mL/min, expected $CL_E = 8.0$ L/hr

By direct calculation:

When $CL_{CR} = 50$ mL/min: $\begin{aligned}CL_R &= (50/100)(12\ \text{L/hr})\\ &= 6.0\ \text{L/hr}\end{aligned}$

Since $CL_{NR} = 2.0$ L/hr: $\begin{aligned}CL_E &= CL_R + CL_{NR}\\ &= 8.0\ \text{L/hr}\end{aligned}$

Part c

The 8-hour dosing interval is maintained.

Adjusted dose $= (8/14)(1\text{g}) = 0.57$ g

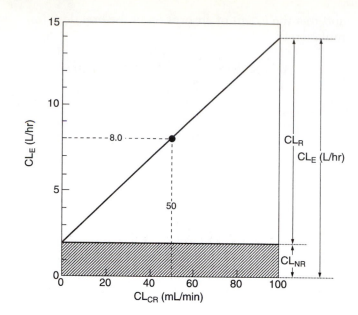

FIGURE II.4 Nomogram for estimating NAPA elimination clearance in patients with impaired renal function. The hypothetical patient described in Part b of the problem has a creatinine clearance of 50 mL/min and would be expected to have a NAPA elimination clearance of 8.0 L/hr.

This would reduce fluctuation between peak and trough levels, but would be awkward if only 0.5 g tablets were available.

Part d

The 1-g dose is maintained and the interval is adjusted.

The usual 8-hour interval corresponds to: 8 hr/6.2 hr = 1.3 half-lives when renal function is normal.

Expected half-life when $CL_{CR} = 50$ mL/min:

$$t_{1/2} = \frac{(\ln 2)V_{d(area)}}{CL_E} = \frac{(\ln 2)(125\ \text{L})}{8.0\ \text{L/hr}} = 10.8\ \text{hr}$$

Adjusted dose interval $= (1.3)(10.8\ \text{hr}) = 14$ hr

In practice, a 12-hour dose interval would be selected to increase patient convenience.

Index